ASTHMA

ASTHMA

COMORBIDITIES, COEXISTING CONDITIONS, AND DIFFERENTIAL DIAGNOSIS

Edited by
Richard F. Lockey, MD

DISTINGUISHED UNIVERSITY HEALTH PROFESSOR
PROFESSOR OF MEDICINE, PEDIATRICS & PUBLIC HEALTH
JOY MCCANN CULVERHOUSE CHAIR OF ALLERGY AND IMMUNOLOGY
DIRECTOR, DIVISION OF ALLERGY AND IMMUNOLOGY
DEPARTMENT OF INTERNAL MEDICINE
UNIVERSITY OF SOUTH FLORIDA COLLEGE OF MEDICINE
JAMES A. HALEY VETERANS' HOSPITAL
TAMPA, FLORIDA

Dennis K. Ledford, MD

PROFESSOR, MEDICINE & PEDIATRICS
MABEL & ELLSWORTH SIMMONS PROFESSOR OF ALLERGY & IMMUNOLOGY
DIVISION OF ALLERGY AND IMMUNOLOGY
DEPARTMENT OF INTERNAL MEDICINE
UNIVERSITY OF SOUTH FLORIDA COLLEGE OF MEDICINE
JAMES A. HALEY VETERANS' HOSPITAL
TAMPA, FLORIDA

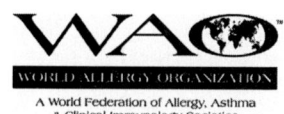

OXFORD
UNIVERSITY PRESS

OXFORD
UNIVERSITY PRESS

Oxford University Press is a department of the University of Oxford.
It furthers the University's objective of excellence in research, scholarship,
and education by publishing worldwide.

Oxford   New York
Auckland   Cape Town   Dar es Salaam   Hong Kong   Karachi
Kuala Lumpur   Madrid   Melbourne   Mexico City   Nairobi
New Delhi   Shanghai   Taipei   Toronto

With offices in
Argentina   Austria   Brazil   Chile   Czech Republic   France   Greece
Guatemala   Hungary   Italy   Japan   Poland   Portugal   Singapore
South Korea   Switzerland   Thailand   Turkey   Ukraine   Vietnam

Oxford is a registered trademark of Oxford University Press
in the UK and certain other countries.

Published in the United States of America by
Oxford University Press
198 Madison Avenue, New York, NY 10016

© World Allergy Organization 2014

All rights reserved. No part of this publication may be reproduced, stored in a
retrieval system, or transmitted, in any form or by any means, without the prior
permission in writing of Oxford University Press, or as expressly permitted by law,
by license, or under terms agreed with the appropriate reproduction rights organization.
Inquiries concerning reproduction outside the scope of the above should be sent to the
Rights Department, Oxford University Press, at the address above.

You must not circulate this work in any other form
and you must impose this same condition on any acquirer.

Library of Congress Cataloging-in-Publication Data
Asthma (Lockey)
Asthma : comorbidities, coexisting conditions, and differential diagnosis / edited by
Richard F. Lockey, Dennis K. Ledford ; with the World Allergy Organization.
p. ; cm.
Includes bibliographical references and index.
ISBN 978–0–19–991806–5 (alk. paper)
I. Lockey, Richard F., editor of compilation.   II. Ledford, Dennis K., 1950– editor of compilation.
III. World Allergy Organization, issuing body.   IV. Title.
[DNLM: 1. Asthma—complications.   2. Asthma—diagnosis.   3. Diagnosis, Differential.   4. Respiratory Tract
Diseases—complications.   5. Respiratory Tract Diseases—diagnosis. WF 553]
RC591
616.2'38—dc23
2013033500

This material is not intended to be, and should not be considered, a substitute for medical or other professional advice.
Treatment for the conditions described in this material is highly dependent on the individual circumstances. And, while
this material is designed to offer accurate information with respect to the subject matter covered and to be current as
of the time it was written, research and knowledge about medical and health issues are constantly evolving and dose
schedules for medications are being revised continually, with new side effects recognized and accounted for regularly.
Readers must therefore always check the product information and clinical procedures with the most up-to-date published product information and data sheets provided by the manufacturers and the most recent codes of conduct and
safety regulation. The publisher and the authors make no representations or warranties to readers, express or implied,
as to the accuracy or completeness of this material. Without limiting the foregoing, the publisher and the authors make
no representations or warranties as to the accuracy or efficacy of the drug dosages mentioned in the material. The
authors and the publisher do not accept, and expressly disclaim, any responsibility for any liability, loss, or risk that
may be claimed or incurred as a consequence of the use and/or application of any of the contents of this material.

1 3 5 7 9 8 6 4 2
Printed in the United States of America
on acid-free paper

Dedication

We dedicate this book to students, physicians, scientists, and colleagues seeking to better understand and treat asthma and its comorbid and coexisting conditions.

CONTENTS

Foreword xi
Preface xiii
Contributors xv

SECTION ONE: IMMUNOLOGIC

1. **Hypersensitivity Pneumonitis—Coexisting and Differential Diagnosis** 3
   David I. Bernstein

2. **Antineutrophil Cytoplasmic Antibody-Positive Vasculitis—Comorbid and Coexisting** 12
   Lanny J. Rosenwasser and Dennis K. Ledford

3. **Allergic Bronchopulmonary Aspergillosis—Comorbid** 21
   Paul A. Greenberger

4. **Immunodeficiency: Innate, Primary, and Secondary—Comorbid and Coexisting** 32
   Jean M. Brown and John W. Sleasman

SECTION TWO: PULMONARY

5. **Sleep Apnea in Children and the Upper Airway—Comorbid and Coexisting** 49
   Athanasios Kaditis

6. **Asthma and Obstructive Sleep Apnea** 63
   Larry M. Ladi and Edward S. Schulman

• vii

7. Chronic Obstructive Pulmonary Disease and Irreversible Airflow Obstruction—Comorbid, Coexisting, and Differential Diagnosis 80
Stephen P. Peters

8. Bronchiectasis—Comorbid, Coexisting, and Differential Diagnosis 92
Nizar Naji and Paul M. O'Byrne

9. Bronchiolitis—Comorbid, Coexisting, and Differential Diagnosis 103
Kelly J. Cowan and Theresa W. Guilbert

10. Genetic Disorders and Asthma—Coexisting and Differential Diagnosis 115
Neetu Talreja and Ronald Dahl

11. Other Pulmonary Abnormalities—Comorbid, Coexisting, and Differential Diagnosis 139
Robert A. Wise and Emily P. Brigham

12. Pneumonia—Comorbid and Coexisting 148
Chrysanthi L. Skevaki, Athanassios Tsakris, and Nikolaos G. Papadopoulos

13. Cough—Comorbid, Coexisting, and Differential Diagnosis 161
Pramod Kelkar, Alan Goldsobel, and Riccardo Polosa

14. Occupational Asthma—Comorbid and Differential Diagnosis 172
Manon Labrecque, Roberto Castaño, Grégory Moullec, Ignacio Ansottegui, and Denyse Gautrin

SECTION THREE: CARDIAC AND CARDIOVASCULAR

15. Adult Cardiac Conditions—Coexisting and Differential Diagnosis 193
Paola Rogliani, Andrea Segreti, and Mario Cazzola

16. Pediatric Cardiac Conditions—Coexisting and Differential Diagnosis 204
Louis I. Bezold

17. Pulmonary Hypertension—Coexisting and Differential Diagnosis 215
Aaron B. Waxman and Kerri Akaya Smith

SECTION FOUR: UPPER/EXTRATHORACIC AIRWAY

18. Allergic Rhinitis—Comorbid 231
Robert M. Naclerio and Ruby Pawankar

19. Nonallergic Rhinopathies and Lower Airway Syndromes—Comorbid 244
James N. Baraniuk, Michael S. Blaiss and Debendra Pattanaik

20. Infectious Comorbidities of Asthma in the Upper Airway 260
Claus Bachert and Griet Vandeplas

21. Nasal Polyps and Chronic Rhinosinusitis—Comorbid 279
Hae-Sim Park, Mario Sánchez-Borges, Seung Youp Shin, and Marek L. Kowalski

22. Vocal Cord Dysfunction and Paradoxical Vocal Fold Motion Disorder—Comorbid, Coexisting, and Differential Diagnosis 288
Roger W. Fox and Mark C. Glaum

SECTION FIVE: GASTROINTESTINAL

23. Gastroesophageal Reflux—Comorbid and Coexisting   299
    Promila Banerjee and Stephen J. Sontag

SECTION SIX: METABOLIC

24. Obesity and Asthma—Comorbid and Coexisting   321
    Erick Forno, Louis-Philippe Boulet, and Juan C. Celedón

25. Endocrine Disorders—Comorbid and Coexisting   334
    Kyriaki Sideri and Adnan Custovic

26. Osteopenia and Osteoporosis—Comorbid and Coexisting   345
    Joshua A. Steinberg and Andrea J. Apter

27. Pregnancy—Comorbid and Coexisting   367
    Jennifer A. Namazy, Michael Schatz, and Sandra Gonzalez-Diaz

SECTION SEVEN: PSYCHOLOGICAL ISSUES

28. Psychological Factors—Comorbid and Coexisting   379
    Fulvio Braido, Tatiana Slavyanskaya, Revaz Sepiashvili, Ilaria Baiardini, and Giorgio Walter Canonica

29. Asthma, Substance Abuse, and Tobacco Use—Comorbid and Coexisting   395
    Riccardo Polosa and Pasquale Caponnetto

SECTION EIGHT: EXERCISE

30. Exercise-Induced Bronchoconstriction and Asthma—Coexisting   409
    Matteo Bonini, André Moreira, and Sergio Bonini

SECTION NINE: ENVIRONMENTAL AND POPULATION EFFECTS

31. Environmental Protective and Risk Factors in Asthma—Comorbid and Coexisting   421
    Tari Haahtela and Ömer Kalayci

SECTION TEN: AGE

32. Asthma Over 65—A Disease About Which Little Is Known   441
    Chelle Pope, Richard D. deShazo, and Monroe James King

SECTION ELEVEN: FOOD

33. Atopic Dermatitis, Food Allergy, and Anaphylaxis—Comorbid and Coexisting   455
    Julie Wang, Hugh A. Sampson, Alessandro Fiocchi, and Scott Sicherer

Index   467

FOREWORD

THIS BOOK, *Asthma: Comorbidities, Coexisting Conditions, and Differential Diagnoses*, edited by Richard Lockey and Dennis Ledford in collaboration with the World Allergy Organization (WAO), provides a centralized, comprehensive clinical reference on the diagnosis and management of asthma, especially as it relates to comorbidities and coexisting conditions, filling a major gap in our current knowledge and understanding in this field of medicine. Comorbid conditions of asthma, an increasingly important health issue, have not previously been addressed in a comprehensive manner, and this book covers the latest research on the theory and practice of asthma, insights into the fundamentals of asthma and its comorbidities, and the most effective advances in the diagnosis and management of asthma and its comorbidities.

This book presents scientifically based information for multiple comorbid conditions as they relate to asthma, including rhinitis, rhinosinusitis, gastroesophageal reflux disease, sleep apnea, vocal cord dysfunction syndrome, obesity, and chronic obstructive pulmonary disease, as well as immunologic, psychological, and endocrine conditions and many others that play a major role in the diagnosis and optimal treatment of asthma. Addressing these comorbid conditions with the appropriate knowledge leads to better disease management. Therefore, a book on this very important subject that provides state-of-the-art information in a single-volume text is most ideal for the practicing physicians who take care of patients with asthma.

While the WAO International Scientific Conference (WISC) 2010 in Dubai on the theme of "Asthma and Co-morbid Conditions, Expanding the Practice of Allergy for Optimal Patient Care" helped to build the foundation for this book, the editors and authors, who are well known worldwide for their contributions to allergy and clinical immunology, have put forward their collective years of experience in the clinical evaluation and treatment of asthma in developing this book.

An estimated 300 million people suffer from asthma worldwide, and the existence of comorbidities is increasingly recognized in clinical practice as a means to achieve better control. This book will help expand the physician's knowledge base while aiding the delivery of optimal patient care because it addresses how those conditions affect asthma. It is a new topic of interest to everyone who cares for patients with asthma and will also provide a good source of knowledge for postgraduate students specializing in this field.

We congratulate and commend the editors for their extensive and dedicated efforts in putting together this excellent, comprehensive, and unique scientific work.

Ruby Pawankar
WAO President, 2012–2013
Lanny J. Rosenwasser
WAO President Elect, 2012–2013
Mario Sánchez-Borges
WAO Secretary General, 2012–2013

PREFACE

THE EDITORS, with their perspective of more than 75 years of combined clinical and research experience with asthma, believe that "asthma is the most treatable of all chronic diseases," a comment they often use when beginning a lecture on this subject to medical students, residents, physicians, and other health care professionals. Yet, data from throughout the world, based on emergency department visits, frequency of hospitalizations, and quality of life, indicate that the diagnosis and treatment of asthma are not optimal and need improvement. The reasons for this paradox are, first, that asthma is not thought of as a complex, heterogeneous disease or syndrome consisting of different phenotypes, defined as "the observable properties of an organism that are produced by the interaction of the genotype and the environment," and endotypes, defined as "conditions characterized by a specific pathobiological process" (2013 Merriam-Webster Dictionary). Second, asthma is variable, particularly in its severity, and is influenced by known, unknown, avoidable, and unavoidable environmental factors. Third, treatment usually requires complex inhalational devices that are difficult for patients to understand and to use, and with which compliance is suboptimal. Patients must be continually educated as to how they should administer and take their medications. Fourth, assessment of asthma is based primarily on symptoms, and at times all symptoms are due to asthma, but also many times some or all symptoms are due to unrecognized and untreated comorbid or coexisting conditions. Too often, asthma is viewed as a disease occurring in isolation, and comorbid and coexisting conditions are not appropriately identified and treated. *Asthma: Comorbidities, Coexisting Conditions, and Differential Diagnosis* addresses this problem.

The concept of "comorbid conditions" may be used to refer to diseases that occur coincidentally, but in this book, the term is used to describe two conditions that influence one another. Thus, a comorbid condition in this context influences asthma. It is sometimes difficult to differentiate a comorbidity from a coexisting condition—the former playing a role in the actual pathophysiology of asthma and its exacerbations, and the latter not necessarily contributing to such a role. Either way, both have to be appropriately diagnosed and treated.

What consequences occur when asthma is not accurately diagnosed and characterized and comorbid conditions are not appropriately identified? First, asthma is often inadequately treated because of a comorbid condition (e.g., acute or chronic sinusitis) that is associated with exacerbations of asthma. Conversely, asthma or suspected asthma may be overtreated when the comorbid or coexisting condition results in symptoms that are attributed to but not due to asthma, such as vocal fold dysfunction, which can result in cough, stridor (often misinterpreted as wheezing), and shortness of breath. Second, control is inadequately assessed because symptoms, and sometimes even lung function, can be influenced by both asthma and comorbid and coexisting illnesses. Examples of the latter include concomitant vocal fold dysfunction, bronchiectasis, and cystic fibrosis. Thus, asthma, particularly moderate to severe asthma, like any other complicated chronic disease, requires a physician with knowledge of and concern for the entire individual, and assessment begins with a complete, very detailed history and physical examination.

Richard F. Lockey, MD
Dennis K. Ledford, MD

CONTRIBUTORS

Ignacio Ansottegui, MD
Head, Department of Allergy and Immunology
Hospital Quirón Bizkaia
Erandio, Spain

Andrea J. Apter, MD
Professor of Medicine
University of Pennsylvania School of Medicine
Penn Presbyterian Medical Center
Philadelphia, Pennsylvania

Claus Bachert, MD, PhD
Chief of Clinic, ENT Department
Ghent University
Ghent, Belgium

Ilaria Baiardini, PhD
Allergy & Respiratory Diseases Clinic—DIMI
University of Genoa
IRCCS San Martino–IST University Hospital
Genova, Italy

Promila Banerjee, MD
Associate Professor of Medicine
Loyola University Medical Center
Department of Gastroenterology
Veterans Affairs Hospital
Hines, Illinois

James N. Baraniuk, MD
Associate Professor of Rheumatology, Immunology and Allergy
Georgetown University
Washington, D.C.

David I. Bernstein, MD
Professor of Medicine and Environmental Health
University of Cincinnati College of Medicine
Cincinnati, Ohio

Louis I. Bezold, MD
Jennifer Gill Roberts Professor in Pediatric
  Cardiology
Vice-Chair of Pediatrics
University of Kentucky College of Medicine
Lexington, Kentucky

Michael S. Blaiss, MD
Clinical Professor of Pediatrics and Medicine
University of Tennessee Health
  Sciences Center
Germantown, Tennessee

Matteo Bonini, MD, PhD
Department of Internal Medicine Lung
  Function Unit
Sapienza University of Rome
Institute of Translational Pharmacology
Rome, Italy

Sergio Bonini, MD
Department of Medicine
Second University of Naples
Institute of Translational Pharmacology
Naples, Italy

Louis-Philippe Boulet, MD
Laval University Heart and Lung Institute
  (IUCPQ)
Québec, Canada

Fulvio Braido, MD
Allergy & Respiratory Diseases Clinic—DIMI
University of Genoa
IRCCS San Martino–IST University Hospital
Genova, Italy

Emily P. Brigham, MD
Department of Pulmonary and Critical Care
Johns Hopkins University School of Medicine
Baltimore, Maryland

Jean M. Brown, MD
Department of Allergy, Immunology &
  Rheumatology
University of South Florida College of
  Medicine
Tampa, Florida

Giorgio Walter Canonica, MD
Allergy & Respiratory Diseases Clinic—DIMI
University of Genoa
IRCCS San Martino–IST University Hospital
Genova, Italy

Pasquale Caponnetto, PhD
University of Catania
Center for the Prevention and Treatment of
  Tobacco Smoking
Policlinico-Vittorio Emanuele University
  Hospital
Catania, Italy

Roberto Castaño, MD, PhD
Department of Otolaryngology Head & Neck
  Surgery
Université de Montréal and Hôpital du Sacré-
  Cœur de Montréal
Montréal, Québec, Canada

Mario Cazzola, MD
Department of System Medicine
University of Rome Tor Vergata
IRCCS San Raffaela Pisana Hospital
Rome, Italy

Juan C. Celedón, MD, DrPH
Neils K. Jerne Professor of Pediatrics
Professor of Medicine
Professor of Human Genetics
University of Pittsburgh School of Medicine
Children's Hospital of Pittsburgh of UPMC
Pittsburgh, Pennsylvania

Kelly J. Cowan, MD
Department of Pulmonology & Sleep
  Medicine
University of Wisconsin School of Medicine
  and Public Health
Madison, Wisconsin

Adnan Custovic, MD, PhD
Professor of Allergy
University Hospital of South Manchester
Manchester, United Kingdom

Ronald Dahl, MD
Professor
Odense University Hospital
Odense, Denmark

Richard D. deShazo, MD
Billy S. Guyton Distinguished Professor
Professor of Medicine and Pediatrics
University of Mississippi Medical Center
Jackson, Mississippi

Alessandro Fiocchi, MD
Chief, Division of Allergy
Department of Pediatrics
Bambino Gesù Hosptial
Rome, Vatican City, Italy

Erick Forno, MD, MPH
Assistant Professor of Pediatrics
University of Pittsburgh School of Medicine
Children's Hospital of Pittsburgh of UPMC
Pittsburgh, Pennsylvania

Roger W. Fox, MD
Professor of Medicine, Pediatrics and Public Health
University of South Florida College of Medicine
Tampa, Florida

Denyse Gautrin, PhD
Professor of Preventative and Social Medicine
University of Montréal
Hôpital du Sacré-Coeur de Montréal
Montréal, Québec, Canada

Mark C. Glaum, MD, PhD
Associate Professor of Medicine and Pediatrics
University of South Florida College of Medicine
Tampa, Florida

Alan Goldsobel, MD
Allergy and Asthma Associates of Northern California
Adjunct Associate Clinical Professor of Pediatrics
Stanford University School of Medicine
Clinical Professor of Medicine
University of California—San Francisco
San Francisco, California

Sandra Gonzalez-Diaz, MD, PhD
Head, Allergy & Clinical Immunology
Hospital Universitario and Medical School
Universidad Autónoma de Nuevo León
Monterrey, Mexico

Paul A. Greenberger, MD
Professor of Medicine-Allergy-Immunology
Northwestern University Feinberg School of Medicine
Chicago, Illinois

Theresa W. Guilbert, MD
Assistant Professor of Pediatric Pulmonology
University of Wisconsin School of Medicine and Public Health
Madison, Wisconsin

Tari Haahtela, MD, PhD
Professor of Medicine, Clinical Allergology
Helsinki University Hospital
Skin and Allergy Hospital
Helsinki, Finland

Athanasios Kaditis, MD
Assistant Professor of Pediatrics and Pediatric Pulmonology
First Department of Pediatrics
Pediatric Pulmonology Unit, Sleep Disorders Laboratory
University of Athens School of Medicine
Aghia Sophia Children's Hospital
Athens, Greece

Ömer Kalayci, MD
Professor of Pediatrics
Pediatric Allergy and Asthma Unit Hacettepe University
Ankara, Turkey

Pramod Kelkar, MD
Founder, National Cough Clinic
Partner, Allergy and Asthma Care, PA
Maple Grove, Minnesota

Monroe James King, DO
Adjunct Clinical Associate Professor of Medicine
University of South Florida College of Medicine
Tampa, Florida

Marek L. Kowalski, MD
Department of Immunology, Rheumatology and Allergy
Medical University of Lodz
Lodz, Poland

Manon Labrecque, MD, MSc
Professor of Medicine
University of Montréal
Hôpital du Sacré-Coeur de Montréal
Montréal, Québec, Canada

Larry M. Ladi, MD
Department of Pulmonary Disease & Critical Care Medicine
Drexel University College of Medicine
Hahnemann University Hospital
Philadelphia, Pennsylvania

André Moreira, MD, PhD
Faculty of Medicine
University of Porto
Centro Hospitalar de São João
Porto, Portugal

Gregory Moullec, PhD
Department of Medicine
Hôpital du Sacré-Coeur de Montréal
Montréal, Québec, Canada

Robert M. Naclerio, MD
Professor of Surgery
The University of Chicago School of Medicine
University of Chicago Medical Center
Chicago, Illinois

Nizar Naji, MB, MRCPI
Department of Medicine
McMaster University
Firestone Institute for Respiratory Disease
St. Joseph's Hospital
Hamilton, Ontario, Canada

Jennifer A. Namazy, MD
Scripps Clinic Medical Group
San Diego, California

Paul M. O'Byrne, MB, FRCP(C), FRSC
Professor of Respirology
Chair, Department of Medicine
McMaster University
Firestone Institute for Respiratory Disease
St. Joseph's Hospital
Hamilton, Ontario, Canada

Nikolaos G. Papadopoulos, MD, PhD
Allergy Department
2nd Pediatric Clinic
University of Athens School of Medicine
Athens, Greece

Hae-Sim Park, MD
Department of Allergy and Clinical Immunology
Ajou University School of Medicine
Suwon, South Korea

Debendra Pattanaik, MD, FAAAAI, FACR
Assistant Professor of Medicine
University of Tennessee Health Science Center
Memphis, Tennessee

Ruby Pawankar, MD, PhD, FRCP
Division of Allergy
Department of Pediatrics
Nippon Medical School
Tokyo, Japan

Stephen P. Peters, MD, PhD, FAAAAI, FACP, FCCP, FCPP
Professor of Internal Medicine, Pediatrics and Translational Science
Associate Director, Center for Genomics and Personalized Medicine Research
Wake Forest School of Medicine
Winston-Salem, North Carolina

Riccardo Polosa, MD, PhD
Professor of Internal Medicine
University of Catania
Center for the Prevention and Treatment of Tobacco Smoking
Policlinico-Vittorio Emanuele University Hospital
Catania, Italy

Chelle Pope, MD
Department of Medicine
University of Mississippi Medical Center
Jackson, Mississippi

Sepiashvili Revaz, MD, PhD
Head of the Department of Allergy &
  Immunology
People's Friendship University of Russia
Director of the Institute of
  Immunophysiology
University of Russia
Moscow, Russia

Paola Rogliani, MD
Professor of System Medicine
University of Rome Tor Vergata
Rome, Italy

Lanny J. Rosenwasser, MD
Dee Lyons/Missouri Endowed Chair in
  Pediatric Immunology Research
Professor of Pediatrics, Allergy/Immunology
  Division
Children's Mercy Hospital
Professor of Pediatrics, Medicine, and Basic
  Science
University of Missouri-Kansas City, School of
  Medicine
Kansas City, Missouri

Hugh A. Sampson, MD
Dean of Translational Biomedical Sciences
Professor of Pediatrics, Allergy and
  Immunology
Icahn School of Medicine at Mount Sinai
New York, New York

Mario Sánchez-Borges, MD
Clinical Immunology
Central University of Venezuela
Allergy/Immunology Service
La Trinidad Medical Center
Caracas, Venezuela

Michael Schatz, MD, MS
Department of Allergy
Kaiser Permanente Medical Center
San Diego, California

Edward S. Schulman, MD
Professor of Medicine
Department of Pulmonary Disease & Critical
  Care Medicine
Drexel University College of Medicine
Director, Allergy and Asthma Center
Hahnemann University Hospital
Philadelphia, Pennsylvania

Andrea Segreti, MD
Department of System Medicine
University of Rome Tor Vergata
Rome, Italy

Seung Youp Shin, MD
Department of Otolaryngology
Kyung Hee University School of Medicine
Seoul, South Korea

Scott Sicherer, MD
Professor of Pediatrics, Allergy and
  Immunology
Icahn School of Medicine at Mount Sinai
New York, New York

Kyriaki Sideri, MD
Allergy Department
University Hospital of South Manchester
Manchester, United Kingdom

Chrysanthi L. Skevaki, MD, PhD
Allergy Department
2nd Pediatric Clinic
University of Athens School of Medicine
Athens, Greece

Tatiana Slavyanskaya, MD, PhD
Professor of the Department of Allergy &
  Immunology
Institute of Immunophysiology
People's Friendship University of Russia
University of Russia
Moscow, Russia

John W. Sleasman, MD
Professor and Chief
Division of Allergy and Immunology
Duke University School of Medicine
Durham, North Carolina

Kerri Akaya Smith, MD
Assistant Professor of Medicine
University of Pennsylvania
Philadelphia, Pennsylvania

Stephen J. Sontag, MD
Associate Professor of Medicine
Loyola University Medical Center
Department of Gastroenterology
Veterans Affairs Hospital
Hines, Illinois

Joshua A. Steinberg, MD
Assistant Professor of Allergy and Immunology
Medical College of Wisconsin
Children's Hospital of Wisconsin
Milwaukee, Wisconsin

Neetu Talreja, MD
Affiliate Assistant Professor of Medicine
Division of Allergy and Immunology
Department of Internal Medicine
University of South Florida College of Medicine
Tampa, Florida

Athanassios Tsakris, MD, PhD
Microbiology Department
University of Athens School of Medicine
Athens, Greece

Griet Vandeplas, MD
ENT Resident, ENT Department
Ghent University
Ghent, Belgium

Julie Wang, MD
Associate Professor of Pediatrics, Allergy and Immunology
Icahn School of Medicine at Mount Sinai
New York, New York

Aaron B. Waxman, MD, PhD
Associate Professor of Medicine
Harvard Medical School
Director, Pulmonary Vascular Disease Program
Brigham and Women's Hospital
Boston, Massachusetts

Robert A. Wise, MD
Professor of Medicine, Pulmonary and Critical Care
Johns Hopkins University School of Medicine
Johns Hopkins Asthma & Allergy Center
Baltimore, Maryland

SECTION ONE

IMMUNOLOGIC

1

HYPERSENSITIVITY PNEUMONITIS

COEXISTING AND DIFFERENTIAL DIAGNOSIS

David I. Bernstein

KEY POINTS

- Hypersensitivity pneumonitis (HP) is diagnosed based on a consistent medical and environmental history, lung function, and radiographic findings.
- There are no validated laboratory biomarkers that establish the diagnosis of HP.
- Patients with HP can present with wheezing and obstructive abnormalities, leading to an incorrect asthma diagnosis. The presence of a gas exchange abnormality, bronchoalveolar lavage lymphocytosis, and characteristic infiltrative changes on high-resolution chest computed tomography can be used to distinguish HP from asthma.
- Asthma and HP can coexist in the same patient.
- Early diagnosis of HP and cessation of exposure to causative antigens result in remission of the disease and no residual impairment.

INTRODUCTION

Hypersensitivity pneumonitis (HP), also referred to as extrinsic allergic alveolitis, is an allergic inflammatory parenchymal lung disease usually caused by inhalational exposure to organic antigens from microbial bioaerosols or animal sources encountered in the work or home environment. Uncommonly, HP is caused by reactive chemicals (e.g., diisocyanates), primarily in an occupational setting. If recognized early in the course of disease, most patients with HP can achieve complete remission after prompt cessation of exposure to causative antigens at home and work. Clinical recognition relies on awareness of HP on the part of the physician evaluating unexplained dyspnea or cough. An astute clinician with a working knowledge of HP, able to administer a directed medical and environmental history, is likely to make the diagnosis. Among the interstitial lung disorders, acute and subacute HP are preeminently treatable and reversible by the timely initiation of measures to avoid exposure to causative antigens.

EPIDEMIOLOGY

The true incidence of HP is uncertain, but the prevalence and incidence are thought to be low. Governmental surveillance systems may be unable to identify new cases mainly because primary physicians are not clinically proficient at recognizing the major presenting features of this condition (Table 1.1). There are some data on the prevalence of HP in exposed worker populations at risk. For example, 420 to 3,000 cases of HP are estimated to occur for every 100,000 members of the general farming population.[1,2] High attack rates of HP have been reported in specific environmental settings. For example, as many as 59% of machine workers exposed to contaminated metalworking fluids and 37% of lifeguards working at public swimming pools contaminated by gram-negative bacteria were reportedly affected with HP.[3,4]

The mean age at diagnosis was 41 years (range, 21 to 65 years), with 8% diagnosed before 15 years of age, in one large series of patients with bird fancier's lung disease. HP

Table 1.1. Distinguishing Clinical Features of Hypersensitivity Pneumonitis and Asthma

	HYPERSENSITIVITY PNEUMONITIS	ASTHMA
Spirometry	Restrictive with reduced forced vital capacity, obstructive pattern, or mixed restrictive/obstructive pattern	Reversible airway obstruction
Diffusion capacity, carbon monoxide (D_{LCO}) or O_2 desaturation with exercise (gas exchange abnormality)	Reduced	Normal
Asthma symptoms (wheezing)	Not uncommon (25%)	Very common
Lung volumes	Reduced total lung capacity (TLC)	Normal or increased TLC and residual volume
Bronchoalveolar lavage (BAL)[20]	Lymphocytosis (>25% of cells), predominance of CD8+ with CD4/CD8 < 1; >1% mast cells; moderate neutrophilia and mild eosinophilia	Eosinophils (1%–4%), lymphocytes (3%), moderate neutrophils
Chest radiograph	Diffuse pulmonary infiltrates with ground-glass appearance or normal radiograph	Normal or hyperinflation
High-resolution computed tomography (HRCT)	Subacute HP: interstitial infiltrative patterns with ground-glass appearance with emphysematous bullae Chronic HP: reticular opacities, honeycombing	Bronchial wall thickening and air trapping

is seldom recognized and therefore may be underdiagnosed in children.[5] A review of 114 cases of HP reported that 18% had a family history of pulmonary fibrosis of unknown cause, perhaps representing a susceptibility factor for HP.[6] There is also epidemiologic evidence suggesting that smokers are at lower risk for developing HP compared with similarly exposed nonsmokers.[7,8]

DIAGNOSIS

Clinical Manifestations

Typically, patients present with acute, subacute, or chronic clinical manifestations. Dyspnea and cough are the most common presenting clinical manifestations.[9] Acute HP presents with flulike symptoms, fever, dyspnea, cough, and oxygen desaturation, typically beginning 4 to 8 hours after inhaled exposure to ambient antigens. These patients can also present with weight loss, fatigue, and anorexia.[10] Such a presentation may be indistinguishable from acute community acquired pneumonia.[11] Acute respiratory failure requiring mechanical ventilation is described.[12] Diffuse pulmonary infiltrates with a ground-glass appearance are typical pulmonary radiographic findings. Pulmonary function assessment usually reveals a restrictive pattern of impairment, and diffusion capacity is reduced in most patients, although obstructive or mixed patterns can also be seen. Altered gas exchange and reduced oxygen desaturation with exercise can be demonstrated.

Subacute and chronic forms of HP are less common than the acute form. In a large series of cases, only 20% of patients were diagnosed in the chronic phase of the disease.[9] Such patients typically present with progressive shortness of the breath and dry cough, presumably caused by a lower level chronic antigen exposure. Fever has been described in the subacute form.[10] In one report of a series of patients with bird fancier's lung, the mean delay from symptoms to diagnosis in all patients was 1.6 years, but it was 3.2 years for those diagnosed with chronic HP.[9] Pulmonary hypertension has been recognized on Doppler examination in about 20% of cases and is an indicator of reduced median survival.[13]

Laboratory findings, including serum precipitins to the suspect causative antigens, are not diagnostic and are unable to differentiate affected patients from similarly exposed patients without symptoms. Serum precipitating antibodies (i.e., precipitins) to suspect antigens are assayed. Testing the patient's serum with standard commercial panels of antigens is usually not useful, but evaluating precipitins to antigens isolated or cultured from a suspected environmental source may be informative. If positive, precipitins should be used primarily as indirect evidence supporting significant exposure to the suspected antigen. Erythrocyte sedimentation rate has been reported to be elevated in approximately 40% and lactate dehydrogenase level in 50% of confirmed cases of HP.[9] Although positive skin test responses with suspect antigens (e.g., avian serum) have been observed in most affected patients with HP, these tests are not useful because positive tests are also detected in asymptomatic similarly exposed individuals. Positive lymphocyte transformation tests to detect causative HP antigens have been reported but not validated; such tests are not commercially available.

Diagnostic Criteria

In a study of 116 patients with confirmed HP, the diagnosis could be established with a high degree of confidence if the following six clinical predictors were present: exposure to a known offending antigen; positive precipitating antibodies to the offending antigen indicating evidence of exposure; recurrent episodes of symptoms; inspiratory crackles on physical examination; symptoms occurring 4 to 8 hours after exposure; and weight loss.[14] Thus clinical criteria are often sufficient to establish a diagnosis of acute HP and, in unusual circumstances, bronchoalveolar lavage (BAL) or lung biopsy can be informative in confirming a suspected diagnosis of HP and differentiating it from other possible lung conditions.[15] Reliable diagnostic criteria, however, have not been clearly defined for subacute and chronic HP. The chest radiograph is normal in as many as 50% of cases, and absent serum precipitins do not exclude the diagnosis of HP. Challenge testing may be necessary in some circumstances. This can be accomplished by allowing patients under close medical monitoring to be reexposed to the suspected antigenic source in the incriminated home or work environment. Laboratory challenge testing with specific antigens bears substantial risks for acute exacerbation of the pneumonitis.

Radiographic Findings

The chest radiograph often reveals patchy or diffuse pulmonary infiltrates but may be normal.[14] In subacute HP, high-resolution computed tomography (HRCT) of the lung reveals interstitial infiltrative patterns with a ground-glass appearance and mosaic patterns, small centrilobular nodules, and emphysematous changes caused by air trapping.[9] HRCT findings characteristic of chronic HP include reticular opacities indicative of pulmonary fibrosis combined with the aforementioned findings of subacute HP.[16] Advanced HRCT fibrotic changes associated with honeycombing and traction bronchiectasis (abnormal airway dilation due to lung fibrosis) are independent radiologic predictors of mortality from chronic progressive HP.[17]

PATHOGENESIS AND HISTOPATHOLOGY

Lung biopsy samples obtained from patients with subacute HP exhibit cellular bronchiolitis, noncaseating granulomas located near bronchioles, and bronchiolocentric lymphocytic interstitial pneumonitis.[16] In contrast, biopsy samples from patients with acute HP reveal neutrophilic infiltrates and fibrin deposition.[18] Peribronchiolar fibrosis and emphysematous changes are often seen in chronic HP.[19] Fibrotic abnormalities observed in biopsy samples of HP may result from inflammatory injury and remodeling associated with recurrent episodes of acute HP or chronic inflammation attributable to persistent antigen exposure over months or years before diagnosis and cessation of antigenic exposure. Less typical patterns consistent with usual interstitial pneumonitis, nonspecific interstitial pneumonitis, and organizing pneumonia have also been recognized in patients diagnosed with chronic HP.

In the BAL, a brisk lymphocytosis is usually observed exceeding 40% of total cells in most patients presenting with acute, subacute, and chronic HP, with neutrophils also detected in BAL of acute HP.[9] Minimal numbers of mast cells and eosinophils are detected in BAL.[20] BAL CD8+ cells predominate over CD4+ cells (i.e., CD4/CD8 ratio < 1) in 60% of affected patients. In alveolar macrophages collected from patients with acute and chronic HP, spontaneous and lipopolysaccharide stimulated production of interleukin-12 (IL-12), IL-18, and tumor necrosis factor-α were increased compared with controls.[21] There is limited evidence from BAL studies suggesting that individuals with HP may have reduced regulatory T-cell function compared with asymptomatic exposed individuals.[22] A murine model of antigen-induced granulomatous lung inflammation associated with HP was thought to be dependent on toll receptor 9 and generation of IL-17–generating CD4+ and γ/δ T cells.[23]

CAUSES

Numerous causes of HP are described, with most discovered to be related to microbial antigen sources (Table 1.2). Causative antigens can often be traced back to chronic exposure to microbial bacterial and fungal spores. Exposure to an offending antigen can be documented by medical history, demonstration of serum antibodies to suspect antigens, and environmental assessment, sometime involving sampling of environmental sources of antigen (e.g., stagnant water) for microbiologic cultures to identify species of fungi or bacteria. A partial review of notable causative substances is presented later.

Atypical Mycobacteria

Human exposure to aerosols generated by hot-water tub sources has led to exposures to nontuberculous bacteria and pneumonia. It is uncertain, however, whether such cases represent primary infection or HP.[24]

Table 1.2. Exposures and Common Causes of Hypersensitivity Pneumonitis

PERSONS AT RISK	SOURCE	CAUSATIVE ANTIGENS
Farmers, food and agricultural workers	Contaminated hay, sugar cane bagasse	Thermophilic actinomycetes (e.g., *Saccharopolyspora rectivirgula*) fungi
Home dwellers	Contaminated humidifiers	Thermophilic actinomycetes, *Klebsiella* spp., amoeba, *Alternaria tenuis*, *Aureobasidium pullulans*, *Penicillium notatum*, and *Aspergillus* species
Home dwellers	Indoor humidity (summer-type pneumonitis)	*Trichosporon cutaneum*
Home dwellers	Hot tubs	*Mycobacterium avium*, *Cladosporium* spp.
Home dwellers	Basement sewage	*Cephalosporium* spp.
Machine workers	Contaminated aerosolized metalworking fluids	Mycobacteria, *Pseudomonas fluorescens*, *Aspergillus niger*, *Staphylococcus capitis*, *Rhodococcus* spp., *Bacillus pumilus*
Home dwellers who are bird fanciers, poultry workers	Bird droppings, feathers	Serum proteins
Diisocyanate-exposed and urethane foam workers	Chemical fumes or vapors	Methylene diphenyl diisocyanate

Atypical mycobacteria from contaminated metalworking fluids have been implicated as causes of HP among machine workers exposed to fluid aerosols generated by machining (e.g., metal grinding); a variety of fungi and gram-positive and gram-negative bacteria have also been cultured from these fluids.[25-28,29]

Fungi

HP has been reported in food production workers exposed to shiitake mushroom spores and in mushroom workers exposed to *Aspergillus glaucus*.[30,31] *Cladosporium* species encountered in a home environment have been implicated in chronic HP.[32] In addition to the thermophilic bacteria, deuteromycetes, including *Alternaria tenuis*, *Aureobasidium pullulans*, *Penicillium notatum*, and aspergilli, have been implicated as causes of humidifier lung disease.[33] *Trichosporon cutaneum* is a fungus linked to contamination of moist indoor environments in residential homes in Japan and an HP syndrome commonly referred to as "summer-type pneumonitis."[34]

Thermophilic Bacteria

Thermophilic bacteria are saprophytic organisms and are common causes of HP. These bacteria grow very well under specific conditions of temperature and moisture and are generally found in moldy hay, silage, sugar cane stalks, and decaying vegetative matter. Farmers and food processing and agricultural workers (e.g., dairy farmers, sugar cane workers, mushroom workers, potato processors) working in contaminated indoor spaces inhale large numbers of spores of thermophilic bacteria and develop HP. Humidifier lung disease is one of the most common nonoccupational forms of HP and is reportedly caused by sensitization to thermophilic spores (thermoactinomycetes) aerosolized into rooms of homes from free-standing contaminated humidifiers that have been poorly maintained. However, other causes of humidifier lung disease have been identified in the absence of identifiable thermophiles, and fungi and yeast have been implicated.[35]

Chemicals

Chemicals are very rare causes of HP in the occupational setting. Nearly all cases reported to date have been attributed to exposure to methylene diphenyl diisocyanate among chemical manufacturing workers and those involved with urethane products and a variety of industrial applications.[36-38]

DIFFERENTIAL DIAGNOSIS

Chronic HP may be very challenging to distinguish histopathologically from idiopathic pulmonary fibrosis, usual interstitial pneumonia, and nonspecific interstitial pneumonia.[39] The clinician must rely ultimately on the clinical presentation, identification of causative antigens, consistent lung function and radiographic features, and resolution of HP following avoidance of exposure to the antigenic source. The diagnosis can be missed if the clinician fails to obtain an adequate medical, occupational, and environmental history. Missing the diagnosis can occur if it is incorrectly assumed that HP is excluded based on inconsistent findings, including a normal chest radiograph, absence of serum precipitating antibodies to suspect antigens, or atypical lung function findings (e.g., obstructive pattern).

Although atypical, HP can occasionally present with lung function most suggestive of an obstructive pattern or a mixed obstructive and restrictive pattern.[40] Obstructive patterns are often reported in cases of HP caused by avian antigens and atypical mycobacteria.[41,42] In this case, the clinician must rely on evidence of reduced gas exchange (e.g., D_{LCO}), radiographic findings, or decreased lung volumes (e.g., total lung capacity) to distinguish HP from asthma.[43] Common reports of wheezing, asthmatic symptoms, and airway obstruction in patients with HP are quite consistent with histopathologic findings demonstrating inflammation in large and peripheral airways.

HP and asthma can coexist in the same patient. This is highlighted by a Japanese patient presenting with hypereosinophilia and confirmed asthma with reversible obstruction triggered by inhalation of an indoor microbial contaminant, *Trichosporon asahii*, a common cause of HP in Japan (i.e., summer-type pneumonitis). Remarkably, typical pathologic changes consistent with HP were confirmed on lung biopsy in the same patient.[44] Thus HP is a complex syndrome that can occur alone or in association with airway disease in the same patient.[45]

Other conditions that can be confused with HP are chronic bronchitis, asthma, and organic toxic dust syndrome. Organic toxic dust syndrome is an acute transient response characterized by fevers, chills, and other flu-like symptoms but no pulmonary infiltrates, lasting 24 to 48 hours after inhalation of mycotoxins or endotoxin contaminants in bioaerosols generated by contaminated humidifiers (i.e., humidifier fever) or from contaminated agricultural dusts.

MANAGEMENT AND PROGNOSIS

Early diagnosis and antigen avoidance remain the cornerstone for successful management of HP. In the home, this may be as simple as removing the contaminated free-standing humidifier. In an occupational setting, this often requires removal of an affected worker with HP from his or her work environment. Complete resolution of lung function and radiologic abnormalities is common with acute forms of HP following reduction or cessation of exposure to offending sources of environmental antigen. Systemic corticosteroids are usually recommended initially but should never be considered a substitute for exposure reduction or cessation. The long-term effectiveness of oral corticosteroids, however, in modifying disease outcomes and the long-term prognosis of HP has not been established in controlled studies.[46,47] For severe disease, 40 to 60 mg of daily oral prednisone, in divided doses, should be given for 1 to 2 weeks and then tapered over subsequent weeks. Maintenance treatment with oral corticosteroids is rarely indicated. Resolution of radiographic ground-glass densities and nodular opacities generally improves after successful avoidance of exposure and can be used along with lung function parameters (forced vital capacity, D_{LCO}) to track avoidance treatment outcomes.[48]

When a sentinel case is identified, all necessary environmental control measures should be instituted to prevent new cases. This includes control measures that reduce exposure to dusts, bioaerosols, and chemicals in occupational environments where HP cases are identified. Wetting down or chemically treating contaminated sugar cane compost has been effective in reducing dispersion of thermophilic bacterial spores that cause HP in sugar cane workers. In work environments, a reduction in indoor humidity and prevention of the accumulation of stagnant water are recommended in heating and ventilation systems where microbial overgrowth can occur. Routine maintenance and cleaning of humidifiers, air-conditioning units, and ventilation systems is also recommended. In the 1990s, widespread HP was recognized in machining workers exposed to aerosolized metalworking fluids contaminated with multiple bacteria and fungi.[28] The declining number of new HP cases reflects discontinuation of the practice of retaining for months large reservoirs of metalworking fluids that over time become biocontaminated with microbial antigens and that are then recirculated from machine to machine.

Clinical diagnoses following diagnosis and modification of exposure are variable. Farmers diagnosed with farmer's lung who remain on the farm and modify their barn exposure do no worse than those who leave the farm environment entirely.[49] Patients with HP caused by avian antigens appear to have worse outcomes than those with farmer's lung, which may be attributed to greater cumulative antigenic exposure. In one study the median survival for patients with chronic pigeon breeder's lung was 134 months, or a median 5-year survival rate of 71%.[50] Progressive symptoms with fatal outcome have been reported in a worker with HP associated with combined exposure to avian proteins and metalworking fluids despite strict avoidance of the causative antigens.[51]

UNMET, FUTURE RESEARCH NEEDS

1. Elucidate risk factors that define those individuals at high risk for the development of HP.
2. Investigate novel laboratory biomarkers that can assist in the diagnosis of HP.
3. Evaluate new treatment modalities (e.g., biologic agents) that can mitigate disease progression in patients with progressive HP that does not improve with environmental control measures.

CONCLUSION

Early recognition of HP is essential to prevent long-term impairment and disability caused by pulmonary fibrosis. Diagnosis is established based on clinical criteria, radiographic features, and lung function, but lung biopsy is sometimes necessary. In general, the prognosis is excellent provided that environmental sources of causative antigen are identified and avoidance is instituted early in the course of the disease. Exposure control measures must be instituted in work or home environments where cases are identified to effectively eliminate the sources of antigen exposure (e.g., contaminated humidifiers or water-cooling systems) in order to prevent new cases of HP.

REFERENCES

1. Gruchow HW, Hoffmann RG, Marx JJ Jr, Emanuel DA, Rimm AA. Precipitating antibodies to farmers lung antigens in a Wisconsin farming population. *Am Rev Respir Dis.* 1981;124:411–415.
2. Madsen D, Klock LE, Wenzel FJ, Robbins JL, Schmidt CD. The prevalence of farmer's lung in an agricultural population. *Am Rev Respir Dis.* 1976;113:171–174.
3. Fox J, Anderson H, Moen T, Gruetzmacher G, Hanrahan L, Fink J. Metal working fluid-associated hypersensitivity pneumonitis: an outbreak investigation and case-control study. *Am J Ind Med.* 1999;35:58–67.
4. Rose CS, Martyny JW, Newman LS, et al. "Lifeguard lung": endemic granulomatous pneumonitis in an indoor swimming pool. *Am J Public Health.* 1998;88:1795–1800.
5. Fan LL. Hypersensitivity pneumonitis in children. *Curr Opin Pediatr.* 2002;14:323–326.

6. Okamoto T, Miyazaki Y, Tomita M, Tamaoka M, Inase N. A familial history of pulmonary fibrosis in patients with chronic hypersensitivity pneumonitis. *Respiration*. 2013;85:384–390.
7. Murin S, Bilello KS, Matthay R. Other smoking-affected pulmonary diseases. *Clin Chest Med*. 2000;21:121–137, ix.
8. Arima K, Ando M. [Smoking and hypersensitivity pneumonitis]. *Ryoikibetsu Shokogun Shirizu*. 1994;No. 3:428–430.
9. Morell F, Roger A, Reyes L, Cruz MJ, Murio C, Munoz X. Bird fancier's lung: a series of 86 patients. *Medicine* (Baltimore). 2008;87:110–130.
10. Navarro C, Mejia M, Gaxiola M, Mendoza F, Carrillo G, Selman M. Hypersensitivity pneumonitis: a broader perspective. *Treat Respir Med*. 2006;5:167–179.
11. Marvisi M, Balzarini L, Mancini C, Mouzakiti P. A new type of hypersensitivity pneumonitis: salami brusher's disease. *Monaldi Arch Chest Dis*. 2012;77:35–37.
12. Deschenes D, Provencher S, Cormier Y. Farmers lung-induced hypersensitivity pneumonitis complicated by shock. *Respir Care*. 2012;57:464–466.
13. Koschel DS, Cardoso C, Wiedemann B, Hoffken G, Halank M. Pulmonary hypertension in chronic hypersensitivity pneumonitis. *Lung*. 2012;190:295–302.
14. Lacasse Y, Selman M, Costabel U, et al. Clinical diagnosis of hypersensitivity pneumonitis. *Am J Respir Crit Care Med*. 2003;168:952–958.
15. Richerson HB, Bernstein IL, Fink JN, et al. Guidelines for the clinical evaluation of hypersensitivity pneumonitis. Report of the Subcommittee on Hypersensitivity Pneumonitis. *J Allergy Clin Immunol*. 1989;84:839–844.
16. Silva CI, Churg A, Muller NL. Hypersensitivity pneumonitis: spectrum of high-resolution CT and pathologic findings. *AJR Am J Roentgenol*. 2007;188:334–344.
17. Walsh SL, Sverzellati N, Devaraj A, Wells AU, Hansell DM. Chronic hypersensitivity pneumonitis: high resolution computed tomography patterns and pulmonary function indices as prognostic determinants. *Eur Radiol*. 2012;22:1672–1679.
18. Hariri LP, Mino-Kenudson M, Shea B, et al. Distinct histopathology of acute onset or abrupt exacerbation of hypersensitivity pneumonitis. *Hum Pathol*. 2012;43:660–668.
19. Selman M, Lacasse Y, Pardo A, Cormier Y. Hypersensitivity pneumonitis caused by fungi. *Proc Am Thorac Soc*. 2010;7:229–236.
20. Caillaud DM, Vergnon JM, Madroszyk A, Melloni BM, Murris M, Dalphin JC. Bronchoalveolar lavage in hypersensitivity pneumonitis: a series of 139 patients. *Inflamm Allergy Drug Targets*. 2012;11:15–19.
21. Ye Q, Nakamura S, Sarria R, Costabel U, Guzman J. Interleukin 12, interleukin 18, and tumor necrosis factor alpha release by alveolar macrophages: acute and chronic hypersensitivity pneumonitis. *Ann Allergy Asthma Immunol*. 2009;102:149–154.
22. Girard M, Israel-Assayag E, Cormier Y. Impaired function of regulatory T-cells in hypersensitivity pneumonitis. *Eur Respir J*. 2011;37:632–639.
23. Bhan U, Newstead MJ, Zeng X, et al. TLR9-dependent IL-23/IL-17 is required for the generation of Stachybotrys chartarum-induced hypersensitivity pneumonitis. *J Immunol*. 2013;190:349–356.
24. Sood A, Sreedhar R, Kulkarni P, Nawoor AR. Hypersensitivity pneumonitis-like granulomatous lung disease with nontuberculous mycobacteria from exposure to hot water aerosols. *Environ Health Perspect*. 2007;115:262–266.
25. Gupta A, Rosenman KD. Hypersensitivity pneumonitis due to metal working fluids: Sporadic or under reported? *Am J Ind Med*. 2006;49:423–433.
26. Bernstein DI, Lummus ZL, Santilli G, Siskosky J, Bernstein IL. Machine operator's lung: a hypersensitivity pneumonitis disorder associated with exposure to metalworking fluid aerosols. *Chest*. 1995;108:636–641.
27. Yadav JS, Khan IU, Fakhari F, Soellner MB. DNA-based methodologies for rapid detection, quantification, and species- or strain-level identification of respiratory pathogens (Mycobacteria and Pseudomonads) in metalworking fluids. *Appl Occup Environ Hyg*. 2003;18:966–975.
28. Kreiss K, Cox-Ganser J. Metalworking fluid-associated hypersensitivity pneumonitis: a workshop summary. *Am J Ind Med*. 1997;32:423–432.
29. Rhodes G, Fluri A, Ruefenacht A, Gerber M, Pickup R. Implementation of a quantitative real-time PCR assay for the detection of Mycobacterium immunogenum in metalworking fluids. *J Occup Environ Hyg*. 2011;8:478–483.
30. Ampere A, Delhaes L, Soots J, Bart F, Wallaert B. Hypersensitivity pneumonitis induced by Shiitake mushroom spores. *Med Mycol*. 2012;50:654–657.
31. Yoshida K, Ando M, Ito K, et al. Hypersensitivity pneumonitis of a mushroom worker due

32. to Aspergillus glaucus. *Arch Environ Health.* 1990;45:245–247.
32. Watanuki Z, Okada S, Chiba S, Kamei K, Suzuki Y, Yamada N. Increased prevalence of high anti-Cladosporium antibody titers in interstitial lung diseases. *Tohoku J Exp Med.* 2012;226:287–291.
33. Baur X, Behr J, Dewair M, et al. Humidifier lung and humidifier fever. *Lung.* 1988;166:113–124.
34. Sugita T, Ikeda R, Nishikawa A. Analysis of Trichosporon isolates obtained from the houses of patients with summer-type hypersensitivity pneumonitis. *J Clin Microbiol.* 2004;42:5467–5471.
35. Suda T, Sato A, Ida M, Gemma H, Hayakawa H, Chida K. Hypersensitivity pneumonitis associated with home ultrasonic humidifiers. *Chest.* 1995;107:711–717.
36. Hara S, Yamamoto K, Yoda A, et al. [Three cases of isocyanate-induced hypersensitivity pneumonitis with different HRCT findings]. *Nihon Kokyuki Gakkai Zasshi.* 2009;47:839–843.
37. Vandenplas O, Malo JL, Dugas M, et al. Hypersensitivity pneumonitis-like reaction among workers exposed to diphenylmethane [correction to piphenylmethane] diisocyanate (MDI). *Am Rev Respir Dis.* 1993;147:338–346.
38. Malo JL, Zeiss CR. Occupational hypersensitivity pneumonitis after exposure to diphenylmethane diisocyanate. *Am Rev Respir Dis.* 1982;125:113–116.
39. Costabel U, Bonella F, Guzman J. Chronic hypersensitivity pneumonitis. *Clin Chest Med.* 2012;33:151–163.
40. Villar A, Munoz X, Cruz MJ, Morell F. [Hypersensitivity pneumonitis caused by Mucor species in a cork worker]. *Arch Bronconeumol.* 2009;45:405–407.
41. Blatman KH, Grammer LC. Chapter 19: Hypersensitivity pneumonitis. *Allergy Asthma Proc.* 2012;33(Suppl 1):S64–66.
42. Marras TK, Wallace RJ Jr, Koth LL, Stulbarg MS, Cowl CT, Daley CL. Hypersensitivity pneumonitis reaction to Mycobacterium avium in household water. *Chest.* 2005;127:664–671.
43. Funke M, Fellrath JM. Hypersensitivity pneumonitis secondary to lovebirds: a new cause of bird fancier's disease. *Eur Respir J.* 2008;32:517–521.
44. Hirakata Y, Katoh T, Ishii Y, Kitamura S, Sugiyama Y. Trichosporon asahii-induced asthma in a family with Japanese summer-type hypersensitivity pneumonitis. *Ann Allergy Asthma Immunol.* 2002;88:335–338.
45. Selman M, Vargas MH. Airway involvement in hypersensitivity pneumonitis. *Curr Opin Pulm Med.* 1998;4:9–15.
46. Selman M, Pardo A, King TE Jr. Hypersensitivity pneumonitis: insights in diagnosis and pathobiology. *Am J Respir Crit Care Med.* 2012;186:314–324.
47. Chan AL, Juarez MM, Leslie KO, Ismail HA, Albertson TE. Bird fancier's lung: a state-of-the-art review. *Clin Rev Allergy Immunol.* 2012;43:69–83.
48. Tateishi T, Ohtani Y, Takemura T, et al. Serial high-resolution computed tomography findings of acute and chronic hypersensitivity pneumonitis induced by avian antigen. *J Comput Assist Tomogr.* 2011;35:272–279.
49. Cormier Y, Belanger J. Long-term physiologic outcome after acute farmers lung. *Chest.* 1985;87:796–800.
50. Perez-Padilla R, Salas J, Chapela R, et al. Mortality in Mexican patients with chronic pigeon breeder's lung compared with those with usual interstitial pneumonia. *Am Rev Respir Dis.* 1993;148:49–53.
51. Zacharisen M, Schoenwetter W. Fatal hypersensitivity pneumonitis. *Ann Allergy Asthma Immunol.* 2005;95:484–487.

2

ANTINEUTROPHIL CYTOPLASMIC ANTIBODY–POSITIVE VASCULITIS

COMORBID AND COEXISTING

Lanny J. Rosenwasser and Dennis K. Ledford

KEY POINTS

- Vasculitis, particularly antineutrophil cytoplasmic antibody–positive vasculitis, may complicate asthma or present with respiratory symptoms that may be interpreted as asthma or sinusitis.
- Asthma with infiltrates or abnormal chest radiographs may suggest vasculitis.
- Abnormal sinus or chest imaging and blood tests such as eosinophil counts, acute phase reactants, and antineutrophil cytoplasmic antibody tests suggest vasculitis, but tissue biopsy is necessary for confirmation.
- Treatment of vasculitis associated with airway disease requires systemic corticosteroids, usually with immunosuppressants such as alkylating agents or antimetabolites. Eosinophilic granulomatosis with polyangiitis is particularly responsive to corticosteroids and in some cases may be treated with corticosteroids alone.

INTRODUCTION

The antineutrophil cytoplasmic antibody (ANCA)-positive vasculitic syndromes are particularly important from the perspective of respiratory disease because they are potential comorbid conditions associated with asthma and other pulmonary diseases. Vasculitis is a pathologic process characterized by inflammation and injury or necrosis of the blood vessel wall. The inflammation may compromise the affected vessel lumen or result in thrombosis, leading to ischemic changes in the tissues as well as hemorrhage and necrosis of the blood vessel. Any size, location, and type of blood vessel may be involved, including large muscular arteries, medium-sized arteries, arterioles, capillaries, and postcapillary veins, although specific syndromes selectively affect certain vessels. The possibility that vasculitic syndromes are related to other comorbid conditions, such as connective tissue diseases, infections, drug reactions that lead to serum sickness–like reactions, or congenital deficiencies of complement, also will influence the clinical impact of vasculitis on respiratory diseases.[1-3]

The spectrum of vasculitis includes unique syndromes, and within syndromes, further subsets of the clinical manifestations may be based on serologic findings such as ANCA (Figure 2.1). The ANCA-positive vasculitides frequently have pulmonary involvement, including eosinophilic granulomatosis with polyangiitis (EGPA), also termed Churg-Strauss syndrome (CSS) and allergic angiitis with granulomatosis (AAG); granulomatosis with polyangiitis (GPA), also known as Wegener's granulomatosis; and microscopic polyangiitis (MPA). The prevalence and specificity of ANCA varies with these syndromes. EGPA is of particular concern as a comorbidity of asthma because it occurs almost exclusively in subjects with preceding asthma, usually for more than 10 years, and is characterized by tissue eosinophilia and chronic sinusitis. GPA often includes upper airway inflammation, such as rhinitis, otitis media with effusion, sinusitis, or mastoiditis, in addition to cough and an abnormal chest radiograph (Figure 2.2). MPA may present with alveolar pulmonary hemorrhage resulting in cough and shortness of breath. The ANCA-positive vasculitides are systemic diseases and affect many other organs and tissues, particularly the skin, neurologic system, gastrointestinal tract, kidney, and heart, but the respiratory manifestations are most likely to present a comorbidity for asthma.

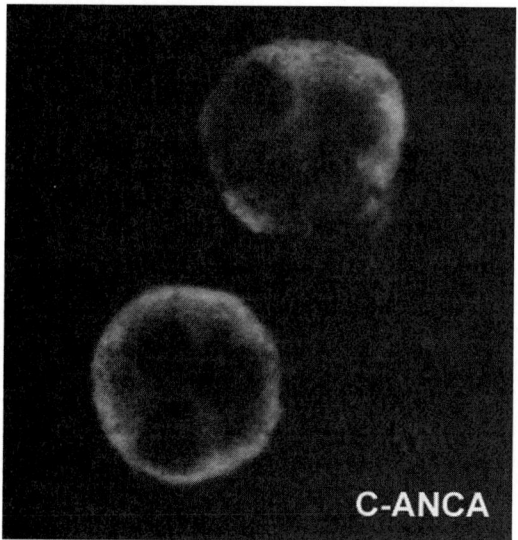

FIGURE 2.1 This is a high-powered fluorescent microscopic view of a slide demonstrating antineutrophil cytoplasmic antibody (ANCA). Dried neutrophils are overlaid with a serum sample from a test subject, followed by antihuman antibody labeled with a fluorescent tag. The typical binding pattern shows fluorescence greater in the peripheral cytoplasm in granulomatosis with polyangiitis (Wegener's granulomatosis), as seen in this figure, and more perinuclear in eosinophilic granulomatosis with polyangiitis (Churg-Strauss syndrome) and microscopic polyangiitis. This immunofluorescent test is more sensitive than identification of specific antibodies, usually for proteinase 3 (granulomatosis with polyangiitis) or myeloperoxidase (microscopic polyangiitis or eosinophilic granulomatosis with polyangiitis), although confirmation of specific antibodies is a more specific test. See Color Plate 1 in insert.

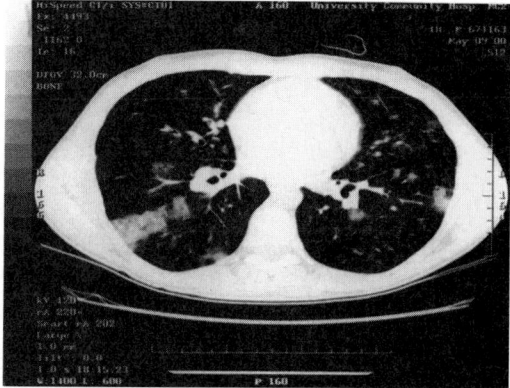

FIGURE 2.2 Computed tomographic chest radiograph without contrast in a young male with granulomatosis with polyangiitis (Wegener's granulomatosis). Cavitary, nodular lesions are the typical manifestations of this vasculitis syndrome in the chest, but infiltrates may also occur, resembling pneumonia. Symptoms may include chest pain, cough, or hemoptysis. Infectious or malignant causes of these findings need to be excluded, as a diagnosis cannot be made with certainty based on radiographs.

ETIOLOGY

The etiology of ANCA-positive vasculitis is unknown, as is true of most of the vasculitis syndromes, and the etiologies of the various ANCA syndromes likely differ. The pathologic mechanisms important in ANCA vasculitis include immune complex disease, mononuclear cell activation, neutrophil activation, and eosinophil recruitment, particularly in EGPA for the latter. The tissue damage from immune complexes is thought to be similar to serum sickness from the point of view of complement activation and damage of blood vessel wall, leading to increased vascular permeability, necrosis of the involved tissue, and hemorrhage and lumen occlusion. The contribution of allergic-like pathology, including increased immunoglobulin E (IgE), eosinophilia and activation of tissue mast cells, is likely in some forms of vasculitis, particularly EGPA. The recruitment and activation of eosinophils and neutrophils in an individual with a history of asthma resembles an allergic reaction, but there is no specific allergen stimulus of EGPA. Cocaine inhalation is associated with eosinophilic airway inflammation, and positive ANCA occurs in subjects with cocaine, induced septal perforation; but the specificity of the ANCA is elastase with cocaine, compared with myeloperoxidase in typical EGPA. Infections that exacerbate chronic respiratory disease also may play a role in vasculitis affecting the respiratory tract. GPA may respond partially or transiently to trimethoprim-sulfamethoxazole, and GPA frequently presents with chronic inflammatory sinus or ear disease, suggesting an infectious etiology. No infectious cause has been identified. MPA may follow respiratory infection or appear as a drug reaction, but neither is confirmed to be important in the pathogenesis.

Granulomatous responses, typical of EGPA and GPA, suggest T-cell–mediated immunity, but such pathology also may be triggered by stimulation of the innate immune system. This observation implies a potential role of T cells, macrophages, and cytokines in the pathogenesis of EGPA and GPA as well as direct, intrinsic, innate immune responses of tissue cells, including dendritic cells and macrophages, in host-defense-type reactions. Another possibility is that components of the respiratory system, including epithelia, endothelia, fibroblasts, myofibroblasts, and muscle cells, may be involved in the generation of respiratory vasculitis, suggesting a form of autoimmune disease. The focus of the inflammation on the respiratory tissue results in abnormal physiology and worsening respiratory function, both of which increase the comorbidity of respiratory dysfunction in ANCA-positive vasculitis.

CLINICAL CHARACTERISTICS

The clinical characteristics of vasculitis reflect the heterogeneity and overlap among the various syndromes. Four major groups of vasculitis are outlined in Table 2.1.

EGPA (also termed CSS and AAG) is the major vasculitic syndrome associated with asthma. Up to 99% of individuals with EGPA have coexistent asthma that precedes the vasculitis.[4-6] Most of these subjects have moderately severe to severe asthma. In addition, about 60% of EGPA subjects have antimyeloperoxidase-positive ANCA, and the individuals with positive ANCA have greater eosinophilia, more intense inflammation, more generalized organ system involvement, and generally a worse prognosis than those with ANCA-negative EGPA.

The identification of EGPA as an asthma comorbidity is critical because systemic complications may occur irrespective of whether the asthma controlled. Unrecognized, untreated EGPA also places the affected individual at increased risk for complications, including myocardial infarction, mononeuritis multiplex, central nervous system complications, and ruptured abdominal viscus. Any subject with persistent asthma is likely to have three of the criteria for the diagnosis of EGPA: peripheral eosinophilia, sinusitis, and asthma. Tissue eosinophilia and vascular or perivascular inflammation are the distinguishing features but would only be detected if EGPA were suspected and biopsies performed. Thus, EGPA should be considered in any individual requiring National Heart Lung Blood Institute Expert Panel Report step 5 or 6 treatment. Also, asthma that is managed well but is associated with

Table 2.1. Classification of Vasculitis

Polyarteritis Nodosa Group
- Polyarteritis nodosa (PAN)
- Microscopic polyarteritis (MPA)
- Eosinophilic granulomatosis with polyangiitis (EGPA)*

Granulomatosis Vasculitis Group
- Granulomatosis with polyangiitis (GPA, or Wegener's granulomatosis)
- Lymphomatoid granulomatosis
- Temporal arteritis (giant cell arteritis)
- Takayasu's arteritis

Hypersensitivity Vasculitis Group
- Serum sickness
- Henoch-Schönlein purpura (HSP)
- Vasculitis associated with infections, malignancy, and connective tissue disease
- Congenital complement deficiency

Miscellaneous
- Kawasaki disease
- Behçet's disease
- Erythema nodosum

*This is also know as allergic angiitis and granulomatosis (AAG) or Churg-Strauss syndrome (CSS). Some experts classify "eosinophilic granulomatosis with polyangiitis" in the "granulomatosis vasculitis" group.

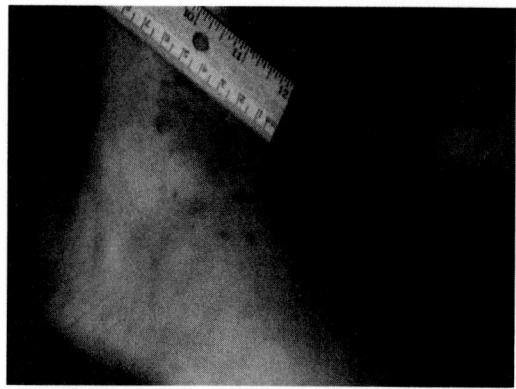

FIGURE 2.3 A skin rash in a young male with eosinophilic granulomatosis with polyangiitis (EGPA, or Churg-Strauss syndrome). EGPA may affect variable-sized blood vessels and in dermatologic manifestations may resemble hypersensitivity vasculitis with palpable purpura. See Color Plate 2 in insert.

increasing eosinophilia and any evidence of systemic complications should raise suspicion for EGPA. Systemic manifestations include a rash suggestive of leukocytoclastic vasculitis or palpable purpura (most likely nonrespiratory feature) (Figure 2.3), footdrop or other peripheral neurologic disease, abdominal pain, or pericardial or myocardial abnormalities. In addition to other organ involvement, asthma with lung infiltrates should raise suspicion for EGPA. Intermittent or chronic systemic corticosteroid therapy, or even very high doses of inhaled corticosteroids, sometimes required for the management of persistent asthma, will mask or partially treat EGPA, resulting in complications of vasculitis when the corticosteroid therapy is tapered or discontinued. Other conditions in the differential diagnosis of an asthmatic patient with EGPA include allergic bronchopulmonary aspergillosis, aspirin- or nonsteroidal anti-inflammatory drug–exacerbated respiratory disease, eosinophilic bronchitis, eosinophilic pneumonia, parasite disease with pulmonary involvement, fungal hypersensitivity sinusitis, eosinophilic otitis media, drug reaction with rash, and hypereosinophilic syndrome.

Several reports have associated the onset of EGPA with the introduction of leukotriene modifiers for the treatment of asthma. The leading explanation is that a reduction of corticosteroid therapy following leukotriene modifier therapy allows the suppressed EGPA to become evident. Other investigators have suggested that EGPA may actually be caused or exacerbated by leukotriene modifiers. No evidence that the leukotriene modifiers are the cause or contribute pathologically to EGPA is available other than a possible increase in the prevalence of CSS since leukotriene modifiers were introduced. Other asthma therapies, including inhaled cromolyn sodium and parenteral omalizumab, and even inhaled corticosteroids, have also been associated with EGPA, although causal roles are not suspected.

Manifestations of GPA are in both the upper airway and lung, with or without renal involvement. Typically the respiratory specialist will encounter patients with respiratory symptoms or findings without renal disease. The upper airway manifestations include severe sinusitis, chronic otitis media with effusion, mastoiditis, nasal cartilage perforation or collapse, tracheal collapse (Figure 2.4), hearing loss, or hoarseness. Lower airway manifestations include pulmonary infiltrates or nodules, shortness of breath, or cough, which may be associated with hemoptysis. Systemic manifestations are protean, with renal involvement being the most common. Renal manifestations include hematuria and decreased renal function with nephritis. The upper airway pathology associated with some lower respiratory symptoms is the most likely scenario in which GPA presents as a comorbidity of suspected asthma. Significant upper respiratory disease, particularly rhinitis or rhinosinusitis, is associated with asthma, making GPA a potential comorbidity for consideration in most patients with persistent asthma symptoms. Asthma is not specifically associated with GPA, but cough and shortness of breath with sinus or nasal complaints are symptoms that are shared between the diseases. The differential diagnosis of GPA includes EGPA, pulmonary tuberculosis, lymphoma, bacterial lung abscess, Goodpasture's disease (antiglomerular basement membrane disease), polychondritis, and lung cancer.

MPA is an ANCA-positive vasculitis associated with small vessel hemorrhage, particularly in the lung. The lung bleeding is likely to result in the presentation of affected individuals with cough and shortness of breath, but wheezing would not be expected. Subtle infiltrates may raise the suspicion of infectious disease or even inflammatory diseases such as hypersensitivity pneumonitis. There is no predilection for MPA in subjects with asthma.

DIAGNOSIS

ANCA-positive vasculitic syndromes may present as a respiratory complaint because of the clinical features shared with asthma and other respiratory diseases or the association of EGPA with asthma. Vasculitis should be suspected in patients with difficult-to-treat asthma or with symptoms that are suggestive of but atypical for asthma or obstructive lung disease. The vasculitic syndromes are protean, systemic illnesses that may present with varied symptoms that are difficult to characterize in a limited review. The overlap of respiratory symptoms with systemic complaints or findings should raise the suspicion of vasculitis. Specific features that may suggest the consideration of vasculitis include anemia, fatigue, nonspecific joint complaints, rash suggestive of hypersensitivity vasculitis (Figure 2.3), hearing loss, nasal bleeding, weight loss, elevation of acute phase reactants, and neurologic complaints, particularly neuropathy or mononeuritis multiplex.

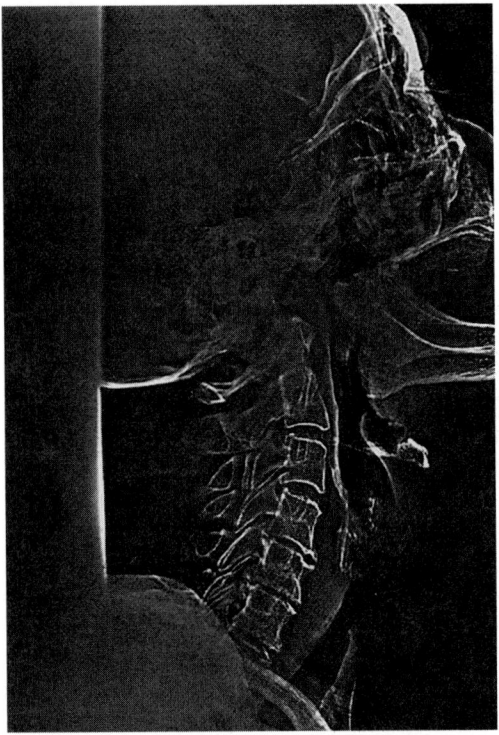

FIGURE 2.4 Collapse of the tracheal cartilage due to granulomatosis with polyangiitis (Wegener's granulomatosis). Typically necrotizing tissue destruction occurs in the upper airway, lung, and kidney, but involvement of only one tissue may occur. In addition to necrosis of the nasal septum, mastoiditis, middle ear disease, sinusitis with bone necrosis, and laryngeal involvement or tracheal collapse may occur in the upper airway. The figure shows the appearance of the trachea during inhalation.

Tests that may assist in making the diagnosis of vasculitis include the following (Table 2.2).

Table 2.2. Diagnosis of Vasculitis

- Chest imaging with posterior-anterior and lateral radiograph or computed tomography (Figure 2.2)
- Serum creatinine
- Complete blood count to assess for anemia and eosinophilia
- Acute phase reactants
    - Erythrocyte sedimentation rate
    - C-reactive protein
    - Platelet count
- Sinus imaging to evaluate bone erosion or atypical sinusitis
- Ear or mastoid imaging
- Hearing/audiology testing
- ANCA with specific antibody for proteinase 3 and myeloperoxidase
- Urine analysis for blood or protein
- Nerve conduction studies
- Biopsy of affected tissues to confirm vasculitis and tissue inflammation

ANCA testing is a useful strategy to assist in the evaluation of suspected vasculitis that is a comorbidity of asthma or other respiratory disease. Immunofluorescence using the serum of the test subject applied to fixed neutrophils,

Table 2.3. Diagnosis of Eosinophilc Granulomatosis with Polyangiitis (Churg-Strauss Syndrome)*

- Asthma or atopy
- Blood eosinophilia > 500/mm³
- Neuritis or neuropathy/mononeuritis multiplex
- Pulmonary infiltrates
- Sinusitis
- Tissue eosinophilia and granuloma associated with vasculitis

*Four of six criteria suggests diagnosis of EGPA.

followed by labeled antihuman IgG, is the most sensitive assay for ANCA but is not as specific as Western blot in identifying antibody specific for myeloperoxidase or proteinase 3 or other granule contents (Figure 2.1). Immunofluorescence is difficult to standardize, and the interpretation is variable based on the experience of the individual viewing the immunofluorescence pattern. Thus, immunofluorescence is a sensitive screening assay that should be confirmed with identification of antibody to specific substances. Using this strategy, about 50% to 60% of EGPA patients have ANCA-positive disease, with more than 75% of those with positive immunofluorescence having myeloperoxidase antibody (Table 2.3). Ninety percent of patients with GPA have a positive ANCA, but the 10% with a negative ANCA are often patients with airway limited disease, clinical presentations more likely to be seen by physicians treating asthma and allergic respiratory disease. GPA limited to the upper airway is ANCA positive in about 60% of cases. Ninety percent of patients with GPA and a positive ANCA have antibody specific for proteinase 3. About 70% of patients with MPA have a positive ANCA, and most of these cases are specific for myeloperoxidase. Identifying subsets of ANCA-positive vasculitic syndromes may predict treatment response. For example, rituximab may be more effective in syndromes with autoantibody specificity for proteinase 3 or myeloperoxidase (see "Treatment").[7-14]

Without tissue confirmation (Figure 2.5), the diagnosis of vasculitis remains tentative. Unfortunately, respiratory tissue biopsies often have too low a yield of sufficient tissue to provide a definitive diagnosis. Typically transbronchial biopsy will not be definitive, and nasal, ear, or sinus biopsies usually must include blood vessels to confirm diagnosis. Malignancy and infection, particularly fungal and mycobacterial infection, also need to be considered in the differential diagnosis, so culture of biopsy material may be helpful.

The major diagnostic criteria of EGPA have changed from the original suggestion made 25 years ago by Lanham, first to a revision of the Lanham criteria in 1990 by the American College of Rheumatology, in which six criteria were used, and four out of the six gave a definite diagnosis of EGPA, and second to the

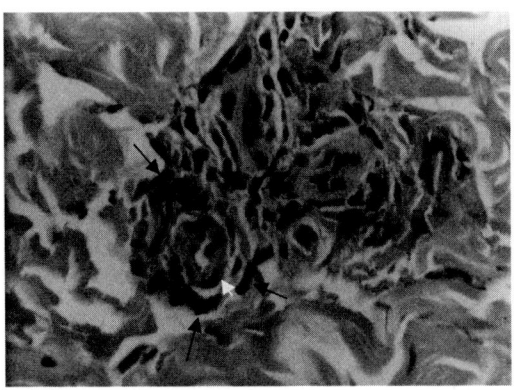

FIGURE 2.5 A skin biopsy from a subject with eosinophilic granulomatosis with polyangiitis (EGPA, or Churg-Strauss syndrome). This is a high-power view with hematoxylin and eosin staining. Eosinophil infiltration of the tissue (*black arrows*) and of the small vessels (*white arrowhead*) in the subcutaneous tissue is seen. Granulomas are not noted, and with early diagnosis, this is often the case. See Color Plate 3 in insert.

Chapel Hill Consensus Conference in 1994, which examined in more detail the potential pathologic findings of EGPA (Table 2.4). Criteria are generally developed for defining subjects for clinical trials, and fulfillment of these criteria is not required for an individual diagnosis.

More than 90% of EGPA (CSS) cases are associated with moderately severe to severe asthma, usually with significant peripheral blood eosinophilia and tissue eosinophilia. A variety of other clinical manifestations associated with EGPA include evidence of atopy; sinus disease and upper airway disease; polyneuropathy or mononeuritis multiplex, usually of an extremity; and pulmonary infiltrates in addition to airway obstruction associated with asthma. Four out of six categories of clinical involvement are required to fulfill criteria of a clinical diagnosis of EGPA, but tissue confirmation of extravascular eosinophil tissue infiltration is required for definitive diagnosis.

PHARMACOLOGIC TREATMENT

Optimal treatment strategies for EGPA or MPA are not established but are based primarily on the more common vasculitic syndromes, such as GPA or polyarteritis nodosa. Thus, EGPA, GPA, and MPA have similar treatments with some variations. Initial treatment for ANCA-positive vasculitis is high-dose (2 mg/kg) systemic corticosteroid coupled with cytotoxic therapy such as cyclophosphamide. With evidence of clinical response, the dose of corticosteroid is gradually reduced to every-other-day treatment, and after 6 to 12 months the cytotoxic therapy is changed to methotrexate, azathioprine, or mycophenolate mofetil. EGPA is more responsive to corticosteroids, and treatment with systemic corticosteroids may minimize or obviate the need for cytotoxic therapy. If less intense treatment is used, vigilance is paramount to recognize any evidence of serious organ dysfunction that would warrant more aggressive cytotoxic or other aggressive immunosuppressive therapy. Such manifestations would include severe abdominal pain, hematuria or change in renal function, chest pain, or neurologic findings (Table 2.4). High-dose intravenous immunoglobulin may also be helpful in EGPA, presumably because of a decrease in eosinophils due to immunomodulation by the immunoglobulin therapy (Table 2.5). Interferon-α has also benefited EGPA. There are reports that targeting eosinophils with anti–interleukin-5 (anti–IL-5) resulted in improvement in refractory EGPA. Anti-IL-5 has not been used for GPA or MPA. Rituximab (anti-CD20, targeting

Table 2.4. Antineutrophil Cytoplasmic Antibody Profile—Eosinophilic Granulomatosis with Polyangiitis (Churg-Strauss Syndrome)

- Anti–proteinase 3 (anti-PR3) antineutrophil cytoplasmic antibody (ANCA); usually not found in Eosinophilic granulomatosis with polyangiitis (Churg-Strauss syndrome)
- Antimyeloperoxidase (anti-MPO) ANCA; positive in approximately 60% of Eosinophilic granulomatosis with polyangiitis
- Anti-MPO ANCA positivity; associated with more eosinophils and inflammation, more organ systems involved, and more symptoms

Table 2.5. Treatments for Eosinophilic Granulomatosis with Polyangiitis other than Corticosteroids and Cytotoxic/Antiproliferative Agents

- Interferon-α
- Intravenous immunoglobulin
- Biologic monoclonals
- Omalizumab (anti–immunoglobulin E)
- Mepolizumab (anti–interleukin-5)
- Reslizumab (anti–interleukin-5)
- Rituximab (anti-CD20)

B lymphocytes) may improve ANCA-positive vasculitis that is refractory to standard therapy or that is associated with side effects limiting the use of other therapies.[16,17] The potential contribution of IL-17 to EGPA is under investigation. Lymphocytes producing IL-17 have been associated with autoimmune disease and variants of asthma. Finally, case reports of clinical response of EGPA to omalizumab (monoclonal anti-IgE) are in the literature.

Long-lasting remission occurs with treatment of EGPA. Following ANCA titers is of no value, but monitoring clinical features, acute phase reactants, and peripheral eosinophil counts, is useful. Complete remission does not generally occur with GPA, and lifelong immunomodulator therapy or immunosuppression is usually required. Less is known about the prognosis of MPA.

UNMET, FUTURE RESEARCH NEEDS

Insight into the etiology and regulation of the pathology of ANCA-associated vasculitis is needed, as is true of most of the systemic vasculitic syndromes. EGPA and MPA are very rare, making controlled trials problematic. GPA is more common, and treatment algorithms are better defined. The absence of a definite cause of ANCA-associated vasculitis makes cure unlikely for most of these diseases. The association of the airway with ANCA-positive syndromes also requires additional understanding.

There is evidence that ANCA activates neutrophils and may play role in the pathogenesis of these diseases. However, a number of patients are ANCA negative but have vasculitis that is very similar, and ANCA titers do not predict their disease course. Thus, alternative pathologic pathways are likely, and insight into these pathways is needed.

CONCLUSION

The ANCA-associated vasculitis syndromes, EGPA (CSS or AAG), GPA (Wegener's granulomatosis), and MPA, are serious comorbidities of asthma or upper respiratory disease, or the symptoms of the vasculitis may resemble asthma or associated upper airway disease. ANCA-associated vasculitis is potentially fatal but is responsive to a variety of treatments if it is recognized before serious organ dysfunction. The role of ANCA in these conditions has not been defined because EGPA, GPA, or MPA may occur without ANCA, and the titer of ANCA does not predict clinical course. Clinical suspicion and consideration of tissue biopsy are important for recognition before irreversible complications occur. Corticosteroid therapy for asthma or suspected asthma may modify the presentations of ANCA-positive vasculitis, particularly EGPA.

REFERENCES

1. Ozaki S. ANCA-associated vasculitis: diagnostic and therapeutic strategy. *Allergol Int.* 2007;56:87–96.
2. Lionaki S, Blyth ER, Hogan SL, et al. Classification of antineutrophil cytoplasmic autoantibody vasculitides: the role of antineutrophil cytoplasmic autoantibody specificity for myeloperoxidase or proteinase 3 in disease recognition and prognosis. *Arthritis Rheum.* 2012;64:3452–3462.
3. Healy B, Bibby S, Steele R, Weatherall M, Nelson H, Beasley R. Antineutrophil cytoplasmic autoantibodies and myeloperoxidase autoantibodies in clinical expression of Churg-Strauss syndrome. *J Allergy Clin Immunol.* 2013;131:571–576.
4. Vaglio A, Buzio C, Zwerina J. Eosinophilic granulomatosis with polyangiitis (Churg-Strauss): state of the art. *Allergy.* 2013;68:261–273.

5. Pagnoux C, Guilpain P, Guillevin L. Churg-Strauss syndrome. *Curr Opin Rheumatol.* 2007;19:25–32.
6. Sable-Fourtassou R, Cohen P, Mahr A, et al. Antineutrophil cytoplasmic antibodies and Churg-Strauss syndrome. *Ann Intern Med.* 2005;143:632–638.
7. Guillevin L, Pagnoux C, Guilpain P, Bienvenu B, Martinez V, Mouthon L. Indications for biotherapy in systemic vasculitides. *Clin Rev Allergy Immunol.* 2007;32:85–96.
8. Mouna Maamar M, Tazi-Mezalek Z, Harmouche H, el Hamany Z, Adnanoui M, Aouni A. Churg-Strauss syndrome associated with AA amyloidosis: a case report. *Pan Afr Med J.* 2012;12:30.
9. Stone JH, Merkel PA, Spiera R, et al. Rituximab versus cyclophosphamide for ANCA-associated vasculitis. *N Engl J Med.* 2010;363:221–232.
10. Jones RB, Cohen Tervaert JW, Hauser T, et al. Rituximab versus cyclophosphamide in ANCA-associated renal vasculitis. *N Engl J Med.* 2010;363;211–220.
11. Falk RJ, Jennette C. Rituximab in ANCA-associated disease. *N Engl J Med.* 2010;363: 285–286.
12. Schonermarck U, Rau S, Fischerder M, Nosssent JC. Rituximab or cyclophosphamide in ANCA-associated renal vasculitis. *N Engl J Med.* 2010;363:21.
13. Goncalves C, Pinaffi JC, Carvalho JF, et al. Antineutrophil cytoplasmic antibodies in chronic rhinosinusitis may be a marker of undisclosed vasculitis. *Am J Rhinol.* 2007;15:691–694.
14. Cartin-Ceba R, Keogh KA, Specks U, Sethi S, Fervenza F. Rituximab for the treatment of Churg-Strauss syndrome with renal involvement. *Nephrol Dial Transplant.* 2011;26: 2865–2871.
15. Shoichi Ozaki S. ANCA-associated vasculitis: diagnostic and therapeutic strategy. *Allergol Int.* 2007;56:87–96.
16. Stone JH, Merkel PA, Speira R, et al. Rituximab versus cyclophosphamide for ANCA-associated vasculitis. *N Engl J Med* 2010;363:221–232.
17. Martinez Del Pero M, Chaudbry A, Jones RB, Sivasotby P, Jani P, Jayne D. B-cell depletion with rituximab for refractory head and neck Wegener's granulomatosis: a cohort study. *Clin Otolaryngol* 2009;34:328–335.

3

ALLERGIC BRONCHOPULMONARY ASPERGILLOSIS

COMORBID

Paul A. Greenberger

KEY POINTS

- Allergic bronchopulmonary aspergillosis (ABPA) may cause increasing severity of asthma, but rarely it presents in the absence of symptomatic asthma with collapse of a lobe, suggesting lymphoma.
- New pulmonary infiltrates are associated with peripheral blood eosinophilia, often from 8% to 35%.
- Oral glucocorticoids are the drug of choice for treatment of ABPA; antifungal therapies are adjunctive. There are case reports of benefit as well as lack of response with the monoclonal antibody omalizumab.
- The total immunoglobulin E concentration varies with disease activity in that it can double or increase 5- to 10-fold at the time of an episode of pulmonary infiltrates with eosinophilia.
- Bronchiectasis can be present in multiple lobes and is irreversible. Because of the presence of calcium salts, the mucus is of high attenuation on computed tomographic scans of the lungs.
- Spores of *Aspergillus fumigatus* are inhaled and grow in bronchial mucus as septate hyphae.
- *A. fumigatus* has 23 standardized allergens, many of which are potent enzymes that damage bronchial epithelium and serve in a proinflammatory manner.
- Genetic susceptibilities support a pattern of helper T-cell type 2 responses and increased responsiveness to interleukin-4.

INTRODUCTION

Allergic bronchopulmonary aspergillosis (ABPA), a disease that complicates asthma and cystic fibrosis, is in the differential diagnosis of pulmonary infiltrates, peripheral blood or sputum eosinophilia, elevated total serum immunoglobulin E (IgE) concentration, and bronchiectasis, any or all of which may occur in patients with established asthma.[1] ABPA may cause increasing severity of asthma, but alternatively it can present in the absence of symptomatic asthma with collapse of a lobe, suggesting lymphoma. Complications of ABPA include bronchiectasis (which is irreversible), collapse of a lobe or lung with resultant permanent fibrotic findings, pulmonary cavities, chronic sputum production consistent with a diagnosis of chronic bronchitis, atypical mycobacteria or gram-negative bacteria with species of *Pseudomonas aeruginosa* or *Burkholderia cepacia* in sputum, hypoxemia, and respiratory failure. Furthermore, use of long-term prednisone can cause adverse effects, and the antifungal azoles have their own adverse effects and drug interactions.[2]

CLINICAL FEATURES

Some of the clinical features of ABPA include (1) tenacious, golden-brown mucous plugs that are expectorated by patients and demonstrate eosinophils, septate hyphae, and growth of *A. fumigatus*; (2) pulmonary infiltrates associated with peripheral blood eosinophilia[3] (often ranging from 8% to 35%); (3) cough; (4) dyspnea associated with worsening of asthma; (5) onset of chronic sputum production in a nonsmoker; and (6) wheezing or post-tussive crackles on auscultation of the lung.

The tenacious mucous plugs may be difficult or impossible to extract during bronchoscopy in a patient with unexplained pulmonary infiltrates. Alternatively, patients may produce plugs readily either at times of new or continuing pulmonary infiltrates or as part of ongoing mucous plugging from ABPA. The plugs demonstrate eosinophils and septate hyphae consistent with *A. fumigatus* that can be recovered in culture either from bronchoscopy samples or from sputum.

Most patients with ABPA have several of the following phenotypes of atopy: allergic rhinitis, immediate skin reactivity to multiple inhalant and mold allergens, food allergy, drug allergy, urticaria, and a family history of allergic diseases.[4] The diagnosis of asthma typically antedates the onset of and diagnosis of ABPA (pulmonary infiltrates with eosinophilia), but ever since a report in 1971, it has been recognized that asthma may become manifest on or after the diagnosis of ABPA.[5] The severity of asthma ranges from intermittent to persistent severe. Although some patients describe acute wheezing dyspnea upon exposure to freshly cut grass, damp basements, raked leaves, or moldy hay or in the vicinity of recently turned compost piles, in a series of 38 patients with ABPA, 4 patients did not report any of these classic triggers of mold-associated wheezing.[4]

ABPA may be suspected in the setting of patients with transient pulmonary infiltrates (often with peripheral blood eosinophilia) (Figure 3.1), but some patients present with homogeneous and dense consolidations that mimic bacterial pneumonia, or lymphoma. The associated clinical symptoms or physical examination findings can be expected to be less intense than if the same radiographic consolidations were the result of a community-acquired pneumonia, when the patient would report severe dyspnea, productive cough, fever, chills, and rigors.

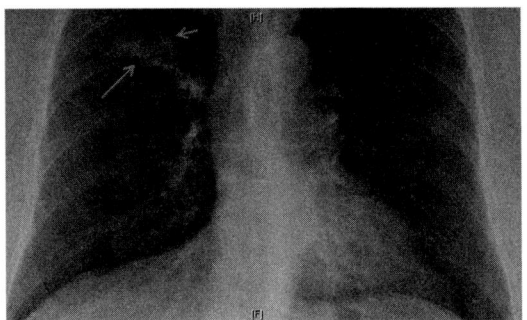

FIGURE 3.1 A 55-year-old patient with stage III ABPA presented with cough but no wheeze. The chest film demonstrates mucoid impaction (*red arrows*) in the right upper lobe consistent with an exacerbation of ABPA. The white blood count was 10,000/μL with 34% eosinophils. The total IgE concentration had increased to 7,020 kU/L, compared with 2,607 kU/L 4 months previously when she was asymptomatic.

HOW TO DIAGNOSE ACCURATELY AND WHAT DIAGNOSTIC TESTS OR STRATEGIES TO EMPLOY

The diagnostic criteria are listed in Table 3.1 for ABPA with central bronchiectasis (ABPA-CB)[1,6-9] and ABPA without bronchiectasis (ABPA-seropositive).[10,11] Nearly all patients have immediate skin reactivity to prick skin testing with a mix of *Aspergillus* species, but if the prick skin test is negative, an intradermal injection of *A. fumigatus* can be expected to be positive. This finding is important from the screening perspective. If a skin-testing process with high sensitivity shows negative results, then ABPA can essentially be ruled out.[8] This observation remains true despite the presence of elevated total immunoglobulin E (IgE) concentrations or of precipitating antibodies to *A. fumigatus*.

The demonstration of immediate cutaneous reactivity to *A. fumigatus* or the in vitro demonstration of anti–*A. fumigatus* IgE antibodies is essential, and elevated total IgE concentration means greater than 417 kU/L (1 kU/L = 1 IU/mL = 2.4 ng/mL). The total IgE concentration varies with disease activity in that it can double or increase 5- to 10-fold at the time of an episode of pulmonary infiltrates with eosinophilia. The baseline total IgE concentration often is elevated and does not return to less than 417 kU/L despite months of daily prednisone in the absence of infiltrates or significant mucous plugging on chest radiographs or high-resolution computed tomography (HRCT) examination of the lungs. Of note, the fraction of total IgE that is reactive with *A. fumigatus* is low. However, diluted sera from patients with ABPA have at least twice the antibodies to *A. fumigatus* when compared with sera from patients with asthma and 3 or 4+ prick skin test reactivity to *Aspergillus* but in which there are not sufficient criteria for a diagnosis of ABPA.[6] The latter observation forms the basis for a useful diagnostic test because about 25% or more of patients with

Table 3.1. Criteria for Diagnosis of Allergic Bronchopulmonary Aspergillosis

CLASSIC CASE WITH BRONCHIECTASIS	MINIMAL ESSENTIAL CRITERIA
Asthma	Yes
Bronchiectasis (proximalinner two-thirds of lung on high-resolution computed tomography)	Yes
Chest radiographic infiltrates (typically upper lobes or middle lobe)	No
Immediate skin reactivity to *Aspergillus* species or *Aspergillus fumigatus*	Yes
Total immunoglobulin E (IgE) concentration > 417 kU/L	Yes
Elevated serum anti–*A. fumigatus* IgE and/or IgG*	Yes
ALLERGIC BRONCHOPULMONARY ASPERGILLOSIS WITHOUT BRONCHIECTASIS (ABPA-SEROPOSITIVE)	
Asthma	Yes
Chest radiographic infiltrates (typically upper lobes or middle lobe)	Yes/no†
Immediate skin reactivity to *Aspergillus* species or *A. fumigatus*	Yes
Total IgE concentration > 417 kU/L	Yes
Elevated serum anti–*A. fumigatus* IgE and IgG*	Yes

* Compared with sera from patients with allergic asthma and skin test reactivity to *A. fumigatus*.
† Minimal essential criteria for ABPA-seropositive did not include current chest radiographic infiltrates when first published in 1993,[10] but by 2012,[11] it was considered a minimal criterion.

persistent asthma have immediate skin reactivity to *Aspergillus* species, yet only about 1% of such patients have ABPA.[8] Furthermore, the same observation occurs with measurement of anti–*A. fumigatus* IgG, whose measurement also can help discriminate between allergic (fungal) asthma and ABPA.[10]

Some diagnostic criteria are not essential, such as precipitating antibodies to *A. fumigatus*. In a series in which 69 of 86 patients (80%) with ABPA (including 50 of 58 with ABPA-CB and 19 of 28 with ABPA-seropositive) had detectable precipitating antibodies, precipitating antibodies to *A. fumigatus* were detected in 84 of 827 patients (10.1%) evaluated for ABPA because of a positive immediate skin test to *Aspergillus* species (prick skin test, and if negative, intradermal).[10]

The chest radiographs occasionally may be free of infiltrates, especially if the patient is not having a pulmonary exacerbation. In ABPA-seropositive (or ABPA-CB), the chest radiograph typically shows mucous plugging, pneumonia, transient upper lobe infiltrates, the finger-in-glove sign of distally occluded bronchi filled with secretions, or no pertinent findings.[10] The HRCT examination findings do not demonstrate bronchiectasis (ABPA-seropositive) but still reveal mucous plugging, infiltrates, or the tree-in-bud pattern.[12] The latter refers to clusters of nodular opacities from inspissated mucoid impaction of bronchioles.[12]

HRCT has been extremely useful in the diagnosis of ABPA and has helped to replace lung biopsies or wedge resections. Bronchiectasis occurs in ABPA in areas of pulmonary infiltrates, especially if the infiltrates have not been treated. The bronchiectasis may be present on the chest radiograph as ring shadows, but often HRCT examination is required. In contrast to the bronchiectasis of patients with cystic fibrosis, bronchiectasis in ABPA is considered "proximal," meaning dilated bronchi are present in the inner two-thirds of the field during HRCT examination.[13] Although some patients with ABPA-CB (and absence of cystic fibrosis) can have areas of proximal and distal bronchiectasis, most patients with ABPA do not. Alternatively, peripheral bronchiectasis was detectable in 33% of lobes if the inner two-thirds rule was used and in 43% of lobes if the inner one-half (from hilum to chest wall) rule was used.[14] In cystic fibrosis, the bronchiectasis extends peripherally so that although it can be "proximal," it also can be "proximal" and "distal."[15] HRCT scanning in ABPA can reveal bronchiectasis if the ratio of the internal diameter of the bronchus to the diameter of the adjacent artery is greater than 1 (Figure 3.2). Terminology for bronchiectasis is as follows: *cylindrical* (normally shaped bronchi with a lumen larger than the adjacent artery), *varicose* (dilatation of bronchi with a beaded pattern longitudinally), or *cystic* (marked saccular dilatation with or without air fluid levels).[13] The distribution of bronchiectasis typically involves multiple lobes,[14,16] and because of the presence of calcium salts, the mucus is of high attenuation.[14,17] The frequent finding of bronchiectasis in the posterior segment of the right upper lobe mimics infection with *Mycobacterium tuberculosum*. HRCT examination also can demonstrate mucoid

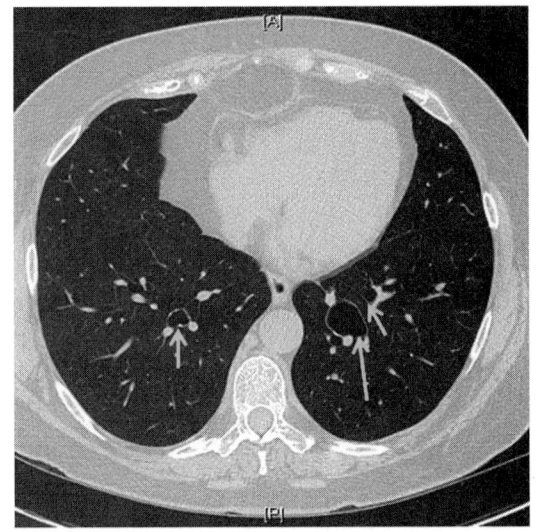

FIGURE 3.2 A 53-year-old patient with long-standing ABPA with chronic productive cough. High-resolution computed tomography illustrates bronchiectasis (*red arrows*). Note that the ratio of the internal diameter of the bronchus to that of the adjacent artery (*solid white circle*) clearly is greater than 1, consistent with bronchiectasis.

impaction, centrilobular nodules, pulmonary fibrosis, a mosaic pattern, air trapping, unsuspected infiltrates, and thickening of the bronchial walls.

The strategies to diagnose ABPA begin with different approaches. One approach is to screen and consider the possibility of ABPA when there is evidence of immediate skin reactivity to *A. fumigatus* (which means prick or "epicutaneous" test and, if negative, an intradermal test). In some reports, this approach leads to as high as a 25% incidence of ABPA, likely from specialist referral patterns.[18-20] Use of a very sensitive fluorescence enzyme immunoassay (FEIA) for anti–*A. fumigatus* IgE as a screening test seemingly should produce similar results. If the results are negative, then that essentially excludes a diagnosis of ABPA. If evidence of other fungi is present, then the patient may have allergic bronchopulmonary mycosis. If the skin test or FEIA is positive, then one should obtain the total serum IgE concentration. If it is elevated, then at the Northwestern University Division of Allergy-Immunology, we determine the anti–*A. fumigatus* IgE and IgG, compared with sera from patients without ABPA but in whom there is a 3 or 4+ prick skin test response to *A. fumigatus*. If this test is positive, then ABPA is often present and is "seropositive" if there is no bronchiectasis on HRCT examination of the lungs. In the absence of such a specialized test, a decision must be made to obtain the HRCT of the lungs when the patient has asthma (and often a history of a pulmonary infiltrate, even if it was diagnosed as a community-acquired pneumonia), positive skin test to *A. fumigatus*, and total IgE concentration of greater than 417 kU/L.

The second approach to diagnose ABPA stems directly from the presence of one of the five diagnostic criteria for ABPA: (1) pulmonary infiltrate with peripheral blood eosinophilia, (2) suspicious mucous plugging or homogeneous consolidation on HRCT obtained in a patient perhaps because of increasingly more severe asthma, (3) proximal bronchiectasis and other radiographic findings identified by the radiologist as consistent with ABPA, (4) unexpected peripheral blood eosinophilia (ranging from 8% to 35%), or (5) recovery of *A. fumigatus* from sputum or from bronchoscopy. If a patient with asthma presents with any of these criteria, then skin testing for *A. fumigatus* (or FEIA) should be performed and the concentration of total IgE determined. HRCT can help to confirm or rule out ABPA-central bronchiectasis.

When making the diagnosis, it is important to consider the five stages of ABPA (Table 3.2) because the patient may be diagnosed with ABPA in the absence of current radiographic infiltrates.[21-23] In stage I (acute), the patient meets the minimal essential criteria listed in Table 3.1 for ABPA-seropositive as well as having the pulmonary infiltrates that indicate ABPA-CB. Peripheral blood eosinophilia is expected but is not an essential criterion for this stage. Administration of prednisone helps to clear the pulmonary infiltrates, decreases symptoms of asthma and sputum production, and results in the decline of peripheral blood eosinophilia. There should be an expected reduction of total IgE concentration of at least 33% in 6 weeks.[24] Prednisone is administered for 2 to 3 months and then discontinued. If the patient remains without new pulmonary infiltrates (unexplained by other causes) and does not require long-term prednisone for control of asthma for 6 months, then the patient is considered to be in stage II (remission). The patient can remain in stage II for months, for years, or permanently. Occasionally, a patient remains in remission for 7 years before having an exacerbation (stage III). The exacerbation stage resembles stage I (acute), with new pulmonary infiltrates, elevation over baseline of total serum IgE (at least double the baseline concentration, which itself can remain elevated, e.g., at 5,000 kU/L), and if measured, peripheral blood eosinophilia. Often, the index diagnosis of ABPA is made in patients who, from a retrospective vantage point, presented in stage III (exacerbation). In these patients, pulmonary infiltrates (see Figure 3.1) are cleared with prednisone. Mucous plugs may or may not be present and often are reduced in number by prednisone (and in some patients by antifungal azole therapy). The total IgE concentration will decline with effective prednisone (and in some patients antifungal azole) therapy.

Table 3.2. Stages of Allergic Bronchopulmonary Aspergillosis with Central Bronchiectasis

STAGE	RADIOGRAPHIC INFILTRATES*	TOTAL IGE CONCENTRATION	INDICATION FOR PREDNISONE†
I (acute)	Yes	> 417 kU/L	Yes
II (remission)	No	> or < 417 kU/L	No
III (exacerbation)	Yes	> 417 kU/L	Yes
IV (corticosteroid-dependent asthma)	Usually not	> or < 417 kU/L	Yes for asthma
V (end-stage fibrocavitary)	Fibrosis, cavities	> or < 417 kU/L	Yes

*Can be present on chest radiographs as mucous plugging, homogeneous infiltrates, consolidation, or cavitation; in addition, can be present on high-resolution computed tomography as bronchiectasis or tree-in-bud bronchiolar infiltrates (see text).

† May supplement with antifungal therapy as adjunctive treatment or potentially other therapies (see text). Prednisone is not indicated for treatment of stage II ABPA even if the total immunoglobulin E is elevated at concentrations greater than 3,000 kU/L.

If there are increasing medication requirements for persistent asthma and, in particular, the need for prednisone administration to control asthma as opposed to all other therapies, the disease is classified as stage IV (corticosteroid-dependent asthma).[21,22] There may or may not be new pulmonary infiltrates with increases in total IgE, compatible with an exacerbation. Stage V (end-stage fibrocavitary asthma) is identified when there is irreversible fibrotic, cavitary, or fibrocavitary lung disease with severe reductions in forced expiratory volume in 1 second (FEV_1), irreversible airways obstruction, and restriction on pulmonary function tests. New pulmonary infiltrates are more likely to be associated with gram-negative pneumonia (P. aeruginosa), atypical mycobacteria (rapidly growing), or other pathogens, but not A. fumigatus.

There are several "false" steps to avoid when diagnosing ABPA: (1) failing to have a high enough index of suspicion for ABPA when a patient with asthma presents with persistent asthma, immediate skin test reactivity to A. fumigatus, and two prior episodes of pneumonia or known and otherwise unexplained bronchiectasis or chronic productive cough; (2) failing to adequately identify or exclude anti–A. fumigatus IgE by performing a prick skin test but, if nonreactive, failing to perform an intradermal test, causing reduced sensitivity in this screening test; (3) devaluing the potential importance of peripheral blood eosinophilia ranging from 8% to 35% or more in a patient with increasingly severe asthma or a new pulmonary infiltrate; and (4) failing to search for ABPA when a patient with asthma presents with collapse of a lung segment or lobe and no malignancy or other explanation is found on bronchoscopy but there is inspissated mucus that is not readily retrieved or removed during bronchoscopy.

ALLERGIC BRONCHOPULMONARY ASPERGILLOSIS IS A COMORBID-COEXISTING SUBTYPE OF ASTHMA

ABPA is referred to as an endotype or subtype of asthma with its own pathophysiology, susceptibilities, and treatment.[25] ABPA complicates asthma and may convert intermittent or persistent mild asthma into persistent severe asthma. Whereas in asthma there is either no detectable bronchiectasis or a few areas of cylindrical bronchiectasis that are not clinically important, in ABPA-CB there can be widespread bronchiectasis with up to three patterns (cylindrical, saccular, or varicose) as previously mentioned. Furthermore, in asthma, remodeling can result in thickened bronchial walls and subepithelial fibrosis, but in ABPA, there can be large areas of mucoid impaction, collapse of a lobe or even lung, pulmonary infiltrates, tree-in-bud bronchiolar infiltrates, atelectasis, frank fibrosis, or bronchiolitis obliterans. Thus, ABPA involves the proximal and distal airways, can destroy lung architecture, and can produce bronchiectasis, pulmonary fibrosis, and cavitary lung disease. A notable feature of ABPA is the saprophytic colonization of the bronchi with hyphae of *A. fumigatus* and production of mucous plugs that clear or are reduced in number with oral glucocorticoids.

The differential diagnosis of ABPA includes conditions that have similarities with aspects of ABPA. Major conditions to be considered include Churg-Strauss syndrome, eosinophilic pneumonia (chronic, simple, acute, tropical), idiopathic hypereosinophilic syndrome, drug allergy, parasitism (such as *Strongyloides stercoralis*), allergic bronchopulmonary mycosis, and hypersensitivity pneumonitis from fungi.[26-28] In Churg-Strauss syndrome, which is a systemic, necrotizing, extravascular, eosinophilic granulomatous vasculitis, there are pulmonary infiltrates, peripheral blood eosinophilia ranging from 20% to 60% on differential, peripheral neuropathy (mononeuritis multiplex), and palpable purpura.[26] The antineutrophil cytoplasmic antibody (perinuclear) test is positive in 60% of patients, and the antineutrophil cytoplasmic antibody (cytoplasmic) is identified in 10% of patients.[26] In ABPA, such results are negative, and there is an absence of mononeuritis multiplex and palpable purpura. Of the four types of eosinophilic pneumonia, chronic eosinophilic pneumonia most closely mimics ABPA. The chest radiographic infiltrates can be bilateral and peripheral, although not always the "photographic negative of pulmonary edema."[27] Peripheral blood eosinophilia should be at least 1,000/μL, and chronic eosinophilic pneumonia responds to low-dosage prednisone.[26] In idiopathic hypereosinophilic syndrome, there must be at least 1,500 eosinophils/μL for 6 months in the absence of other explanations. The chest radiographic findings often consist of pulmonary edema, interstitial infiltrates, and pleural effusions.[27] In drug allergy, the radiographic findings can include consolidation, hilar adenopathy, diffuse infiltrates, pleural effusions, ground-glass opacities, and reticulonodular densities.[27] In parasitic infections with *S. stercoralis* in patients without immunocompromise, there can be pulmonary opacities and nodules with a skin rash (serpiginous, linear pruritic lesions, or maculopapular erythematous rash).[27] In immunocompromised patients, *S. stercoralis* can cause life-endangering respiratory failure and sepsis. Allergic bronchopulmonary mycosis represents rare syndromes when species of *Aspergillus* are not etiologic, but other fungi are. Usually, there is repeated recovery of the incriminated fungus in sputum, and there is evidence of immunologic hypersensitivity by skin and laboratory tests. Lastly, hypersensitivity pneumonitis can be attributable to multiple fungi, including species of *Aspergillus*.[28]

LIFESTYLE AND BEHAVIOR MODIFICATION STRATEGIES

It is advisable to inform patients with ABPA that direct exposure to moldy mulches, in which the aerosolized spore burden can increase up to 30-fold, can cause acute severe asthma (status asthmaticus) and exacerbations (stage III). Because of its ability to survive warm temperatures, in contrast to most other fungi, there is the example of a compost pile that heats organically and sustains *A. fumigatus*. Exposure to such shoveled compost provides a large burden of respirable spores that can trigger acute severe asthma or an exacerbation of ABPA. Other sources of fungi, such as from moldy basements, moisture-damaged building materials,[29] areas in the living or working environments with visible and presumably respirable fungi, and outdoor hobbies or occupational exposures to fungi, should be avoided and remediated, if feasible. Although not performed in patients with ABPA, studies have reported beneficial interventions from remediation of indoor environments in patients with fungal asthma.[11] The use of impermeable encasings for pillows reduced dust mites and β-(1,3)-glucan, a proinflammatory fungal cell wall component, after 6 weeks.[30] It is suggested that dust mite encasings be placed on the mattress as well to reduce exposure to fungi in the bedroom.

Physicians and other health care professionals caring for patients with ABPA should ensure that the patients understand the benefits and risks associated with oral glucocorticosteroid use. I have consulted on a number of patients who refuse to use prednisone or methylprednisone for exacerbations of ABPA, which results in new areas of bronchiectasis and lung damage, all of which is irreversible. For many patients with ABPA, oral glucocorticoids are not indicated "perpetually" but can be administered for 2 to 3 months to treat exacerbations. Smoking cigarettes and marijuana (which can harbor spores of A. fumigatus) must be discontinued. Furthermore, azoles that may be considered for adjunctive therapy have known drug–drug interactions and adverse effects (usually transient).

PHARMACOLOGIC TREATMENT

Prednisone is the drug of choice to resolve mucoid impactions and related pulmonary infiltrates that characterize stage I, III, and IV ABPA. One approach is to administer prednisone at 0.5 mg/kg/day (a single morning dose) for 1 to 2 weeks and then convert to alternate-day use for 2 to 3 months.[1,7,9] Longer courses of daily prednisone occasionally are required[11] to clear the infiltrates, especially if exposure continues and new collapse occurs. Administration of a single morning dose of prednisone is my choice, based on the literature and on long-term experience indicating its effectiveness in the absence of a controlled trial. The half-life of prednisone (determined as its metabolite, prednisolone) is about 3 hours in serum, and the pharmacologic (therapeutic) effect can be as long as 36 hours for maintenance of pulmonary function in stable patients. Some physicians choose to administer prednisone in a dose of 15 to 20 mg three times a day for the first week in an effort to clear the pulmonary infiltrates and improve respiratory status. Chest HRCT can be repeated after 2 to 3 months, and if the lungs are clear of infiltrates, the prednisone can be tapered and discontinued. The total IgE concentration should decrease by at least 33% in 6 weeks,[24] unless there are new infiltrates or the patient does not adhere to the prescribed dosage. If the emergence of ABPA has caused worsening of the patient's asthma such that control cannot be achieved without scheduled prednisone, despite inhaled glucocorticoids, long-acting $ß_2$-adrenergic receptor agonists, a leukotriene receptor antagonist, and treatment of comorbidities (e.g., allergic rhinitis, rhinosinusitis, or gastroesophageal reflux disease, any of which may be present), the patient is determined to have stage IV (corticosteroid-dependent) ABPA. Usually, alternate-day prednisone is effective in such patients, and the major side effects of prednisone can be avoided. Patients should be informed about controlling dietary intake of calories to avoid weight gain, possible sleep disturbance, and mood change from alternate-day prednisone; the need for good bone health; and the need for yearly ophthalmologic examinations. Alternatively, if the patient does not require additional daily or alternate-day prednisone and there are no new pulmonary exacerbations of ABPA for at least 6 months, the patient has entered stage II (remission). Asthma is managed as indicated, but long-term scheduled prednisone is not required. The total IgE concentration can be determined every 3 to 6 months initially to search for subclinical exacerbation. Stage V (end-stage fibrocavitary) ABPA is treated with as little scheduled prednisone as required, either alternate-day or single morning administration, and other antiasthma medications. Antimicrobial agents may be indicated for gram-negative bacteria, atypical mycobacteria, or fungi. Devices and medications to assist with chronic sputum expectoration should be considered. In some patients, daily oxygen is required.

Antifungal therapy is adjunctive and has yet to be associated with reliable clearing of mucoid impactions and pulmonary infiltrates. However, the literature describes the benefits of antifungal therapy (itraconazole or posaconazole) for reducing the exacerbations of asthma that occur in patients with ABPA, sputum eosinophilia and eosinophilic cationic protein, total IgE concentration and anti–A. fumigatus IgE antibodies, and dosage requirements of prednisone.[31–37] A trial of antifungal therapy should be for a minimum of 6 months.

Itraconazole, voriconazole, and posaconazole have recognized adverse effects, drug–drug interactions, and drug–age pharmacokinetic issues.[2,38] Some adverse effects include nausea, elevated liver function tests (usually reversible), and photosensitivity. Proton pump inhibitors and histamine-2 receptor antagonists reduce absorption of itraconazole because of their suppression of acid. However, proton pump inhibitors can increase concentrations of voriconazole. Coadministration of the enzyme inducer phenytoin or rifampin reduces voriconazole concentrations because much of its elimination is by cytochrome P450 2C19.[2]

Some experience with omalizumab, a monoclonal antibody to IgE, in ABPA has been published in patients with asthma[39] or with coexisting cystic fibrosis.[40,41] The improvements consist of reductions in exacerbations of asthma and oral glucocorticosteroid requirements, which is similar to what is known for patients with persistent severe asthma who receive omalizumab. A case report of lack of a sustained benefit after initial improvement with omalizumab in ABPA and cystic fibrosis provides a different perspective.[41] When omalizumab is administered to patients with ABPA and persistent asthma, a trial should be for 4 to 6 months, as suggested for patients without ABPA. It remains to be demonstrated whether mepolizumab, an antibody to interleukin-5, a cytokine that supports growth of eosinophils, will be effective in reducing the numbers of ABPA exacerbations (new pulmonary infiltrates with increases in total IgE concentration), and whether the beneficial responses that occur with mepolizumab in patients with persistent severe eosinophilic asthma also will occur in patients with ABPA. Mepolizumab is not available commercially at this time.

UNMET, FUTURE RESEARCH NEEDS

1. Understanding the virulence of the genus *Aspergillus*, and in particular that of *A. fumigatus*, of which many of the 23 characterized allergens produce potent enzymes[11] that can damage epithelium and serve in a proinflammatory manner

2. Learning what and how genetic susceptibilities[42] favor the intense immunologic helper T-cell type 2 response and emergence of ABPA in patients with asthma

3. Determining why innate host defenses are insufficient in ABPA but not asthma to ward off saprophytic growth of *A. fumigatus* hyphae in bronchial mucus

4. Identifying the basis for the remarkable 2- to 10-fold increases in total IgE concentration at the time of exacerbations of ABPA, including why the anti–*A. fumigatus* IgE antibodies do not surge in parallel fashion

5. Learning how prednisone can help resolve the pulmonary infiltrates and clinical symptoms while reducing the total IgE concentration

6. Studying whether administration of vitamin D can help patients with ABPA and prevent new infiltrates or help clear current ones

7. Developing the most predictive and discriminative diagnostic tools to differentiate patients with ABPA from patients with mild or severe fungal asthma[43]

8. Establishing how frequently and with what novel and safe methodology radiologic examinations can contribute to early diagnosis of ABPA exacerbations and recognition of irreversible findings

9. Identifying the most optimal treatments of current exacerbations and how to prevent future mucoid impactions so as to avoid emergence of irreversible bronchiectasis

10. Studying how to implement new advances in the diagnosis and treatment of ABPA into the health care system so that patients will be identified early and treated effectively before excessive bronchiectasis and other aspects of irreversible lung damage occur

CONCLUSION

ABPA is one of the most important comorbid, coexisting subtypes of asthma because it results in irreversible lung destruction and may convert intermittent or persistent mild asthma into persistent severe asthma. The fact that the treatment of choice to clear pulmonary infiltrates and sputum eosinophilia is an oral glucocorticosteroid but not antifungal therapy remains true after 50 years of attempts to improve our understanding and treatment of ABPA. It remains to be established whether monoclonal antibodies will contribute to meaningful improvement in management of patients or what combination therapy will be optimum instead of relying on oral glucocorticoids. Certainly, innovative, safe, and effective approaches to treatment are needed to decrease the harmful impact that untreated or inadequately treated ABPA can have on patients with asthma.

REFERENCES

1. Greenberger PA. Allergic bronchopulmonary aspergillosis. *Allergy Asthma Proc.* 2012:33:S61–S63.
2. Dolton MJ, Ray JE, Chen SC-A, Ng K, Pont LG, McLachlan AJ. Multicenter study of voriconazole pharmacokinetics and therapeutic drug monitoring. *Antimicrob Agents Chemother.* 2012;56:4793–4799.
3. Rosenberg M, Patterson R, Mintzer R, Cooper BJ, Roberts M, Harris, KE. Clinical and immunologic criteria for the diagnosis of allergic bronchopulmonary aspergillosis. *Ann Intern Med.* 1977;86:405–414.
4. Ricketti AJ, Greenberger PA, Patterson R. Immediate-type reactions in patients with allergic bronchopulmonary aspergillosis. *J Allergy Clin Immunol.* 1983;71:541–545.
5. McCarthy DS, Pepys J. Allergic bronchopulmonary aspergillosis. Clinical immunology: (1) clinical features. *Clin Allergy.* 1971;1:261–286.
6. Greenberger PA, Liotta JL, Roberts M. The effects of age on isotypic antibody responses to Aspergillus fumigatus: implications regarding in vitro measurements. *J Lab Clin Med.* 1989;114:278–284.
7. Greenberger PA. Allergic bronchopulmonary aspergillosis. In: Grammer LC, Greenberger PA, eds. *Patterson's Allergic Diseases*, 7th ed. Philadelphia: Wolters Kluwer, Lippincott, Williams & Wilkins; 2009:439–456.
8. Greenberger PA, Patterson R. Allergic bronchopulmonary aspergillosis and the evaluation of the patient with asthma. *J Allergy Clin Immunol.* 1988;81:646–650.
9. Greenberger PA. Allergic bronchopulmonary aspergillosis. *J Allergy Clin Immunol.* 2002;110:685–692.
10. Greenberger PA, Miller TP, Roberts M, Smith LL. Allergic bronchopulmonary aspergillosis in patients with and without evidence of bronchiectasis. *Ann Allergy.* 1993;70:333–338.
11. Knutsen AP, Bush RK, Demain JG, et al. Fungi and allergic lower respiratory tract diseases. *J Allergy Clin Immunol.* 2012;129:280–291.
12. Devakonda A, Raoof S, Sung A, Travis WD, Naidich D. Bronchiolar disorders: a clinical-radiological diagnostic algorithm. *Chest.* 2010;137:938–941.
13. Neeld DA, Goodman LR, Gurney JW, Greenberger PA, Fink JN. Computerized tomography in the evaluation of allergic bronchopulmonary aspergillosis. *Am Rev Respir Dis.* 1990;142:1200–1205.
14. Agarwal R, Khan A, Garg M, Aggarwal AN, Gupta D. Chest radiographic and computed tomographic manifestations in allergic bronchopulmonary aspergillosis. *World J Radiol.* 2012;4:141–150.
15. Brody AS, Klein JS, Molina PL, Quan J, Bean JA, Wilmott RW. High-resolution computed tomography in young patients with cystic fibrosis: Distribution of abnormalities and correlation with pulmonary function tests. *J Pediatr.* 2004;145:32–38.
16. Mitchell TAM, Hamilos DL, Lynch DA, Newell JD. Distribution and severity of bronchiectasis in allergic bronchopulmonary aspergillosis (ABPA). *J Asthma.* 2000;37:65–72.
17. Martinez S, Heyneman LE, McAdams HP, Rossi SE, Restrepo CS, Eraso A. Mucoid impactions: finger-in-glove sign and other CT and radiographic features. *RadioGraphics.* 2008;28:1369–1382.
18. Schwartz HJ, Greenberger PA. The prevalence of allergic bronchopulmonary aspergillosis in patients with asthma, determined by serologic and radiologic criteria in patients at risk. *J Lab Clin Med.* 1991;117:138–142.
19. Maurya V, Gugnani HC, Sarma PU, Madan T, Shah A. Sensitization to Aspergillus antigens and occurrence of allergic bronchopulmonary aspergillosis in patients with asthma. *Chest.* 2005;127:1252–1259.
20. Sarkar A, Mukherjee A, Ghoshal AG, Kundu S, Mitra S. Occurrence of allergic bronchopulmonary mycosis in patients with asthma: an Eastern India experience. *Lung India.* 2010;27:212–216.
21. Patterson R, Greenberger PA, Radin RC, Roberts M. Allergic bronchopulmonary aspergillosis: staging of disease. *Ann Intern Med.* 1982;96:286–291.

22. Patterson R, Greenberger PA, Lee TM, et al. Prolonged evaluation of patients with corticosteroid-dependent asthma stage of allergic bronchopulmonary aspergillosis. *J Allergy Clin Immunol*. 1987;80:663–668.
23. Lee TM, Greenberger PA, Patterson R, Roberts M, Liotta JL. Stage V (fibrotic) allergic bronchopulmonary aspergillosis: a review of 17 cases followed from diagnosis. *Arch Intern Med*. 1986;146:319–343.
24. Ricketti AJ, Greenberger PA, Patterson R. Serum IgE as an important aid in management of allergic bronchopulmonary aspergillosis. *J Allergy Clin Immunol*. 1984;74:68–71.
25. Lotvall J, Akdis CA, Bacharier LB, et al. Asthma endotypes: a new approach to classification of disease entities within the asthma syndrome. *J Allergy Clin Immunol*. 2011;127:355–360.
26. Greenberger PA, Grammer LC. Pulmonary disorders, including vocal cord dysfunction. *J Allergy Clin Immunol*. 2010;125:S248–S254.
27. Jeung YJ, Kim K-I, Seo IJ, et al. Eosinophilic lung diseases: a clinical, radiologic and pathologic overview. *RadioGraphics*. 2007;27:617–639.
28. Greenberger PA. Mold-induced hypersensitivity pneumonitis. *Allergy Asthma Proc*. 2004;25:219–223.
29. Torvinen E, Meklin T, Torkko P, et al. Mycobacteria and fungi in moisture-damaged building materials. *Appl Environ Microbiol*. 2006;72:6822–6824.
30. Siebers R, Parkes A, Miller JD, Crane J. Effect of allergen-impermeable covers on β-(1,3)-glucan content of pillows. *Allergy*. 2007;62:451–454.
31. Pasqualotto AC, Powell G, Niven R, Denning DW. The effects of antifungal therapy on severe asthma and allergic bronchopulmonary aspergillosis. *Respirology*. 2009;14:1121–1127.
32. Chishimba L, Niven RM, Cooley J, Denning DW. Voriconazole and posaconazole improve asthma severity in allergic bronchopulmonary aspergillosis and severe asthma with fungal sensitization. *J Asthma*. 2012;49:423–433.
33. Wark PA, Hensley MJ, Saltos N, et al. Anti-inflammatory effect of itraconazole in stable allergic bronchopulmonary aspergillosis: a randomized controlled trial. *J Allergy Clin Immunol*. 2003;111:952–957.
34. Stevens DA, Schwartz HJ, Lee JY, et al. A randomized controlled trial of itraconazole in allergic bronchopulmonary aspergillosis. *N Engl J Med*. 2000;342:756–762.
35. Glackin L, Leen G, Elnazer B, Greally P. Voriconazole in the treatment of allergic bronchopulmonary aspergillosis in cystic fibrosis. *Ir Med J*. 2009;102:29.
36. Patterson K, Strek ME. Allergic bronchopulmonary aspergillosis. *Proc Am Thorac Soc*. 2010;7:237–244.
37. Mahdavinia M, Grammer LC. Management of allergic bronchopulmonary aspergillosis: a review and update. *Ther Adv Respir Dis*. 2012;6:173–187.
38. Baxter CG, Marshall A, Roberts M, Felton TW, Denning DW. Peripheral neuropathy in patients on long-term triazole antifungal therapy. *J Antimicrob Chemother*. 2011;66:2136–2139.
39. Tillie-Leblond I, Germaud P, Leroyer C, et al. Allergic bronchopulmonary aspergillosis and omalizumab. *Allergy*. 2011;66:1252–1259.
40. ElMallah MK, Hendeles L, Hamilton RG, Capen C, Schuler PM. Management of patients with cystic fibrosis and allergic bronchopulmonary aspergillosis using anti-immunoglobulin E therapy (omalizumab). *J Pediatr Pharmacol Ther*. 2012;17:88–92.
41. Brinkmann F, Schwerk N, Hansen G, Ballmann M. Steroid dependency despite omalizumab treatment of ABPA in cystic fibrosis. *Allergy*. 2010;65:130–139.
42. Knutsen AP, Slavin RG. Allergic bronchopulmonary aspergillosis in asthma and cystic fibrosis. *Clin Develop Immunol*. 2011;2011:843763.
43. Denning DW, O'Driscoll BR, Powell G, et al. Randomized controlled trial of oral antifungal treatment for severe asthma with fungal sensitization: the Fungal Asthma Sensitization Trial (FAST) study. *Am J Respir Crit Care Med*. 2009;179:11–18.

4

IMMUNODEFICIENCY: INNATE, PRIMARY, AND SECONDARY

COMORBID AND COEXISTING

Jean M. Brown and John W. Sleasman

KEY POINTS

- In the United States, an estimated 750,000 individuals could have primary immune deficiency, whereas 56 million receive therapy with agents that significantly impair immunity.
- Immune deficiencies are often associated with asthma and other forms of chronic lung disease.
- Children with cellular or humoral immune deficiency with persistent viral respiratory tract infections are predisposed to asthma or have clinical manifestations that mimic asthma.
- The underlying diagnosis of immune deficiency should be considered in patients with interstitial pneumonitis, which can be difficult to differentiate from asthma.
- The diagnosis of immune deficiency should involve a rational diagnostic evaluation based on the clinical presentation and pattern of infections.
- Treatment of immunodeficiency includes prevention of infection with antibiotics, immune prophylaxis with gammaglobulin replacement therapy, or possibly hematopoietic stem cell transplantation.

INTRODUCTION

Patients with immunodeficiency disease present with recurrent infections, and sinopulmonary conditions are the predominant clinical manifestation.[1] Immune deficiencies also result in immune dysregulation, with asthma as a common feature. Furthermore, many immune deficiencies can lead to chronic pulmonary infections that mimic asthma and remain unrecognized (Table 4.1). The physician recognizes and properly treats these disorders on the basis of a rational use of the clinical clues, imaging, and laboratory studies that lead to an accurate diagnosis. Unrecognized,

Table 4.1. Pulmonary Conditions That Mimic Asthma

Pneumonia
Bronchiolitis
Bronchiectasis
Interstitial lung disease
Chronic obstructive pulmonary disease

---

many of these conditions can lead to chronic disease with high morbidity.

Immunodeficiency disorders, based on their etiology, are classified as primary or secondary. Primary immunodeficiency diseases (PIDDs) are usually due to heritable defects in innate or adaptive immunity resulting in distinct susceptibility to certain types of infections, immune dysregulation, or increased risk for malignancy. Certain immune deficiencies, such as Wiskott-Aldrich syndrome, are particularly prone to symptoms of allergy and asthma because of skewed T-cell responses toward helper T-cell type 2 cytokine patterns with increased production of immunoglobulin E (IgE), eosinophilia, and eczema. In contrast, defects in T-cell and B-cell development, such as severe combined immune deficiency (SCID), result in the increased susceptibility to interstitial pneumonitis caused by opportunistic infections that can mimic asthma. Chronic sinopulmonary infections, due to viral, bacterial, or fungal infections, can also mimic allergic rhinitis and asthma with persistent upper airway inflammation, a common comorbid condition associated with asthma or worsening asthma.

Secondary immunodeficiencies are acquired conditions that occur in otherwise normal individuals and can lead to similar clinical manifestations, such as chronic sinopulmonary infection. Examples of secondary immune diseases include human immunodeficiency virus (HIV) infection and acquired immunodeficiency syndrome (AIDS), exposure to immune-suppressing drugs, extremes of age, and malnutrition, all of which result in predisposition to opportunistic infections. Similar to primary immune deficiency disorders, secondary defects in immunity also impair distinct components of the immune response. Children younger than 2 years cannot respond to T-cell–independent antigens, such as bacterial cell wall polysaccharide, so pathogens such as *Haemophilus influenzae* and *Streptococcus pneumoniae* are major worldwide causes of infant mortality. With advanced age, cell-mediated and antibody function wanes, rendering elderly people at increased risk for varicella-zoster virus and pneumococcal pneumonia. Malnutrition has a profound adverse impact on adaptive immunity, whereas chemotherapy severely compromises phagocytic cell function. HIV-1 infection results in loss of memory T-cell function early in infection; without antiretroviral therapy, there is continued loss of CD4 T-cell function until AIDS develops.

EPIDEMIOLOGY OF IMMUNE DEFICIENCY

Based on a 2007 survey of more than 10,000 households, the Immune Deficiency Foundation estimates the prevalence of clinically significant PIDD to be about 1 in 1,200 individuals living in the United States. A National Institutes of Health consensus panel extrapolated these results and proposed that there are at least 250,000 individuals with known PIDD in the United States and an estimated 500,000 undiagnosed cases.[2] When less severe clinical phenotypes of PIDD, such as selective IgA and mannose-binding lectin deficiency, are considered, PIDD could affect more than 5% of the population.[3] Half of all PIDD patients are diagnosed after age 30 years, and the primary clinical manifestation is chronic infection before diagnosis. About 16% of patients with PIDD have concomitant asthma.[2]

PIDD is heterogeneous in its etiology and clinical manifestations. The clinical phenotypes can be defined by the parts of the immune system most affected, that is, the innate, cellular, humoral, or phagocytic components. The International Union of Immunological Societies (IUIS) Expert Committee on Primary Immunodeficiency classified the distinct categories illustrated in Table 4.2,[4] providing guidelines to better facilitate disease understanding

Table 4.2. The IUIS Classification of Human Primary Immunodeficiencies

Combined immunodeficiencies
Well-defined syndromes with immunodeficiency
Predominantly antibody deficiencies
Diseases of immune dysregulation
Congenital defects of phagocyte number, function, or both
Defects in innate immunity
Autoinflammatory disorders
Complement deficiencies

and recognition. Because many forms of PIDD are rare, the relative prevalence is illustrated in broader categories in Figure 4.1. Antibody deficiency disorders make up the most common category at 50%; combined cellular and antibody deficiencies, 20%, isolated cellular deficiencies, 10%; phagocyte deficiencies, 18%; and complement deficiencies, 2%.[1]

About 56 million individuals living in the United States receive therapy with agents that significantly impair immunity. Cancer chemotherapy is most prevalent, but the use of immune suppression for treatment of autoimmune disease and for the prevention of organ transplant rejection is increasing. However, these numbers are eclipsed by malnutrition, which affects 925 million people worldwide.

HIV infection has emerged as one of the leading causes of secondary immunodeficiency disease that also is associated with asthma. HIV-associated immune deficiency begins within the first few weeks of infection as a result of massive loss of memory CD4 T cells within the gastrointestinal system, with impairment of T-cell and B-cell responses to antigens.[5] Loss of CD4 T cells leads to AIDS, characterized by profound susceptibility to opportunistic infections and cancer. HIV infection also is associated with an increased risk for asthma. The Joint United Nations Programme on HIV/AIDS reported that at the end of 2010, an estimated 34 million people worldwide and 1.2 million in the United States were infected with HIV.[6] Gingo and colleagues, in 2012, reported a physician-diagnosed asthma prevalence of 21% in HIV-infected adults; however, only 9% of the patients studied demonstrated bronchodilator reversibility (≥12% increase in forced expiratory volume in 1 second [FEV_1] or forced vital capacity [FVC]).[7] Increased risk factors for HIV-associated asthma include female gender, high body mass index, family history of asthma, previous history of bacterial or *Pneumocystis* pneumonia, and not receiving antiretroviral therapy.

ASTHMA AS A PROMINENT CLINICAL FEATURE ASSOCIATED WITH IMMUNE DEFICIENCY

Children with cellular or humoral immune deficiency develop persistent viral respiratory tract infections, most commonly with respiratory syncytial virus (RSV), rhinovirus, and parainfluenza, which predispose to asthma or have clinical manifestations that mimic asthma. In addition, these viral infections and *Pneumocystis jiroveci* can cause severe pneumonia and respiratory failure. Comorbid conditions, such as pneumonia, bronchiolitis, bronchiectasis, interstitial lung disease (ILD), and chronic obstructive pulmonary disease (COPD), need to be considered in PIDD patients presenting with asthma-like symptoms.[2] The diagnostic characteristics of asthma and other lung disorders are outlined in Table 4.3.

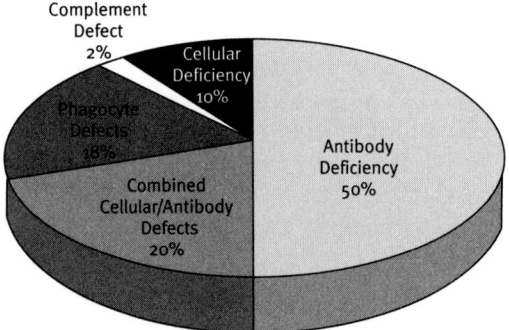

FIGURE 4.1 Primary immune deficiencies and relative prevalence in the United States. (Adapted from Morbidity and Mortality Weekly Report (MMWR); 2004.)

Table 4.3. Diagnostic Characteristics of Asthma and Other Lung Disorders

	ARTERIAL BLOOD GASES (PH, PAo$_2$, PAco$_2$)	BRONCHODILATOR REVERSIBILITY	CHEST CXR or CT	ASSOCIATED PIDD
Asthma	All normal to low	++++	CXR: Normal or hyperinflation	DOCK8 Deficiency CVID Specific antibody deficiency Th1 Selective IgA deficiency IgG subclass deficiency HIV
Bronchiectasis	pH: Normal to low Pao$_2$: Normal to low Paco$_2$: Normal to high	++	CXR: Persistent focal infiltrate CT: Airway dilatation and thickening, mucous plugs	CVID XLA ARAG
Interstitial lung disease	All normal to low	+/−	CXR: Normal or bibasilar reticular, nodular, or mixed pattern	CVID HIV SCID
Pneumonia	All normal to low	−	CXR: Infiltrate; possible consolidation or pleural effusion	Combined immunodeficiencies Well-defined syndromes with immunodeficiency Antibody deficiencies Diseases of immune dysregulation Congenital defects of phagocyte Defects in innate immunity Complement deficiencies

ABG, arterial blood gas; ARAG, autosomal recessive agammaglobulinemia; CT, computed tomography scan; CVID, common variable immune deficiency; CXR, chest x-ray; HIV, human immunodeficiency virus; Paco$_2$, partial pressure of carbon dioxide in arterial blood; Pao$_2$, partial pressure of oxygen in arterial blood; PIDD, primary immunodeficiency diseases; SCID, severe combined immunodeficiency; THI, transient hypogammaglobulinemia of infancy; XLA, X-linked agammaglobulinemia.

Pneumonia and Bronchiolitis

Infectious bronchiolitis and pneumonia usually present with fever, tachycardia, and tachypnea. However, in PIDD patients, the severity and duration are usually greater, and the disease requires more aggressive treatment. Bacterial infections usually require prolonged intravenous antibiotic treatment. Empyema is a common complication of patients with antibody deficiency.[8] When an immune deficiency is suspected, a chest radiograph is indicated to determine the extent of pulmonary disease, such as the degree of hyperinflation, peribronchial cuffing typical of bronchiolitis, or pneumatoceles, a pathognomonic finding seen in hyper-IgE syndrome.

Infants with SCID are at high risk for acute interstitial pneumonitis and infections with opportunistic pathogens. Typically these include viruses, atypical mycobacteria, and fungi such as *P. jiroveci* pneumonia (PCP). The clinical presentation usually begins with a fever, nonproductive cough, and tachypnea, and the patient may be hypoxemic. PCP commonly occurs in HIV-infected children and adults and is an AIDS-defining illness associated with advanced CD4 T-cell depletion. In HIV-infected adults, the onset of PCP can be insidious, occurring over several weeks with increasing respiratory symptoms, whereas HIV-infected infants and children can present with acute respiratory failure.[9] The chest radiograph shows interstitial disease with diffuse perihilar infiltrates and ground-glass opacities, even in early stages. It also demonstrates hyperinflation that can mimic bronchiolitis. Distinguishing laboratory findings for PCP include a reduced arterial oxygen pressure (Pa_{O_2}), increased alveolar-arterial oxygen gradient ($PA_{O_2} - Pa_{O_2}$), and elevated serum lactate dehydrogenase (LDH) level. Diagnosis of PCP in the bronchial alveolar lavage (BAL) fluid or sputum is made by direct histologic examination using a silver stain or direct fluorescent antibody (DFA). DNA and messenger RNA amplification of PCP, using polymerase chain reaction (PCR), is also highly sensitive; however, it is difficult to distinguish colonization from invasive disease in many cases.[10]

Nontuberculosis atypical mycobacterium (NTM) is also associated with invasive ILD in patients with cellular immune deficiency and phagocytic disorders. Radiographic findings include infiltrates in the mid-lung fields associated with a reticular nodular pattern and hilar adenopathy. Disseminated NTM is more typical in patients with phagocytic disorders, including defects in interferon-γ, the interleukin-2 receptor, or signal transduction and transcription 1. Noninvasive NTM is associated with pulmonary epithelial defects that occur in diseases such as chronic bronchiectasis, COPD, primary ciliary dyskinesia, and cystic fibrosis.[11] Clinical progression with persistent cough, fever, and fatigue can be slow, occurring over months to years. Identification of the organism by culture or PCR analysis of the sputum or BAL can diagnose NTM. Because NTM can cross-react with mycobacterial tuberculosis (MTB), a tuberculin skin test can be positive in such patients if they have intact cellular immunity. The commercially available quantiferon release assay used to diagnose MTB cannot be used to diagnose NTM.[12]

Pneumonia in infants and children with chronic granulomatous disease (CGD) is commonly due to infection with catalase-positive organisms such as *Staphylococcus aureus*, *Nocardia* species, and *Aspergillus* species.[13] The chest radiograph typically demonstrates reticular nodular infiltrates consistent with MTB or NTM, with clinical findings of fever, adenopathy, and noncaseating granulomas.

EVALUATION

The evaluation of opportunistic infections in a patient with pulmonary symptoms suspected of having an immune deficiency should include a complete blood count, lymphocyte subset analysis, LDH, and quantitative immunoglobulin levels. The BAL and sputum analysis should include a Gram stain, potassium hydroxide (KOH) preparation for fungal elements, acid-fast bacillus (AFB) stain, bacterial culture for aerobic and anaerobic organisms, fungal culture and DFA for PCP, and DFA for RSV. PCR can be used to detect viruses in BAL fluid such as cytomegalovirus, adenovirus, herpes simplex virus 1 and 2, human herpesvirus 6, Epstein-Barr virus, influenza, parainfluenza, human metapneumovirus, rhinovirus, and enterovirus. It can also be used to diagnose *Mycoplasma pneumoniae* and toxoplasmosis. A modified AFB stain can be applied in the diagnosis of *Nocardia* species, whereas an *Aspergillus* galactomannan antigen detects *Aspergillus* infection.

THERAPY

Treatment of pulmonary infections in immune-compromised patients should not be delayed while awaiting diagnostic tests, even if treatment interferes with the results of antigen-based assays. Suspected PCP is treated with trimethoprim-sulfamethoxazole (TMP-SMX). Dosing for children older than 2 months of age and adults is 15 to 20 mg/kg/day in three or four doses for 21 days. Alternative antiparasitic agents include pentamadine, primaquine plus clindamycin, dapsone plus trimethoprim, and atovaquone. Corticosteroids can be prescribed at 1 mg/kg every 12 hours for 5 to 7 days, followed by a tapering dose during the next 7 to 12 days in children to decrease pulmonary inflammation and minimize the risk for respiratory failure.[8] Children older than 13 years and adults receive prednisone at 40 mg twice a day for 5 days, then 40 mg a day for 5 days, and then 20 mg a day for 11 days. Broad-spectrum antibiotics, antifungal agents such as voriconazole, and antiviral therapy should be initiated empirically, as indicated, until the source of infection is confirmed. Mycobacterium-avium complex should also be empirically treated with a multidrug regimen.

Chronic Interstitial Lung Disease

Not all pulmonary disease seen in immune deficiency patients is caused by infections. ILD, characterized by nonmalignant, noninfectious inflammation of the lung parenchyma resulting in fibrosis or granulomatous reaction, can be seen in patients with secondary immune deficiency who have received chemotherapy or radiation either as treatment for malignancy or as myeloablation before hematopoietic stem cell transplantation (HSCT). ILD is also a manifestation of chronic graft-versus-host disease following HSCT.[14]

Granulomatous-Lymphocytic Interstitial Lung Disease

Granulomatous-lymphocytic interstitial lung disease (GLILD) is a pulmonary condition almost exclusively associated with common variable immunodeficiency (CVID). The chest imaging scan shows widespread pulmonary micronodules with a lower lung zone predominance, smooth interlobular septal thickening, and thoracic and abdominal lymphadenopathy that can mimic sarcoidosis, *Mycobacteria* species infection, or malignancy. Hepatomegaly and splenomegaly with noncaseating granulomas are common within both organs.[15] Patients with suspected pulmonary sarcoidosis should have quantitative immunoglobulin levels performed as part of their evaluation. Many patients with GLILD have bronchiectasis and multifocal pulmonary consolidation typical of CVID. Over time, the pulmonary nodules and lymphadenopathy commonly wax and wane. Clinical symptoms include progressive dyspnea and nonproductive cough associated with fatigue and weight loss. Fifteen percent to 20% of patients with CVID also have common autoimmune findings, including thrombocytopenia, neutropenia, and hemolytic anemia. Other laboratory features include low T-cell counts with inverted CD4/CD8 T-cell ratios and low numbers of memory B cells. The etiology of this condition is unclear but may be associated with persistent viral infections such as human herpesvirus 8.[16] Studies show that treatment with anti-CD20 monoclonal antibody, prednisone, and azathioprine is effective in controlling progression of the disease.[17]

Bronchiectasis

Bronchiectasis is common in many PIDDs that manifest with chronic recurrent pyogenic infections that destroy lung parenchyma. This is typically seen with a primary antibody deficiency, such as CVID, and may be more progressive because of delayed diagnosis. Bronchiectasis, defined as permanent dilatation of bronchi and bronchioles, should be suspected in patients with PIDD who have recurrent pneumonia and chronic cough with mucopurulent sputum production. Most patients experience dyspnea and wheezing, and nearly half have pleuritic chest pain. Wheezes, crackles, and rhonchi are commonly heard on auscultation. Digital clubbing, rarely seen in patients with asthma, should alert physicians to the possibility of bronchiectasis. Diagnostic evaluation for bronchiectasis should include a noncontrast, high-resolution computed tomography (CT) scan of the chest. Bronchiectatic changes include airway lumen dilatation greater than 1.5 times the width of nearby vessels, lack of airway tapering in the periphery, varicose constrictions along airways, and ballooned cysts at the end of bronchi. Location is also helpful diagnostically because bronchiectasis in the lower lung fields is commonly seen in immunodeficiency-associated infections. However, airway dilatation is not specific for bronchiectasis because this can be seen on chest CT in patients with asthma and chronic bronchitis. If arterial blood gas analysis is performed in a patient with bronchiectasis, the pH and Pa_{O_2} may be normal; subtle elevation in Pa_{CO_2} is common. Spirometry usually demonstrates a decreased FEV_1/FVC ratio with a normal to slightly decreased FVC and FEV_1. Bronchial hyperresponsiveness is present in 40% of patients, as demonstrated by spirometry following the administration of a β-adrenergic receptor agonist. The mainstay of antibiotic therapy is based on identification of the bacteria and its sensitivity.[18] In patients with immune deficiency and bronchiectasis, organisms such as *Pseudomonas* species, *Streptococcus pneumoniae*, *Moraxella catarrhalis*, and nontypeable *H. influenzae* are commonly found in sputum and BAL fluid.[19]

SPECIFIC IMMUNODEFICIENCIES WITH PULMONARY DISEASE AS A PREDOMINANT MANIFESTATION

Although not all primary immunodeficiencies involve the pulmonary system, many patients with PIDD have asthma and conditions that mimic asthma as a predominant clinical presentation. Immune deficiencies associated with asthma are summarized in Table 4.4.

Combined T-Cell and B-Cell Deficiencies

HIV infection and SCID are two of the most common cellular immune deficiencies associated with interstitial pneumonitis either due to opportunistic infections or from lymphocytic infiltrates. SCID is a heterogeneous group of primary immune deficiencies that share a common origin of defective T-cell development. They can be further defined based on the extent of B-cell and natural killer (NK) cell dysfunction. Typically, children with SCID have failure to thrive and severe, life-threatening opportunistic infections. Most die within the first 2 years of life unless diagnosed and treated. Although asthma is not associated with SCID, both AIDS and SCID patients can develop wheezing when infected with common pulmonary pathogens, including PCP, parainfluenza 3, RSV, adenovirus, and cytomegalovirus.[8]

The diagnostic evaluation of a patient suspected of having defective cellular immunity should consist of screening laboratory tests that include a complete blood count to measure the white blood cell count and the different white blood cell types; lymphocyte subset analysis by flow cytometry to enumerate T, B, and NK cells; quantitative immunoglobulins to measure IgG, IgA, and IgM; and HIV antibody to detect HIV infection. The diagnosis of SCID is suspected if total T-cell counts are significantly lower than age-adjusted norms. The most common SCID variant is X linked, resulting from a mutation in the common γ chain of the interleukin-2 receptor. These patients have no detectable T cells but have normal B-cell counts and low to absent NK cell numbers. Total absence of lymphocytes (T, B, and NK cells) is characteristic of adenosine deaminase deficiency, another common SCID variant. Absence of T and B cells but presence of normal NK cells occurs in patients with defects in the recombination activating gene.

Clinical management of children suspected of having SCID should be considered a medical emergency for diagnostic confirmation and

Table 4.4. Laboratory Findings in Common Antibody Deficiencies Associated with Pulmonary Disease

	IgG	IgA	IgM	IgE	IgG SUBCLASS	VACCINE TITERS	T CELLS	B CELLS	NATURAL KILLER CELLS	OTHER
XLA	Absent	Absent	Absent	Absent	Absent	Absent	Normal	Absent	Normal	
ARAG	Low	Low	Low	Low	Low	Low				
DOCK8	Normal High	Variable	Low	Normal High	Low	Poor	Low	Low	Low	
CVID	Low	Low Normal	Low Normal	Variable	Low Normal	Absent	Low Normal	Normal	Normal	
SAD	Normal	Normal	Normal	Normal	Normal	Poor	Normal	Normal	Normal	
THI	Low	Low Normal	Low Normal	Normal High	Low Normal	Normal	Low to normal CD4	Normal High	Normal	
sIgA	Normal	Low	Normal	Normal	Low Normal	Normal	Normal	Normal	Normal	
WAS	Normal	High	Low	High	Low Normal IgG2	Poor polysaccharide response	Low CD3 and CD4; variable CD8	Normal	Normal High Quantity; Low Function	Low platelet number and volume
AT	Normal	Low Normal	Normal Normal	Low Normal	Low Normal	Poor	Low Normal	Normal	Normal	High α-fetoprotein

XLA, X-linked agammaglobulinemia; ARAG, autosomal recessive agammaglobulinemia; DOCK8, dedicatory of cytokinesis 8 deficiency; CVID, common variable immune deficiency; SAD, specific antibody deficiency; THI, transient hypogammaglobulinemia of infancy; sIgA, selective IgA deficiency; WAS, Wiskott-Aldrich syndrome; AT, ataxia-telangiectasia.

therapy with HSCT.[20] Patients should receive PCP prophylaxis with TMP-SMX, replacement gammaglobulin therapy, and reverse isolation to minimize pathogen exposure. They should not receive immunizations with live vaccines, including rotavirus, Bacillus Calmette-Guérin, varicella, or measles, mumps, and rubella. HSCT is successful in 95% of patients who receive definitive therapy before 3 months of age.

Antibody Deficiency Disorders

Humoral immunodeficiencies are the most common clinically significant PIDD with sinopulmonary infections as the predominant manifestation.

CONGENITAL AGAMMAGLOBULINEMIA

X-linked agammaglobulinemia (XLA) and autosomal recessive agammaglobulinemia (ARAG) share common features of absence of all immunoglobulin isotypes and no detectable B lymphocytes. Affected patients usually develop serious bacterial infections early in life because maternal antibody is lost after 6 to 12 months of age. They have recurrent pneumonia that is frequently complicated by empyema. Males with XLA have a mutation in the Bruton tyrosine kinase protein that results in arrest of B-cell development. ARAG is less common and variable in the genetic defects that lead to the arrest of B-cell maturation. Patients have no circulating B cells as measured by using flow cytometry pan B-cell markers such as CD20 and CD19. T-cell enumeration and function are normal. Treatment consists of lifelong immunoglobulin replacement therapy.[21]

COMMON VARIABLE IMMUNODEFICIENCY

CVID is a phenotype of hypogammaglobulinemia defined as at least two immunoglobulin isotypes that are greater than 2 standard deviations below normal range for age. Most patients also have poor antibody function, as defined by failure to respond to immunizations. In contrast to congenital agammaglobulinemia, B cells are detectable and often are present in normal numbers. CVID is an acquired immune deficiency because patients have normal antibody function in infancy and childhood but lose B-cell function capacity. The diagnosis is usually made during the third decade of life when recurrent sinopulmonary infections develop, and as a result, bronchiectasis is common. Autoimmunity and chronic gastrointestinal conditions, such as autoimmune cytopenias, inflammatory bowel disease, and arthritis, are common comorbidities.[22] As mentioned previously, 10% to 15% of patients develop GLILD with lymphadenopathy, splenomegaly, and autoimmune cytopenias. About 15% of patients with CVID also have asthma; however, COPD with bronchiectasis occurs in more than half of patients with CVID. Treatment of CVID involves regular administration of gammaglobulin to maintain IgG levels at a minimum of 500 mg/dL.[23]

SPECIFIC ANTIBODY DEFICIENCY

Specific antibody deficiency (SAD) is defined by isolated poor vaccine responses, especially to pneumococcal immunization in patients with recurrent sinopulmonary infections. SAD is also associated with refractory asthma phenotypes.[24] Intravenous immunoglobulin therapy decreases asthma morbidity, number of hospitalizations, and requirement for glucocorticoid therapy, perhaps by decreasing the frequency of respiratory tract infections. Patients with asthma and recurrent sinopulmonary infections should be evaluated for SAD. The diagnosis is usually made on the basis of normal to low immunoglobulin levels but failure to produce protective antibody titers to at least 70% of the vaccinated serotypes of pneumococcal polysaccharide in patients greater than 6 years of age, or to at least 50% in children 2 to 5 years of age.[25] Management is controversial because there are not well-controlled clinical trials indicating the best treatment options for these patients, which include prophylactic antibiotics and immunoglobulin replacement therapy.[26,27]

TRANSIENT HYPOGAMMAGLOBULINEMIA OF INFANCY

Transient hypogammaglobulinemia of infancy (THI) is an accentuation of the normal, physiologic decline in IgG as maternal antibody wanes with delayed immunoglobulin synthesis by the infant. The IgG nadir occurs between the third and ninth months of life, but IgG levels are restored by 3 years of age.[28] THI involves one or more immunoglobulin isotypes that are 2 standard deviations below the mean values for age. Common clinical manifestations include recurrent upper respiratory tract infections, lower respiratory tract infections, and asthma. The prevalence of asthma among children with THI is as high as 70%. The diagnosis of THI is based on transiently low immunoglobulin levels but normal response to immunization and normal B-cell numbers.[29] THI should be considered as a diagnosis in infants with asthma and recurrent respiratory tract infections. THI is an accentuation of the normal ontogeny of humoral immunity. The use of antibiotics for acute infection is usually the sole therapy.

SELECTIVE IMMUNOGLOBULIN A DEFICIENCY

Selective IgA deficiency is the most common antibody immunodeficiency, with a prevalence estimated at 1 in 400 individuals. It is defined by IgA serum levels of less than 0.05 g/L with normal IgG and IgM in a patient older than 4 years. Although two-thirds of selective IgA deficiency cases are asymptomatic, one-third of patients have recurrent respiratory and gastrointestinal infections, atopy, and autoimmune disorders.[30] Asthma is the most common atopic condition and may be attributed to dust mite sensitization.[31] Nearly one-third of selective IgA–deficient patients also have IgG subclass deficiency, and there is a common association between selective IgA deficiency and IgG2 and IgG4 deficiency. Many of these patients also have poor polysaccharide vaccine responses. Assessment of IgA should be carried out in patients with asthma and recurrent respiratory infections. However, unlike other antibody deficiencies, selective IgA deficiency should *not* be treated with replacement gammaglobulin.

There are several other well-defined immunodeficiency syndromes whose clinical manifestations involve pulmonary symptoms.

DiGeorge Syndrome (22q11.2 Deletion)

DiGeorge syndrome, or 22q11.2 deletion, is a chromosomal abnormality that results in abnormal migration of neural crest cells to the third and fourth pharyngeal pouches during embryogenesis. DiGeorge syndrome has a broad range of clinical features that include conotruncal cardiac defects, palatal abnormalities, hypoparathyroidism with hypocalcemia, and thymic hypoplasia. The clinical spectrum can be partial or complete, defined as a total absence of T cells. Some form of T-cell lymphopenia is seen in more than 75% of patients, creating a higher risk for recurrent sinopulmonary infections including PCP and viral pneumonia.[32] In addition, palatal abnormalities may lead to aspiration pneumonia. Except in the case of complete DiGeorge syndrome, T-cell lymphopenia resolves in most children, and they no longer require prophylaxis for PCP by the time they enter school. Children with DiGeorge syndrome are at risk for developing autoimmune cytopenias, antibody deficiency, and neuropsychiatric disorders, whereas the asthma prevalence is the same as in the general population. Children with very low T-cell counts should be placed on PCP prophylaxis. Complete DiGeorge syndrome has been successfully treated with thymic transplantation.

Wiskott-Aldrich Syndrome

Wiskott-Aldrich syndrome (WAS) has the clinical manifestations of thrombocytopenia, immune deficiency, and eczema. It is an X-linked condition caused by mutations in the WAS protein that play a role in relaying signals from the cell surface to the actin cytoskeleton of hematopoietic cells. Recurrent otitis media, bacterial pneumonia, and food allergy are common, but asthma is not commonly associated with WAS. Patients have a characteristic immunoglobulin profile of normal IgG, elevated IgA and IgE, and low IgM. Risk for bleeding and stroke due to thrombocytopenia is the greatest morbidity, and patients with WAS should be considered for HSCT.[33]

Ataxia-Telangiectasia

Ataxia-telangiectasia is a rare autosomal recessive neurocutaneous syndrome manifested by oculocutaneous telangiectasia, immunodeficiency with sinopulmonary infections, progressive neurodegeneration, and cerebellar ataxia. The disorder is due to improper DNA breakage repair and radiosensitivity, leading to an increased risk for malignancy.

Immune deficiency is characterized by selective IgA deficiency, poor pneumococcal antibody response, and T-cell lymphopenia due to thymus hypoplasia. Elevated serum α-fetoprotein is characteristic and can be used as a screening test for the diagnosis.[34] Lung disease develops in 70% of patients due to recurrent pulmonary infections, ineffective cough, abnormal airway secretion clearance, and oropharyngeal dysphagia with recurrent aspiration. As a result, pneumonia and malignancy are the leading causes of mortality.[35]

Hyper–Immunoglobulin E Syndrome

Hyper-IgE syndrome is characterized by staphylococcal pneumonia with pneumatoceles, severe eczema, and elevated IgE levels greater than 2,000 IU/mL. It is inherited as an autosomal dominant immunodeficiency, the result of mutations in the transcriptional factors STAT3 and tyrosine kinase 2. Despite the elevations in IgE, asthma is not associated with hyper-IgE syndrome.[36]

Dedicator of cytokinesis 8 (DOCK8) deficiency has features similar to those of hyper-IgE syndrome but is clinically distinct because of a higher incidence of viral cutaneous infections, sepsis, neurologic complications, asthma, and other atopic disease. It is autosomal recessive and has a more severe phenotype and higher mortality rate. Therefore, an evaluation for DOCK8 deficiency should be considered in a patient with asthma, pneumonia, and elevated IgE.[37]

Chronic Granulomatous Disease

The most common defect in phagocytosis associated with recurrent pulmonary infections is CGD. Because of defects in NADPH oxidase, these groups of disorders share the common feature of failure to generate microbial killing within the white cell phagosome. Patients are susceptible to infection with catalase-positive bacteria and fungi, including *S. aureus* and Burkholderia, Candida, Serratia, Nocardia, Chromobacterium, and *Aspergillus* species. Biopsies of infections in the lung, lymphoid tissues, liver, spleen, and bone show granuloma formation. CGD patients with pneumonia have chest radiographs that typically reveal a pattern similar to MTB with associated hilar adenopathy, particularly when caused by *Aspergillus*. Although pulmonary infections are common in CGD, asthma prevalence is the same as in the general population. There are multiple defects in the NADPH pathway that lead to CGD. The most common form is X linked due to a mutation in gp91phox, but autosomal recessive forms occur in 40% of cases due to defects in cytochrome proteins p47, p67, and p22. The diagnosis of CGD is made using a flow cytometry–based assay of granulocyte respiratory burst activity with dihydrorhodamine assay. Antibiotic therapy should be targeted to treat catalase-positive organisms, particularly *S. aureus* and *Aspergillus* species. Subcutaneous interferon-γ improves granulocyte function and is used in the long-term treatment of patients with CGD.[38]

Hereditary Angioedema

Complement deficiencies are rare and often are more likely to be associated with autoimmune disease than asthma. However, hereditary angioedema is characterized by recurrent nonpruritic subcutaneous and submucosal edema of the upper airway and gastrointestinal tract that can be confused with anaphylaxis. It is inherited as an autosomal dominant disorder resulting from insufficiency of C1 esterase inhibitor activity. Episodes are triggered by trauma, infections, medications, stress, and surgical manipulation. Edema is self-limited but affects the face, extremities, gastrointestinal tract, upper respiratory tract, and larynx. Laryngeal swelling may lead to asphyxiation. Symptoms may be described as "difficulty breathing," so clinical evaluation must differentiate between upper airway and lower airway symptoms. Hereditary angioedema leads to the overproduction of bradykinin levels, which results in increased vascular permeability and leakage of fluid into the interstitial space of subcutaneous or submucosal tissues. Laboratory findings during acute attacks show low C4 levels and decreased C1 esterase inhibitor levels. The lower airways are not involved, so asthma is not commonly seen. Antihistamines and bronchodilators are not effective in acute attacks. C1 esterase inhibitor, kallikrein inhibitor, bradykinin, β_2-adrenergic receptor antagonist, danazol, and 17-α-alkylated androgen are the most effective therapies used to treat and prevent attacks.[39]

Mannose-Binding Lectin Deficiency

Mannose-binding lectin (MBL) deficiency involves a serum protein that plays a major role in opsonization and complement activation. Low MBL levels are associated with increased risk for recurrent upper respiratory infections, particularly in early childhood before maturation of the adaptive immunity occurs. However, the clinical significance of MBL deficiency is controversial because the gene frequency is very high, and 2% to 5% of individuals carry defective alleles but are otherwise healthy.[40] Both higher and lower levels of MBL are reported with asthma, contributing to the overall confusion about its role in asthma pathogenesis. MBL deficiency should be considered in children with asthma and recurrent upper respiratory infections.

CLINICAL EVALUATION OF SUSPECTED IMMUNODEFICIENCIES

The initial evaluation for suspected immunodeficiency should involve a detailed history, a thorough assessment of infection patterns, interpretation of clinical and laboratory findings in the context of the patient's age, and determination of whether these findings are associated with a particular immune deficiency. Common laboratory findings in immune deficiencies associated with asthma are summarized in Table 4.5. Recurrent pulmonary disease, disease severity, and infections with opportunistic pathogens require a more detailed evaluation, including imaging studies, arterial blood gas determination, and pulmonary function testing to define the pathogenesis of the underlying lung disease. These studies are critical to developing a rational diagnostic assessment for underlying immunodeficiency.

Children with pneumonia and ILD should be evaluated for defects in cellular immunity. Screening assays for PIDD should include a complete blood count, lymphocyte subset analysis, HIV antibody, and quantitative immunoglobulins. Screening tests for children and adults with recurrent bacterial sinopulmonary infections should include quantitative immunoglobulins, total IgE levels, and assessment of antibody function by obtaining preimmunization and postimmunization titers to T-cell–dependent antigens such as tetanus and diphtheria and T-cell–independent antigens through the administration of 23-valent Pneumovax. Pneumococcal responses are considered protective if there is antibody to 70% of the immunizing serotypes in older children and adults or to 50% of serotypes in children younger than 5 years.[25] Other diagnostic tests for children with recurrent sinopulmonary infections include MBL levels and tests for nonimmunologic causes such as sweat chloride for cystic fibrosis and ciliary biopsy to evaluate for ciliary dyskinesia (see Chapter 10).

If cultures of sputum or BAL show organisms suggestive of specific defects in immune function, such as infection with catalase-positive organisms, evaluation of granulocyte function using dihydrorhodamine assay is necessary to evaluate for CGD. Less than 10% of children or adults with recurrent sinopulmonary infections will have an underlying PIDD because most patients will have symptoms due to environmental exposure or allergic disease as the primary cause of the infection. However, the diagnosis in patients with PIDD is often delayed, sometimes for decades, because of the failure to include PIDD in the differential diagnosis.

Table 4.5. Laboratory Findings in Common Cellular Deficiencies Associated with Pulmonary Disease

	IMMUNOGLOBULIN PROFILE	T CELLS	B CELLS	NATURAL KILLER CELLS	OTHER
T-B+ SCID					
γC deficiency	Low	Markedly low	Normal or high	Markedly low	
JAK3 deficiency	Low	Markedly low	Normal or high	Markedly low	
IL-7Rα deficiency	Low with variable IgM	Markedly low	Normal or high	Normal	
T-B- SCID					
RAG 1/2 deficiency	Low	Markedly low	Markedly low	Normal	
DCLRE1C (Artemis) deficiency	Low	Markedly low	Markedly low	Normal	
T-B- SCID					
Reticular dysgenesis	Low	Markedly low	Low or normal	Low	
Adenosine deaminase deficiency	Low	Markedly low or absent	Markedly low or absent	Low	
HIV	Variable with normal to high IgE	Low CD4	Normal or high	Variable	Positive HIV ELISA
DiGeorge syndrome	Low to normal IgG and IgA; normal IgM; normal to high IgE	Low CD8; low to normal CD3 and CD4	Normal	Normal	22q11.2 chromosomal deletion on FISH or chromosomal microarray

ELISA, enzyme-linked immunosorbent assay; HIV, human immunodeficiency virus; FISH, fluorescence in situ hybridization; SCID, severe combined immunodeficiency; T-, no detectable T cells; B-, no detectable B cells; T+, T cells present; B+, B cells present.

PHARMACOLOGIC TREATMENT FOR IMMUNE DEFICIENCIES WITH ASTHMA

The mainstay of treatment for patients with immunodeficiency is the prevention of infection by the use of antibiotics or immune prophylaxis with gammaglobulin replacement therapy for antibody deficiencies. PIDD involving cellular immunity must be recognized quickly because HSCT is most successful if initiated in the first 3 months of life.

Gammaglobulin replacement can be administered as a monthly intravenous infusion of 400 to 600 mg/kg or as a weekly subcutaneous infusion given at 100 to 200 mg/kg per week to ensure serum steady-state IgG levels. The immunoglobulin dose is titrated to prevent recurrent infection with a minimal trough level of 500 mg/dL.[23] Acute infections require a longer duration of therapy to ensure clearance. Patients with CGD should be treated with antibacterial and fungal prophylaxis and benefit from interferon-γ therapy. Asthma in patients with PIDD is generally easier to manage with bronchodilator therapy if recurrent infections are minimized.

Lifestyle and behavioral modification strategies should include minimizing exposure to other people with infections as well as receiving routine care and vaccinations as appropriate. Discussing general health, nutrition, and emotional well-being is also important in patients with chronic medical conditions. If applicable, genetic counseling and carrier detection are important for future family planning.

UNMET, FUTURE RESEARCH NEEDS

1. There is an urgent need to develop readily available laboratory-based diagnostic tools for the effective and rapid diagnosis of newer immune deficiency diseases.
2. Furthermore, there is a lack of evidence-based clinical pathways to treat even the most common immune disorders such as antibody deficiency conditions.
3. As genetic screening becomes more practical, it may be possible to effectively screen for PIDD at birth so that definitive therapy can be initiated before the onset of infection and secondary complications.
4. As more patients with immune deficiency are diagnosed, the need for safe and effective pharmaceutical options is essential for improved quality of life.
5. Advances in transplantation research such as less toxic chemotherapy are critical for decreasing mortality associated with severe primary immune deficiency.

CONCLUSION

Immune deficiencies are rare conditions that cover a broad category of immune dysfunction in the humoral, adaptive, and innate immune systems. They are often underdiagnosed and misdiagnosed, especially when pulmonary manifestations are involved. Clinical suspicion, in conjunction with laboratory tests, pulmonary function tests, and chest imaging, is critical for proper diagnosis and management of these diseases.

REFERENCES

1. Lindegren ML, Kobrynski L, Rasmussen SA, et al. Applying public health strategies to primary immunodeficiency diseases: a potential approach to genetic disorders. *MMWR Recomm Rep*. 2004;53(RR-1):1–29.
2. Immune Deficiency Foundation. Primary immunodeficiency diseases in America: 2007. May 1, 2009. http://primaryimmune.org/wp-content/uploads/2011/04/Primary-Immunodeficiency-Diseases-in-America-2007The-Third-National-Survey-of-Patients.pdf
3. Turner MW. Deficiency of mannan binding protein: a new complement deficiency syndrome. *Clin Exp Immunol*. 1991;86(Suppl 1):53–56.
4. Al-Herz W, Bousfiha A, Casanova JL, et al. Primary immunodeficiency diseases: an update on the classification from the International Union of Immunological Societies Expert Committee for Primary Immunodeficiency. *Front Immunol*. 2011;2:54.
5. Sleasman JW, Goodenow MM. HIV-1 infection. *J Allergy Clin Immunol*. 2003;111(2 Suppl):S582–S592.
6. UNAIDS. World Aids Day Report: 2011. http://www.unaids.org/en/media/unaids/contentassets/documents/unaidspublication/2011/jc2216_worldaidsday_report_2011_en.pdf
7. Gingo MR, Wenzel SE, Steele C, et al. Asthma diagnosis and airway bronchodilator response in HIV-infected patients. *J Allergy Clin Immunol*. 2012;129(3):708–714, e8.
8. Buckley RH. Pulmonary complications of primary immunodeficiencies. *Paediatr Respir Rev*. 2004;5(Suppl A):S225–S233.
9. Sleasman JW, Hemenway C, Klein AS, Barrett DJ. Corticosteroids improve survival of children with AIDS and *Pneumocystis carinii* pneumonia. *Am J Dis Child*. 1993;147(1):30–34.
10. Carmona EM, Limper AH. Update on the diagnosis and treatment of Pneumocystis pneumonia. *Ther Adv Respir Dis*. 2011;5(1):41–59.
11. Griffith DE, Aksamit T, Brown-Elliott BA, et al. An official ATS/IDSA statement: diagnosis, treatment, and prevention of nontuberculous mycobacterial diseases. *Am J Respir Crit Care Med*. 2007;175(4):367–416.
12. Kobashi Y, Mouri K, Yagi S, et al. Clinical evaluation of the QuantiFERON-TB Gold test in patients with non-tuberculous mycobacterial disease. *Int J Tuberc Lung Dis*. 2009;13(11):1422–1426.

13. Winkelstein JA, Marino MC, Johnston RB Jr, et al. Chronic granulomatous disease: report on a national registry of 368 patients. *Medicine.* 2000;79(3):155–169.
14. American Thoracic Society and the European Respiratory Society. Idiopathic pulmonary fibrosis: diagnosis and treatment. *Am J Respir Crit Care Med.* 2000;161(2):646–664.
15. Park JH, Levinson AI. Granulomatous-lymphocytic interstitial lung disease (GLILD) in common variable immunodeficiency (CVID). *Clin Immunol.* 2010;134(2):97–103.
16. Wheat WH, Cool CD, Morimoto Y, et al. Possible role of human herpesvirus 8 in the lymphoproliferative disorders in common variable immunodeficiency. *J Exp Med.* 2005;202(4):479–484.
17. Chase NM, Verbsky JW, Hintermeyer MK, et al. Use of combination chemotherapy for treatment of granulomatous and lymphocytic interstitial lung disease (GLILD) in patients with common variable immunodeficiency (CVID). *J Clin Immunol.* 2013;33(1):30–39.
18. Barker AF. Bronchiectasis. *N Engl J Med.* 2002;346(18):1383–1393.
19. Tarzi MD, Grigoriadou S, Carr SB, Kuitert LM, Longhurst HJ. Clinical immunology review series: an approach to the management of pulmonary disease in primary antibody deficiency. *Clin Exp Immunol.* 2009;155(2):147–155.
20. Cowan MJ, Neven B, Cavazanna-Calvo M, Fischer A, Puck J. Hematopoietic stem cell transplantation for severe combined immunodeficiency diseases. *Biol Blood Marrow Transplant.* 2008;14(1 Suppl 1):73–75.
21. Conley ME, Rohrer J, Minegishi Y. X-linked agammaglobulinemia. Clinical reviews in allergy & immunology. 2000;19(2):183–204.
22. Cunningham-Rundles C. How I treat common variable immune deficiency. *Blood.* 2010;116(1):7–15.
23. Bonilla FA, Bernstein IL, Khan DA, et al. Practice parameter for the diagnosis and management of primary immunodeficiency. *Ann Allergy Asthma Immunol.* 2005;94(5 Suppl 1):S1–S63.
24. Schwartz HJ, Hostoffer RW, McFadden ER Jr, Berger M. The response to intravenous immunoglobulin replacement therapy in patients with asthma with specific antibody deficiency. *Allergy Asthma Proc.* 2006;27(1):53–58.
25. Kamchaisatian W, Wanwatsuntikul W, Sleasman JW, Tangsinmankong N. Validation of current joint American Academy of Allergy, Asthma & Immunology and American College of Allergy, Asthma and Immunology guidelines for antibody response to the 23-valent pneumococcal vaccine using a population of HIV-infected children. *J Allergy Clin Immunol.* 2006;118(6):1336–1341.
26. Orange JS, Ballow M, Stiehm ER, et al. Use and interpretation of diagnostic vaccination in primary immunodeficiency: a working group report of the Basic and Clinical Immunology Interest Section of the American Academy of Allergy, Asthma & Immunology. *J Allergy Clin Immunol.* 2012;130(3 Suppl):S1–S24.
27. Boyle RJ, Le C, Balloch A, Tang ML. The clinical syndrome of specific antibody deficiency in children. *Clin Exp Immunol.* 2006;146(3):486–492.
28. Dorsey MJ, Orange JS. Impaired specific antibody response and increased B-cell population in transient hypogammaglobulinemia of infancy. *Ann Allergy Asthma Immunol.* 2006;97(5):590–595.
29. Keles S, Artac H, Kara R, et al. Transient hypogammaglobulinemia and unclassified hypogammaglobulinemia: "similarities and differences." *Pediatr Allergy Immunol.* 2010;21(5):843–851.
30. Aghamohammadi A, Cheraghi T, Gharagozlou M, et al. IgA deficiency: correlation between clinical and immunological phenotypes. *J Clin Immunol.* 2009;29(1):130–136.
31. Papadopoulou A, Mermiri D, Taousani S, et al. Bronchial hyper-responsiveness in selective IgA deficiency. *Pediatr Allergy Immunol.* 2005;16(6):495–500.
32. Sullivan KE, Jawad AF, Randall P, et al. Lack of correlation between impaired T cell production, immunodeficiency, and other phenotypic features in chromosome 22q11.2 deletion syndromes. *Clin Immunol Immunopathol.* 1998;86(2):141–146.
33. Ochs HD. The Wiskott-Aldrich syndrome. *Springer Semin Immunopathol.* 1998;19(4):435–458.
34. Nowak-Wegrzyn A, Crawford TO, Winkelstein JA, Carson KA, Lederman HM. Immunodeficiency and infections in ataxia-telangiectasia. *J Pediatr.* 2004;144(4):505–511.
35. McGrath-Morrow S, Lefton-Greif M, Rosquist K, et al. Pulmonary function in adolescents with ataxia telangiectasia. *Pediatr Pulmonol.* 2008;43(1):59–66.
36. Sowerwine KJ, Holland SM, Freeman AF. Hyper-IgE syndrome update. *Ann N Y Acad Sci.* 2012;1250:25–32.
37. Zhang Q, Davis JC, Lamborn IT, et al. Combined immunodeficiency associated with DOCK8 mutations. *N Engl J Med.* 2009;361(21):2046–2055.
38. Holland SM. Chronic granulomatous disease. *Clin Rev Allergy Immunol.* 2010;38(1):3–10.
39. Hsu D, Shaker M. An update on hereditary angioedema. *Curr Opin Pediatr.* 2012;24(5):638–646.
40. Staley KG, Stover C, Strippoli MP, Spycher BD, Silverman M, Kuehni CE. Mannan-binding lectin in young children with asthma differs by level of severity. *J Allergy Clin Immunol.* 2007;119(2):503–505.

SECTION TWO

PULMONARY

5

SLEEP APNEA IN CHILDREN AND THE UPPER AIRWAY

COMORBID AND COEXISTING

Athanasios Kaditis

KEY POINTS

- Obstructive sleep apnea (OSA) is the most severe form of obstructive sleep-disordered breathing (SDB), a spectrum of abnormal respiratory patterns during sleep characterized by snoring and increased respiratory effort due to increased upper airway resistance and pharyngeal collapsibility. Adenotonsillar hypertrophy and obesity are the most frequent causes of OSA in children.
- The clinical manifestations of OSA include obstructive sleep apneas (cessation of oronasal airflow) and hypopneas (reduction of airflow) accompanied by arousals from sleep, restless sleep, daytime symptoms (sleepiness, inattention, hyperactivity), and academic difficulties.
- Asthmatic children have a higher prevalence of SDB than nonasthmatic children, and tonsillar hypertrophy mediates, at least in part, this epidemiologic association.
- Cysteinyl leukotrienes contribute to the pathogenesis of both asthma and OSA in childhood. Cysteinyl leukotrienes have also been implicated in the pathogenesis of adenotonsillar hypertrophy.
- Preliminary evidence suggests that treatment of sleep apnea with adenotonsillectomy results in improved control of coexisting asthma.
- Taking under consideration the epidemiologic association between OSA and asthma, when one of the two disorders is diagnosed, the possibility of the other disease being present should be entertained.

INTRODUCTION

Obstructive sleep-disordered breathing (SDB) frequently coexists with asthma.[1] Both disorders are accompanied by airway inflammation and diurnal and nocturnal symptoms,[2,3] and they may affect quality of life,[4] behavior, and cognition.[5] When obstructive SDB and asthma coexist in a child, they can have cumulative effects on morbidity; therefore, they should be recognized and treated promptly.

The term *obstructive SDB* refers to a spectrum of abnormal breathing patterns during sleep of variable severity, including snoring and increased respiratory effort.[6] Depending on the severity of upper airway obstruction, SDB may range from primary snoring to upper airway resistance syndrome, obstructive hypoventilation, and obstructive sleep apnea (OSA). OSA is the most severe form of obstructive SDB, and it is characterized by intermittent partial or complete upper airway obstruction (hypopnea or obstructive apnea, respectively) that impairs normal ventilation and sleep pattern.

Patency of the upper airway during sleep is maintained by complex interactions between upper airway resistance, pharyngeal collapsibility, tone of the pharyngeal dilator muscles, and negative intraluminal pressure generated by the inspiratory muscles.[6] This fine balance of mechanical forces can be impaired by one or more abnormalities affecting components of the upper airway, including adenotonsillar hypertrophy, allergic rhinitis, obesity, craniofacial anomalies, abnormal muscle tone; and abnormal control of breathing (Table 5.1).

Adenotonsillar hypertrophy and obesity are the most frequent abnormalities that are related to increased resistance to airflow and pharyngeal collapsibility during inspiration.[7] When upper airway resistance increases, inspiratory intrapharyngeal pressure becomes more negative than usual in order to maintain normal airflow and alveolar ventilation. Reflex activation of the pharyngeal dilator muscles prevents collapse of the pharyngeal airway under the influence of negative intraluminal pressure.[6] In children with OSA, abrupt, intermittent reductions in the tone of the pharyngeal dilator muscles during sleep lead to episodic partial or complete airway collapse (hypopneas or apneas, respectively) and intermittent hypoxemia and hypercapnia. Pharyngeal airway patency is restored by electroencephalographic (EEG) arousals or frank awakenings and increased sympathetic tone, which activate the pharyngeal dilator muscles.

Table 5.1. Conditions Predisposing to Obstructive Sleep Apnea in Childhood

I. Adenotonsillar hypertrophy and/or allergic rhinitis
II. Obesity
III. Craniofacial abnormalities
    Mild mandibular prognathism
    Mild mandibular hypoplasia
    Marked midfacial deficiency (e.g., Apert's syndrome, Crouzon's syndrome, Pfeiffer's syndrome, repaired cleft palate)
    Marked mandibular hypoplasia (e.g., Pierre Robin sequence, Treacher Collins syndrome, Nager's syndrome, Stickler's syndrome)
IV. Abnormal neuromotor tone and/or control of breathing
    Cerebral palsy
    Duchenne's muscular dystrophy
V. Combinations of abnormalities
    Down syndrome
    Achondroplasia
    Prader-Willi syndrome
    Mucopolysaccharidoses

CLINICAL FEATURES

Nocturnal Symptoms

Snoring is the cardinal symptom of obstructive SDB. It is produced from vibration of the upper airway soft tissues related to the high inspiratory airflow through the partially obstructed pharyngeal airway. In most studies, prevalence of habitual snoring (>3 nights/week) in the pediatric population ranges from 7% to 15% of the pediatric population based on parental report.[8] The prevalence of parent-reported apneas varies from 0.2% to 4%.[8] Other nocturnal clinical manifestations of obstructive SDB include *labored breathing, restless sleep*, and *mouth breathing*. During inspiration, paradoxic inward movement of the chest wall under the influence of the extremely negative intrathoracic pressure is frequently observed. Overall, parents underreport SDB symptoms, and as a result, the sensitivity of reported snoring for the diagnosis of OSA is 50% or compared with polysomnography, the diagnostic gold standard.[9] Despite this limitation, children who are reported to snore frequently are 3.5 times more likely to have OSA compared with those without snoring.[9]

EEG (cortical) arousals, subcortical arousals (i.e., movements without EEG changes), or frank awakenings that accompany obstructive events increase the neuromotor tone of the pharyngeal dilator muscles, and this change contributes to the relief of upper airway obstruction. Although sleep macrostructure is not disturbed (i.e., there are no changes in the percentage of different sleep stages), there is preliminary evidence that obstructive SDB is actually characterized by "micro-disruption" of the sleep pattern. Respiratory-related EEG arousals, as well as intermittent hypoxemia, possibly contribute to the increased neurocognitive morbidity associated with obstructive SDB.[10] EEG arousals affect adversely the prefrontal cortex, predisposing to behavioral problems (inattention, hyperactivity, impulsivity, aggression) and cognitive dysfunction in children with SDB.[11] Repetitive arousals also upregulate the synthesis of proinflammatory mediators that are involved in the pathogenesis of daytime sleepiness.[12]

Diurnal Symptoms

Most clinical symptoms during the day either are associated with the cause of increased upper airway resistance or are consequences of poor sleep quality (OSA morbidity). For example, children with OSA frequently have nasal congestion, upper respiratory tract infections, and mouth breathing secondary to adenoidal hypertrophy or allergic rhinitis. Tonsillar hypertrophy may be accompanied by dysfunction in chewing, swallowing, articulation, and voice, which improve after treatment of OSA with adenotonsillectomy.

Physical Examination Findings

Obesity and adenotonsillar hypertrophy are frequent findings in children with OSA. Nasal mucosa edema, nasal septum deviation, and polyps can contribute to increased upper airway resistance, which predisposes to obstructive SDB. Retrognathia, a hypoplastic mandible, or midface hypoplasia may also be present. On examination of the oropharynx, not only hypertrophic tonsils but also a high-arched palate and small oropharyngeal opening can be identified. A careful neurologic examination may reveal abnormal skeletal muscle tone (hypertonia or hypotonia), which can lead to abnormal function of the pharyngeal dilator muscles during inspiration in the sleeping child.

Obstructive Sleep Apnea–Associated Morbidity

The presence of habitual snoring is associated with increased risk for *primary nocturnal enuresis*. Several pathophysiologic mechanisms (e.g., increased plasma levels of atrial and brain natriuretic peptides) have been proposed to explain this association. Uncontrolled studies have shown a decrease in the frequency or complete resolution of enuresis after adenotonsillectomy. Inadequate weight or even height gain is an adverse consequence of OSA, especially in infancy. In a meta-analysis, it was concluded that age- and gender-adjusted height and weight increase significantly after adenotonsillectomy.[13]

Poor sleep quality is the most likely cause of daytime morbidity from the central nervous system. In the Tucson Children's Assessment of Sleep Apnea Study (population based), *excessive daytime sleepiness* was reported by parents in 24.3% and learning problems in 11.3% of children with OSA compared with 13.7% and 4.1%, respectively, of those without OSA.[9] Moreover, children with habitual snoring are three times more likely to have *hyperactive behavior* and increased risk for *inattentive behavior* compared with subjects without snoring.[2] Obstructive SDB correlates with deficits in academic abilities, language comprehension, and planning and organizational skills.

OSA has been associated with systemic and pulmonary hypertension. Reports based on 24-hour ambulatory blood pressure measurements indicate that the higher the severity of OSA, the higher the risk for *blood pressure over the 90th percentile*, adjusted for gender, age, and height.[14] *Pulmonary hypertension* and *cor pulmonale* have been reported in cases of severe OSA.

ALLERGIC RHINITIS, OBSTRUCTIVE SLEEP-DISORDERED BREATHING, AND SLEEP DISTURBANCE

Of interest, sleep disturbance, daytime fatigue and hypersomnolence, decreased cognitive functioning, and impaired quality of life are symptoms shared by OSA and allergic rhinitis.[15] Hence, it is possible that obstructive SDB due to nasal mucosa edema and nasal obstruction contributes to the reported sleep disturbance in subjects with allergic rhinitis. Nevertheless, limited evidence indicates a role for allergic rhinitis and atopy in the pathogenesis of obstructive SDB.[16]

DIAGNOSIS

Overnight polysomnography in a pediatric sleep laboratory is the objective (gold standard) method used to determine the presence and severity of intermittent upper airway obstruction during sleep and to diagnose OSA. The following parameters are usually recorded: EEG; right and left oculogram; submental and tibial electromyogram; body position; electrocardiogram; thoracic and abdominal wall motion; oronasal airflow (oronasal thermistor, nasal pressure transducer, end-tidal CO_2 sensor); oxygen saturation of hemoglobin; and video recording.[17] Scoring of sleep stages (wake, non-REM 1-2-3, and REM), arousals, and respiratory events is usually based on the recommendations of the American Academy of Sleep Medicine.[17]

Obstructive-type sleep apnea is defined as absent oronasal airflow for at least two breaths in duration, in the presence of chest and abdominal wall motion. *Central-type sleep apnea* is characterized by the absence of both airflow and respiratory effort, whereas *mixed-type apnea* has a central and an obstructive component. *Hypopnea* is a reduction in the airflow signal amplitude of at least 50% compared with baseline, accompanied by oxygen desaturation of hemoglobin equal to or greater than 3% or by an arousal or awakening. *apnea-hypopnea index (AHI)* is defined as the average number of apneas and hypopneas per hour of sleep time.

Children with reported snoring who undergo polysomnography may or may not have apneas or hypopneas, gas exchange abnormalities, or arousals from sleep because obstructive SDB includes a spectrum of abnormal respiratory patterns of variable severity. OSA is diagnosed in the presence of consistent clinical manifestations (especially snoring and increased respiratory effort) and abnormal polysomnography findings. Nevertheless, many parents may be unaware of the presence of OSA symptoms in their child. Furthermore, there is no consensus regarding cut-off values of polysomnography parameters that define OSA. In recent studies, the threshold value that has been applied to define abnormal AHI is 1 episode/hour.[7] Published evidence reveals that AHI of more than 5 episodes/hour is associated with increased risk for blood pressure elevation, and AHI of more than 1 episode/hour is related to increased frequency of clinical manifestations from the central nervous system, such as excessive daytime sleepiness and academic difficulties.

Primary snoring is defined as habitual snoring without apneas, hypopneas, frequent arousals from sleep, or gas exchange abnormalities. Children with *upper airway resistance syndrome* have snoring, increased work of breathing during sleep, frequent arousals, and daytime sleepiness, but no apneas, hypopneas, or gas exchange abnormalities at night. In *obstructive hypoventilation*, end-tidal CO_2 greater than 50 mm Hg is measured for more than 20% of the total sleep time duration, although apneas, hypopneas, or arousals are not recorded.

Although polysomnography is the gold standard tool for the diagnosis of OSA, pediatric sleep laboratories are not widely available. Therefore, when a child with habitual snoring and adenotonsillar hypertrophy cannot undergo polysomnography in a sleep laboratory, alternative simpler diagnostic methods such as nocturnal oximetry or video recording may be used to objectively evaluate severity of SDB.

COMORBID, COEXISTING, AND DIFFERENTIAL DIAGNOSES

Coexistence of Sleep Apnea and Asthma: Evidence From Epidemiologic Studies

Obstructive SDB and recurrent wheezing or asthma frequently coexist in children, as suggested by several epidemiologic studies (Table 5.2). Increased prevalence of snoring or abnormal polysomnography findings occur in children with history of wheezing or physician-diagnosed asthma.[18-29] In addition, children with persistent wheezing or frequent episodes of wheezing a higher risk for increased AHI or snoring than those with less severe symptoms.[23,26]

The association between recurrent asthma and sleep apnea is bidirectional because children with elevated AHI also have increased risk for wheezing (see Table 5.1).[30] SDB is a significant predictor of the presence of severe asthma, and thus an important research question is whether treatment of upper airway obstruction improves asthma morbidity.[31]

Similarities and Differences in Symptoms of Obstructive Sleep Apnea and Asthma in Childhood

The main pathophysiologic abnormality of OSA is nocturnal, intermittent upper airway obstruction, whereas asthma symptoms are due to relatively stable lower airway obstruction that deteriorates during nocturnal sleep. Hence, the mechanical effects and the associated symptoms and signs in OSA are different from those in asthma, although both disorders have similar adverse effects on sleep quality (Table 5.3). The detrimental consequences of OSA on sleep and the central nervous system have already been discussed (see "Nocturnal Symptoms" and "Obstructive Sleep Apnea–Associated Morbidity"). Childhood asthma has a negative impact on sleep quality, which gets worse with increased disease severity, poorer asthma control, and lower respiratory function.[32] Similar to sleep apneic children, children with mild to moderate asthma experience nocturnal awakenings.[33]

The relative proportion of different sleep stages (sleep macro-structure) is not affected in asthmatic children, but reduced sleep efficiency occurs relative to control subjects, probably as a result of frequent nocturnal awakenings.[34] The number of missed school days, presence of daytime sleepiness or tiredness, and memory and concentration deficits in asthmatic children are often correlated with the frequency of nocturnal awakenings.[35] Control of asthma results in improved sleep quality.[36]

The epidemiologic association of asthma with poor sleep quality persists even if coexisting OSA is taken under consideration.[20] More specifically, in a cross-sectional study, children with parental report of wheezing in the last 12 months had a two fold higher risk for difficulty falling asleep, a four fold higher risk for restless sleep, and a five fold higher risk for daytime sleepiness than children without wheezing after statistical adjustment for the presence of snoring.[20]

Table 5.2. Epidemiologic Studies Supporting an Association between Recurrent Wheezing or Asthma and Obstructive Sleep-Disordered Breathing in Childhood

FIRST AUTHOR, COUNTRY	AGE (YR)	NO. OF SUBJECTS	RISK FACTORS	OUTCOME MEASURE	OR (95% CI)	REF. NO.
Ross, USA	9.1 ± 3.4	108	Habitual loud snoring (≥3–4 times/wk) and ≥3 desaturations/hr in nocturnal oximetry	Severe asthma at 12-mo follow-up	3.6 (1.3–10.4)	31
Sulit, USA	8–11	835	Obstructive apnea-hypopnea index ≥5 episodes/hr or obstructive apnea index ≥1 episode/hr	Wheezing apart from colds in the last year or treatment with asthma medications in the last 3 mo	1.9 (1.3–2.9)	30
Chng, Singapore	4–7	10,279	Physician-diagnosed asthma	Snoring	1.3 (1.1–1.6)	18
Corbo, Italy	6–13	1,615	Cough and phlegm without cold	Snoring often	1.8 (1.1–3.0)	19
Desager, Belgium	7–14	943	Wheezing in the last 12 mo	Snoring in the last 6 mo	1.9 (1.0–3.9)	20
Ersu, Turkey	5–13	2,147	History of asthma	Snoring always or frequently	2.0 (1.1–3.6)	21
Kaditis, Greece	7.6 ± 3.6	442	Physician-diagnosed wheezing requiring treatment in the past 12 mo	Snoring ≥1 night/wk over the last 6 mo	1.7 (1.1–2.7)	22
Kuehni, UK	1–5	6,811	1–10 attacks of wheeze	Snoring almost always over the last 12 mo	1.4 (1.1–1.7)	23
			>10 attacks of wheeze		2.6 (1.5–4.7)	
Lu, Australia	2–5	974	Physician-diagnosed asthma	Snoring ≥4 nights/wk in the absence of a cold	2.0 (1.3–3.1)	24

Marshall, Australia	5	516	Wheezing in the last 12 mo and either an asthma diagnosis between 18 mo and 5 yr of age or >12% increase in FEV_1 after a bronchodilator	Snoring	2.7 (1.2–5.9)	25
				Snoring ≥3 nights/wk	3.4 (1.6–7.2)	
Redline, USA	2–18	399	Physician-diagnosed asthma	Apnea-hypopnea index >10 episodes/hr	3.8 (1.4–10.6)	26
			Occasional wheezing		3.3 (1.2–8.9)	
			Persistent wheezing		7.5 (2.0–27.4)	
Teculescu, France	5–6.4	190	Exercise-induced bronchospasm	Snoring often	8.7 (2.8–26.4) [relative risk]	27
Valery, Australia	0–17	1,650	Ever had wheezing	Snoring >1 night/wk over last 6 mo	2. (1.4–3.2)	28
			Wheezing in the last 12 mo		5.4 (3.6–8.1)	
			Ever had asthma		3.2 (2.2–4.7)	
			Wheezing during or after exercise in the last 12 mo		4.7 (2.8–7.8)	
Verhulst, Sri Lanka	6–12	652	Wheezing in the last 12 mo	Snoring	2.8 (1.6–4.7)	29

FEV_1, forced expiratory volume in 1 second.

Table 5.3. Comparison of Obstructive Sleep Apnea and Asthma Symptoms and Signs

	OBSTRUCTIVE SLEEP APNEA (OSA)	ASTHMA
Cardinal nocturnal symptoms	Snoring, apneas, and hypopneas with increased respiratory effort during sleep	Cough, increased respiratory effort in severe asthma, deterioration at night
Cardinal diurnal symptoms	Related to the cause of OSA, e.g., mouth breathing when adenoidal hypertrophy or allergic rhinitis is present	Cough, increased respiratory effort in severe asthma
Characteristics of increased respiratory effort	Increased inspiratory effort, intercostal retractions	Increased expiratory effort (and in severe cases inspiratory) with intercostal retractions and contraction of abdominal muscles on expiration
Effects on sleep	No effects on sleep macro-structure but frequent arousals and awakenings	No effects on sleep macro-structure, frequent awakenings
Effects on the central nervous system	Excessive daytime sleepiness, hyperactive behavior, inattentive behavior, deficits in language, spatial and organizational skills, academic difficulties	Excessive daytime sleepiness, tiredness, memory and concentration deficits, academic difficulties

Pathogenetic Mechanisms Linking Obstructive Sleep-Disordered Breathing and Recurrent Wheezing or Asthma

The epidemiologic association of recurrent wheezing or asthma with obstructive SDB is probably the result of common pathogenetic pathways, as has been proposed in a review article.[1] Airway inflammation related to leukotrienes and airway oxidative stress are potential mechanisms implicated in the pathogenesis of both disorders.

Elevated concentrations of leukotriene B4, cysteinyl leukotrienes, and markers of oxidative stress (8-isoprostane) have been detected in the exhaled breath condensate collected from both asthmatic children[37] and sleep apneic children.[38] These compounds are probably synthetized and released by cells in the alveoli and airways such as alveolar macrophages, neutrophils, eosinophils, and bronchial epithelial cells. A speculative series of events is presented in Table 5.4, explaining how OSA and associated intermittent alveolar hypoxia during sleep may contribute to symptoms of asthma.

Asthma could also worsen symptoms of obstructive SDB. We speculate that adenotonsillar tissue is exposed to exhaled reactive oxygen metabolites released from the asthmatic airway that upregulate activity of 5-lipoxygenase (Table 5.4). Hydrogen peroxide, for example, can penetrate biomembranes. Enhanced activity of cysteinyl leukotrienes has been found in hypertrophic adenoid and tonsils of sleep apneic children.[39] Cysteinyl leukotrienes, which induce a proliferative response in tonsillar cell cultures, probably contribute to adenotonsillar tissue hypertrophy, increased upper airway resistance, and sleep apnea.[40]

Table 5.4. Speculative Mechanisms Explaining the Association Between Obstructive Sleep-Disordered Breathing and Asthma in Children

OBSTRUCTIVE SLEEP-DISORDERED BREATHING PROMOTES ASTHMA SYMPTOMS	ASTHMA PROMOTES OBSTRUCTIVE SLEEP-DISORDERED BREATHING SYMPTOMS
A. Apneas and hypopneas during sleep are accompanied by episodic alveolar hypoxia, which promotes release of oxygen free radicals (airway oxidative stress)	Oxygen free radicals released from the asthmatic airway upregulate 5-lipoxygenase activity in pharyngeal lymphoid tissues, promoting synthesis of cysteinyl leukotrienes and adenotonsillar hypertrophy
B. Oxidative stress upregulates activity of 5-lipoxygenase (key enzyme in leukotriene synthesis) in epithelial and other airway wall cells and in neutrophils found at increased numbers in the airway lumen of sleep apneic children	RSV infection (wheezing illness) enhances synthesis of cysteinyl leukotrienes and neurotrophins in the lower airway and in the adenotonsillar tissue, leading to adenotonsillar enlargement
C. Leukotriene B4 synthetized in the airway recruits more neutrophils, which further release leukotrienes and oxygen free radicals	Coexisting allergic rhinitis in asthmatic children increases upper airway resistance and the risk for obstructive sleep-disordered breathing
D. Cysteinyl leukotrienes and oxygen free radicals released in the lower airway trigger airway inflammation, bronchial hyperresponsiveness, and bronchospasm	Coexisting obesity in asthmatic children predisposes to obstructive sleep-disordered breathing

Respiratory syncytial virus (RSV) is one of the triggers of virus-induced wheezing in early life. Pharyngeal lymphoid tissue is the primary site of proliferation of respiratory viruses, where RSV may enhance expression of neurotrophins and cysteinyl leukotrienes and ultimately induce adenotonsillar hypertrophy.[41] This speculation provides an interpretation of the increased prevalence of tonsillar hypertrophy and sleep apnea in children with wheezing.[22] In addition, there is some evidence that allergic rhinitis, which frequently coexists with asthma, and the associated nasal mucosa edema increase nasal resistance and the risk for obstructive SDB.[42] Finally, obesity is a risk factor for both obstructive SDB and asthma, and mechanisms related to overweight may exacerbate both conditions.[26]

Lifestyle and Behavior Modification Strategies

Regular physical exercise along with a balanced diet should be implemented in all children with obstructive SDB and especially in those who are obese. Weight loss in severely obese children with OSA may lead to improvement in the severity of intermittent upper airway obstruction during sleep. Nevertheless, appreciable weight reduction is difficult to achieve and sustain. Avoidance of passive and exposure to indoor allergens other lifestyle modification measure that may reduce upper airway inflammation, resistance to airflow, and the tendency for apneas and hypopneas.

MEDICAL AND SURGICAL TREATMENT

Indications for Treatment of Obstructive Sleep Apnea

There is no evidence clarifying whether OSA symptoms, abnormal findings on polysomnography, or morbidity related to OSA are indications for treatment. Although AHI of more than 5 episodes/hour in children is considered a standard indication for adenotonsillectomy in the presence of adenotonsillar hypertrophy, there is evidence that even habitual snoring without apneas (AHI of less than 1 episode/hour) is associated with neurocognitive deficits.[43]

Based on limited published evidence and on clinical experience regarding the efficacy of OSA treatment, some indications for therapeutic intervention are the following:

- Children with OSA of at least moderate severity (AHI > 5 episodes/hour), irrespective of the presence of morbidity
- Subjects with AHI of 1 to 5 episodes/hour (mild OSA) but with OSA-related morbidity (e.g., enuresis, inadequate somatic growth, poor academic performance, systolic or diastolic blood pressure > 95th percentile for gender, age, and height or pulmonary hypertension)
- Subjects with increasing body mass index percentile and preadolescent males (risk factors for persistent OSA)
- Children with neuromuscular disorders and craniofacial abnormalities (risk factors for development of pulmonary hypertension)

It is unclear whether children with primary snoring, upper airway resistance syndrome, or obstructive hypoventilation should be treated. A *stepwise treatment approach* for OSA, moving from less invasive to more invasive therapeutic intervention, can include one or more of the following modalities:

- Weight control
- Administration of anti-inflammatory medications (intranasal corticosteroids, leukotriene modifiers)
- Adenotonsillectomy
- Application of orthodontic appliances
- Application of nasal continuous positive airway pressure (nCPAP)
- Craniofacial surgery (midface and mandibular distraction osteogenesis)
- Tracheostomy

If a child needs treatment, the applied therapeutic modalities should address all abnormalities potentially contributing to upper airway dysfunction.[7] For example, a child with adenotonsillar hypertrophy and midface hypoplasia will most likely benefit from the combination of adenotonsillectomy and an orthodontic appliance or craniofacial surgery. Successful treatment of OSA is accompanied by improvement in quality of life, acceleration of somatic growth rate, resolution or decrease in the frequency of enuresis, and reversal of cor pulmonale and pulmonary hypertension.[7] Moreover, treated children have less daytime sleepiness, hyperactivity, and aggression and less health care use after treatment.[7]

Specific Treatment Modalities for Obstructive Sleep-Disordered Breathing

The value of *weight control* as a therapeutic intervention for OSA was discussed in a previous section (see "Lifestyle and Behavior Modification Strategies"). When *intranasal corticosteroids* are administered for 4 to 8 weeks to children with mild OSA and adenoidal hypertrophy, they can improve symptoms of nasal obstruction and polysomnography indices.[44] Reduction in the upper airway resistance and severity of obstructive SDB is probably the result of a decrease in adenoidal tissue volume because addition of corticosteroids in tonsillar cell cultures induces cellular apoptosis. Topical corticosteroids have also been used with benefit for those children with residual OSA after adenotonsillectomy. Preliminary studies reveal that leukotriene modifiers (e.g., montelukast) could be useful in the treatment of sleep apneic children with adenotonsillar hypertrophy.

Surgical excision of the hypertrophic pharyngeal and palatine tonsils (*adenoidectomy* and *tonsillectomy*, respectively) is the standard treatment for OSA in childhood. This procedure reduces upper airway resistance and pharyngeal collapsibility. In a recent controlled trial of adenotonsillectomy for sleep apnea in childhood (CHAT), children 5 to 9 years of age with OSA were randomized to early adenotonsillectomy or a strategy of watchful waiting. Adenotonsillectomy did not significantly improve attention or executive function but it decreased symptoms and improved behavior, quality of life, and polysomnographic outcomes.[45] Of note, 46% of untreated children had also normalization of the AHI over a period of 7 months and some improvement in symptoms behavior and quality of life. A retrospective, multicenter study demonstrated postoperatively significant reduction in AHI and respiratory arousal index and increase in oxygen saturation of hemoglobin nadir.[46] Only 30% of all studied subjects had a normal AHI (<1 episode/hour) after adenotonsillectomy, a finding that emphasizes the need for applying more than one treatment modality and addressing all abnormalities that predispose to upper airway dysfunction.

Children with OSA and obesity who do not respond to weight loss, those with moderate to severe SDB after adenotonsillectomy, and sleep apneic children with neuromuscular disorders or craniofacial abnormalities may improve with the application of nCPAP (i.e., continuous airflow delivered through a nasal mask during sleep) in order to "stent" the pharyngeal airway and prevent collapse of its walls during inspiration.

Small randomized, controlled trials support the use of *orthodontic appliances* in otherwise healthy children with dental malocclusion, mandibular hypoplasia, and OSA. These devices move the mandible and tongue forward and increase the size of the pharyngeal airway lumen. Craniofacial procedures may be indicated in cases of profound craniofacial abnormalities accompanied by OSA. *Mandibular distraction osteogenesis* is used for the treatment of OSA in children with severe mandibular hypoplasia. *Rapid maxillary expansion and distraction osteogenesis of the midface* can relieve upper airway obstruction in children with midfacial deficiency. Finally, children with moderate to severe OSA unresponsive to other measures are candidates for *tracheostomy*.

Does Treatment of Obstructive Sleep-Disordered Breathing Improve Recurrent Wheezing and Asthma, and Vice Versa?

Although obstructive SDB increases the risk for recurrent wheezing or asthma, and vice versa, very few studies have explored the hypothesis that alleviating symptoms of one of the two disorders results in improvement of the other. Small studies with adult participants have concluded that treatment of OSA by nCPAP is accompanied by improvement in nocturnal asthma symptoms and quality of life, but not always by a change in respiratory function and bronchial hyperresponsiveness.[47,48]

Three studies have evaluated the effect of adenotonsillectomy—as a treatment intervention for OSA in children—on concomitant asthma symptoms.[49-51] Busino and colleagues recorded a reduced number of hospital visits and use of systemic steroids and asthma medications in a cohort of 93 asthmatic children 1 year after adenotonsillectomy, and these findings were confirmed in a smaller cohort by Saito and colleagues.[49,50]

In a published cohort by Kheirandish-Gozal and colleagues, children with poorly controlled asthma and OSA underwent adenotonsillectomy and follow-up evaluation for asthma symptoms 1 year after surgery. After adenotonsillectomy, annual number of asthma exacerbations, weekly rescue use of bronchodilators, and symptom score decreased significantly, whereas forced expiratory volume in 1 second (FEV_1) increased significantly.

The effects of improved asthma control on the severity of coexisting obstructive SDB have not been studied. However, in a multicenter, retrospective review of children who were subjected to adenotonsillectomy, presence of asthma was identified as a significant predictor of residual SDB in nonobese subjects.[46] It is thus possible that lower airway inflammation related to asthma promotes intermittent upper airway obstruction during sleep.

UNMET, FUTURE RESEARCH NEEDS

1. Does treatment of OSA improve asthma and vice versa?
2. What is the role of leukotriene modifiers in the treatment of children with OSA and adenotonsillar hypertrophy?
3. What is the contribution of allergic rhinitis to increased upper airway resistance and obstructive SDB?
4. Do therapeutic interventions for allergic rhinitis decrease the severity of obstructive SDB significantly?

CONCLUSION

OSA and recurrent wheezing or asthma frequently coexist in childhood. When one of the two disorders is diagnosed, the possibility of the other disorder being present should be entertained. Both OSA and asthma have adverse effects on sleep quality. Cysteinyl leukotrienes contribute to the pathogenesis of adenotonsillar hypertrophy, which is an important risk factor for OSA. Airway oxidative stress and inflammation related to leukotrienes in the upper and lower respiratory tract could be the pathogenetic links explaining the epidemiologic association between asthma and OSA in children. A series of therapeutic interventions, such as weight loss, intranasal corticosteroids, adenotonsillectomy, orthodontic devices, and nCPAP, may be necessary for complete resolution of OSA in childhood. Preliminary evidence indicates that adenotonsillectomy as a treatment for OSA improves control of coexistent asthma.

REFERENCES

1. Malakasioti G, Gourgoulianis K, Chrousos G, Kaditis A. Interactions of obstructive sleep-disordered breathing with recurrent wheezing or asthma and their effects on sleep quality. *Pediatr Pulmonol.* 2011;46(11):1047–1054.
2. Schechter MS. Technical report: diagnosis and management of childhood obstructive sleep apnea syndrome. *Pediatrics.* 2002;109(4):e69.
3. National Heart Lung and Blood Institute, National Asthma Education and Prevention Program. *Expert Panel Report: Guidelines for the Diagnosis and Management of Asthma 2007.* Bethesda, MD: National Heart Lung and Blood Institute; 2007.
4. Ekici A, Ekici M, Kurtipek E, et al. Association of asthma-related symptoms with snoring and apnea and effect on health-related quality of life. *Chest.* 2005;128(5):3358–3363.
5. Garetz SL. Behavior, cognition, and quality of life after adenotonsillectomy for pediatric sleep-disordered breathing: summary of the literature. *Otolaryngol Head Neck Surg.* 2008;138(1 Suppl):S19–26.
6. Katz ES, D'Ambrosio CM. Pathophysiology of pediatric obstructive sleep apnea. *Proc Am Thorac Soc.* 2008;5(2):253–262.
7. Kaditis A, Kheirandish-Gozal L, Gozal D. Algorithm for the diagnosis and treatment of pediatric OSA: a proposal of two pediatric sleep centers. *Sleep Med.* 2012;13(3):217–227.
8. Lumeng JC, Chervin RD. Epidemiology of pediatric obstructive sleep apnea. *Proc Am Thorac Soc.* 2008;5(2):242–252.
9. Goodwin JL, Kaemingk KL, Mulvaney SA, Morgan WJ, Quan SF. Clinical screening of school children for polysomnography to detect sleep-disordered breathing: the Tucson Children's Assessment of Sleep Apnea Study (TuCASA). *J Clin Sleep Med.* 2005;1(3):247–254.
10. Blunden SL, Beebe DW. The contribution of intermittent hypoxia, sleep debt and sleep disruption to daytime performance deficits in children: consideration of respiratory and non-respiratory sleep disorders. *Sleep Med Rev.* 2006;10(2):109–118.
11. Beebe DW, Gozal D. Obstructive sleep apnea and the prefrontal cortex: towards a comprehensive model linking nocturnal upper airway obstruction to daytime cognitive and behavioral deficits. *J Sleep Res.* 2002;11(1):1–16.
12. Hatipoglu U, Rubinstein I. Inflammation and obstructive sleep apnea syndrome pathogenesis: a working hypothesis. *Respiration.* 2003;70(6):665–671.
13. Bonuck KA, Freeman K, Henderson J. Growth and growth biomarker changes after adenotonsillectomy: systematic review and meta-analysis. *Arch Dis Child.* 2009;94(2):83–91.
14. Amin R, Somers VK, McConnell K, et al. Activity-adjusted 24-hour ambulatory blood pressure and cardiac remodeling in children with sleep disordered breathing. *Hypertension.* 2008;51(1):84–91.
15. Storms W. Allergic rhinitis-induced nasal congestion: its impact on sleep quality. *Prim Care Respir J.* 2008;17(1):7–18.

16. McColley SA, Carroll JL, Curtis S, Loughlin GM, Sampson HA. High prevalence of allergic sensitization in children with habitual snoring and obstructive sleep apnea. Chest. 1997;111(1):170–173.
17. Iber C, Ancoli-Israel S, Chesson A, Quan SF, for the American Academy of Sleep Medicine. The AASM Manual for the Scoring of Sleep and Associated Events: Rules, Terminology and Technical Specifications, 1st ed. Westchester, IL: American Academy of Sleep Medicine; 2007.
18. Chng SY, Goh DY, Wang XS, Tan TN, Ong NB. Snoring and atopic disease: a strong association. Pediatr Pulmonol. 2004;38(3):210–216.
19. Corbo GM, Fuciarelli F, Foresi A, De Benedetto F. Snoring in children: association with respiratory symptoms and passive smoking. BMJ. 1989;299(6714):1491–1494.
20. Desager KN, Nelen V, Weyler JJ, De Backer WA. Sleep disturbance and daytime symptoms in wheezing school-aged children. J Sleep Res. 2005;14(1):77–82.
21. Ersu R, Arman AR, Save D, et al. Prevalence of snoring and symptoms of sleep-disordered breathing in primary school children in Istanbul. Chest. 2004;126(1):19–24.
22. Kaditis AG, Kalampouka E, Hatzinikolaou S, et al. Associations of tonsillar hypertrophy and snoring with history of wheezing in childhood. Pediatr Pulmonol. 2010;45(3):275–280.
23. Kuehni CE, Strippoli MP, Chauliac ES, Silverman M. Snoring in preschool children: prevalence, severity and risk factors. Eur Respir J. 2008;31(2):326–333.
24. Lu LR, Peat JK, Sullivan CE. Snoring in preschool children: prevalence and association with nocturnal cough and asthma. Chest. 2003;124(2):587–593.
25. Marshall NS, Almqvist C, Grunstein RR, Marks GB. Predictors for snoring in children with rhinitis at age 5. Pediatr Pulmonol. 2007;42(7):584–591.
26. Redline S, Tishler PV, Schluchter M, Aylor J, Clark K, Graham G. Risk factors for sleep-disordered breathing in children: associations with obesity, race, and respiratory problems. Am J Respir Crit Care Med. 1999;159(5 Pt 1):1527–1532.
27. Teculescu DB, Caillier I, Perrin P, Rebstock E, Rauch A. Snoring in French preschool children. Pediatr Pulmonol. 1992;13(4):239–244.
28. Valery PC, Masters IB, Chang AB. Snoring and its association with asthma in Indigenous children living in the Torres Strait and Northern Peninsula Area. J Paediatr Child Health. 2004;40(8):461–465.
29. Verhulst SL, Vekemans K, Ho E, et al. Is wheezing associated with decreased sleep quality in Sri Lankan children? A questionnaire study. Pediatr Pulmonol. 2007;42(7):579–583.
30. Sulit LG, Storfer-Isser A, Rosen CL, Kirchner HL, Redline S. Associations of obesity, sleep-disordered breathing, and wheezing in children. Am J Respir Crit Care Med. 2005;171(6): 659–664.
31. Ross KR, Storfer-Isser A, Hart MA, et al. Sleep-disordered breathing is associated with asthma severity in children. J Pediatr. 2012;160(5):736–742.
32. Dean BB, Calimlim BC, Sacco P, Aguilar D, Maykut R, Tinkelman D. Uncontrolled asthma among children: impairment in social functioning and sleep. J Asthma. 2010;47(5):539–544.
33. Strunk RC, Sternberg AL, Bacharier LB, Szefler SJ. Nocturnal awakening caused by asthma in children with mild-to-moderate asthma in the childhood asthma management program. J Allergy Clin Immunol. 2002;110(3):395–403.
34. Stores G, Ellis AJ, Wiggs L, Crawford C, Thomson A. Sleep and psychological disturbance in nocturnal asthma. Arch Dis Child. 1998;78(5):413–419.
35. Diette GB, Markson L, Skinner EA, Nguyen TT, Algatt-Bergstrom P, Wu AW. Nocturnal asthma in children affects school attendance, school performance, and parents' work attendance. Arch Pediatr Adolesc Med. 2000;154(9):923–928.
36. Mahajan P, Pearlman D, Okamoto L. The effect of fluticasone propionate on functional status and sleep in children with asthma and on the quality of life of their parents. J Allergy Clin Immunol. 1998;102(1):19–23.
37. Zanconato S, Carraro S, Corradi M, et al. Leukotrienes and 8-isoprostane in exhaled breath condensate of children with stable and unstable asthma. J Allergy Clin Immunol. 2004;113(2):257–263.
38. Goldbart AD, Krishna J, Li RC, Serpero LD, Gozal D. Inflammatory mediators in exhaled breath condensate of children with obstructive sleep apnea syndrome. Chest. 2006;130(1):143–148.
39. Kaditis AG, Ioannou MG, Chaidas K, et al. Cysteinyl leukotriene receptors are expressed by tonsillar T cells of children with obstructive sleep apnea. Chest. 2008;134(2):324–331.
40. Dayyat E, Serpero LD, Kheirandish-Gozal L, et al. Leukotriene pathways and in vitro adenotonsillar cell proliferation in children with obstructive sleep apnea. Chest. 2009;135(5):1142–1149.
41. Goldbart AD, Mager E, Veling MC, et al. Neurotrophins and tonsillar hypertrophy in

children with obstructive sleep apnea. *Pediatr Res.* 2007;62(4):489–494.
42. Mansfield LE, Diaz G, Posey CR, Flores-Neder J. Sleep disordered breathing and daytime quality of life in children with allergic rhinitis during treatment with intranasal budesonide. *Ann Allergy Asthma Immunol.* 2004;92(2):240–244.
43. Emancipator JL, Storfer-Isser A, Taylor HG, et al. Variation of cognition and achievement with sleep-disordered breathing in full-term and preterm children. *Arch Pediatr Adolesc Med.* 2006;160(2):203–210.
44. Zhang L, Mendoza-Sassi RA, Cesar JA, Chadha NK. Intranasal corticosteroids for nasal airway obstruction in children with moderate to severe adenoidal hypertrophy. *Cochrane Database Syst Rev.* 2008(3):CD006286.
45. Marcus CL, Moore RH, Rosen CL, et al. A randomized trial of adenotonsillectomy for childhood sleep apnea. *N Engl J Med* 2013;368:2366–2376.
46. Bhattacharjee R, Kheirandish-Gozal L, Spruyt K, et al. Adenotonsillectomy outcomes in treatment of obstructive sleep apnea in children: a multicenter retrospective study. *Am J Respir Crit Care Med.* 2011;182(5):676–683.
47. Ciftci TU, Ciftci B, Guven SF, Kokturk O, Turktas H. Effect of nasal continuous positive airway pressure in uncontrolled nocturnal asthmatic patients with obstructive sleep apnea syndrome. *Respir Med.* 2005;99(5):529–534.
48. Lafond C, Series F, Lemiere C. Impact of CPAP on asthmatic patients with obstructive sleep apnoea. *Eur Respir J.* 2007;29(2):307–311.
49. Busino RS, Quraishi HA, Aguila HA, Montalvo E, Connelly P. The impact of adenotonsillectomy on asthma in children. *Laryngoscope.* 2010;120(Suppl 4):S221.
50. Saito H, Asakura K, Hata M, Kataura A, Morimoto K. Does adenotonsillectomy affect the course of bronchial asthma and nasal allergy? *Acta Otolaryngol Suppl.* 1996;523: 212–215.
51. Kheirandish-Gozal L, Dayyat EA, Eid NS, Morton RL, Gozal D. Obstructive sleep apnea in poorly controlled asthmatic children: effect of adenotonsillectomy. *Pediatr Pulmonol.* 2011;46(9):913–918.

6

ASTHMA AND OBSTRUCTIVE SLEEP APNEA

Larry M. Ladi and Edward S. Schulman

KEY POINTS

- Obstructive sleep apnea syndrome (OSAS) affects 26% of U.S. adults and is undiagnosed in 90%. Children are increasingly affected by OSAS and frequently undiagnosed. The incidence of OSAS continues to increase, in part because of the rise in obesity. Parallel increases have occurred in asthma prevalence.
- Adipose tissue is metabolically active, releasing leptin and other adipokines as well as cytokines that can intensify asthmatic inflammation and airway hyperresponsiveness.
- OSAS-induced pathophysiologic conditions may lead to the worsening of asthma. These conditions include pulmonary mechanical effects, neural and hypoxic reflexes, pulmonary blood pooling, gastroesophageal acid reflux, local and systemic anti-inflammatory effects, angiogenesis, diminished cardiac function, weight gain, and sleep disruption.
- Continuous positive airway pressure, the first line of therapy for OSAS, reverses a number of these pathophysiologic changes and exerts a positive impact on asthma outcomes in patients with both disorders.
- The 2007 National Asthma Education and Prevention Program Expert Panel Report 3 recommends that clinicians evaluate symptoms that suggest OSAS in unstable, poorly controlled asthmatic patients, particularly those who are overweight or obese.
- The ability of the asthma specialist to recognize, diagnose, and treat OSAS-exacerbated asthma represents a significant opportunity to control a major comorbidity and improve outcomes, especially in difficult-to-control cases.

INTRODUCTION

Obstructive sleep apnea syndrome (OSAS), the most common type of sleep disorder, affects approximately 26% of U.S. adults, of whom about 90% are undiagnosed. This disease results from obstruction of the upper airway with resultant brief periods of breathing cessation of at least 10 seconds (apnea) or marked reductions in flow (hypopnea) during sleep insufficient to meet the definition of apnea. This pattern is accompanied by oxyhemoglobin desaturation, persistent inspiratory efforts against the occluded airway, and arousal from sleep. Clinically, the condition is recognized by recurrent sleep interruptions, snoring, choking and gasping spells on awakening, and daytime drowsiness caused by loss of normal sleep (Table 6.1),[1] and the diagnosis is confirmed and graded on overnight polysomnography criteria (Tables 6.2 and 6.3). When uncorrected, the disorder often leads to hypertension, respiratory failure, and cardiac abnormalities.

In 1993, a study conducted on middle-aged workforce subjects estimated that 4% of men and 2% of women met the criteria for sleep apnea syndrome: an apnea-hypopnea index (AHI) of five or more events per hour and hypersomnolence.[2] Reports suggest that the prevalence of OSAS is increasing in part because of the rise in obesity, a major risk factor for OSAS. For example, the Centers for Disease Control and Prevention report that every state in the United States has an obesity rate that exceeds 15%, and in nine states, the rate is more than 30%.[3] Hence, obesity has steadily become a major health concern. A survey of 4,115 adult men and women that was conducted in 2009 and 2010 as part of the National Health and Nutrition Examination Survey (NHANES), a nationally representative sample of the U.S. population, further attests to this increase. The age-adjusted prevalence of overweight (body mass index [BMI] > 25) was 64.5% in 2009–2010, compared with 55.9% in NHANES III (1988–1994; $P < .01$). Extreme obesity (BMI > 40) also increased significantly in the population, from 2.9% to 4.7% ($P = .002$).[4] Children are also increasingly overweight, and the prevalence of overweight in children has more than doubled in the past 20 years. As a major risk factor for OSAS, the role of obesity is clear. In both men and women whose BMI exceeds 40, OSAS is at least 10 times more common. In addition, the number of patients diagnosed with OSAS between 1990 and 1998 increased 12-fold, from 108,000 to more than 1.3 million.[5]

As the prevalence of OSAS has increased, so too has the prevalence of asthma. About 7.5% of adults in the United States have this disease. Even though the precise prevalence of OSAS in asthma patients has not yet been elucidated, several studies report

Table 6.1. History, Physical Examination, and Laboratory Features of Obstructive Sleep Apnea Syndrome

Daytime hypersomnolence	Crowded airway, high Mallampati score (3 or 4)
Witnessed apneas	Tonsillar, uvular hypertrophy; polyps
Snoring	Systemic hypertension
Choking, snorting, gasping causing awakenings	Pulmonary hypertension, cor pulmonale
Nonrestorative sleep	Atrial fibrillation, cardiac dysrhythmias
Morning headaches	Cardiovascular and cerebrovascular disease
Difficulty concentrating, memory loss	Hypercapnia
Obesity (body mass index > 30)	Falling asleep while asleep reading, watching TV, driving
Large collar size: male >17"; female >16"	Gastroesophageal reflux
Macroglossia, retrognathia, micrognathia	Hypothyroidism

" = inches.

Table 6.2. Diagnostic Criteria for Confirmation of Obstructive Sleep Apnea

Either of these two conditions exists:
- The number of obstructive events (i.e., apneas, hypopneas, or respiratory effort–related arousals per hour of sleep) is more than 15 in an asymptomatic patient. More than 75% of the apneas and hypopneas must be obstructive.
- Five or more obstructive apneas, obstructive hypopneas, or respiratory effort–related arousals per hour of sleep (i.e., an apnea hypopnea index or respiratory disturbance index of ≥5 events per hour) in a patient who reports any of the following: unintentional sleep episodes during wakefulness; daytime sleepiness; nonrestorative sleep; fatigue; insomnia; waking up holding breath, gasping, or choking; or the bed partner describing loud snoring, breathing interruptions, or both during the patient's sleep. More than 75% of the apneas and hypopneas must be obstructive.

From Epstein LJ, Kristo D, Strollo PJ Jr, et al. Clinical guideline for the evaluation, management and long-term care of obstructive sleep apnea in adults. Adult Obstructive Sleep Apnea Task Force of the American Academy of Sleep Medicine. *J Clin Sleep Med.* 2009;5(3):263–276.

an increased prevalence of OSAS symptoms in such patients. However, other studies also show that symptoms of OSAS, such as snoring and witnessed apneas, are common in the asthmatic population.[6] Other investigators have found a similar relationship between asthma and witnessed apneas and have noted increased daytime sleepiness in young adult asthmatic patients, suggesting the presence of a sleep disorder.[7] In addition, there is a high prevalence of snoring in young women with atopy and a significant association of snoring with asthma. Because snoring and daytime sleepiness are common symptoms in OSAS, a possible association between asthma and OSAS is suggested.[8]

The 2007 National Asthma Education and Prevention Program Expert Panel Report 3 recommends that clinicians evaluate symptoms that suggest OSAS in patients with unstable, poorly controlled asthma, particularly those who are overweight or obese. Symptoms in asthmatic patients that should prompt consideration of a sleep evaluation are listed in Table 6.4. Continuous positive airway pressure (CPAP), the first line of therapy for OSAS, has been shown in prospective clinical studies to have a positive impact on asthma outcomes in patients with both disorders. The beneficial effect may occur because of the ability of CPAP to reverse many of the OSAS-induced pathophysiologic conditions that can lead to the worsening of asthma (Table 6.5). Such mechanisms of reversal include leptin and other adipokine suppression; mechanical and nonmechanical effects; gastroesophageal acid reflux suppression; local and systemic anti-inflammatory effects, including suppression of increased serum levels of inflammatory cytokines, chemokines, and vascular

Table 6.3. Diagnostic Criteria and Severity Grading for Obstructive Sleep Apnea

Mild OSA: AHI >5–15 events per hour
Moderate OSA: AHI 16–30 events per hour
Severe OSA: AHI >30 events per hour

AHI, apnea-hypopnea index; OSA, obstructive sleep apnea.

Table 6.4. Symptoms That Should Prompt a Sleep Evaluation

Witnessed apneic episodes, gasping, or choking at night
Excessive sleepiness
Nocturia
Morning headaches
Decreased concentration or memory loss
Decreased libido
Nocturnal diaphoresis

Table 6.5. Pathophysiologic Features of Obstructive Sleep Apnea Impacted by Continuous Positive Airway Pressure Therapy

Upper airway collapse

Expression of leptin and proinflammatory adipokines, cytokines, or free radicals

Angiogenesis, vascular endothelial growth factor generation

Enhanced vagal tone

Sympathetic surges of blood pressure

Irritating stimulation of glottis and laryngeal neural receptors; Mueller maneuver

Desaturation, organ hypoxia, and carotid body stimulation

Decreased functional residual capacity, small airway closure

Smooth muscle stiffness

Increased pulmonary capillary blood volume

Airway edema

Gastroesophageal reflux

Insulin resistance

Weight gain

---

endothelial growth factor (VEGF); angiogenesis; cardiac function improvements; weight reduction; and sleep restoration. Clarifying the potential benefits of CPAP treatment for patients with both disorders has important implications for optimal asthma therapeutic outcomes.[9]

Asthma is a common chronic disorder characterized by episodic airflow obstruction, hyperresponsiveness, and airway inflammation. The airway inflammation is frequently associated with infiltration of eosinophils and cluster of differentiation 4 (CD4) lymphocytes. The latter express helper T-cell type 2 cytokines, including interleukin (IL)-4, IL-5, and IL-13. The airways histopathologically show denudation of the airway epithelium, thickening of basement membranes, increased mucus generation, and smooth muscle hypertrophy. We will explore what is known about how characteristic changes in asthmatic airways are influenced by mechanisms operative in OSAS noted to worsen asthma control and how CPAP may improve those changes (see Table 6.3).

EXPLORING OBESITY AND THE LEPTIN HYPOTHESIS

Adipose tissue serves as an endocrine organ helping to regulate metabolism and immune functions. Excess adipose tissue produces an increased risk for metabolic disorders including type 2 diabetes and steatohepatitis. Leptin is a hormone produced by adipocytes that circulates systemically and acts on the hypothalamus to induce satiety and to increase the basal metabolic rate.[10,11] In the lean state, leptin is secreted in low levels, accompanied by the anti-inflammatory adipokine adiponectin, secreted in high levels. In obesity, serum leptin levels are increased, and adiponectin levels are decreased. This increase in leptin suggests that there is leptin resistance, perhaps at the receptor level, similar to the insulin resistance observed in patients with type 2 diabetes.[12] However, leptin's role in the parallelism between obesity and asthma is yet unknown. Leptin is a member of the IL-6 cytokine family. Therefore, it is considered proinflammatory, further stimulating the release of other proinflammatory cytokines from adipocytes such as IL-6, IL-8, and tumor necrosis factor-α (TNF-α). Lung cells, including airway epithelial and hematopoietic cells, express leptin receptors, and monocytes and macrophages respond to leptin with increased lipopolysaccharide-stimulated production of cytokines.[13,14] CD4 T cells exposed to leptin also demonstrate increased proliferative responses to T-cell mitogens. Furthermore, starvation and malnutrition are associated with immune dysfunction, and leptin administration reverses the immunosuppressive effects of acute starvation.[15] Obesity, in general, is associated with markers of systemic inflammation, including increases in peripheral blood leukocytes, levels of C-reactive protein, TNF-α, IL-6, and markers of lipid peroxidation.[16] Therefore, a greater understanding of the underlying inflammatory mechanisms operative in obesity may help provide insights into common denominators in OSAS and asthma.

A novel hypothesis is emerging for the role of leptin in the pathogenesis of asthma. Even after the BMI had been controlled for, leptin was noted to be increased in the serum of male asthmatic compared with nonasthmatic children.[17] In a murine model, the administration of leptin to mice increased both airway hyperresponsiveness (AHR) to inhaled methacholine and serum immunoglobulin E (IgE) levels, the latter suggesting a role for leptin to increase the activation of mast cells.[18]

Obese male patients with OSAS exhibit leptin levels approximately 50% higher than those of similarly obese men without OSAS, supported clinically by several case-control studies.[19,20] In addition, a significant correlation ($r = -.76$, $P < .001$) independent of BMI was found between plasma-soluble leptin receptor levels and the AHI.[21] Although the exact mechanism is not yet understood, the increased leptin levels may be driven by the hypoxic stimuli characteristic of OSAS.[22] Also, OSAS may lead to leptin resistance. A leptin resistance mechanism has been described in the brain that involves upregulation of suppressors of cytokine signaling 3 in the hypothalamus, which blocks leptin-induced signal transduction and limits leptin receptor signaling.[23] Leptin resistance, coupled with increased levels of serum leptin observed in OSAS and the known proinflammatory effects of leptin, suggests that this hormone may be relevant to asthma exacerbations in OSAS. The relationship between the elevated leptin levels in OSAS and AHR could suggest an important additional link between the morbidities of OSAS and asthma.

CPAP treatment prevents the OSAS-induced hypoxic stimuli, which might explain why CPAP is effective in decreasing serum leptin levels in OSAS patients.[24] In addition, CPAP may lead to a reduction in the proinflammatory effects of elevated leptin and to a suppression of the hypothesized increased AHR associated with elevated hormone levels.

WEIGHT GAIN MECHANISMS IN OBSTRUCTIVE SLEEP APNEA SYNDROME

The repetitive episodes of hypoxia and sleep fragmentation that occur in OSAS induce glucose intolerance and increase insulin resistance.[9,25,26] Some studies show that the severity of OSAS correlates with the degree of insulin resistance.[27,28] This increase in insulin resistance in OSAS may be related to stimulation of the sympathetic nervous system, stimulation of the hypothalamic-pituitary-adrenal axis, and release of the adipocyte-derived inflammatory cytokines IL-6, TNF-α, and leptin. Insulin resistance may cause patients to continue to gain weight as a result of the circulating insulin, which stimulates the appetite and storage of fat. Patients with OSAS have a decrease in growth hormone secretion.[29-31] Because of the lipolytic activity of growth hormone, the suppression of growth hormone in untreated OSAS results in impaired lipolysis and thereby promotes fat storage and weight gain. Finally, daytime sleepiness and fatigue are sequelae of untreated OSAS and result from both the hypoxia and the fragmented sleep occurring when the termination of apneas and hypopneas causes brief arousals.[32] The effects of daytime sleepiness may undermine efforts toward weight management. Sleepiness also negatively affects cognition, general activity, and mood.[33,34] These negative effects have detrimental consequences on health and motivation toward a more healthy lifestyle, such as participating in energetic activities and choosing healthy meal options. These factors influence the individual's ability to lose and maintain weight. In addition, sleepiness may be a large contributing factor to overeating, which further exacerbates a sedentary lifestyle. All of these negative habits, over time, result in a continual cycle of obesity, which worsens sleep apnea, which in turn leads to an increased severity of both OSAS and asthma.

The use of CPAP in OSAS patients is reported to lead to weight loss through a decrease in insulin resistance and an increase in growth hormone secretion, with a subsequent increase in its lipolytic action and a decrease in visceral body fat.[24,35-37] In addition, CPAP improves daytime wakefulness, with consequent improvements in cognition, functioning, and health-promoting activities essential for weight loss. Successful weight loss with CPAP in asthmatic patients with concomitant OSAS may therefore help improve patient outcomes.

Airway Smooth Muscle

Factors that modulate the interaction of actin and myosin within airway smooth muscle can alter the smooth muscle response. In obese individuals, the airway smooth muscles are more likely to have less tension. This results in part from the decreased functional residual capacity (FRC) produced by breathing patterns marked by higher rates and lower tidal volumes (TV) than in lean individuals.[38] The decreased FRC shortens smooth muscle length and thereby decreases its tension. The tidal stretch of smooth muscle in the airway is an extremely potent bronchodilator. The stretch of airway smooth muscle detaches actin–myosin cross-bridges and leads to reduced shortening and force generation. Therefore, in an obese individual, decreased FRC and decreased TV lead to smooth muscle stiffness with impairment of stretch resulting in increased shortening and hyperresponsiveness.[39]

Indeed, studies show in human subjects and mice that obesity appears to predispose individuals to AHR.[40] Hence, asthma is more prevalent in obese individuals, and obesity appears to make a pertinent contribution to the severe asthma phenotype. For example, obese or overweight patients account for 75% of emergency department visits for this disease. Longitudinal studies indicate that obesity antedates asthma and that the relative risk for or incidence of asthma increases with increasing obesity.[41] Morbidly obese asthmatic subjects studied after weight loss demonstrated decreased severity and symptoms of asthma.[42] For example, Litonjua and colleagues reported an association between increased BMI and the onset of AHR in a longitudinal study of aging male subjects in the United States.[43] Two other large cross-sectional studies confirm these findings.[44,45] However, although the association between BMI and AHR is not universally observed in epidemiologic studies, obese mice also demonstrate innate AHR.[46] Thus, it appears that OSAS and the frequently associated weight gain may play a significant role in worsening asthma outcomes.

Local Airway Inflammation

OSAS is associated with inflammation of both the upper and lower respiratory tracts. Inflammatory and oxidative stress markers, including pentane, exhaled nitric oxide, and IL-6 and 8-isoprostane, are noted in expired air of OSAS patients and may provide evidence for the presence of airway inflammation in OSAS.[47]

One proposed mechanism for airway inflammation in OSAS is the mechanical stress exerted on the mucosa by the high negative pressure transmitted against a closed airway passage as a result of the strong inspiratory effort produced by snoring and obstructive apneas. This repeated mechanical trauma on the upper airway triggers local inflammation of the nasal and pharyngeal mucosa.[48] Increases in polymorphonuclear leukocytes and inflammatory mediators such as bradykinin and vasoactive intestinal peptide are found in the local nasal mucosa of OSAS patients.[49] Chronic inflammation of the soft palate, with increased interstitial edema, has also been noted.[50] The uvula demonstrates mucous gland hypertrophy and infiltration of the lamina propria with T cells,[51,52] and inflammatory changes of the upper airway musculature are described.[53] In a fashion analogous to asthma, in which the upper and lower airways are considered a continuum, in OSAS, bronchial inflammation with elevated levels of neutrophils in induced sputum is demonstrated similar to the nasal mucosa.[54,55]

One additional point is that airway inflammation can affect not only the airway caliber and flow rates but also the underlying bronchial hyperresponsiveness, a cardinal feature of asthma. Therefore, local airway inflammation present in OSAS may trigger asthma pathophysiology.[56,57]

Neural Receptors and Mechanical Effects

Patients with OSAS have an increased vagal tone during sleep as a consequence of partial or complete airway obstruction during sleep apneas. The mechanics of potent vagal stimulation are similar to those that occur during the Muller maneuver, which consists of an inspiratory effort against a closed glottis.[47,58] The increase in vagal tone that occurs during apnea episodes could be a trigger for nocturnal asthma attacks in sleep apnea patients. In fact, several studies show that an increase in vagal tone stimulates the muscarinic receptors located in the central airways, leading to bronchoconstriction and causing nocturnal asthma.[56,59] Furthermore, suppression of the increased vagal tone by inhaled anticholinergic medications leads to improvement in the forced expiratory flow, reduction in early-morning decreases in peak expiratory flow, and protection against nocturnal asthma symptoms.[60,61]

Another factor in the neural reflex mechanism involves the neural receptors at the glottic inlets and in the laryngeal region, which have powerful bronchoconstrictive reflex activity. Nadel and Widdicombe showed in anesthetized cats that mechanical irritation of the laryngeal mucosa increased total lung resistance distal to the larynx.[62] The afferent limb of the reflex is localized to the superior laryngeal nerve, and the efferent limb through the vagus nerve. Stimulation of the larynx also increases activity in efferent parasympathetic nerve fibers going to the trachea and bronchi. As a result, the repeated stimulation of these neural receptors during periods of heavy snoring and obstructive apneas could stimulate neural reflex–induced bronchoconstriction. In addition, it can follow the more negative intrathoracic pressure generated during obstructive apneas that intensifies pulmonary capillary blood volume. Hence, intrapulmonary pooling of blood displacing air could further decrease lung volumes in sleep apnea patients. These changes in lung volumes from blood pooling were observed during sleep in asthmatic subjects with nocturnal bronchoconstriction.[63,64]

Moreover, an additional postulated trigger for reflex bronchoconstriction is from stimulation of the carotid body due to hypoxia, which results from obstructive apneas.[65] Denjean and colleagues report that mild hypoxia enhances the bronchial responsiveness to methacholine in sheep and that this effect is abolished in all animals after carotid chemodenervation.[66] Additional investigators have shown a hypoxia-potentiated bronchoconstricting reflex in response to histamine in anesthetized dogs and in response to aerosolized histamine in awake sheep.[51,52] Furthermore, a hypoxia-induced increase in bronchial responsiveness to methacholine is reported in asthmatic subjects.[66] Evidence indicates that hypoxia may modulate the airway response to constricting stimuli through the vagal pathway, likely initiated by stimulation of the peripheral carotid body chemoreceptors.[50,53,54]

Neuromechanical and Mechanical Effects of Continuous Positive Airway Pressure

CPAP effects include increasing mean airway pressure, recruiting underventilated alveoli, increasing minute ventilation, and stabilizing and preventing collapse of the upper airway.[67,68] In addition, several studies show that CPAP improves the bronchial smooth muscle hyperreactivity response to methacholine in patients with bronchial asthma and enhances the effect of bronchodilators on methacholine-induced bronchoconstriction.[69,70]

Wang and colleagues[70] suggest that CPAP may alter the intrinsic property of airway smooth muscle in response to stimuli and may decrease airway edema through a pressuring effect mechanism on the airway mucosa. This effect attenuates the exaggerated responsiveness to methacholine in the airways of asthmatic patients.[71,72] Furthermore, CPAP also decreases airway resistance by creating a pneumatic splinting effect that opposes airway smooth muscle contraction.[72] However, a counteractive effect on airway smooth muscle contraction may fade quickly after the pressure is removed. A reduction in the load on inspiratory muscles by CPAP is another hypothesis that has been suggested to decrease airway resistance.[70] The increase in residual volume results from a dynamic airway collapse in asthma, which may increase the load on inspiratory muscle. CPAP reduces the load on the inspiratory muscles, improving their efficiency and decreasing the energy cost of their work.[73] The improvement occurs not only in the inspiratory phase but also in the expiratory muscular pressure on which maximal expiratory flow is dependent.[74,75]

Furthermore, lung inflation may contribute to the mechanism of action of CPAP. The closure of the peripheral airways can be prevented by applying positive pressure, which leads to an increase in an end-expiratory lung volume and in FRC, resulting in an increase in total lung capacity (lung inflation).[76]

According to Flenley and colleagues, lung inflation decreases airway resistance and increases expiratory muscle function.[77] The recruitment of closed small airways in the lower portions of the lungs is suggested as an explanation for the improvement in gas exchange seen with CPAP.[78,79] Carr and Essex initially reported a 33% to 71% increase in the diameter of large conducting airways of anesthetized, spontaneously breathing dogs given 20 cm H_2O CPAP, thereby suggesting a significant bronchodilatory effect.[80] Barach and Swenson observed similar findings in humans with asthma given positive airway pressure; the application of CPAP caused dilation of smaller bronchi by 1 mm and larger bronchi by 2 mm, leading to interest in its use in patients with acute asthma.[81] Shivaram and colleagues report a reduction in respiratory rate and dyspnea when using CPAP in patients with acute asthma.[82] CPAP also reduced pulmonary resistance and the work of inspiratory muscles in asthmatic subjects in whom bronchospasm was induced by histamine.[73]

The immediate effects of CPAP on the nocturnal breathing pattern, sleep structure, and oxygen saturation curve traditionally are attributed to the mechanical splinting of the nasopharynx, oropharynx, and hypopharynx. Preventing the vagal stimulation, including the Muller maneuver during apneas, prevents the mechanical irritation of the neural receptors of the laryngeal mucosa and the hypoxia-inducing carotid body chemoreceptor-mediated reflex bronchoconstriction.[59,62,63,83] Furthermore, with free passage of air, the more negative intrathoracic pressure and intensified pulmonary capillary blood volume in OSAS are mitigated. Hence, such an increase was observed during sleep in asthmatic subjects with nocturnal symptoms and could contribute to the deleterious effect of decreased lung volume in the development of nocturnal bronchoconstriction in OSAS patients.[57,64,84]

Obstructive Sleep Apnea Syndrome and Systemic Inflammation

Even in the absence of an overt inflammatory insult, chronic low-grade systemic inflammation in individuals with OSAS is characterized by increased serum concentrations of cytokines, cytokine receptors, chemokines, and acute phase proteins.[85] The origin of this inflammation appears to be at least in part, the oxidative stress induced by oxygen desaturation during sleep apneas.[86] Importantly, systemic inflammatory markers correlate with the presence of diseases common to OSAS, including atherosclerosis. However, with respect to airway smooth muscle, OSAS-related increases in serum TNF-α are of particular interest. TNF receptors are expressed on airway smooth muscle, and as exogenous TNF-α increases in vitro, so does the contractility of mouse airways in response to a variety of contractile agonists.[87,88] OSAS-induced oxidative stress also results in elevation of IL-6, which might contribute to bronchial inflammation.[89] Finally, this cytokine may mix with and enhance multiple additional proinflammatory mediators to produce endothelial activation for leukocyte recruitment.

VASCULAR ENDOTHELIAL GROWTH FACTOR AND AIRWAY ANGIOGENESIS

VEGF is a hypoxia-sensitive glycoprotein that stimulates vessel growth.[90] In addition, VEGF is essential for neoangiogenesis during embryonic development, wound healing, and tumor growth. Furthermore, an increasing body of evidence indicates that VEGF may play an important role in the pathogenesis of bronchial asthma and contribute to bronchial inflammation, AHR, and vascular remodeling.[20] A correlation between increased VEGF levels in asthmatic patients and the degree of airway obstruction also is described.[91,92] OSAS patients have elevated concentrations of VEGF that correlate with the severity of the syndrome as reflected by the AHI and the degree of nocturnal oxygen desaturation.[92] The most likely trigger of VEGF release in OSAS is hypoxia through hypoxia-inducible factor–mediated gene expression as a result of repetitive nighttime hypoxia. Patients with OSAS, with repetitive oxygen deprivation, also are reported to have elevated free oxygen radicals and endothelin-1, which in turn may enhance gene expression of VEGF.[93] Also, the inhibitory effect of nitric oxide on VEGF gene induction may be weakened through the downregulation of nitric oxide synthesis found in OSAS.[94,95] Although highly likely, no conclusive data yet exist implicating the elevated VEGF levels in OSAS patients with the bronchial inflammation and the hyperresponsiveness fundamental to asthmatic airway inflammation.

Anti-inflammatory Effects of Continuous Positive Airway Pressure on Blood and Airways

Even in the absence of an overt inflammatory insult, chronic, low-grade systemic inflammation in individuals with OSAS is characterized by increased serum concentrations of cytokines, chemokines, and acute phase proteins.[96] Because asthma is an inflammatory airway disorder and because OSAS may act as an inflammatory stimulus, coexistent OSAS may potentially augment airway inflammation, leading to further deterioration of the respiratory status.[97] Treatment with CPAP eliminates or reduces OSAS-induced chronic intermittent hypoxia, which is a potent trigger for oxidative stress and development.[87] Schulz and colleagues report that neutrophil superoxide generation is markedly enhanced in OSAS before treatment with CPAP and that effective CPAP therapy leads to a rapid long-lasting decrease in superoxide release.[88] In addition, CPAP reduces plasma levels of C-reactive protein and proinflammatory cytokines. Treatment of OSAS with CPAP is effective in reducing VEGF concentrations, which may play a role in the pathogenesis of asthma.[91]

The effect of CPAP treatment on inflammation of the lower airways has been evaluated. Using induced sputum, Devouassoux and colleagues found that neutrophils, IL-8, and nitric oxide production are not significantly modified after 1 and 4 weeks of CPAP treatment in patients with OSAS.[98] The authors suggest that the persistence of inflammation may have resulted from the short duration of treatment. However, further studies are necessary to analyze bronchial inflammation over a longer period and should include sequential evaluation of lower airway structure and function as well as cytokine and oxidative stress markers (Figure 6.1).

Gastroesophageal Reflux

The prevalence of gastroesophageal reflux (GER) (see Chapter 23) is increased in patients with OSAS.[99] Green and Broughton and Valipour and colleagues report that GER was a complication in 62% and 58% of patients with OSAS, respectively.[84,85] It is suggested that obesity contributes to the same risk factors for OSAS and GER; however, OSAS patients exhibit significantly more GER than do members of the average population even when one controls for alcohol intake and BMI.[100] This relative increase in GER is thought to be created by the increased trans-diaphragmatic pressure and decreased intrathoracic pressure occurring during apneic episodes.[101] Other plausible mechanisms include stomach dilatation, decreased gastric motility, and transient lower esophageal sphincter relaxation caused by the autonomic nervous abnormality induced by apneic episodes.[102]

GER, occurring during sleep, is a known trigger for nocturnal asthma and can provoke asthma symptoms through vagal reflexes induced by exposure of the esophagus to stomach acid.[103] In fact, acid instillation into the mid-esophagus results in a significant increase in the airway resistance in adults with asthma.[104] Studies in canines show that airway resistance is similarly affected by acid instillation into the esophagus, a response ablated by vagotomy.[105] Another mechanism induced by GER is micro-aspiration of gastric content, which causes bronchoconstriction.[106] OSAS-induced acid reflux may play a causative role in triggering asthma symptoms.

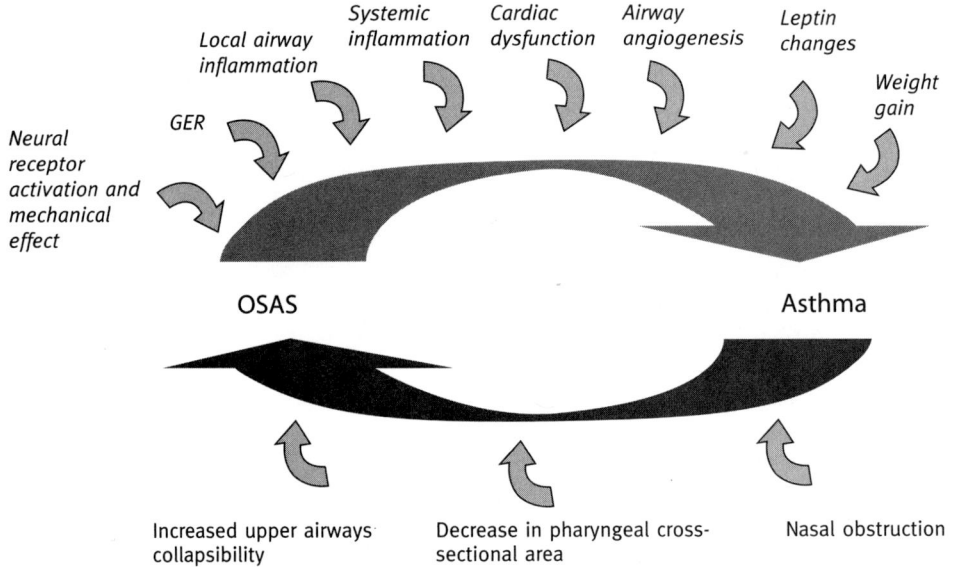

FIGURE 6.1 Interrelationship between obstructive sleep apnea and asthma. GER, gastroesophageal reflux. (From Alkhalil M, Schulman E, Getsy J. Obstructive sleep apnea syndrome and asthma: what are the links? *J Clin Sleep Med.* 2009;5[1]:71–78.)

Anti–Acid Reflux Effect of Continuous Positive Airway Pressure

It is well documented that CPAP treatment of OSAS improves GER.[84,99-101,107] The CPAP effect is thought to be the result of passive elevation of intraesophageal pressure, constriction of the lower esophageal sphincter reflex, and stabilization of the autonomic nervous abnormalities induced by the apneic episodes. Previous studies show that the effective treatment of GER, by either medication or surgery, leads to an improvement in asthma symptoms.[108–110] Therefore, CPAP may help improve acid reflux and consequently improve asthma symptoms triggered by OSAS.[103,111,112]

Cardiac Dysfunction in Obstructive Sleep Apnea Syndrome

OSAS leads to many cardiovascular consequences, which may complicate a coexisting airway obstruction in asthmatic patients. OSAS increases the risk for ischemic heart disease and congestive heart failure (CHF).[113] Moreover, dogs in which obstructive sleep apnea is induced develop left ventricular dysfunction.[114] This situation is thought to be caused by several mechanisms. Animal and human intervention studies indicate that OSAS contributes to the development of systemic hypertension, a precursor of CHF.[115,116] Recurrent hypoxemia, hypercapnia, and baroreflex inhibition resulting from repetitive surges in nocturnal blood pressure may contribute to elevated sympathetic nerve activity, known to be cardiotoxic in patients with CHF.[117-119] Hypoxemia may also independently lead to oxidative vascular wall injury.[120,121]

Both clinical and experimental data indicate that CHF causes airway obstruction, and accumulating clinical evidence indicates that one crucial component of bronchial narrowing of CHF is hyperresponsiveness to cholinergic stimuli with subsequent constriction of airway smooth muscles.[122,123] Various mechanisms are proposed to be involved in the AHR associated with CHF, including downregulation of pulmonary β-adrenergic receptors with concomitant decreases in adenylyl cyclase activity, which results in significant attenuation of cyclic adenosine monophosphate–mediated airway relaxation.[124] Other mechanisms include pulmonary edema–induced airway constriction by vagal reflexes, nonspecific bronchial C-fiber activation, thickening of bronchial walls, changes in epithelial sodium and water transport, and increased endothelin levels.[125] OSAS, by aggravating cardiac dysfunction, could further stimulate AHR in asthmatic patients.

Improving Cardiac Function

Several studies confirm the beneficial effect of CPAP on cardiac dysfunction. For example, in patients with idiopathic cardiomyopathy, treatment of OSAS with CPAP leads to significant improvement in heart function.[126] Kaneko and coworkers demonstrated significant improvement in cardiac function associated with a fall in systemic blood pressure with 1 month of CPAP in patients with idiopathic and ischemic cardiomyopathy.[127] The mechanism underlying this improvement in left ventricle ejection fraction is thought to be due to a decrease in sympathetic nerve activity related to abolition of hypoxemia after CPAP treatment.[128] OSAS treatment with CPAP also may improve the left ventricle ejection fraction by inducing a decrease in blood pressure and a reduction of the left ventricular transmural pressure gradient.[116,129] The resulting improvement in cardiac function will decrease CHF-induced AHR and associated pulmonary symptoms.

Restoring Normal Sleep Patterns

Sleep deprivation blunts the arousal response to bronchoconstriction, hypoxia, and hypercapnia. Ballard and colleagues investigated the effect of sleep deprivation in asthmatic patients and its effect on airway resistance, arousal response to bronchoconstriction, and ventilation.[130] They induced bronchoconstriction with aerosolized methacholine while the patients were awake, during normal sleep, and after 36 hours of sleep deprivation, and then measured inspiratory pressure, supraglottic pressures, TV, respiratory rate, and minute ventilation. They found that prior sleep deprivation raised the airway resistance and the arousal threshold to induced bronchoconstriction but did not affect ventilatory and occlusion pressure responses. The blunted arousal response to bronchoconstriction found in the Ballard study may contribute significantly to fatal nocturnal asthma caused by delayed awareness of symptoms and a delay in seeking treatment.

OSAS induces hypoxia and fragmented sleep secondary to repeated episodes of apneas and hypopneas that cause brief periods of arousal.[32] CPAP works as a pneumatic splint to effectively eliminate upper airway obstruction and thus improve sleep fragmentation by reducing the number of hypoxia- and hypopnea-apnea–related arousals. Therefore, CPAP may help to prevent the deleterious effect of OSAS-induced sleep fragmentation on asthma outcomes.

UNMET, FUTURE RESEARCH NEEDS

1. Pathophysiologic mechanisms tying together obesity, OSAS, and asthma require increased research.
2. Better definition is needed of adipokines and other cytokine mediators produced by adipose tissue that may underlie OSAS-exacerbated asthma.
3. Within the group of OSAS-exacerbated asthmatic patients, there are likely different phenotypes and endotypes that require better understanding because each may require more targeted therapies.[131-133]
4. New approaches to the treatment of OSAS-exacerbated asthma beyond CPAP are needed (e.g., novel appliances, bariatric surgery) because CPAP therapy may be poorly tolerated.
5. Education programs among physicians, especially asthma specialists, are needed to increase awareness and understanding of treatment of OSAS, especially in patients with poorly controlled asthma.

CONCLUSION

OSAS and asthma are both increasing in the general population and are detrimental to each other. Furthermore, obesity appears to increase the risk for both diseases. Data suggest that OSAS is an independent risk factor for asthma exacerbations and that OSAS symptoms are more common in asthmatic patients than in the general population, hence linking these two major diseases.[134] Both conditions share mechanical, hormonal, and immunologic reasons for their effects. However, studies show that CPAP might modify airway smooth muscle function and asthma control in patients with both disorders. Despite the ever-increasing population of patients presenting with both disorders, large prospective, randomized controlled studies are still necessary to more fully evaluate OSAS therapeutics and asthma outcomes.

REFERENCES

1. Young T, Palta M, Dempsey J, et al. Burden of sleep apnea: rationale, design, and major findings of the Wisconsin Sleep Cohort study. *WMJ*. 2009;108(5):246.
2. Young T, Dempay J, Weber S. The occurrence of sleep disordered breathing among middle-aged adults. *N Engl J Med*. 1993;328:1230–1235.
3. Centers for Disease Control and Prevention. Vital signs, adult obesity. http://www.cdc.gov/vitalsigns/AdultObesity/index.html. Accessed March 31, 2013.
4. Flegal KM, Carroll MD, Kit BK, Ogden CL. Prevalence of obesity and trends in the distribution of body mass index among US adults, 1999-2010. *JAMA*. 2012;307(5):491–497.
5. Namen AM, Dungen DP, Fleischer A, et al. Increased physician-reported sleep apnea: the national ambulatory medical care survey. *Chest*. 2002;121:1741–1747.
6. Auckley D, Moallem M, Shaman Z, et al. Findings of Berlin Questionnaire survey: comparison between patients seen in an asthma clinic versus internal medicine clinic. *Sleep Med*. 2008;9(5):494–499.
7. Janson C, De Backer W, Gislason T, et al. Increased prevalence of sleep disturbances and daytime sleepiness in subjects with bronchial asthma: a population study of young adults in three European countries. *Eur Respir J*. 1996;9:2131–2138.
8. Alkhalil M, Schulman ES, Getsy J. Obstructive sleep apnea syndrome and asthma: the role of continuous positive airway pressure treatment. *Ann Allergy Asthma Immunol*. 2008;101(4):350–357.
9. Alkhalil M, Schulman E, Getsy J. Obstructive sleep apnea syndrome and asthma: what are the links? *J Clin Sleep Med*. 2009;5(1):71–78.
10. Considine RV, Sinha MK, Heiman ML, et al. Serum immunoreactive-leptin concentrations in normal-weight and obese humans. *N Engl J Med*. 1996;334:292–295.
11. O'Donnell C, Tankersley C, Polotsky V, et al. Leptin, obesity and respiratory function. *Respir Physiol*. 2000;119:163–170.
12. Maffei M, Halaas J, Ravussin E, et al. Leptin levels in human and rodent: measurement of plasma leptin and ob RNA in obese and weight reduced subjects. *Nat Med*. 1995;1:1155–1161.
13. Bergen HT, Cherlet TC, Manuel P, Scott JE. Identification of leptin receptors in lung and isolated fetal type II cells. *Am J Respir Cell Mol Biol*. 2002;27:71–77.
14. Torday JS, Sun H, Wang L, Torres E, Sunday ME, Rubin LP. Leptin mediates the parathyroid hormone-related protein paracrine stimulation of fetal lung maturation. *Am J Physiol Lung Cell Mol Physiol*. 2002;282:L405–L410.
15. Lord GM, Matarese G, Howard JK, Baker RJ, Bloom SR, Lechler RI. Leptin modulates the T-cell immune response and reverses starvation-induced immunosuppression. *Nature*. 1998;394:897–901.
16. Rajala MW, Scherer PE. Minireview. The adipocyte: at the crossroads of energy homeostasis, inflammation and atherosclerosis. *Endocrinology*. 2003;144:3765–3773.
17. Guler N, Kirerleri E, Ones U, et al. Leptin: does it have any role in childhood asthma? *J Allergy Clin Immunol*. 2004;114:254–259.
18. Shore SA, Schwartzman IN, Mellama MS, et al. Effect of leptin on allergic airway responses in mice. *J Allergy Clin Immunol*. 2005;115:103–109.
19. Philips B, Kato M, Narkiewicz K, et al. Increases in leptin levels, sympathetic drive and weight gain in obstructive sleep apnea. *Am J Physiol Heart Circ Physiol*. 2000;279:H234–H237.
20. Imagawa S, Yamaguchi Y, Higuchi M, et al. Levels of vascular endothelial growth factor are elevated in patients with obstructive sleep apnea-hypopnea syndrome. *Blood*. 2001;98:1255–1257.
21. Manzella D, Prillo M, Razzino T, et al. Soluble leptin receptor and insulin resistance as determinant of sleep apnea. *Int J Obes Relat Metab Disord*. 2002;26:370–375.
22. Tatsumi K, Kasahara Y, Kurosu K, et al. Sleep oxygen desaturation and circulating leptin in obstructive sleep apnea-hypopnea syndrome. *Chest*. 2005;127:716–721.
23. Bjorbaek C, Elmquist JK, Frantz JD, Shoelson SE, Flier JS. Identification of SOCS-3 as a potential mediator of central leptin resistance. *Mol Cell*. 1998;1:619–625.
24. Harsch IA, Konturek PC, Koebnick C, et al. Leptin and ghrelin levels in patients with

obstructive sleep apnea: effect of CPAP treatment. *Eur Respir.* 2003;22:251–257.
25. Punjabi NM, Ahmad MM, Polotsky VY, et al. Sleep-disordered breathing, glucose intolerance, and insulin resistance. *Respir Physiol Neurobiol.* 2003;136:167–178.
26. Punjabi NM, Sorkin JD, Katzel LI, et al. Sleep-disordered breathing and insulin resistance in middle-aged and overweight men. *Am J Respir Crit Care Med.* 2002;165;677–682.
27. Nagai Y, Nakatsumi Y, Abe T, et al. Is the severity of obstructive sleep apnea associated with the degree of insulin resistance? *Diabet Med.* 2003;20:80–82.
28. Tiihonen M, Partinen M, Narvanen S. The severity of obstructive sleep apnea is associated with insulin resistance. *J Sleep Res.* 1993;2:56–61.
29. Gianotti L, Pivetti S, Lanfranco F, et al. Concomitant impairment of growth hormone secretion and peripheral sensitivity in obese patients with obstructive sleep apnea syndrome. *J Clin Endocrinol Metab.* 2002;87:5052–5057.
30. Clark RW, Schmidt HS, Malarkey WB. Disordered growth hormone and prolactin secretion in primary disorders of sleep. *Neurology.* 1979;29:855–861.
31. Nieminen P, Lopponen T, Tolonen U, et al. Growth and biochemical markers of growth in children with snoring and obstructive sleep apnea. *Pediatrics.* 2002;109:e55.
32. Dinges DF, Maislin G, Stanley B, et al. Sleepiness and neurobehavioral functioning in relation in apnea severity in a cohort of commercial motor vehicle operators. *Sleep.* 1998;21(Suppl):83.
33. Engleman HM, Cheshire KE, Deary IJ, et al. Daytime sleepiness, cognitive performance and mood after continuous positive airway pressure for sleep apnea/hypopnea syndrome. *Thorax.* 1993;48:911–914.
34. Gooneratne NS, Weaver TE, Cater JR. Functional outcomes of excessive daytime sleepiness in older adults. *J Am Geriatr Soc.* 2003;51:642–649.
35. Harsch IA, Konturek PC, Koebnick C, et al. Leptin and ghrelin levels in patients with obstructive sleep apnea: effect of CPAP treatment. *Eur Respir J.* 2003;22:251–257.
36. Cooper BG, White JE, Ashworth LA, et al. Hormonal and metabolic profiles in subjects with obstructive sleep apnea syndrome and the acute efforts of nasal continuous positive airway pressure treatment. *Sleep.* 1995;18:172–179.
37. Chin K, Shimizu K, Nakamura T, et al. Changes in intraabdominal visceral fat and serum leptin level in patients with obstructive sleep apnea syndrome following nasal continuous positive airway pressure therapy. *Circulation.* 1999;100:706–712.
38. Fredberg JJ, Inouye DS, Mijailovich SM, Butler JP. Perturbed equilibrium of myosin binding in airway smooth muscle and its implications in bronchospasm. *Am J Respir Crit Care Med.* 1999;159:959–967.
39. Thomson CC, Clark S, Camargo CA Jr. Body mass index and asthma severity among adults presenting to the emergency department. *Chest.* 2003;124:795–802.
40. Camargo CA Jr, Weiss ST, Zhang S, et al. Prospective study mass index, weight change, and risk of adult-onset asthma in women. *Arch Intern Med.* 1999;159:2582–2588.
41. Guerra S, Wright AL, Morgan WJ, et al. Persistence of asthma symptoms during adolescence: role of obesity and age at the onset of puberty. *Am J Respir Crit Care Med.* 2004;170:78–85.
42. Aaron SD, Fergusson D, Dent R, et al. Effect of weight reduction on respiratory function and airway reactivity in obese women. *Chest.* 2004;125:2046–2052.
43. Litonjua AA, Sparrow D, Celedon JC, et al. Association of body mass index with the development of methacholine AHR in men: the normative aging study. *Thorax.* 2002;57:581–585.
44. Chinn S, Jarvis D, Burney P. Relation of bronchial responsiveness to body mass index in the ECRHS. European Community Respiratory Health Survey. *Thorax.* 2002;57:1028–1033.
45. Celedon JC, Palmer LJ, Litonjua AA, et al. Body mass index and asthma in adults in families of subjects with asthma in aging, China. *Am J Respir Crit Care Med.* 2001;164:1835–1840.
46. Shore SA, Rivera-Sanchez YM, Schwartzman IN, et al. Responses to ozone are increased in obese mice. *J Appl Physiol.* 2003;95:938–945.
47. Guilleminault C, Winkle R, Melvin K, et al. Cyclical variation of the heart rate in sleep apnea syndromes: mechanism and usefulness of 24 hr electrocardiography as a screening technique. *Lancet.* 1984;1:126–136.
48. Naykayama K. Surgical removal of carotid body for bronchial asthma. *Chest.* 1961;40;595–604.
49. Sullivan CE. Bilateral carotid body resection in asthma: vulnerability to hypoxic death in sleep. *Chest.* 1980;78:354.
50. Denjean A, Canet E, Praud JP, et al. Hypoxia-induced bronchial responsiveness in awake sheep: role of carotid chemoreceptors. *Respir Physiol.* 1991;83:201–210.

51. Vidruk EH, Sorkness RL. Histamine-induced reflex tracheal constriction is attenuated by hyperoxia and exaggerated by hypoxia. *Am Rev Respir Dis.* 1985;32:287–291.
52. Ahmed T, Marchette B. Hypoxia enhances nonspecific bronchial reactivity. *Am Rev Respir Dis.* 1985;132:287–291.
53. Nadel JA, Widdicombe JG. Effects of changes in blood gas tensions and carotid sinus pressure on tracheal volume and total lung resistance to airflow. *J Physiol.* 1962:163:13–33.
54. Green M, Widdicombe JG. The effects of ventilation of dogs with different gas mixtures on airway calibre and lung mechanics. *J Physiol.* 1966;186;363–381.
55. Vidruk EH. Hypoxia potentiates, oxygen attenuates deflation-induced reflex tracheal constriction. *J Appl Physiol.* 1985;59:941–946.
56. Boushey HA, Holtzman MJ, Sheller JR, et al. State of the art: bronchial hyperreactivity. *Am Rev Respir Dis.* 1980;121:389–413.
57. Morrison JF, Pearson SB. The parasympathetic nervous system and the diurnal variation of lung mechanics in asthma. *Respir Med.* 1991;85:285–289.
58. Guilleminault C, Tilkian A, Lehrman K, et al. Sleep apnea syndrome: state of sleep and autonomic dysfunction. *J Neurol Neurosurg Psychiatry.* 1977;40:718–725.
59. Morrison JF, Pearson SB, Dean HG. Parasympathetic nervous system in nocturnal asthma. *BMJ.* 1988;296:1427–1429.
60. Cropp GJ. The role of the parasympathetic nervous systems in the maintenance of chronic airway obstruction in asthmatic children. *Am Rev Respir Dis.* 1975:112:599–605.
61. Coe CI, Barnes PJ. Reduction of nocturnal asthma by an inhaled anticholinergic drug. *Chest.* 1986;90:485–488.
62. Nadel JA, Widdicombe JG. Reflex effects of upper airway irritation on total lung resistance and blood pressure. *J Appl Physiol.* 1962;17:861–865.
63. Desjardin JA, Sutarik JM, Suh B, et al. Influence of sleep on pulmonary capillary volume in normal and asthmatic subjects. *Am J Respir Crit Care Med.* 1995;152;193–198.
64. Ballard RD, Irvin CG, Martin RJ, et al. Influence of sleep on lung volumes in asthmatic patients and normal subjects. *J Appl Physiol.* 1990;68:2034–2041.
65. Nakayama K. Surgical removal of the carotid body for bronchial asthma. *Chest.* 1961;40:595–604.
66. Denjean A, Roux C, Herve P, et al. Mild isocapnic hypoxia enhances the bronchial response to methacholine in asthmatic subjects. *Am Rev Respir Dis.* 1988;138:789–793.
67. British Thoracic Society Standards of Care Committee. Non-invasive ventilation in acute respiratory failure. *Thorax.* 2002;57:192–211.
68. Wysocki M, Antonelli M. Noninvasive mechanical ventilation in acute hypoxemic respiratory failure. *Eur Respir J.* 2001;18:209–220.
69. Lin H, Wang C, Yang C, et al. Effect of nasal continuous positive airway pressure on methacholine-induced bronchoconstriction. *Respir Med.* 1995;89:121–128.
70. Wang CH, Lin HC, Huang TJ, et al. Differential effects of nasal continuous positive airway pressure on reversible or fixed upper and lower airway obstruction. *Eur Respir J.* 1996;9:952–959.
71. Cabanes L, Weber SN, Matran R, et al. Bronchial hyperresponsiveness to methacholine in patients with impaired left ventricular function. *N Engl J Med.* 1989;320:1317–1322.
72. Martin RJ, Pak J. Nasal CPAP in nonapneic nocturnal asthma. *Chest.* 1991;100(4):1024–1027.
73. Martin JG, Shore SA, Engel LA. Effect of continuous positive airway pressure on respiratory mechanics and pattern of breathing in induced asthma. *Am Rev Respir Dis.* 1982;126:812–817.
74. Martin JG, Shore SA, Engel L. Mechanical load and inspiratory muscle action during induced asthma. *Am Rev Respir Dis.* 1983;128:455–460.
75. Hyatt RE, Schilder DP, Fry DL. Relationship between maximum expiratory flow and degree of lung inflation. *J Appl Physiol.* 1958;13:331–336.
76. Verbraecken J, Willemen M, De Cock W, et al. Continuous positive airway pressure and lung inflation in sleep apnea patients. *Respiration.* 2001;68(4):357–364.
77. Flenly DC, Pengelly LD, Milic-Emili J. Immediate effects of positive-pressure breathing on the ventilatory response to CO2. *J Appl Physiol.* 1971;30:7–11.
78. Lopata M, Onal E. Mass loading, sleep apnea, and the pathogenesis of obesity hypoventilation. *Am Rev Respir Dis.* 1982;126:640–645.
79. Douglas FC, Chong PY. Influence of obesity on peripheral airways patency. *J Appl Physiol.* 1972;33:559–563.
80. Carr DT, Essex HE. Certain effects of positive pressure respiration on the circulatory and respiratory systems. *Am Heart J.* 1946;31:53–73.
81. Barach A, Swenson P. Effect of breathing gases under positive pressure on lumens of small

and medium sized bronchi. *Arch Intern Med.* 1939;63:946–948.
82. Shivaram U, Miro Am, Cash ME, et al. Cardiopulmonary responses to continuous positive airway pressure in acute asthma. *J Crit Care.* 1993;8:87–92.
83. Hoffstein V, Viner S, Mateika S, et al. Treatment of obstructive sleep apnea with nasal continuous positive airway pressure: patient compliance, perception of benefits, and the side effects. *Am Rev Respir Dis.* 1992;145: 841–845.
84. Green BT, Broughton WA. Marked improvement in nocturnal gastroesophageal reflux in a large cohort of patients with obstructive sleep apnea treated with continuous positive airway pressure. *Arch Intern Med.* 2003;163:41–45.
85. Valipour A, Makker HK, Hardy R, et al. Symptomatic gastroesophageal reflux in subjects with a breathing sleep disorder. *Chest.* 2002;121:1748–1753.
86. Shamsuzzamann AS, Winnicki M, Lanfranchi P, et al. Elevated C-reactive protein in patients with obstructive sleep apnea. *Circulation.* 2002;105:2462–2464.
87. Xu W, Chi L, Row BW, et al. Increased oxidative stress is associated with chronic intermittent hypoxia-mediated brain cortical neuronal cell apoptosis in a mouse model of sleep apnea. *Neuroscience.* 2004;126:313–323.
88. Schulz R, Mahmoudi S, Hattar K, et al. Enhanced release of superoxide from polymorphonuclear neutrophils in obstructive sleep apnea: impact of continuous positive airway pressure therapy. *Am J Respir Crit Care Med.* 2000;162:566–570.
89. Yokoe T, Minoguchi K, Matsuo H, et al. Elevated levels of C-reactive protein and IL-6 in patients with obstructive sleep apnea syndrome are decreased by nasal continuous positive airway pressure. *Circulation.* 2003;107:1129–1134.
90. Lavie L, Kraicizi H, Hefetz A, et al. Plasma vascular endothelial growth factor in sleep apnea syndrome: effects of nasal continuous positive air pressure treatment. *Am J Respir Crit Care Med.* 2002;165:1624–1628.
91. Asai K, Kabazawa H, Kamoni H, et al. Increased levels of vascular endothelial growth factor in induced sputum in asthmatic patients. *Clin Exp Allergy.* 2003;33:595–599.
92. Schulz R, Hummel C, Heinemann S, et al. Serum levels of vascular endothelial growth factor are elevated in patients with obstructive sleep apnea and severe nighttime hypoxia. *Am J Respir Crit Care Med.* 2002;165:67–70.
93. Kuroki M, Voest EE, Amano S, et al. Reactive oxygen intermediates increase vascular endothelial growth factor expression in vitro and in vitro. *J Clin Invest.* 1996;98:1667–1675.
94. Schulz R, Schmidt D, Blum A, et al. Decreased plasma levels of nitric oxide derivatives in obstructive sleep apnea: response to CPAP therapy. *Thorax.* 2000;55:1046–1051.
95. Liu Y, Christoy H, Morita T, et al. Carbon monoxide and nitric oxide suppress the hypoxic induction of vascular endothelial growth factor gene via the 5 enhancer. *J Biol Chem.* 1998;273:15257–15262.
96. Dyugovskaya L, Lavie P, Lavie L. Increased adhesion molecules expression and production of reactive oxygen species in leukocytes of sleep apnea patients. *Am J Respir Crit Care Med.* 2002:165:934–939.
97. Sabato R, Guido P, Salerno FG, et al. Airway inflammation in patients affected by obstructive sleep apnea. *Monaldi Arch Chest Dis.* 2006;65(2):102–105.
98. Devouassoux G, Levy P, Rossini E, et al. Sleep apnea is associated with bronchial inflammation and continuous, positive airway pressure-induced airway hyperresponsiveness. *J Allergy Clin Immunol.* 2007;119:597–603.
99. Penzel T, Becker HF, Brandenburg U, et al. Arousal in patients with gastroesophageal reflux and sleep apnoea. *Eur Respir J.* 1999;14:1266–1270.
100. Ing AJ, Ngu MC, Breslin AB. Obstructive sleep apnea and gastroesophageal reflux. *Am J Med.* 2000;108:120S–125S.
101. Kerr P, Shoenut JP, Steens RD, et al. Nasal continuous positive airway pressure: a new treatment for nocturnal gastroesophageal reflux? *J Otolaryngol.* 1995;24:238–241.
102. Urata M, Fukuno H, Nomura M, et al. Gastric motility and autonomic activity during obstructive sleep apnea. *Aliment Pharmacol Ther.* 2006;24:132–140.
103. Avidan B, Sonnenberg A, Schnell TG, et al. Temporal associations between coughing or wheezing and acid reflux in asthmatics. *Gut.* 2001;49:767–772.
104. Schan CA, Harding SM, Haile JM, et al. Gastroesophageal reflux-induced bronchoconstriction: an intraesophageal acid infusion study using state of the art technology. *Chest.* 1994;106:731–737.
105. Mansfield LE, Hameister HH, Spaudling HS, et al. The role of the vagus nerve in airway

narrowing caused by intraesophageal hydrochloric acid provocation and esophageal distention. *Am Allergy*. 1981;47:431–434.
106. Chernow B, Johnson LF, Janowitz WR, et al. Pulmonary aspiration as a consequence of gastroesophageal reflux: a diagnostic approach. *Dig Dis Sci*. 1979;24:839–844.
107. Kerr P, Shoenut JP, Millar T, et al. Nasal CPAP reduces gastroesophageal reflux in obstructive sleep apnea syndrome. *Chest*. 1992;101:1539–1544.
108. Field SK, Sutherland LR. Does medical antireflux therapy improve asthma in asthmatics with gastroesophageal reflux? A critical review of the literature. *Chest*. 1998;114:275–283.
109. Perrin-Fayolle M, Gormand F, Braillon G, et al. Long-term results of surgical treatment for gastroesophageal reflux in asthmatic patients. *Chest*. 1989;96:40–45.
110. Komatsu Y, Hoppo T, Jobe BA. Proximal reflux as a cause of adult-onset asthma: the case for hypopharyngeal impedance testing to improve the sensitivity of diagnosis. *JAMA Surg*. 2013;148(1):50–58.
111. Cibella F, Cuttitta G. Nocturnal asthma and gastroesophageal reflux. *Am J Med*. 2001;111:31–36.
112. Davis RS, Larsen GL, Grunstein MM. Respiratory response to intraesophageal acid infusion in asthmatic children during sleep. *J Allergy Clin Immunol*. 1983;72:393–398.
113. Shahar E, Whitney CW, Redline S, et al. Sleep-disordered breathing and cardiovascular disease: cross-sectional results of Sleep Heart Health Study. *Am J Respir Care Med*. 2001;163:19–25.
114. Parker JD, Brooks D, Kozer LF, et al. Acute and chronic effects of airway obstruction on canine left ventricular performance. *Am J Respir Crit Care Med*. 1999;160:1888–1896.
115. Brooks D, Horner RL, Kozar LF, et al. Obstructive sleep apneas cause of systemic hypertension: evidence from canine model. *J Clin Invest*. 1997;99:106–109.
116. Becker HF, Jerrentrup A, Ploch T, et al. Effect of nasal continuous positive airway pressure treatment on blood pressure in patients with obstructive sleep apnea. *Circulation*. 2003;107:68–73.
117. Morgan BJ, Crabtree DC, Palta M, et al. Combined hypoxia and hypercapnia evokes long-lasting sympathetic activation in humans. *J Appl Physiol*. 1995;79:205–213.
118. Carlson JT, Hedner JA, Sellgren J, et al. Depressed baroreflex sensitivity in patients with obstructive sleep apnea. *Am J Respir Crit Care Med*. 1996;154:1490–1496.
119. Mann DL, Kent RL, Parsons B, et al. Adrenergic effects on the biology of the adult mammalian cardiocyte. *Circulation*. 1992;85:790–804.
120. Prabhakar NR. Sleep apneas: an oxidative stress? *Am J Respir Crit Care Med*. 2002;165:859–860.
121. Ip MS, Lam B, Chan LY, et al. Circulating nitric oxide is suppressed in obstructive sleep apnea and is reversed by nasal continuous positive airway pressure. *Am J Respir Crit Care Med*. 2000;162:2166–2171.
122. Snashall PD, Chung KF. Airway obstruction and bronchial hyperresponsiveness in left ventricular failure and mitral stenosis. *Am Rev Respir Dis*. 1991;144:945–956.
123. Brunnee T, Graf K, Kastens B, et al. Bronchial hyperreactivity in patients with moderate pulmonary circulation overload. *Chest*. 1993;103:1477–1481.
124. Borst MM, Beuthien W, Schwencke C, et al. Desensitization of the pulmonary adenylyl cyclase system: a cause of airway hyperresponsiveness in congestive heart failure. *J Am Coll Cardiol*. 1999;34:848–856.
125. Levin ER. Endothelins. *N Engl J Med*. 1999;333:356–363.
126. Malone S, Liu PP, Holloway R, et al. Obstructive sleep apnoea in patients with dilated cardiomyopathy: effects of continuous positive airway pressure. *Lancet*. 1991;338:1480–1484.
127. Kaneko Y, Floras JS, Usui K, et al. Cardiovascular effects of continuous positive airway pressure in patients with heart failure and obstructive sleep apnea. *N Engl J Med*. 2003;348:1233–1241.
128. Mansfield DR, Gollogly NC, Kaye DM, et al. Controlled trial of continuous positive airway pressure in obstructive sleep apnea and heart failure. *Am J Respir Crit Care Med*. 2004;169:361–366.
129. Naughton MT, Rahman MA, Hara K, et al. Effect of continuous positive airway pressure on intrathoracic and left ventricular transmural pressures in patients with congestive heart failure. *Circulation*. 1995;91:1725–1731.
130. Ballard RD, Tan WC, Kelly PL, et al. Effect of sleep and sleep deprivation on ventilatory response to bronchoconstriction. *J Appl Physiol*. 1990;69:490–497.

131. Corren J, Lemanske RF, Hanania NA, et al. Lebrikizumab treatment in adults with asthma. *N Engl J Med.* 2011;365:1088–1098.
132. Holguin F, Bleecker ER, Busse WW, et al. Obesity and asthma: an association modified by age of asthma onset. *J Allergy Clin Immunol.* 2011;127:1486–1493.
133. Sutherland ER, Goleva E, King TS, et al. Cluster analysis of obesity and asthma phenotypes. *PLoS ONE.* 2012;7:e36631.
134. Ten Brinke A, Sterk PJ, Masclee AA, et al. Risk factors of frequent exacerbations in difficult to treat asthma. *Eur Respir J.* 2005;26:812–818.

7

CHRONIC OBSTRUCTIVE PULMONARY DISEASE AND IRREVERSIBLE AIRFLOW OBSTRUCTION

COMORBID, COEXISTING, AND DIFFERENTIAL DIAGNOSIS

Stephen P. Peters

KEY POINTS

- Asthma and chronic obstructive pulmonary disease (COPD) have a number of elements in common, including airway obstruction (which is variably reversible) and airway inflammation (of different types), that are dependent on the interplay of genetic and environmental factors.
- A particularly important subgroup of patients with both diseases display irreversible airflow obstruction, which broadly defined implies the inability to reverse airway obstruction through environmental, behavior modification, or pharmacologic means.
- Phenotypes and endotypes at the convergence of asthma and COPD occur in patients from both disease categories with irreversible airflow obstruction. In addition, particularly problematic are patients with asthma who smoke.
- Patients with irreversible airflow obstruction demonstrate increased symptoms, a reduced quality of life, and increased exacerbations and health care utilization compared with those without this characteristic.
- The treatment of patients with irreversible airflow obstruction includes environmental and behavior modification (smoking cessation, weight loss if appropriate, and exercise and pulmonary rehabilitation) and pharmacologic interventions.
- Both bronchodilators and anti-inflammatory agents play an important role in managing patients with irreversible airflow obstruction. Advances in therapeutics include the realization that drugs once thought effective only in COPD, such as the anticholinergic agent tiotropium, can also play an important role in managing some patients with asthma. In addition, it is important to identify the patient with fixed airflow

obstruction who is "less inflamed," and therefore corticosteroid insensitive, thereby avoiding high doses of these medications, which are both ineffective and associated with adverse side effects.
- Many of the same genes are associated with abnormal lung function in both asthma and COPD, providing clues to the pathogenesis of fixed airflow obstruction. Such information could identify targets for therapeutic intervention.

INTRODUCTION

Asthma and chronic obstructive pulmonary disease (COPD) are usually thought of as distinct entities. However, the current asthma and COPD guidelines that define these conditions contain a number of similar elements. The National Asthma Education and Prevention Program Expert Panel Report 3 asthma guidelines[1] define asthma as "a chronic inflammatory disorder of the airways in which many cells and cellular elements play a role: in particular, mast cells, eosinophils, neutrophils (especially in sudden onset, fatal exacerbations, occupational asthma, and patients who smoke), T lymphocytes, macrophages, and epithelial cells. In susceptible individuals, this inflammation causes recurrent episodes of coughing (particularly at night or early in the morning), wheezing, breathlessness, and chest tightness. These episodes are usually associated with widespread but variable airflow obstruction that is often reversible either spontaneously or with treatment." The Global Strategy for the Diagnosis, Management, and Prevention of Chronic Obstructive Pulmonary Disease[2] defines COPD as "a common preventable and treatable disease...characterized by persistent airflow limitation that is usually progressive and associated with an enhanced chronic inflammatory response in the airways and the lung to noxious particles or gases. Exacerbations and comorbidities contribute to the overall severity in individual patients." The definitions of asthma and COPD in these guidelines describe inflammation as an important etiologic factor, the presence of exacerbations as an important comorbid condition, and the importance of airflow limitation, which is less reversible in COPD. A major difference is that COPD is considered to be largely "preventable" because of its major associations with cigarette smoking.

These definitions implicitly support the "Dutch hypothesis" put forth by Orie and colleagues[3] that asthma and COPD (emphysema and chronic bronchitis) are different manifestations of one disease, a chronic nonspecific lung disease, in which both the host and environmental factors play a role in the phenotype that is manifest in individual patients. This hypothesis should be particularly applicable for asthma that manifests as irreversible airflow obstruction.

This review focuses on this intersection between asthma and COPD and its clinical and diagnostic features, the morbidities associated with it, current approaches to investigate pathogenesis, and current and future approaches to treatment.

MAKING THE DIAGNOSIS

Definitions of Airway Obstruction and Bronchodilator Reversibility

Asthma and COPD, like a number of diseases of disordered airway function, including bronchiectasis, bronchiolitis, cystic fibrosis, and allergic bronchopulmonary aspergillosis, have airway obstruction as an important component of their pathogenesis. However, the criteria used to determine whether airway obstruction is present are different in asthma than in COPD. For example, asthma guidelines use a fixed ratio of forced expiratory volume in 1 second (FEV_1) to forced vital capacity (FVC), which is age corrected, to define a ratio below which airway obstruction is considered to be present (i.e., a "normal" FEV_1/FVC for a person 8 to 19 years of age is ≥85%; 20 to 39 years of age, ≥80%; 40 to 59 years of age, ≥75%; and 60 to 80 years of age, ≥70%) (Table 7.1).[1] In COPD, an FEV_1/FVC of less than 70% after administration of a short-acting bronchodilator (e.g., 4 puffs of albuterol through a spacer) is considered to indicate airway obstruction.[2] Both of these norms are different from that suggested by pulmonologists who interpret pulmonary function tests. The American Thoracic Society–European Respiratory Society

Table 7.1. Definitions of Airway Obstruction

GROUP	DEFINITION	REFERENCE NO.
NAEPP-ERP3	FEV_1/FVC < age-related norm: 8–19 years of age, <85%; 20–39 years of age, <80%; 40–59 years of age, <75%; 60–80 years of age, <70%	1
Global Strategy for the Diagnosis, Management and Prevention of COPD	FEV_1/FVC < 70% after administration of a short-acting bronchodilator	2
American Thoracic Society–European Respiratory Society Task Force	FEV_1/FVC (or FEV_1/VC) < lower limits of normal (i.e., <5th percentile predicted)	4

Task Force on the Standardisation of Lung Function Testing uses a purely statistical approach to define airway obstruction, that is, an FEV_1/FVC (or FEV_1/VC) ratio that is less than the lower limits of normal, defined as less than the fifth percentile predicted.[4]

Just as there are a variety of definitions of "airway obstruction," there are also a variety of definitions of bronchodilator "reversibility" (reviewed by Hanania[5]). Although the most commonly used standard for bronchodilator reversibility testing is the administration of 4 puffs of albuterol (90 to 100 μg each at 15-second intervals through a spacer), other bronchodilators, such as ipratropium bromide, are also used for this purpose.[6,7]

The American Thoracic Society defines reversibility as an FEV_1 or FVC improvement from pre-dose value of >12% and >200 mL[8] (Table 7.2). The Global Initiative for Chronic Obstructive Lung Disease guidelines define reversibility as an FEV_1 improvement from pre-dose value of more than 12% and more 200 mL.[2] The European Respiratory Society defines reversibility as a percentage of predicted FEV_1 improvement from pre-dose value of ≥10%.[9] The American College of Chest Physicians defines reversibility as an FEV_1 improvement from pre-dose value of ≥15%.[10] And finally, the American Thoracic Society–European Respiratory Society Consensus Statement defines reversibility as FEV_1 and/or FVC improvement from pre-dose value of more than 12% and more than 200 mL.[4]

Therefore, airway obstruction that does not meet one of these definitions of reversibility could be considered to have at least an element of irreversible airflow obstruction. A 2012 National Institutes of Health–National Heart, Lung and Blood Institute Asthma Phenotype Workshop suggests a different definition of irreversible airflow limitation in asthma (Peters, personal communication). That definition includes an FEV_1/FVC ratio below the lower limit of normal for age (8 to 19 years: 85%; 20 to 39 years: 80%; 40 to 59 years: 75%; 60 to 80 years: 70% [Expert Panel Report 3, 2007]) and FEV_1 less than 90% predicted in a patient taking corticosteroids (4 weeks of medium- to high-dose inhaled corticosteroids or 2 weeks of systemic corticosteroids [≥0.5 mg/kg prednisone]) after administration of a rapid-onset bronchodilator (4 puffs of albuterol).

Although different in detail, these definitions suggest that the presence of abnormal lung function that does not normalize, either spontaneously or, more typically, after treatment, is the hallmark of irreversible airflow obstruction.

Differentiating asthma from COPD when irreversible airflow obstruction is present can be difficult. Older age, lack of symptoms in childhood, and cigarette smoking suggest the possibility of COPD, but these factors are not unique to COPD.[11] Spirometry can only confirm the presence of airway obstruction, present in both, and bronchodilator reversibility testing can determine whether the obstruction is

Table 7.2. Definitions of Bronchodilator Reversibility

GROUP	DEFINITION	REFERENCE NO.
American Thoracic Society	FEV_1 or FVC improvement from pre-dose value by ≥12% and ≥200 mL	8
Global Strategy for the Diagnosis, Management and Prevention of COPD	FEV_1 improvement from pre-dose value by ≥12% and ≥200 mL	2
European Respiratory Society	Percentage predicted FEV_1 improvement from pre-dose value of ≥10%	9
American College of Chest Physicians	FEV_1 improvement from pre-dose value by ≥15%	10
American Thoracic Society–European Respiratory Society Task Force	FEV_1 and/or FVC improvement from pre-dose value by ≥12% and ≥200 mL	4

reversible or irreversible. However, more complete pulmonary function testing can help to differentiate asthma from COPD. In asthma, the diffusing capacity should be normal (or perhaps elevated during an acute exacerbation); in emphysema, the diffusing capacity is often decreased.[12] Hyperinflation, *not occurring during a period of an acute exacerbation*, as defined by an increased total lung capacity (TLC), residual volume (RV), or RV/TLC ratio when measuring lung volumes, is more suggestive of emphysema than asthma, as is reduced elastic recoil, although both also are observed in some patients with asthma, particularly in patients with irreversible airflow obstruction.[11,13]

Just as lung physiology shows differences when comparing asthma and COPD, the patterns of airway inflammation are considered to be different. Sutherland and Martin consider the eosinophil to be the most prominent inflammatory cell in asthma, with mast cells, lymphocytes, and macrophages also playing important roles, whereas neutrophils, macrophages, and lymphocytes are considered to be more important in COPD, with the eosinophil playing a minor role, except in the setting of exacerbations.[14] Bafadhel and colleagues paint a more complex picture and report that airway eosinophilic and neutrophilic inflammation is present in 48% and 35% of patients with asthma and in 45% and 59% of COPD subjects, respectively.[15] Similar complexity was reported by Hastie and colleagues, who also state that patients with asthma with both an eosinophilic and a neutrophilic airway inflammatory phenotype are higher health care utilizers than asthmatic patients with other airway inflammatory phenotypes (eosinophilic, neutrophilic, and pauci cellular).[16] In profiling inflammatory mediators in the sputum of patients with asthma and COPD, Bafadhel and colleagues found that there is a higher expression of interleukin-8 (IL-8), tumor necrosis factor receptor I, and tumor necrosis factor receptor II in asthma than in COPD.[15] They also report that within the airway inflammatory sub-phenotypes, there is a differential pattern of mediator expression that is independent of disease (asthma vs. COPD).

CLINICAL FEATURES
Incidence and Associations
INCIDENCE

Vonk and colleagues report that 16% of asthmatic patients have irreversible airflow limitation, defined as an FEV_1 of less than 80% predicted and reversibility less than 9% predicted, after 26 years of follow-up.[17] Forty percent were nonsmokers during the years of evaluation, and smoking was not associated with the development of irreversible airflow limitation.

ASSOCIATIONS IN ADULTS

Asthmatic patients with severe persistent airflow obstruction, defined as an FEV_1 of less than 50% predicted after bronchodilator, are older, have asthma of longer duration, display increased expired nitric oxide and peripheral blood eosinophils, and show more abnormalities on computed tomography scanning compared with asthmatic patients without persistent airflow obstruction, that is, FEV_1 of more than 80% predicted.[18] Duration of disease, increased age, and severity of asthma are also associated with irreversible airflow obstruction in studies by Brown and colleagues.[19] The importance of airway eosinophilic inflammation is stressed by ten Brinke and colleagues.[20] In addition, using other definitions of irreversible airflow obstruction, similar patients are reported to have increased sputum neutrophils[21] and serologic evidence of *Chlamydia pneumoniae* infection.[22] Shaw and colleagues report an inverse association of both eosinophilic and neutrophilic airway inflammation with pre-bronchodilator FEV_1, but only airway neutrophilia with post-bronchodilator FEV_1.[23]

The association of irreversible airflow obstruction and long duration of asthma was confirmed by Cassino and colleagues.[24] Only 18% of nonsmoking asthmatic patients with prolonged disease (>26 years) display a normal FEV_1 (>80% predicted) after bronchodilator administration, whereas 50% of asthmatic patients with short-duration disease (<26 years) have normal FEV_1 after bronchodilator administration.[24]

In patients with asthma and COPD, bronchodilator reversibility (to albuterol and ipratropium bromide and prednisone [30 mg/day for 7 days]) is associated with increased survival.[25]

IRREVERSIBLE AIRFLOW LIMITATION IN CHILDREN

Reports describe the characteristics of lung function in asthmatic children, including a longitudinal evaluation of changes that occur over time.[26-30] However, there are limited data concerning the proportion of patients who either develop or have persistent airflow limitation. Attempts to apply any definition of persistent airflow obstruction to children is confounded by the fact that children with asthma often demonstrate preserved lung function, even in cases of more severe disease.

Covar and colleagues report that 25.7% of the Childhood Asthma Management Program (CAMP) subjects had a significant decrease in post-bronchodilator FEV_1 over 4 to 6 years of observation, defined as more than 1% reduction in FEV_1 per year, and that the patients who demonstrated this decrease were not affected by treatment with either nedocromil or budesonide.[31] However, as a group, these children still displayed a normal FEV_1. Studies in children appear to be confounded by the fact that in classifying asthma severity in children, there is a mismatch among symptoms, medication use, and lung function; that is, lung function is preserved even when symptoms and medication use would classify asthma as severe.[32] Consistent with these suggestions, Jenkins and colleagues report a similar finding in that children with severe asthma had less severe airflow obstruction when compared with adults with severe asthma, and their lymphocytes displayed a greater responsiveness to glucocorticosteroids in vitro.[33]

Phenotypes of Irreversible Airflow Obstruction

A number of different phenotypes can be defined in patients with irreversible airflow obstruction.

IRREVERSIBLE AIRFLOW OBSTRUCTION IN PATIENTS WITH CHRONIC OBSTRUCTIVE PULMONARY DISEASE

Data from a number of sources demonstrate that the presence of COPD is higher in smokers and ex-smokers than in nonsmokers, higher in those older versus younger than 40 years, and higher in men than in women.[2] In the Latin American Project for the Investigation of Obstructive Lung Disease (PLATINO), the prevalence of COPD in five major Latin American cities ranged from

7.8% in Mexico City, Mexico, to 19.7% in Montevidea, Urugay.[34] However, the Burden of Obstructive Lung Disease program also reported a substantial prevalence of COPD in never-smokers, ranging from approximately 3% to 11%.[35] Continued smoking is the most important risk factor for the progressive loss in lung function in these subjects. Sustained quitters in the Lung Health Study lost 72 mL of FEV_1 and continual smokers lost 301 mL of FEV_1 in the 5 years of observation of patients with mild COPD.[36]

IRREVERSIBLE AIRFLOW OBSTRUCTION IN NONSMOKING PATIENTS WITH ASTHMA

Moore and colleagues also identified a phenotype of asthma in nonsmoking patients (<5 pack-years), using an unbiased cluster analysis, that appears "COPD like."[37] Sixteen percent (80% of whom met the American Thoracic Society criteria for severe asthma) of their 726 subjects from a nonrandomized sample were located in "cluster 5," which has the most severe airflow limitation at baseline (mean FEV_1 of 43% predicted), and despite some response to maximal bronchodilator testing (up to 8 puffs of albuterol), 94% of subjects remained with an FEV_1 of less than 80% predicted. Nearly half of the subjects reported three or more oral corticosteroid bursts, and an additional 25% reported an inpatient hospitalization in the past year for a severe asthma exacerbation.[37] Nearly 40% of subjects also reported a history of a prior intensive care unit admission for asthma in their lifetime. Asthma in older adults is recognized as an important and understudied entity because it is underdiagnosed, undertreated, and often confused with or merged into COPD.[38,39]

THE PROBLEM OF THE ASTHMATIC PATIENT WHO SMOKES CIGARETTES

It is estimated that as many of 25% of patients with asthma in developed countries smoke cigarettes.[40] Thompson and colleagues report that current smokers have poorer asthma control, more unscheduled health care visits and oral glucocorticosteroid courses, and higher levels of anxiety and depression than nonsmokers and ex-smokers.[40] Lower levels of both sputum eosinophils and expired nitric oxide were present in current smokers compared with nonsmokers.[41]

The interactions of long-standing asthma, smoking, and atopy were examined by Perret and colleagues, who reported data from a 37-year follow-up of children from Tasmania, Australia.[42] They report that a history of both asthma and smoking is associated with persistent airway obstruction at age 45 years. In addition, the deleterious effects of smoking and asthma on the FEV_1/FVC ratio are worse in atopic versus nonatopic individuals.

COPD Gene investigators compared patients with COPD alone with patients with COPD and coexisting asthma.[43] Patients with COPD and a history of physician-diagnosed asthma were younger (61.3 vs. 64.7 years old), with a higher proportion of African Americans having asthma than non–African Americans (33.6% vs. 15.6%). Despite a lower lifetime smoking intensity (43.7 vs. 55.1 pack-years), subjects with COPD and asthma demonstrated greater gas trapping on chest computed tomography and experienced a lower disease-related quality of life. Finally, they were more likely to have had a severe COPD exacerbation in the past year and more frequent exacerbations.

LIFESTYLE AND BEHAVIOR MODIFICATION STRATEGIES

Lifestyle and behavior modification strategies should play an important role in managing patients with irreversible airway obstruction. The most important of these is smoking cessation, the only proven method to alter the natural history of the progressive loss in patients with COPD who smoke.[36] However, other interventions are also efficacious. For example, pulmonary rehabilitation is a proven benefit that increases the quality of life of patients with COPD.[38,44,45] Finally, dietary modification and weight loss benefit patients with a variety of diseases, including patients with irreversible airflow obstruction.[36,46,47]

PHARMACOLOGIC TREATMENT

The patient with irreversible airflow obstruction appears to lie somewhere near the interface of asthma and COPD, and treatment approaches include medications used to treat each of these diseases. Because no pharmacologic therapeutic approach alters the natural history of either asthma or COPD, treatment is undertaken to reduce symptoms and exacerbations and improve lung function and quality of life. Although anti-inflammatory agents are the cornerstone in treating patients with asthma[1] and bronchodilators are the cornerstone in treating patients with COPD,[2] both classes of agents are used for both diseases.

Inhaled corticosteroids are effective across many domains of asthma and improve symptoms, quality of life, and pulmonary function and reduce exacerbations and asthma-related deaths.[1] In contrast, inhaled corticosteroids in COPD are used mainly to reduce exacerbations.[2] In the 3-year TORCH study, a combination of fluticasone and salmeterol, compared with placebo, reduced mortality in COPD, but not significantly ($P = .052$), and was not different from the active comparator, salmeterol.[48]

Symptomatic treatment with a long-acting bronchodilator, either a long-acting β-agonist or an anticholinergic agent, is used to treat patients with COPD who have daily symptoms.[2] An attempt to decrease the progressive decline in FEV_1 observed in patients with COPD by adding tiotropium bromide to existing medications, was unsuccessful in the 4-year UPLIFT study.[49] Long-acting β-agonists, without the concomitant use of an inhaled corticosteroid, are contraindicated in patients with asthma, largely based on the GlaxoSmithKline SMART trial.[50] Because of the concern about the safety of using long-acting β-agonists to treat patients with asthma, the U.S. Food and Drug Administration has commissioned a long-term safety study of these agents in patients with asthma that is being conducted by the four U.S. manufacturers of these agents.[51]

Because of the similarity of asthma with persistent airflow obstruction and COPD, agents unapproved for treating asthma but approved for treating COPD have been tried in patients with asthma. The most important of these medications is tiotropium bromide, a long-acting anticholinergic agent.[52] This agent was reported to show benefit in patients with COPD and concomitant asthma in 2008.[53] Other studies show benefit in patients with moderate asthma uncontrolled by an inhaled corticosteroid alone[54] and in patients with severe asthma uncontrolled by a combination inhaled corticosteroid and long-acting β-agonist.[55]

Treating an asthmatic patient who smokes cigarettes is particularly problematic. Patients with asthma who smoke demonstrate a reduced response to inhaled corticosteroids,[56-58] hypothesized to be caused by a more neutrophilic, and therefore less corticosteroid-sensitive, type of inflammation. Whether other mechanisms are also important, such as a reduced vasoconstrictor response to glucocorticoids, is not clear.[59] Smoking cessation is the most important intervention shown to alter both airway function (improved FEV_1) and the type of airway inflammation (less neutrophilic).[60] Some classes of drugs appear to work better in smokers with asthma. Lazarus and colleagues, for example, demonstrated an improved response to a leukotriene receptor antagonist in patients with asthma who smoke.[58]

An important but underappreciated concept for patients with persistent airflow obstruction, particularly those labeled as having "asthma," is to not overtreat those who have a corticosteroid-insensitive phenotype with these medications. Treating them with high doses of corticosteroids provides little benefit and produces unwanted side effects. Therefore, monitoring the effects of such treatment with objective and reproducible measures, including lung function, validated questionnaires, frequency of exacerbations, and quality of life measures, is essential.

UNMET, FUTURE RESEARCH NEEDS

1. Key gaps in our knowledge base concerning patients with irreversible airflow obstruction are the following:

    a. To identify the mechanisms that produce irreversible airflow obstruction;

b. To devise effective interventions to either prevent or reverse irreversible airflow obstruction.

2. Genetic association studies provide clues to the following possible mechanisms:

a. A number of genes reported to regulate lung function in normal individuals also are associated with lung function abnormalities in patients with asthma.[61] These include hedgehog interacting protein (*HHIP*); family with sequence similarity 13, member A (*FAM13A*); patched homolog 1 (*PTCH1*); thrombospondin, type I, domain containing 4 (*THSD4*); glutathione S-transferase, C-terminal domain containing (*GSTCD*); advanced glycosylation end-product-specific receptor (*AGER-NOTCH4*); retinoic acid receptor, beta (*RARB*); and zinc finger protein 323 (*ZNF323*).[61]

b. In addition, T_H1 or IL-12–cytokine family genes interleukin 12A (*IL12A*), interleukin 12 receptor, beta 1 (*IL12RB1*), signal transducer and activator of transcription 4 (*STAT4*), and interferon regulatory factor 2 (*IRF2*) are associated with lung function abnormalities in patients with asthma.[62]

3. We propose a two-step model for asthma[62]:

a. T_H2 pathway genes (interleukin 13 [*IL13*], thymic stromal lymphopoietin [*TSLP*], interleukin 33 [*IL33*], and interleukin 1 receptor-like 1 [*IL1RL1*]) confer *asthma susceptibility* and are not associated with lung function abnormalities.

b. Genes listed previously affect *lung function* (Figure 7.1).

4. Several lung function genes in asthma are associated with fixed airflow obstruction in COPD[63] (Figure 7.2), including *HHIP, FAM13A, PITCH1, THSD4, GSTCD, AGER-NOTCH4, RARB,* and *ZKSCAN3-ZNF323*.[62,63]

5. Common genetic abnormalities in asthma and COPD suggest a similar mechanism for the development of fixed airflow obstruction, with different environmental influences (atopy in asthma and smoking in COPD) modifying the expression of these genetic elements.

6. Understanding how these elements interact and work to produce the final common pathway of fixed airflow obstruction should provide opportunities for environmental, genetic, and pharmacologic intervention.

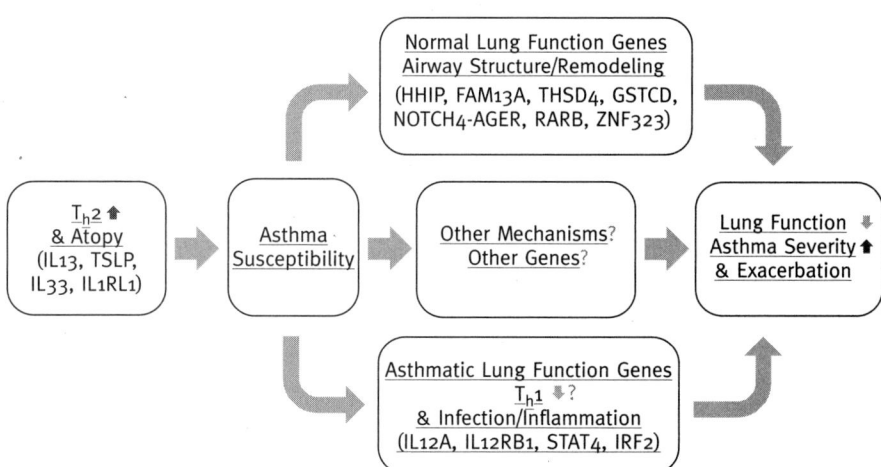

FIGURE 7.1 A two-step model for the development and progression of asthma. This model includes one set of genes associated with asthma susceptibility and another set of genes associated with abnormal lung function in patients with asthma. *Up arrows* indication upregulation of the gene or gene product, and *down arrows* indicate downregulation of the gene or gene product. *Question marks* indicate an uncertain relationship. (From Li X, Hawkins GA, Ampleford EJ, et al. Genome-wide association study identifies Th1 pathway genes associated with lung function in asthma. *J Allergy Clin Immunol.* 2013;132[2]:313–320.)

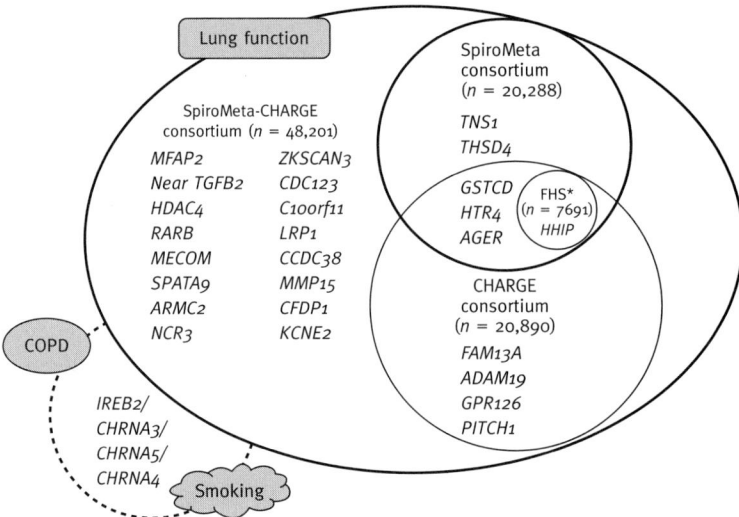

FIGURE 7.2 Genes associated with the development of chronic obstructive pulmonary disease (COPD). Key genes associated with fixed airflow limitation in COPD are shown. Also shown (in the dashed lines to the left) are genes associated with smoking and COPD. (From Wain LV, Soler Artigas M, Tobin MD. What can genetics tell us about the cause of fixed airflow obstruction? *Clin Exp Allergy.* 2012;42[8]:1176–1182.)

CONCLUSION

Patients with fixed airflow obstruction, whether from asthma or COPD, or an overlap phenotype, represent an especially difficult group of patients to both categorize and manage. Many of the current research activities in both asthma and COPD, particularly through research networks, such as the Severe Asthma Research Program (SARP), COPDGene, and the Subpopulations and Intermediate Outcome Measures in COPD Study (SPIROMICS), are designed to subclassify patients with asthma and COPD into different endotypes and phenotypes with the hope that the results will have implications for both the natural history of disease and the response to different therapies. Data outlined in this review, particularly the genetic findings, help strengthen the "Dutch hypothesis" Orie put forth more than 50 years ago about the commonalities of obstructive airways diseases operating under a variety of environmental influences.[3] The identification of targets distinct from inflammation in both asthma and COPD, through different mechanisms—atopy, important in asthma, and smoking, important COPD—could lead to novel treatments for both of these diseases with fixed airflow obstruction. In the meantime, bronchodilators, anti-inflammatory agents, environmental control, and interventions including smoking cessation, weight loss and control, and exercise and pulmonary rehabilitation remain the foundation of the therapeutic approach to these diseases, regardless of their origin.

REFERENCES

1. National Asthma Education and Prevention Program. Expert Panel Report 3. Guidelines for the diagnosis and management of asthma: summary report 2007. http://www.nhlbi.nih.gov/guidelines/asthma/asthsumm.pdf. Accessed March 7, 2013.
2. Global Strategy for the Diagnosis, Management and Prevention of COPD, Global Initiative for Chronic Obstructive Lung Disease (GOLD) 2013. http://www.goldcopd.org/. Accessed March 7, 2013.
3. Orie NGM, Sluiter HJ, de Vries K, et al. The host factor in bronchitis. In: Orie NGM, Sluiter HJ, eds. *Bronchitis*. Assen, the Netherlands: Royal van Gorcum, 1961:43–59.
4. Pellegrino R, Pellegrino R, Viegi G, et al., for the ATS/ERS Task Force. Standardisation of lung function testing: interpretative

strategies for lung function tests. *Eur Respir J.* 2005;26(5):948–968.
5. Hanania NA, Celli BR, Donohue JF, Martin UJ. Bronchodilator reversibility in COPD. *Chest.* 2011;140(4):1055–1063.
6. Miller MR, Hankinson J, Brusasco V, et al., for the ATS/ERS Task Force. Standardisation of spirometry. *Eur Respir J.* 2005;26(2):319–338.
7. Tepper RS, Wise RS, Covar R, et al. Asthma outcomes: pulmonary physiology. *J Allergy Clin Immunol.* 2012;129(3 Suppl):S65–S87.
8. American Thoracic Society. Lung function testing: selection of reference values and interpretative strategies. *Am Rev Respir Dis.* 1991;144(5):1202–1218.
9. Siafakas NM, Vermeire P, Pride NB, et al., for the European Respiratory Society Task Force. Optimal assessment and management of chronic obstructive pulmonary disease (COPD). *Eur Respir J.* 1995;8(8):1398–1420.
10. Report of the Committee on Emphysema American College of Chest Physicians. Criteria for the assessment of reversibility in airways obstruction. *Chest.* 1974;65(5):552–553.
11. Chang J, Mosenifar Z. Differentiating COPD from asthma in clinical practice. *J Intensive Care Med.* 2007;22(5):300–309.
12. Peters SP. When the chief complaint is (or should be) dyspnea in adults. *J Allergy Clin Immunol.* 2013;1(2):129–136.
13. Gelb AF, Zamel N, Krishnan A. Physiologic similarities and differences between asthma and chronic obstructive pulmonary disease. *Curr Opin Pulm Med.* 2008;14(1):24–30.
14. Sutherland ER, Martin RJ. Airway inflammation in chronic obstructive pulmonary disease: comparisons with asthma. *J Allergy Clin Immunol.* 2003;112(5):819–827.
15. Bafadhel M, McCormick M, Saha S, et al. Profiling of sputum inflammatory mediators in asthma and chronic obstructive pulmonary disease. *Respiration.* 2012;83(1):36–44.
16. Hastie AT, Moore WC, Meyers DA, et al., for the National Heart, Lung, and Blood Institute Severe Asthma Research Program. Analyses of asthma severity phenotypes and inflammatory proteins in subjects stratified by sputum granulocytes. *J Allergy Clin Immunol.* 2010;125(5):1028–1036.
17. Vonk JM, Jongepier H, Pahhuysen CIM, et al. Risk factors associated with the presence of irreversible airflow limitation and reduced transfer coefficient in patients with asthma after 26 years of follow up. *Thorax.* 2003;58(4):322–327.
18. Bumbacea D, Campbell D, Nguyen L, et al. Parameters associated with persistent airflow obstruction in chronic severe asthma. *Eur Respir J.* 2004;24(1):122–128.
19. Brown PJ, Greville HW, Finucane KE. Asthma and irreversible airflow obstruction. *Thorax.* 1984;39(2):131–136.
20. ten Brinke A, Zwinderman AH, Sterk PJ, Rabe KF, Bel EH. Factors associated with persistent airflow limitation in severe asthma. *Am J Respir Crit Care Med.* 2001;164(5):744–748.
21. Little SA, MacLeod SJ, Chalmers GW, et al. Association of forced expiratory volume with disease duration and sputum neutrophils in chronic asthma. *Am J Med.* 2002;112(6):446–452.
22. ten Brinke A, van Dissel JT, Sterk PJ, Zwinderman AH, Rabe KF, Bel EH. Persistent airflow limitation in adult-onset nonatopic asthma is associated with serologic evidence of Chlamydia pneumonia infection. *J Allergy Clin Immunol.* 2001;107(3):449–454.
23. Shaw DE, Berry MA, Hargadon B, et al. Association between neutrophilic airway inflammation and airflow limitation in adults with asthma. *Chest.* 2007;132(6):1871–1875.
24. Cassino C, Berger KI, Goldring RM, et al. Duration of asthma and physiologic outcomes in elderly nonsmokers. *Am J Respir Crit Care Med.* 2000;162(4 Pt 1):1423–1428.
25. Hansen EF, Phanareth K, Laursen LC, Kok-Jensen A, Dirksen A. Reversible and irreversible airflow obstruction as predictor of overall mortality in asthma and chronic obstructive pulmonary disease. *Am J Respir Crit Care Med.* 1999;159(4 Pt 1):1267–1271.
26. Morgan WJ, Stern DA, Sherrill DL, et al. Outcome of asthma and wheezing in the first 6 years of life: follow-up through adolescence. *Am J Respir Crit Care Med.* 2005;172(10):1253–1258.
27. Fuhlbrigge AL, Weiss ST, Kuntz KM, Paltiel AD, for the CAMP Research Group. Forced expiratory volume in 1 second percentage improves the classification of severity among children with asthma. *Pediatrics.* 2006;118(2):e347–355.
28. Strunk RC, Weiss ST, Yates KP, Tonascia J, Zeiger RS, Szefler SJ, for the CAMP Research Group. Mild to moderate asthma affects lung growth in children and adolescents. *J Allergy Clin Immunol.* 2006;118(5):1040–1047.
29. Strunk RC, for the Childhood Asthma Management Program Research Group. Childhood Asthma Management Program: lessons learned. *J Allergy Clin Immunol.* 2007;119(1):36–42.

30. Stern DA, Morgan WJ, Wright AL, Guerra S, Martinez FD. Poor airway function in early infancy and lung function by age 22 years: a non-selective longitudinal cohort study. *Lancet.* 2007;370(9589):758–764.
31. Covar RA, Cool C, Szefler SJ. Progression of asthma in childhood. *J Allergy Clin Immunol.* 2005;115(4):700–707.
32. Bacharier LB, Strunk RC, Mauger D, White D, Lemanske RF Jr, Sorkness CA. Classifying asthma severity in children: mismatch between symptoms, medication use, and lung function. *Am J Respir Crit Care Med.* 2004;170(4):426–432.
33. Jenkins HA, Cherniack R, Szefler SJ, Covar R, Gelfand EW, Spahn JD. A comparison of clinical characteristics of children and adults with severe asthma. *Chest.* 2003;124(4):1318–1324.
34. Menezes AM, Perez-Padilla R, Jardim JR, for the PLATINO Team. Chronic obstructive pulmonary disease in five Latin American cities (the PLATINO study): a prevalence study. *Lancet.* 2005;366(9500):1875–1881.
35. Buist AS, McBurnie MA, Vollmer WM, et al., for the BOLD Collaborative Research Group. International variation in the prevalence of COPD (the BOLD Study): a population-based prevalence study. *Lancet.* 2007;370(9589):741–750.
36. Anthonisen NR, Connett JE, Kiley JP, et al., for the Lung Health Study Research Group. Effects of smoking intervention and the use of an inhaled anticholinergic bronchodilator on the rate of decline of FEV_1: the Lung Health Study. *JAMA.* 1994;272(19):1497–1505.
37. Moore WC, Meyers DA, Wenzel SE, et al., for the National Heart, Lung, and Blood Institute's Severe Asthma Research Program. Identification of asthma phenotypes using cluster analysis in the Severe Asthma Research Program. *Am J Respir Crit Care Med.* 2010;181(4):315–323.
38. Gibson PG, McDonald VM, Marks GB. Asthma in older adults. *Lancet.* 2010;376(9743):803–813.
39. Hanania NA, King MJ, Braman SS, et al., for the Asthma in Elderly Workshop participants. Asthma in the elderly: current understanding and future research needs. A report of a National Institute on Aging (NIA) workshop. *J Allergy Clin Immunol.* 2011;128(3 Suppl):S4–S24.
40. Thomson NC, Chaudhuri R, Livingston E. Asthma and cigarette smoking. *Eur Respir J.* 2004;24(5):822–833.
41. Thomson NC, Chaudhuri R, Heaney LG, et al. Clinical outcomes and inflammatory biomarkers in current smokers and exsmokers with severe asthma. *J Allergy Clin Immunol.* 2013;131(4):1008–1016.
42. Perret JL, Dharmage SC, Matheson MC, et al. The interplay between the effects of lifetime asthma, smoking, and atopy on fixed airflow obstruction in middle age. *Am J Respir Crit Care Med.* 2013;187(1):42–48.
43. Hardin M, Silverman EK, Barr RG, et al., for the COPDGene Investigators. The clinical features of the overlap between COPD and asthma. *Respir Res.* 2011;12:127.
44. Berry MJ, Rejeski WJ, Adair NE, Zaccaro D. Exercise rehabilitation and chronic obstructive pulmonary disease stage. *Am J Respir Crit Care Med.* 1999;160(4):1248–1253.
45. Foglio K, Bianchi L, Bruletti G, et al. Long-term effectiveness of pulmonary rehabilitation in patients with chronic airway obstruction. *Eur Respir J.* 1999;13(1):125–132.
46. Lugogo NL, Kraft M, Dixon AE. Does obesity produce a distinct asthma phenotype? *J Appl Physiol.* 2010;108(3):729–734.
47. Noria SF, Grantcharov T. Biological effects of bariatric surgery on obesity-related comorbidities. *Can J Surg.* 2013;56(1):47–57.
48. Calverley PM, Anderson JA, Celli B, et al., for the TORCH investigators. Salmeterol and fluticasone propionate and survival in chronic obstructive pulmonary disease. *N Engl J Med.* 2007;356(8):775–789.
49. Tashkin DP, Celli B, Senn S, et al., for the UPLIFT Study Investigators. A 4-year trial of tiotropium in chronic obstructive pulmonary disease. *N Engl J Med.* 2008;359(15):1543–1554.
50. Nelson HS, Weiss ST, Bleecker ER, Yancey SW, Dorinsky PM, for the SMART Study Group. The Salmeterol Multicenter Asthma Research Trial: a comparison of usual pharmacotherapy for asthma or usual pharmacotherapy plus salmeterol. *Chest.* 2006;129(1):15–26. Erratum in: *Chest.* 2006;129(5):1393.
51. Chowdhury BA, Seymour SM, Levenson MS. Assessing the safety of adding LABAs to inhaled corticosteroids for treating asthma. *N Engl J Med.* 2011;364(26):2473–2475.
52. Bel EH. Tiotropium for asthma: promise and caution. *N Engl J Med.* 2012;367(13):1257–1259.
53. Magnussen H, Bugnas B, van Noord J, Schmidt P, Gerken F, Kesten S. Improvements with tiotropium in COPD patients with concomitant asthma. *Respir Med.* 2008;102(1):50–56.
54. Peters SP, Kunselman SJ, Icitovic N, et al., for the National Heart, Lung, and Blood Institute Asthma Clinical Research Network. Tiotropium bromide step-up therapy for adults with uncontrolled asthma. *N Engl J Med.* 2010;363(18):1715–1726.

55. Kerstjens HA, Engel M, Dahl R, et al. Tiotropium in asthma poorly controlled with standard combination therapy. *N Engl J Med.* 2012;367(13):1198–1207.
56. Chalmers GW, Macleod KJ, Little SA, Thomson LJ, McSharry CP, Thomson NC. Influence of cigarette smoking on inhaled corticosteroid treatment in mild asthma. *Thorax.* 2002;57(3):226–230.
57. Livingston E, Thomson NC, Chalmers GW. Impact of smoking on asthma therapy: a critical review of clinical evidence. *Drugs.* 2005;65(11):1521–1536.
58. Lazarus SC, Chinchilli VM, Rollings NJ, et al., for the National Heart Lung and Blood Institute's Asthma Clinical Research Network. Smoking affects response to inhaled corticosteroids or leukotriene receptor antagonists in asthma. *Am J Respir Crit Care Med.* 2007;175(8):783–790.
59. Livingston E, Chaudhuri R, McMahon AD, Fraser I, McSharry CP, Thomson NC. Systemic sensitivity to corticosteroids in smokers with asthma. *Eur Respir J.* 2007;29(1):64–71.
60. Chaudhuri R, Livingston E, McMahon AD, et al. Effects of smoking cessation on lung function and airway inflammation in smokers with asthma. *Am J Respir Crit Care Med.* 2006;174(2):127–133.
61. Li X, Howard TD, Moore WC, et al. Importance of hedgehog interacting protein and other lung function genes in asthma. *J Allergy Clin Immunol.* 2011;127(6):1457–1465.
62. Li X, Hawkins GA, Ampleford EJ, et al. Genome-wide association study identifies Th1 pathway genes associated with lung function in asthma. *J Allergy Clin Immunol.* 2013;132(2):313–320.
63. Wain LV, Soler Artigas M, Tobin MD. What can genetics tell us about the cause of fixed airflow obstruction? *Clin Exp Allergy.* 2012;42(8):1176–1182.

8

BRONCHIECTASIS

COMORBID, COEXISTING, AND DIFFERENTIAL DIAGNOSIS

Nizar Naji and Paul M. O'Byrne

KEY POINTS

- The prevalence of bronchiectasis is increasing worldwide.
- The diagnosis of bronchiectasis may be missed because of comorbidities.
- Patients with long-standing uncontrolled asthma and those with recurrent severe exacerbations are at greatest risk for developing bronchiectasis.
- A significant percentage of patients with bronchiectasis have airway reversibility to bronchodilators and demonstrate methacholine airway hyperresponsiveness.
- Allergic bronchopulmonary aspergillosis (ABPA) is the most common clinical entity that associates asthma and bronchiectasis.
- Radiologic, microbiologic, and clinical correlation are important to make the diagnosis of ABPA.
- Colonization with *Pseudomonas aeruginosa* is a predictor of recurrent exacerbations of bronchiectasis and gradual decline in lung function.
- The optimal management of patients with asthma and bronchiectasis requires bronchial hygiene, often fixed-dose inhaled corticosteroids and long-acting β-agonist combinations, and, for some patients, systemic corticosteroids. Antibiotic use should be based on sputum microbiology during acute exacerbations.

INTRODUCTION

Bronchiectasis is one of the most debilitating chronic respiratory diseases and affects people of all ages, with significant morbidity and mortality. It is recognized clinically by chronic persistent daily cough, productive of mucopurulent sputum. The defining characteristic is permanent abnormal dilatation and destruction of bronchial walls, involving both the major bronchi and bronchioles. It is a major contributor to progressive lung function decline and functional disability, especially in patients with respiratory comorbidities. Early diagnosis and treatment are essential to control the disease and slow its progression.

The prevalence of bronchiectasis varies significantly across the world and is often underestimated. The differences in prevalence likely result from the differences in the incidence of the disorders that can lead to bronchiectasis. The 2005 prevalence data for the United States indicate that there were 52 cases per 100,000, ranging from 4.2 in young adults to as many as 272 cases per 100,000 in patients older than 75 years.[1] In addition, the prevalence is higher in women. The disease may be missed because of comorbidities and a variety of etiologic factors, or it may be diagnosed late in the course of the disease. However, in recent decades, the number of diagnosed cases has increased in the developed world, likely because of the wide availability of computed tomography (CT) scanning, which has contributed to early detection, even in asymptomatic individuals, and because of increased awareness of the most common and difficult-to-eradicate microorganisms that are often cultured in bronchiectasis (such as *Pseudomonas aeruginosa*).

Patients with long-standing pulmonary disease, especially with severe persistent and refractory asthma, and smokers with asthma or chronic obstructive pulmonary disease (COPD) are at higher risk for developing bronchiectasis because of persistent tissue injury associated with frequent exacerbations, impairment of host response, and subsequent structural airway damage. Long-term airway distortion and bronchiectasis also can result from even one episode of severe pneumonia during childhood because lungs that are still growing are at a higher risk for scarring from chest infections.

PATHOGENESIS OF BRONCHIECTASIS

The most commonly identified causes of bronchiectasis are airway obstruction (e.g., foreign body aspiration), defective host defenses, cystic fibrosis, Young's syndrome (similar to cystic fibrosis [CF], but without increased sweat chlorides, pancreatic insufficiency, or abnormal CF mutations), autoimmune diseases (particularly rheumatic diseases), dyskinetic cilia syndrome, severe pulmonary infections, allergic bronchopulmonary aspergillosis (ABPA), and cigarette smoking.

Bronchiectasis usually results from an initial infection and secondary inflammation or microbial colonization of the airways, which leads to recruitment of inflammatory cells, particularly neutrophils and macrophages; release of reactive oxygen species; and damaging mediators, such as myeloperoxidase and neutrophil elastase, which cause airway damage, parenchymal destruction, and airway dilatation. These cycles of repeated insults with various pathogens and subsequent inflammation lead to impairment of mucociliary clearance and mucus retention and changes in airway structure, which manifest as chronic cough, profuse sputum production, and clinical features of airflow obstruction.

Bronchiectasis is classically subdivided, according to histopathologic appearance, into *cylindrical bronchiectasis*, characterized by thickening and widening of the airways without gradual peripheral tapering (Figure 8.1), and *constrictive bronchiectasis*, which results from defects in the airway wall leading to areas of focal constriction along the dilated airways and giving the airways a tortuous and varicose appearance (see Figure 8.1). The most severe form is *saccular* or *cystic bronchiectasis*, which is associated with progressive destruction of the airways and results in fluid-filled cystic dilatation of the bronchi and bronchioles, giving the airways a honeycomb appearance (see Figure 8.1).

CLINICAL FEATURES

Presentation of patients with bronchiectasis is variable; some patients may have few symptoms, whereas others may present with rapidly progressive disease and worsening airflow obstruction. The primary etiologic factor and comorbidities play an important role in defining the course of the disease. Also, the frequency of exacerbations and type of pathogenic microorganism significantly affect long-term prognosis.

The initial clinical presentation is a troublesome and persistent cough that is

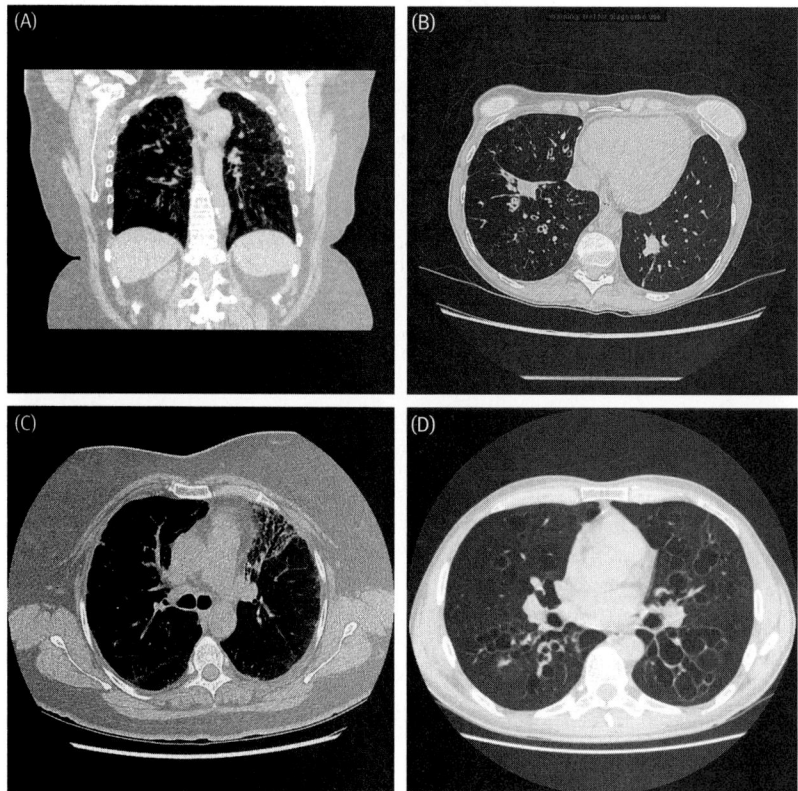

FIGURE 8.1 Three cases of bronchiectasis diagnosed by chest computed tomography. **A, B,** Both axial and coronal views of constrictive bronchiectasis. **C,** Traction bronchiectasis with cylindrical bronchial dilation in association with ground-glass opacity and interlobular septal thickening in the left upper lobe. **D,** Extensive bilateral cystic bronchiectasis.

productive of purulent sputum or episodes identified as recurrent exacerbations of acute bronchitis requiring multiple courses of antibiotics within a short period (2 to 3 months). A history of previous severe childhood infections, such as tuberculosis, mumps, whooping cough, or severe pneumonia, may also be reported by the patient. The patient may describe disturbed sleep, increased dyspnea, exercise limitation, and pleuritic chest pain, in addition to other systemic symptoms, particularly tiredness and weight loss. Hemoptysis can be the lone presenting symptom in some patients, particularly those with invasive disease, fungal infections, or preexistent cavitary lesions.

Clinical examination of the chest may reveal focal or scattered course crepitations or late inspiratory high-pitched wheezing, and examination of the hands can occasionally show digital clubbing, if the patient has had recurrent severe infections.

Allergic Bronchopulmonary Aspergillosis

ABPA is the most commonly encountered clinical entity that associates asthma with bronchiectasis. This is usually identified in asthmatic patients with uncontrolled disease and recurrent asthma exacerbations that are not managed by an inhaled corticosteroid (ICS) alone or combination therapy with ICS and a long-acting inhaled β_2-agonist (LABA). There is often a history of a rapid response to short courses of oral corticosteroid, but this is followed by early and recurrent exacerbations when the corticosteroid is discontinued. Sputum cultures often isolate *Aspergillus fumigatus,* and allergy skin testing for fungus

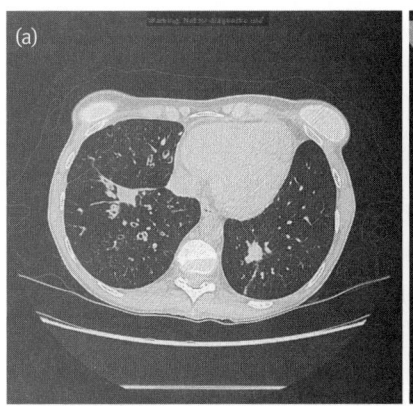 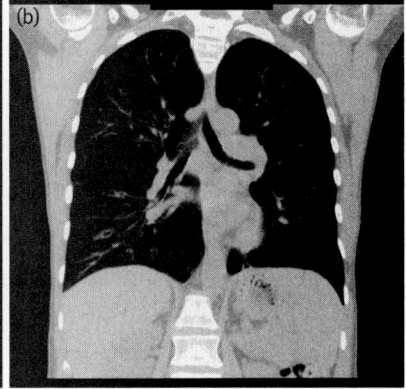

FIGURE 8.2 Axial and coronal views of a chest computed tomographic scan in a patient with allergic bronchopulmonary aspergillosis.

extract is positive in most patients. Certain chest x-ray (CXR) and high-resolution computed tomography (HRCT) changes are characteristic of ABPA (Figure 8.2). In addition, there is usually a peripheral blood eosinophilia, very high serum immunoglobulin E (IgE) levels (>1,000 IU/mL), and serum precipitin antibody level to *Aspergillus* species that indicate an exaggerated helper T-cell immune response.

DIAGNOSIS

Given the diversity of the etiologic factors responsible for the development of bronchiectasis, all patients should be evaluated for potential risks and contributing factors. Information that can be useful in establishing the etiology of bronchiectasis includes the age at onset of symptoms; history of childhood infections; cigarette smoking; comorbidities such as asthma or COPD; frequency of infective exacerbations; allergy to antigens (particularly *Aspergillus* species); history of or concomitant chronic rhinosinusitis; gastroesophageal reflux; recurrent upper respiratory tract infections; or a clinical history suggestive of immune deficiencies, congenital abnormalities, or autoimmune diseases, such as rheumatoid arthritis or Churg-Strauss syndrome (Table 8.1).

The investigations that can assist in establishing the diagnosis and possible etiology are detailed next.

Blood Tests

A complete blood count with differential for peripheral eosinophilia, neutrophilia, or lymphocytosis is useful. The presence of peripheral blood eosinophilia should merit further workup for ABPA, although this is not specific, and a normal eosinophil count does not exclude ABPA. Patients with severe asthma may have a slightly elevated eosinophil count, but in ABPA, levels are usually above 3% but less than 10%. Levels higher than 10% may require investigations to rule out other hypereosinophilic conditions, such as Churg-Strauss syndrome and idiopathic hypereosinophilic syndrome.

Immunoglobulins

Immunoglobulin tests are done to identify patients with humoral immune deficiency or conditions associated with hyperimmune responses. Serum IgE level and *Aspergillus*-specific IgE and IgG antibodies are usually elevated in ABPA. *Aspergillus* species infection should be suspected if the skin test for this organism is positive and associated with elevated IgE levels, classically (>1,000 ng/mL) in a patient who is not receiving corticosteroid therapy, because normal IgE levels in treated patients do not exclude ABPA.

α_1-Antitrypsin Level and Cystic Fibrosis Conductance Regulator Gene Mutation Analysis

The α_1-antitrypsin level and cystic fibrosis conductance regulator (CFTR) gene mutation

Table 8.1. Diseases Associated with Bronchiectasis

Chronic pulmonary disease	Asthma
	Chronic obstructive pulmonary disease
	Bronchomalacia
	Idiopathic pulmonary fibrosis
	Diffuse panbronchiolitis
Hyperimmune response	Allergic bronchopulmonary aspergillosis
	Hypersensitivity pneumonitis
Genetic	Ciliary dyskinesia (primary and secondary)
	α_1-Antitrypsin deficiency
	Cystic fibrosis
	Young's syndrome
	Ehlers-Danlos syndrome
	Mounier-Kuhn syndrome
Systemic diseases	Rheumatoid arthritis
	Sjögren's syndrome
	Yellow nail syndrome
	Inflammatory bowel disease
Immunodeficiency	Hypogammaglobulinemia (acquired and congenital)
	Chronic granulomatous disease
	Immunosuppression (chemotherapy)

analysis investigations may be useful to evaluate coexistent emphysema or CF, particularly in young patients. Both diseases are associated with bronchiectasis, particularly in patients with rapidly progressive disease and in those who demonstrate sputum isolates of unusual pathogens.

Sputum Analysis

Sputum analysis is required for microscopy and culture and sensitivity of bacteria, fungi, viruses, and mycobacteria. The most commonly encountered pathogens in bronchiectasis are *Haemophilus influenzae* and *P. aeruginosa*, followed by *Streptococcus pneumoniae*, *Staphylococcus aureus*, nontuberculous mycobacterium, and enterococci.[2] *H. influenza* and *P. aeruginosa* have been identified in about two-thirds of patients with bronchiectasis. *P. aeruginosa* is the most notorious organism associated with bronchiectasis because of its ability to survive in the airways for a long time and to resist eradication with antibiotics. Colonization with these pathogens is recognized as a predictor of recurrent exacerbations and gradual decline in lung function.[3,4] Sputum microscopy may show evidence of leukocytosis or neutrophilia, common in bronchiectasis,[5] whereas sputum eosinophilia suggests coexistent asthma or ABPA.

Chest X-Ray

A CXR is usually the initial radiographic study undertaken in patients with suspected bronchiectasis, but it is not sensitive enough to identify early changes or confirm the diagnosis of bronchiectasis. The CXR is more useful during infective exacerbations, in advanced bronchiectasis, or for follow-up of patients. The CXR may show evidence of hyperinflation, scarring, or linear atelectasis (due to mucous plugging) and, as the disease progresses, tramlike linear densities or ring shadows that vary in size from a few millimeters to clearly visible cystic shadows, reflecting chronically thickened and dilated airways.

High-Resolution Computed Tomography

HRCT is the gold standard test to confirm the diagnosis of bronchiectasis and is considered more sensitive and more specific than CXR. Bronchiectasis is usually evidenced by widened airways, representing dilated bronchi and bronchioles, and ring shadows with a diameter that is greater than that of adjacent blood vessels. HRCT studies in patients with asthma show evidence of air trapping on expiration and thickened airway walls, lumen narrowing, decreased vascularity, and low attenuation on inspiration.[6] Dilated airways on HRCT with absence of peripheral airway tapering suggest coexistent bronchiectasis. One study shows evidence of bronchial wall thickening, small centrilobular opacities, and decreased lung attenuation in asthmatic patients; additional bronchiectasis was diagnosed in 28.5% of those patients.[7] Another study shows that the prevalence of bronchiectasis in patients with severe asthma is even higher, at 40%.[8]

Mucous plugging on HRCT correlates with airflow obstruction.[9] Mucous plugging involving peripheral airways may manifest on HRCT as irregular distal branching lines (tree-in-bud appearance). However, in more severe and destructive disease, distal or proximal, multiple, thin- or thick-walled cysts appearing in clusters may give the airways a honeycombing appearance. In ABPA, HRCT may show evidence of areas of increased attenuation, air trapping, ground-glass opacities, bronchial thickening, and proximal cylindrical bronchiectasis that predominantly involve the upper lobes. Central bronchiectasis with preservation of airway tapering may indicate ABPA, but this feature is neither sensitive nor specific[10] because 24% of patients with ABPA do not have evidence of central bronchiectasis on HRCT.[11] For this reason, both laboratory and clinical correlation are required to make the diagnosis of ABPA.

Pulmonary Function Tests

Airflow obstruction with or without reversibility is frequently seen in patients with bronchiectasis. Obstructive lung function may reflect air trapping from thickened peripheral airways that are plugged with mucus. Mucous plugging may also contribute to the reduction in vital capacity. In general, airway responses to inhaled bronchodilators in bronchiectasis may be partial or complete, with up to 39% of patients having full reversibility after an inhaled β_2-agonist.[12] In addition, up to two-thirds of patients with bronchiectasis who have normal baseline spirometry show evidence of airway hyperresponsiveness to inhaled methacholine or histamine.[13,14] Therefore, it is important to perform lung function testing to identify those who would most likely benefit from inhaled bronchodilators and to identify the subclass of patients who may have comorbid asthma. Lung volumes and diffusion capacity should also be performed to evaluate the presence of COPD and interstitial lung disease. However, lung volumes may be increased in asthma and bronchiectasis as a result of increased air trapping.

COMORBID DISEASES AND DIFFERENTIAL DIAGNOSIS

Asthma

The occurrence of bronchiectasis in asthma patients is sometimes missed. Thus, patients with bronchiectasis may be treated with inhaled bronchodilators for many years without a formal diagnosis of asthma being made; similarly, asthma patients may present several times with recurrent exacerbations and receive multiple courses of antibiotics and corticosteroids, without a diagnosis of bronchiectasis. The prevalence of bronchiectasis in asthma is estimated to be between 3% and 40%,[7,8,15] and it is highest among patients with severe asthma.[8]

Airway wall thickening is associated with airway inflammation in asthma and has been identified in 82% of asthmatic patients using HRCT, whereas the diagnosis of bronchiectasis was evident in 28.5% of these subjects.[7]

By contrast, another study examined a cohort of 1,680 asthmatic patients and found that only 3% of patients had coexistent bronchiectasis.[16] Previous reports show significant associations between chronicity and severity of asthma and fixed airflow limitation, the degree of airway wall thickness, airway inflammation, and development of bronchiectasis.[8,9]

Allergic Bronchopulmonary Aspergillosis

The prevalence of ABPA in chronic asthma varies worldwide. Some estimates suggest that the prevalence is between 1% and 2%,[11] whereas a large meta-analysis estimates it to be as high as 13%.[17] ABPA has been documented in 32% of asthmatic patients who have a positive allergy skin test to *Aspergillus* species,[18] whereas bronchiectasis was found in up to 76% of patients with ABPA.[11]

ABPA is caused by inhalation of airborne *Aspergillus* spores, which usually cause no significant problem in normal individuals. Immunologic host responses and tissue injury in asthmatic patients play an important role in the development of ABPA, although it is not clear yet whether individual genetic predisposition plays any significant additional role. Patients with ABPA present with a history of severe asthma and recurrent exacerbations that are resistant to ICS or fixed-dose combinations of ICS and LABA. The immunologic response in ABPA is predominantly a helper T-cell type 2 (T_H2) response, which leads to the release of cytokines (interleukin-4 [IL-4], IL-5, and IL-13) that regulate the allergic inflammatory response and lead to eosinophil activation and recruitment and IgE production. Cross-linking of IgE on mast cells leads to mast cell degranulation and the release of the bronchoconstrictor mediators histamine and cysteinyl leukotrienes as well as proinflammatory mediators. The combination of T_H2-mediated eosinophilic and IL-8–mediated neutrophilic inflammation is responsible for tissue injury, structural airway damage, and the development of bronchiectasis. Other conditions associated with a high risk for ABPA are CF, acquired or congenital immune deficiency, immune suppression, and chronic granulomatous disease.[19,20]

Chronic Obstructive Pulmonary Disease

COPD is an irreversible airway disease that is largely caused by smoking. It is associated with chronic inflammation and release of a variety of different mediators, such as neutrophil elastase and myeloperoxidase, that lead to permanent airway damage. Patients with moderate to severe COPD have a high risk for developing bronchiectasis. The prevalence of bronchiectasis in moderate to severe COPD patients is reported to be as high as 50%[3,21] and is closely related to the severity of airflow obstruction, previous hospital admissions, and the presence of potentially pathogenic microorganisms (e.g., *P. aeruginosa*).[3] COPD patients demonstrate a predominance of lower lobe bronchiectasis, higher bacterial colonization, and slower time to recovery from exacerbations.[21]

α_1-Antitrypsin deficiency is a recognized cause of bronchiectasis, either indirectly through the development of emphysema or through a direct effect of the enzyme deficiency. One study identified radiologic evidence of bronchiectasis in 95% of patients with emphysema caused by this enzyme deficiency.[22] Cigarette smoking at an early age can accelerate the disease process, resulting in higher morbidity and mortality. Such patients may require lung transplantation as the disease progresses and have a higher risk for developing respiratory failure and early death.

Gastroesophageal Reflux Disease

Acid reflux and micro-aspiration, particularly at night and in obese individuals, may contribute to the development of bronchiectasis.[23] Gastroesophageal reflux disease (GERD) is also a known risk factor for poor asthma control and exacerbations. Treatment with histamine-2 receptor blockers or proton pump inhibitors may confer some prevention and symptomatic relief.

MANAGEMENT OF BRONCHIECTASIS

Treatment of patients with bronchiectasis should be focused on controlling symptoms, reducing the frequency of exacerbations, and maintaining good functional status. The primary etiology and comorbidities should be identified and treated appropriately.

Bronchial Hygiene

Bronchial hygiene and measures to loosen bronchial secretion are important when patients are not able to expectorate the often thick and large volume of sputum and mucous plugs. Both mechanical and medical measures can improve mucus clearance and ciliary function, reducing the bacterial load and the possibility of infection. Approaches that may help to improve clearance of mucus include physiotherapy techniques (postural drainage and breathing exercises),[24] nebulized hypertonic saline,[25] mucolytic agents,[26] and oscillatory positive expiratory pressure devices.[27]

Inhaled β_2-Agonists

Inhaled β_2-agonists not only have direct effects on relaxing airway smooth muscles to relieve bronchospasm but also mobilize airway secretions. Previous studies show that asthmatic patients with coexistent bronchiectasis demonstrate similar improvement in forced expiratory volume in 1 second (FEV$_1$) following inhaled β_2-agonists compared with asthmatic patients who do not have this disease.[16] Other studies of bronchiectasis show that up to 39% of patients demonstrate full reversibility of bronchoconstriction after inhaled β_2-agonist treatment.[12] Thus, as in asthma, inhaled β_2-agonists should be considered as a rescue treatment to relieve symptoms in patients with bronchiectasis, even if asthma is not considered a comorbid condition.

Inhaled Corticosteroids

Bronchiectasis is a disease that is largely associated with neutrophil-mediated inflammation but can occur in the context of eosinophilic asthma or ABPA. ICS treatment benefits asthma through its anti-inflammatory effect and, in particular, its ability to resolve eosinophilic airway inflammation. Several studies suggest that ICS use can reduce cough, sputum volume, dyspnea scores, and the requirement for inhaled rescue use and improve airflow limitation in bronchiectasis,[28-31] but in contrast to asthma, without bronchiectasis, ICS use does not reduce the frequency of acute exacerbation.[28,32]

Inhaled Corticosteroid and Long-Acting β-Agonist Combinations

Therapy with fixed-dose ICS and LABA combinations is effective in patients with moderate to severe asthma. One study using the combination of budesonide and formoterol, which included patients with noncystic fibrosis bronchiectasis and airflow obstruction (but with no evidence of asthma or COPD), demonstrates that the combination, at doses of 640 μg/day, was superior to high-dose budesonide alone (1,600 μg/day) in improving symptoms of cough, the dyspnea index, and health-related quality of life, with no negative change in sputum microorganisms.[33] The study also shows a reduction in the use of a short-acting β-agonist as a rescue medication and reduction in overall side effects compared with high-dose ICS. However, once again, there was no significant effect on the number of exacerbations with the treatment. Thus, maintenance combination ICS and LABA therapy may have a beneficial effect in patients with bronchiectasis, even without asthma.

Oral Corticosteroids

Oral corticosteroids (usually prednisone) are the drugs usually required for the management of patients with ABPA.[34] The treatment should be started as soon as the diagnosis is made to prevent or postpone disease deterioration and progression to severe bronchiectasis. Prednisone (0.5 to 1 mg/kg daily) should be given for 1 to 2 weeks, followed by dose tapering over the subsequent 4 to 6 months, depending on the clinical response and serial measurement of IgE levels. A maintenance dose of 5 to 10 mg may be considered for long-term use. Other treatments for ABPA include antifungal agents, such as itraconazole, for 4 to 6 months; these are currently recommended as an add-on therapy to allow reduction of glucocorticoid use, particularly in recurrent ABPA, when higher doses of glucocorticosteroids may be necessary.[34,35]

Antibiotics

Antibiotics are used to treat acute exacerbation of bronchiectasis; however, the role of antibiotics as maintenance therapy in preventing recurrent exacerbation of bronchiectasis is less certain. In acute exacerbations of bronchiectasis, patients should be treated with broad-spectrum antibiotics or an antibiotic based on sputum microbiology or response to previous antibiotics. Ideally, the antibiotic used should be based on the results of the sputum culture. Again, the most common organisms associated with bronchiectasis include *H. influenzae* and *P. aeruginosa*, followed by *S. pneumoniae*, *S. aureus*, and nontuberculous mycobacterium.[2] *S. aureus* is more prevalent in patients with CF. *P. aeruginosa* is found in one-third of patients with bronchiectasis and is considered a predictor of lung function decline and a high rate of exacerbations.[3,4]

During exacerbations, oral antibiotics should be prescribed for a minimum of 7 to 10 days.

Quinolones are regarded as the first antibiotics of choice to treat exacerbations. In one study, oral administration of levofloxacin was compared with intravenous ceftazidime in treating exacerbations. Both were equally effective in improving 24-hour sputum volume, sputum purulence, cough, and dyspnea scores.[36] Another study showed that oral ciprofloxacin was as effective as the combination of oral ciprofloxacin and tobramycin nebulization for the treatment of acute exacerbations due to *P. aeroginosa*.[37] Other treatment options include erythromycin, azithromycin, and intravenous gentamycin.

The management of patients with both asthma and bronchiectasis should follow the same treatment plan, which includes optimizing asthma treatment, usually with combined ICS and LABA, and systemic corticosteroid during acute exacerbation, together with oral antibiotics for a minimum of 7 to 10 days with their choice based on sputum culture and sensitivity. In addition, efforts must be made to encourage expectoration with postural drainage or the use of saline nebulization, or both.

UNMET, FUTURE RESEARCH NEEDS

1. Bronchiectasis treatment guidelines highlight the lack of randomized controlled trials, of studies to establish the link between bronchiectasis and other COPDs, and of studies to further assess the role of current and emerging therapies to manage bronchiectasis.[38]

2. Studies in children demonstrate that the early diagnosis and treatment of bronchiectasis are effective to prevent disease progression and reduce the decline in lung function.[39] The radiologic appearance of bronchiectasis can completely resolve.[40] However, studies investigating this concept in adults are lacking.

3. An oral vaccine against inactivated nontypeable *H. influenza* demonstrates safety and efficacy to reduce moderate to severe exacerbations and to reduce the bacterial load in patients with severe COPD.[41] However, it is yet to be investigated and approved for use in patients with bronchiectasis.

4. Biomarkers to identify patients at risk for tissue injury and progression to bronchiectasis are needed. An example is the subgroup of patients with severe persistent neutrophilic asthma, which has similar characteristics to bronchiectasis in the predominance of neutrophilic airway response and an attenuated treatment response to ICS.

CONCLUSION

Bronchiectasis is a common and debilitating chronic airway disease that is associated with a variety of comorbid conditions. It is described in up to 40% of patients with severe refractory asthma. The co-occurrence of severe asthma, ABPA, and bronchiectasis is a well-recognized clinical entity. Bronchial hygiene, to clear airway secretions, is the basis of management. Bronchodilators and fixed-dose combination therapy with ICS and LABA provide clinical benefit but do not reduce the risk for acute exacerbations. The airways of patients with bronchiectasis are often colonized with pathologic bacteria, and acute exacerbations require antibiotic therapy. ABPA often requires daily oral corticosteroids for management.

REFERENCES

1. Weycker DEJ, Oster G, Tino G. Prevalence and economic burden of bronchiectasis. *Clin Pulm Med.* 2005;12:205–209.
2. Angrill J, Agusti C, de Celis R, et al. Bacterial colonisation in patients with bronchiectasis: microbiological pattern and risk factors. *Thorax.* 2002;57:15–19.
3. Martinez-Garcia MA, Soler-Cataluna JJ, Donat Sanz Y, et al. Factors associated with bronchiectasis in patients with COPD. *Chest.* 2011;140:1130–1137.
4. Martinez-Garcia MA, Soler-Cataluna JJ, Perpina-Tordera M, Roman-Sanchez P, Soriano J. Factors associated with lung function decline in adult patients with stable non-cystic fibrosis bronchiectasis. *Chest.* 2007;132:1565–1572.
5. Drost N, D'Silva L, Rebello R, Efthimiadis A, Hargreave FE, Nair P. Persistent sputum cellularity and neutrophils may predict bronchiectasis. *Can Respir J.* 2011;18:221–224.
6. Laurent F, Latrabe V, Raherison C, Marthan R, Tunon-de-Lara JM. Functional significance of air trapping detected in moderate asthma. *Eur Radiol.* 2000;10:1404–1410.
7. Grenier P, Mourey-Gerosa I, Benali K, et al. Abnormalities of the airways and lung parenchyma in asthmatics: CT observations in 50 patients and inter- and intraobserver variability. *Eur Radiol.* 1996;6:199–206.
8. Gupta S, Siddiqui S, Haldar P, et al. Qualitative analysis of high-resolution CT scans in severe asthma. *Chest.* 2009;136:1521–1528.
9. Sheehan RE, Wells AU, Copley SJ, et al. A comparison of serial computed tomography and functional change in bronchiectasis. *Eur Respir J.* 2002;20:581–587.
10. Reiff DB, Wells AU, Carr DH, Cole PJ, Hansell DM. CT findings in bronchiectasis: limited value in distinguishing between idiopathic and specific types. *Am J Radiol.* 1995;165:261–267.
11. Agarwal R. Allergic bronchopulmonary aspergillosis. *Chest.* 2009;135:805–826.
12. Murphy MB, Reen DJ, Fitzgerald MX. Atopy, immunological changes, and respiratory function in bronchiectasis. *Thorax.* 1984;39:179–184.
13. Pang J, Chan HS, Sung JY. Prevalence of asthma, atopy, and bronchial hyperreactivity in bronchiectasis: a controlled study. *Thorax.* 1989;44:948–951.
14. Bahous J, Cartier A, Pineau L, et al. Pulmonary function tests and airway responsiveness to methacholine in chronic bronchiectasis of the adult. *Bull Eur Physiopathol Respir.* 1984;20:375–380.
15. Shiba K, Kasahara K, Nakajima H, Adachi M. Structural changes of the airway wall impair respiratory function, even in mild asthma. *Chest.* 2002;122:1622–1626.
16. Oguzulgen IK, Kervan F, Ozis T, Turktas H. The impact of bronchiectasis in clinical presentation of asthma. *Southern Med J.* 2007;100:468–471.
17. Agarwal R, Aggarwal AN, Gupta D, Jindal SK. Aspergillus hypersensitivity and allergic bronchopulmonary aspergillosis in patients with bronchial asthma: systematic review and meta-analysis. *Int J Tubercul Lung Dis.* 2009;13:936–944.
18. Greenberger PA. Allergic bronchopulmonary aspergillosis and fungoses. *Clin Chest Med.* 1988;9:599–608.
19. Eppinger TM, Greenberger PA, White DA, Brown AE, Cunningham-Rundles C. Sensitization to Aspergillus species in the congenital neutrophil disorders chronic granulomatous disease and hyper-IgE syndrome. *J Allergy Clin Immunol.* 1999;104:1265–1272.
20. Stevens DA, Moss RB, Kurup VP, et al. Allergic bronchopulmonary aspergillosis in cystic fibrosis: state of the art. Cystic Fibrosis Foundation Consensus Conference. *Clin Infect Dis.* 2003;37(Suppl 3):S225–S264.
21. Patel IS, Vlahos I, Wilkinson TM, et al. Bronchiectasis, exacerbation indices, and inflammation in chronic obstructive pulmonary disease. *Am J Respir Crit Care Med.* 2004;170:400–407.
22. Parr DG, Guest PG, Reynolds JH, Dowson LJ, Stockley RA. Prevalence and impact of bronchiectasis in alpha1-antitrypsin deficiency. *Am J Respir Crit Care Med.* 2007;176:1215–1221.
23. Tsang KW, Lam WK, Kwok E, et al. Helicobacter pylori and upper gastrointestinal symptoms in bronchiectasis. *Eur Respir J.* 1999;14:1345–1350.
24. Flude LJ, Agent P, Bilton D. Chest physiotherapy techniques in bronchiectasis. *Clin Chest Med.* 2012;33:351–361.

25. Kellett F, Robert NM. Nebulised 7% hypertonic saline improves lung function and quality of life in bronchiectasis. *Respir Med.* 2011;105:1831–1835.
26. Nair GB, Ilowite JS. Pharmacologic agents for mucus clearance in bronchiectasis. *Clin Chest Med.* 2012;33:363–370.
27. Myers TR. Positive expiratory pressure and oscillatory positive expiratory pressure therapies. *Respir Care.* 2007;52:1308–1326.
28. Tsang KW, Tan KC, Ho PL, et al. Inhaled fluticasone in bronchiectasis: a 12 month study. *Thorax.* 2005;60:239–243.
29. Elborn JS, Johnston B, Allen F, Clarke J, McGarry J, Varghese G. Inhaled steroids in patients with bronchiectasis. *Respir Med.* 1992;86:121–124.
30. Tsang KW, Ho PL, Lam WK, et al. Inhaled fluticasone reduces sputum inflammatory indices in severe bronchiectasis. *Am J Respir Crit Care Med.* 1998;158:723–727.
31. Kharitonov SA, Wells AU, O'Connor BJ, et al. Elevated levels of exhaled nitric oxide in bronchiectasis. *Am J Respir Crit Care Med.* 1995;151:1889–1893.
32. Martinez-Garcia MA, Perpina-Tordera M, Roman-Sanchez P, Soler-Cataluna JJ. Inhaled steroids improve quality of life in patients with steady-state bronchiectasis. *Respir Med.* 2006;100:1623–1632.
33. Martinez-Garcia MA, Soler-Cataluna JJ, Catalan-Serra P, Roman-Sanchez P, Tordera MP. Clinical efficacy and safety of budesonide-formoterol in non-cystic fibrosis bronchiectasis. *Chest.* 2012;141:461–468.
34. Walsh TJ, Anaissie EJ, Denning DW, et al. Treatment of aspergillosis: clinical practice guidelines of the Infectious Diseases Society of America. *Clin Infect Dis.* 2008;46:327–360.
35. Stevens DA, Schwartz HJ, Lee JY, et al. A randomized trial of itraconazole in allergic bronchopulmonary aspergillosis. *N Engl J Med.* 2000;342:756–762.
36. Tsang KW, Chan WM, Ho PL, Chan K, Lam WK, Ip MS. A comparative study on the efficacy of levofloxacin and ceftazidime in acute exacerbation of bronchiectasis. *Eur Respir J.* 1999;14:1206–1209.
37. Bilton D, Henig N, Morrissey B, Gotfried M. Addition of inhaled tobramycin to ciprofloxacin for acute exacerbations of Pseudomonas aeruginosa infection in adult bronchiectasis. *Chest.* 2006;130:1503–1510.
38. Pasteur MC, Bilton D, Hill AT. British Thoracic Society guideline for non-CF bronchiectasis. *Thorax.* 2010;65(Suppl 1):i1–58.
39. Chang AB, Byrnes CA, Everard ML. Diagnosing and preventing chronic suppurative lung disease (CSLD) and bronchiectasis. *Paed Respir Rev.* 2011;12:97–103.
40. Gaillard EA, Carty H, Heaf D, Smyth RL. Reversible bronchial dilatation in children: comparison of serial high-resolution computer tomography scans of the lungs. *Eur J Radiol.* 2003;47:215–220.
41. Tandon MK, Phillips M, Waterer G, Dunkley M, Comans P, Clancy R. Oral immunotherapy with inactivated nontypeable Haemophilus influenzae reduces severity of acute exacerbations in severe COPD. *Chest.* 2010;137:805–811.

9

BRONCHIOLITIS

COMORBID, COEXISTING, AND DIFFERENTIAL DIAGNOSIS

Kelly J. Cowan and Theresa W. Guilbert

KEY POINTS

- Viral respiratory infections are the most common causes of wheezing in infants and young children and are closely linked to the development of recurrent wheezing and asthma and asthma exacerbations.
- Respiratory syncytial virus (RSV) is the most common cause of bronchiolitis in children younger than 12 months, and human rhinovirus (HRV) is the most common cause of wheezing in children older than 12 months. Viral infections are also the most common cause of asthma exacerbations in older children, with HRV being the most common viral etiology.
- The age of the patient, time course of illness, response to treatment, symptom pattern, and presence of asthma risk factors may influence the diagnosis of bronchiolitis versus exacerbation of asthma in early life.
- RSV or HRV lower respiratory tract infection and early aeroallergen sensitization are important independent risk factors for the development of asthma. Of these, wheezing with HRV infection in the first years of life is the strongest risk factor, and children with early-life aeroallergen sensitization and HRV wheezing are even at higher risk for asthma.
- The management of infants and children with bronchiolitis typically involves supportive care. A trial of asthma therapies may be considered for select patients.

INTRODUCTION

Bronchiolitis is a clinical syndrome in infants and children younger than 2 years characterized by airway obstruction and wheezing caused by lower respiratory tract infection (LRTI) and resulting in inflammation of the small airways (bronchioles). The definition of bronchiolitis may be strictly narrowed to the first episode of wheezing in a child younger than 12 months with physical findings of LRTI and no other etiologies or risk factors associated with wheezing. In young children, symptoms and physical findings of bronchiolitis may overlap with virus-induced wheezing and acute asthma exacerbation. There is a complex relationship between LRTI, wheezing, development of asthma, and asthma exacerbation that varies with age, genetic, and environmental risk factors.

Bronchiolitis and *bronchiolitis obliterans* are also nonspecific terms used to describe inflammatory injury to the small airways from various infectious, chemical, immunologic, and idiopathic causes.[1] This chapter will focus on the causes of bronchiolitis that are comorbid with asthma or associated with an increased risk for asthma.

ETIOLOGIES AND EPIDEMIOLOGY OF INFECTIOUS BRONCHIOLITIS

Typically, inflammation of the small airways and wheezing is due to primary viral infection or reinfection and is less commonly caused by bacterial infection. The viruses most studied in relation to bronchiolitis, the development of asthma, and exacerbation of asthma are respiratory syncytial virus (RSV) and human rhinovirus (HRV). RSV is the most common cause of LRTI and wheezing in children younger than 2,[2,3] followed by HRV.[4] The less common human respiratory viruses that lead to bronchiolitis include parainfluenza, metapneumovirus, adenovirus, influenza, coronaviruses, bocavirus, and enteroviruses.[5] In addition, viral coinfection occurs in about one-third of young children hospitalized with bronchiolitis.

Viral bronchiolitis is common, with 18% to 32% of children experiencing it during the first year of life,[6] and RSV is responsible for about half of the cases.[7] The peak incidence of bronchiolitis is between 2 and 6 months of age. It remains a significant cause of respiratory disease during the first 5 years of life, with 40% of children experiencing a wheezing illness by age 3 years and almost half of all children by age 6 years.[8] Each year in the United States, RSV is associated with approximately 132,000 to 172,000 hospitalizations among children younger than 5 years,[9] with the rate of hospitalization highest in children younger than 3 months. RSV is also a significant cause of LRTI in elderly and immunosuppressed patients.[10]

Two RSV subtypes, A and B, are present in most outbreaks, with A subtypes typically causing more severe disease. The infection rate is about 70% in the first year of life, and almost all children are infected at least once by 2 years of age. RSV infections generally occur in the late fall and winter and in the early spring months, with epidemic peaks depending on the global location. The dominant strains of RSV shift yearly. In contrast to many other viruses, the same strain of RSV can reinfect the same individual throughout life.[11] Reinfection illnesses are generally milder, usually consisting of upper respiratory tract symptoms in healthy individuals. The risk for reinfection is decreased by higher levels of serum antibodies and increasing age.

After the first 12 months of age, HRV surpasses RSV as the dominant infection in hospitalized wheezing children. The prevalence of HRV bronchiolitis is between 20% and 40% in emergency department and hospital settings.[6] HRV is also the most common cause of respiratory illness in all ages. It is the main cause of the common cold and can cause both upper and lower respiratory illnesses in children and adults. HRV LRTI is more likely to occur in high-risk groups, including infants and children and adults with asthma. In children with asthma, 85% of asthma exacerbations are linked to viral illness, and two-thirds of those illnesses are caused by HRV.[12] A similar pattern is also seen in adults, with half of asthma exacerbations triggered by viral respiratory infections, typically HRV.[13]

Approximately 100 HRV serotypes and more than 150 distinct HRV strains are identified[14] that can result in repeated infections with different strains in an individual. Up to 20 strains of HRV circulate throughout a community in a season, and the predominant strains differ by season and location, shifting almost completely every year.[7] HRV-C is closely associated with LRTI[15] and is more frequently detected than other HRVs during exacerbations of asthma in children. HRV infections are typically seen in the fall and spring but can occur throughout the year. In children, asthma exacerbation peaks occur regularly in the fall and spring, correlating with HRV prevalence in the community.[15]

CLINICAL FEATURES OF INFECTIOUS BRONCHIOLITIS

Bronchiolitis usually begins with an upper respiratory tract prodrome, including rhinorrhea and cough and intermittent fever. The illness then progresses to LTRI with small airway inflammation. LRTI symptoms typically begin on days 2 to 3 of illness and peak on days 5 to 7 before slowly resolving. Depending on the severity of illness, the physical examination findings may include any combination of the following: diffuse polyphonic expiratory wheezing; prolonged expiratory phase; coarse and fine crackles; tachypnea; intercostal, subcostal, and supraclavicular retractions; grunting; nasal flaring; and various degrees of hypoxemia. The physical examination and severity of symptoms may fluctuate through the course of the illness. The diagnosis of bronchiolitis can be made in the appropriate clinical and epidemiologic setting. The possibility of coinfection with other viruses or bacteria should be considered in severe cases of bronchiolitis. The duration of illness depends on age, presence of high-risk conditions, and causative agent. The typical duration of wheezing in uncomplicated bronchiolitis is between 1 and 2 weeks, with about 10% of patients continuing to have symptoms for at least 4 weeks. A prolonged course is more likely in younger infants and those with comorbid conditions, such as lung disease of prematurity or cardiovascular disease. Complications, severity, and duration of bronchiolitis have mostly been studied in infants with RSV infections.

RSV bronchiolitis is a self-limited illness that resolves without complications in most otherwise healthy infants. Risk factors for severe disease and complications, including apnea and respiratory failure, include gestational age less than 37 weeks, age less than 12 weeks, chronic pulmonary disease, congenital heart disease, immunodeficiency, congenital and anatomic defects of the airways, and neurologic disease.[16] Environmental and other risk factors, such as passive smoking, a crowded household, urban setting, daycare attendance, concurrent birth siblings, older siblings, and high altitude, can increase the risk for severe disease.[17] The clinical manifestations of RSV infection vary with age, health status, and whether the infection is primary or secondary. In addition to the previous risk factors for severe bronchiolitis, other risk factors for lower respiratory tract disease include infants younger than 6 months, particularly if they are born during the first half of the RSV season,[18] male gender, patients of any age group with significant asthma, adults with cardiopulmonary disease, institutionalized elderly patients, and elderly patients with pulmonary disease or functional disability.[10]

DIAGNOSIS

Chest radiographs can support the diagnosis of bronchiolitis but are not routinely necessary. Radiographs may be normal or may show nonspecific abnormalities indistinguishable from those seen with other conditions, including an asthma exacerbation or pneumonia. Abnormalities may include any combination of hyperinflation, peribronchial thickening, infiltrates, and focal or patchy atelectasis due to airway narrowing and mucous plugging.

Virologic studies for common respiratory viruses are also not routinely necessary. If they are positive, they support the diagnosis of viral bronchiolitis but do not exclude coexisting asthma exacerbation or even bacterial coinfection. Furthermore, if negative, because of the limited number of viruses tested on current panels, virologic studies cannot exclude viral illness. Virologic studies for RSV in particular are unlikely to change acute management or outcomes for most children with bronchiolitis diagnosed clinically. Depending on the clinical picture, there may be some utility in specific viral detection because it may lead to decreased use of antibiotics and may aid in the prediction of recurrent wheezing.

DIFFERENTIAL DIAGNOSIS

Bronchiolitis must be differentiated from other acute and chronic respiratory disorders in the infant or child presenting with wheezing or cough. The differential diagnosis can be broad and age dependent and includes virus-triggered wheezing or asthma exacerbation, pneumonia, chronic lung disease, foreign body aspiration, gastroesophageal reflux disease and/or dysphagia leading to aspiration, congenital heart disease, heart failure, immunodeficiency, and congenital and anatomic defects of the airways (Table 9.1).[19] Chronic underlying conditions should be suspected in children with prolonged, severe, or recurrent symptoms and/or poor growth. Evaluation of the patient should be guided by the history and physical examination. Additional studies, such as imaging, bronchoscopy, and laboratory studies, may be needed to distinguish some of these conditions from bronchiolitis if there is a high level of suspicion or if the clinical course is inconsistent with bronchiolitis.

Of course, bronchiolitis may be superimposed on any underlying condition, increasing the risk for severity and duration of the illness.

Exacerbation of asthma triggered by viral infection should be strongly considered in the differential diagnosis of acute wheezing and bronchiolitis presentation. This is especially true in children older than 24 months and those with a history of recurrent wheezing. In addition, suspicion for asthma exacerbation should be higher in infants and children with risk factors for asthma, including those with a family history of asthma and/or a personal or family history of allergy or eczema. Predictive indices, such as the modified asthma predictive index, are developed that incorporate risk factors to help estimate prognosis of infants with recurrent wheezing and potential responders to inhaled corticosteroids (Table 9.2).[19-23] Children with asthma may demonstrate improvement in symptoms after acute asthma therapy, such as bronchodilators and systemic corticosteroids. Furthermore, the time course of illness, response to treatment,

Table 9.1. Age-Related Differential Diagnosis for Wheezing

CONDITION	RELATIVE FREQUENCY OF OCCURRENCE		
	INFANCY	CHILDHOOD	ADOLESCENCE
Asthma	+	+++	+++
Airway malacia	++	+	−
Cystic fibrosis	+++	+	±
Foreign body	++	+++	±
Airway infection	+++	++	+
Bronchopulmonary dysplasia	+++	+	−
Primary ciliary dyskinesia	+	++	+
Bronchiectasis	+	+	+
Congenital anomalies (Vascular ring)	+++	+	−
Vocal cord dysfunction	−	±	++
Tumors	±	±	±
Aspiration syndromes	+	±	±
Pulmonary edema	+	+	+

−, Unlikely to present in this age group; +, likely to present in this age group.

Reprinted with permission from Bacharier[22] and originally modified with permission from Bierman CW, Pearlman DS, eds. *Allergic Diseases From Infancy to Adulthood.* 2nd ed. Philadelphia: WB Saunders; 1988.

Table 9.2. Modified Asthma Predictive Index versus Original Asthma Predictive Index[20]

1. A history of 4 or more wheezing episodes with at least one physician diagnosed
2. In addition, the child must meet at least one of the following major criteria or at least 2 of the following minor criteria

Modified Asthma Predictive Index	Original Asthma Predictive Index
Major Criteria	Major Criteria
• Parental history of asthma	• Parental history of asthma
• MD-diagnosed atopic dermatitis	• MD-diagnosed atopic dermatitis
• **Allergic sensitization to at least one aeroallergen**	
Minor Criteria	Minor Criteria
• **Allergic sensitization to milk, egg, or peanut**	• **MD-diagnosed allergic rhinitis**
• Wheezing unrelated to colds	• Wheezing unrelated to colds
• Blood eosinophils $\geq$ 4%	• Blood eosinophils $\geq$ 4%

Differences in indices are shown in boldface.
Reproduced with permission from Guilbert.[23]

and symptom pattern may influence the diagnosis of bronchiolitis versus exacerbation of asthma (Figure 9.1).

INFECTIOUS BRONCHIOLITIS AND THE DEVELOPMENT OF WHEEZING AND ASTHMA IN CHILDREN

Viral respiratory infections, particularly RSV and HRV, are the most common causes of wheezing in infants and young children and have important influences on the development of recurrent wheezing and asthma and asthma exacerbations in some individuals. About one-third of infants with an acute wheezing illness go on to develop recurrent wheezing.[7] Wheezing with respiratory infections decreases with age for most infants. However, wheezing in early life marks the inception of asthma in certain infants. It remains unclear whether certain viral respiratory infections in early life cause asthma or whether wheezing with these infections reveals a preexisting tendency for asthma and severe LRTI secondary to impaired lung physiology or antiviral responses.[7] A combination of factors is likely involved in the development of asthma, such as genetic predisposition to airway reactivity, exposure to environmental pollutants or allergens, immunologic mechanisms, and disruption of lung growth and development due to viral infections in early childhood.

Infants hospitalized with severe bronchiolitis are at increased risk for developing recurrent wheezing, asthma, and reduced pulmonary function in childhood, particularly during the first decade of life. Multiple studies have linked RSV bronchiolitis in infancy to the development of recurrent wheeze[2,3,24,25] and asthma.[25-27] After bronchiolitis, the highest risk for recurrent wheezing is in the subsequent year or preschool years,[24] with about two-thirds having recurrent wheezing episodes[28] in early life. Infants hospitalized with bronchiolitis also have a two- to three-fold increased risk for developing asthma later in childhood.[7,29]

In one of the largest studies of severe RSV bronchiolitis, there was a nearly 50% prevalence of asthma at age 7 years after severe RSV bronchiolitis in infancy, higher than previously described.[3,25,30] However, most studies find that children with severe RSV bronchiolitis

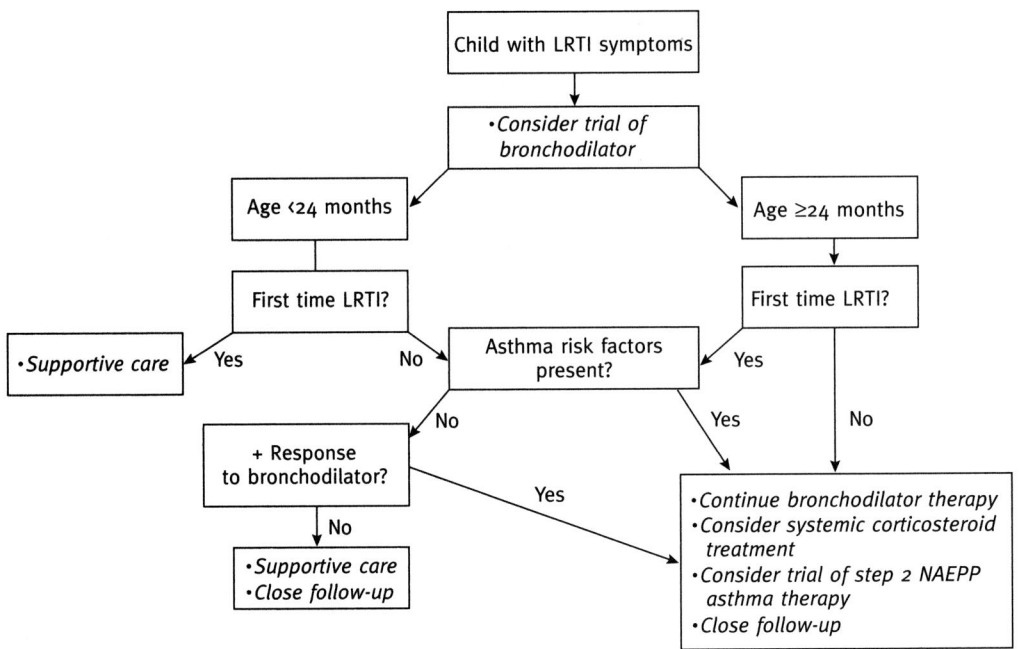

FIGURE 9.1 Suggested approach to a child with lower respiratory tract infection (LRTI) symptoms. NAEPP, National Asthma Education Prevention Program.

in infancy are at significantly increased risk for asthma during the first 6 years of life and that symptoms generally resolve in adolescence.[20,25,28] Severity of bronchiolitis may play a role in increasing the risk for recurrent wheezing[29,31] and development of asthma.[32] Timing of birth and subsequent exposure to peak bronchiolitis in the RSV season may also influence the development of asthma.[33] Adult outcomes are less clear, with one study showing increased risk for asthma in early adulthood after bronchiolitis in infancy,[26] conflicting with other data showing no difference in adolescents.[2] Differences in outcomes of various studies may be due to the severity of bronchiolitis, population size, asthma risk of the cohort, incidence of allergic sensitization, and prevalence of asthma in control populations.

Increased airway hyperresponsiveness is common after severe RSV bronchiolitis, with about two-thirds of children having increased airway hyperresponsiveness, at least when school aged.[28,34] However, this is not necessarily linked to a diagnosis of asthma. Because airway hyperresponsiveness at age 6 years is a risk factor for newly diagnosed asthma in early adulthood,[35] there may be implications for lingering effects in adulthood. Abnormalities in spirometry are more common in young adults who were hospitalized for RSV bronchiolitis in infancy.[36] Similar to that in children, RSV infection in healthy adults may cause short-term airway hyperreactivity.[37] How RSV infection affects long-term pulmonary function in adults with asthma remains unknown.

Children who develop asthma after RSV infection usually have a history of more severe bronchiolitis and/or other asthma risk factors, such as repeated wheezing episodes in early life, maternal history of asthma, aeroallergen sensitization, and high immunoglobulin E levels.[28] Risk for asthma is also increased by blood eosinophilia, male gender, and lower birth length.[7] Aeroallergen sensitization at age 3 years is also associated with asthma diagnosis after severe RSV bronchiolitis.[28,38,39] However, most infants and young children who wheeze with RSV infection are non-atopic.[40] Many of these children demonstrate reduced lung function shortly after birth, which may predispose them to wheezing with respiratory infections.[8,41] Furthermore, infants with lower lung function are at increased risk for airflow obstruction as young adults.[42]

In addition to wheezing with RSV infection, wheezing with HRV respiratory infection and early aeroallergen sensitization are important independent risk factors for the development of asthma. Of these, wheezing with HRV infection in early life gives the highest risk for recurrent wheezing and ultimately developing childhood asthma, with 90% of children with HRV-induced wheezing at age 3 years having asthma by age 6 years.[38,39,43,44] Many children with isolated HRV infection do not wheeze in the absence of allergic cofactors; this is most likely to occur in those who have HRV infection with atopic disease or eosinophilic airway inflammation.[45] Children with early sensitization to aeroallergens are at greater risk for developing viral wheeze and asthma than nonsensitized children.[38] The risk for developing asthma is greatest for infants and toddlers who both wheeze with HRV infection and develop allergen sensitization before age 2 years[7] because these factors are synergistic.[38,39] In addition, early allergic sensitization precedes HRV-triggered wheezing.[46] RSV bronchiolitis does not have the same relationship with allergic sensitization.[46,47] Most nonatopic children with wheezing in early life have resolution of these symptoms by school age and normal lung function at puberty.[48] HRV bronchiolitis carries a higher risk for asthma, at least until adolescence.[6,49,50] If early-childhood wheezing persists until age 6 years and the child has atopic disease, then the child is at high risk for continuing to have chronic asthma through childhood.[51] In a long-term post-bronchiolitis hospitalization follow-up, asthma was more common after HRV (52%) than RSV (15%) bronchiolitis at school age.[49] Recurrent wheezing, childhood asthma, and asthma continuing into adulthood are more common after non-RSV bronchiolitis, most likely HRV, in infancy compared with RSV bronchiolitis.[52] HRV wheezing illnesses in young children are also the most significant predictors of decreased lung function up until age 8 years.[53] It is not known whether this is a cause or an effect of HRV wheezing illnesses. HRV bronchiolitis is also associated with bronchial hyperresponsiveness in childhood and at least into adolescence.[54] There are no conclusive data that tie viral infection to causation of asthma in previously healthy adults.

IMPACT OF THE IMMUNE RESPONSE TO INFECTIOUS BRONCHIOLITIS AND THE DEVELOPMENT OF ASTHMA EXACERBATIONS

Allergic sensitization, allergen exposure, and viral infections also synergistically increase the risk for acute exacerbations and hospitalization in children and adults.[45,55-59] They are the most significant risk factors for exacerbations leading to acute care visits or hospitalization. HRV is found in about 70% of children older than 2 years with acute asthma exacerbations. Other factors that contribute to acute exacerbation include allergy, allergen exposure, indoor and outdoor pollutants, stress, and other infections. Allergic sensitization and eosinophilia are the strongest risk factors for developing virus-induced asthma exacerbations.[7] Children and adults with asthma do not have more colds than other individuals, but they do have greater duration and severity of lower respiratory symptoms,[60,61] particularly those with allergic sensitization.

There are several likely mechanisms for synergy between allergic inflammation and viral infections to cause wheezing and asthma exacerbation, in general involving impaired inflammatory regulation, defective immune response to viruses and allergens, or deficiencies in the epithelium that predispose to allergy, asthma, and increased severity of viral infections.[5,7] Genetic or acquired abnormalities can lead to either underproduction of interferons[62,63] (weak helper T-cell type 1 [T_H1] response) or dysregulation of T_H1 and T_H2 cells of the immune system.[58,64,65] Variation in innate immune response to respiratory viruses in early life may lead to suboptimal antiviral responses, increased risk for respiratory allergies, and changes in airway structure to promote asthma.[5] Viral infections could also enhance allergic inflammation, which in turn may directly inhibit host antiviral responses and promote prolonged infection.

Both viral infections and allergic inflammation can compromise the barrier function of the airway epithelium, which can lead to enhanced absorption of allergens, irritants, and pollutants across the airway wall. This may result in increased allergic inflammation, greater viral replication, and more severe illness. In addition, these effects could be compounded in asthma by defective epithelial repair processes[66] and pollutant triggers such as tobacco smoke. The airway epithelium in asthma has distinct features associated with airway remodeling, including increased numbers of mucus-secreting goblet cells, whereby HRV replication may be enhanced.[7] Respiratory viral infections also increase synthesis of factors that can influence lung growth, development, and repair.[7]

Viruses and bacteria may interact in determining risk for onset of asthma and lead to acute exacerbations. Colonization of the upper airway with bacterial pathogens during the first 3 months of life is linked to virus-induced wheezing and increased risk for subsequent asthma.[67] During exacerbations, the neutrophilic responses to viral infection may be enhanced,[68] especially in the lower airways. Increased severity of infection or greater inflammatory response to infection could lead to airway edema and respiratory smooth muscle contraction and thus aggravate asthma.[15] HRV can also cause enhanced eosinophilic response to allergen challenge in allergic individuals, which, along with T_H2-biased immune responses associated with allergic sensitization, may enhance severity of illness with HRV infection.[15]

In contrast to studies linking early-life infections with respiratory morbidity, the hygiene hypothesis proposes that infections, including respiratory infections in early life, are protective toward the eventual development of allergic diseases and possibly asthma.[69] There is a lower prevalence of allergies and asthma in children in daycare or with older siblings. The proposed protective effect is related to more frequent infections, including respiratory viruses, and stimulation of protective (T_H1) immunity. However, this is likely a complex interaction between susceptibility, age of the host, and type of virus.

TREATMENT OF BRONCHIOLITIS

The management of healthy infants with bronchiolitis typically involves supportive care to ensure hydration, good oxygenation, and stability. Typical asthma therapies are not useful, such as bronchodilators,[70] systemic corticosteroids,[71] and inhaled corticosteroids to treat the acute illness, particularly the first episode of bronchiolitis. In addition, inhaled corticosteroids in this scenario do reduce subsequent wheezing episodes. No treatment to date prevents asthma development in susceptible patients. A problem with trials evaluating bronchodilators in infants and children with bronchiolitis is the difficulty of distinguishing bronchiolitis alone from asthma exacerbation or bronchiolitis combined with asthma exacerbation. With asthma exacerbation, mainstays of acute therapy are inhaled bronchodilators and systemic corticosteroids. Many clinicians believe a subset of infants and children with bronchiolitis improve clinically with bronchodilator use. The American Academy of Pediatrics guidelines indicate that, although it should not be used routinely in the management of bronchiolitis, a monitored trial of bronchodilator medication is an option, with continuation only if there is a documented objective clinical response.[72] If a child has a recurrent pattern of bronchiolitis or a high suspicion for asthma based on persistent symptoms, other asthma risk factors, or response to asthma therapy, acute and chronic asthma therapy according to the Global Initiative for Asthma or the National Asthma Education and Prevention Program guidelines should be considered (Box 9.1).

Immunoprophylaxis with palivizumab decreases the risk for hospitalization because of RSV illness in infants with bronchopulmonary dysplasia, prematurity, and congenital heart disease. RSV immunoprophylaxis with palivizumab administered to preterm infants reduces the relative risk for recurrent wheezing by 80% in children without a family history of atopy but has no effect in children from atopic families.[73]

BRONCHIOLITIS OBLITERANS

Bronchiolitis obliterans is a rare lung disease caused by epithelial injury to the bronchioles and leading to obstruction and obliteration of the distal airways. Potential causes include chemical, infectious, immunologic, or

> **Box 9.1**
>
> Step 2 National Asthma Education Prevention Program (NAEPP) asthma therapy: Inhaled corticosteroid, leukotriene receptor antagonist, cromolyns
> Other considerations:
> With recurrent LRTI—consider evaluation for other causes of recurrent wheezing or cough if low suspicion for asthma or not responding to asthma therapy
> Consider asthma or other underlying disease in children with atypical course of illness, severe illness, or recurrent wheezing with history of severe LRTI
> Consider the viral etiology by testing or seasonal prevalence of viruses in the community because rhinovirus-induced wheezing in children raises suspicion for asthma

idiopathic injury. Bronchiolitis obliterans can be a consequence of chronic lung transplant rejection and hematopoietic cell transplantation. Outside of lung transplantation, postviral injury, most often due to adenovirus, is the most common cause. Although bronchiolitis obliterans may present as asthma, including tachypnea, shortness of breath, cough, wheeze, and sometimes hypoxemia, symptoms are not responsive to bronchodilators. Patients may also have crackles, not typical for asthma, in addition to wheezing on physical examination. Chest radiographs may be normal or yield nonspecific findings such as hyperinflation, atelectasis, or interstitial infiltrates. Spirometry may show airway obstruction without significant response to bronchodilators. To definitively diagnose bronchiolitis obliterans, lung biopsy is the gold standard. However, high-resolution chest computed tomography showing a mosaic pattern with hypolucency caused by air trapping may be helpful in supporting the diagnosis, lessening the need for biopsy in some patients. Treatment of bronchiolitis obliterans varies depending on the cause of disease. Anti-inflammatory therapies may be helpful in some patients, and lung transplantation may be an option for progressive disease unresponsive to therapy.[1]

UNMET, FUTURE RESEARCH NEEDS

1. The relationship between the development of asthma and mild RSV bronchiolitis or upper respiratory tract infection is not well understood.
2. Knowledge regarding the associations between LRTI, allergy, and viral infection leading to asthma is incomplete.
3. It is unclear how less common viral etiologies of LRTI affect the development of asthma.
4. New immune-modulating or antiviral therapies are greatly needed.
5. It is unclear whether preventing RSV infection in children with other risk factors for asthma will prevent the subsequent development of asthma.

CONCLUSION

Viral respiratory infections are the most common causes of wheezing in infants and young children and have important influences on the development of recurrent wheezing and asthma and asthma exacerbations. Underlying disease, including asthma, may coexist with bronchiolitis. The age of the patient, time course of illness, response to treatment, symptom pattern, and presence of asthma risk factors may influence the diagnosis and management of bronchiolitis versus exacerbation of asthma.

REFERENCES

1. Fakhoury K. Wheezing illnesses other than asthma in children. *Up to Date.* 2012–2013.
2. Stein RT, Sherrill D, Morgan WJ, et al. Respiratory syncytial virus in early life and risk

of wheeze and allergy by age 13 years. *Lancet.* 1999;354(9178):541–545.
3. Sigurs N, Bjarnason R, Sigurbergsson F, Kjellman B. Respiratory syncytial virus bronchiolitis in infancy is an important risk factor for asthma and allergy at age 7. *Am J Respir Crit Care Med.* 2000;161(5):1501–1507.
4. Kusel MM, de Klerk NH, Holt PG, Kebadze T, Johnston SL, Sly PD. Role of respiratory viruses in acute upper and lower respiratory tract illness in the first year of life: a birth cohort study. *Pediatr Infect Dis J.* 2006;25(8):680–686.
5. Kloepfer KM, Gern JE. Virus/allergen interactions and exacerbations of asthma. *Immunol Allergy Clin North Am.* 2010;30(4):553–563, vii.
6. Jartti T, Korppi M. Rhinovirus-induced bronchiolitis and asthma development. *Pediatr Allergy Immunol.* 2011;22(4):350–355.
7. Gavala ML, Bertics PJ, Gern JE. Rhinoviruses, allergic inflammation, and asthma. *Immunol Rev.* 2011;242(1):69–90.
8. Martinez FD, Wright AL, Taussig LM, Holberg CJ, Halonen M, Morgan WJ. Asthma and wheezing in the first six years of life. The Group Health Medical Associates. *N Engl J Med.* 1995;332(3):133–138.
9. Stockman LJ, Curns AT, Anderson LJ, Fischer-Langley G. Respiratory syncytial virus-associated hospitalizations among infants and young children in the United States, 1997–2006. *Pediatr Infect Dis J.* 2012;31(1):5–9.
10. Falsey AR, Walsh EE. Respiratory syncytial virus infection in adults. *Clin Microbiol Rev.* 2000;13(3):371–384.
11. Wu P, Hartert TV. Evidence for a causal relationship between respiratory syncytial virus infection and asthma. *Expert Rev Anti-infective Ther.* 2011;9(9):731–745.
12. Johnston SL, Pattemore PK, Sanderson G, et al. Community study of role of viral infections in exacerbations of asthma in 9-11 year old children. *BMJ.* 1995;310(6989):1225–1229.
13. Nicholson KG, Kent J, Ireland DC. Respiratory viruses and exacerbations of asthma in adults. *BMJ.* 1993;307(6910):982–986.
14. Gern JE. Rhinovirus and the initiation of asthma. *Curr Opin Allergy Clin Immunol.* 2009;9(1):73–78.
15. Kim WK, Gern JE. Updates in the relationship between human rhinovirus and asthma. *Allergy Asthma Immunol Res.* 2012;4(3):116–121.
16. Meissner HC. Selected populations at increased risk from respiratory syncytial virus infection. *Pediatr Infect Dis J.* 2003;22(2 Suppl):S40–S44; discussion S44–S45.
17. McConnochie KM, Roghmann KJ. Parental smoking, presence of older siblings, and family history of asthma increase risk of bronchiolitis. *Am J Dis Child.* 1986;140(8):806–812.
18. Houben ML, Bont L, Wilbrink B, et al. Clinical prediction rule for RSV bronchiolitis in healthy newborns: prognostic birth cohort study. *Pediatrics.* 2011;127(1):35–41.
19. Bacharier LB, Guilbert TW. Diagnosis and management of early asthma in preschool-aged children. *J Allergy Clin Immunol.* 2012;130(2):287–296; quiz 297–298.
20. Castro-Rodriguez JA, Holberg CJ, Wright AL, Martinez FD. A clinical index to define risk of asthma in young children with recurrent wheezing. *Am J Respir Crit Care Med.* 2000;162(4 Pt 1):1403–1406.
21. Caudri D, Wijga A, CM AS, et al. Predicting the long-term prognosis of children with symptoms suggestive of asthma at preschool age. *J Allergy Clin Immunol.* 2009;124(5):903–910, e901–e907.
22. Bacharier LB. Evaluation of the child with recurrent wheezing. *J Allergy Clin Immunol.* 2011;128(3):690, e691–e695.
23. Guilbert TW, Morgan WJ, Zeiger RS, et al. Atopic characteristics of children with recurrent wheezing at high risk for the development of childhood asthma. *J Allergy Clin Immunol.* 2004;114(6):1282–1287.
24. Schauer U, Hoffjan S, Bittscheidt J, et al. RSV bronchiolitis and risk of wheeze and allergic sensitisation in the first year of life. *Eur Respir J.* 2002;20(5):1277–1283.
25. Henderson J, Hilliard TN, Sherriff A, Stalker D, Al Shammari N, Thomas HM. Hospitalization for RSV bronchiolitis before 12 months of age and subsequent asthma, atopy and wheeze: a longitudinal birth cohort study. *Pediatr Allergy Immunol.* 2005;16(5):386–392.
26. Sigurs N, Aljassim F, Kjellman B, et al. Asthma and allergy patterns over 18 years after severe RSV bronchiolitis in the first year of life. *Thorax.* 2010;65(12):1045–1052.
27. Sigurs N, Gustafsson PM, Bjarnason R, et al. Severe respiratory syncytial virus bronchiolitis in infancy and asthma and allergy at age 13. *Am J Respir Crit Care Med.* 2005;171(2):137–141.
28. Bacharier LB, Cohen R, Schweiger T, et al. Determinants of asthma after severe respiratory syncytial virus bronchiolitis. *J Allergy Clin Immunol.* 2012;130(1):91–100, e103.
29. Carroll KN, Wu P, Gebretsadik T, et al. The severity-dependent relationship of infant bronchiolitis on the risk and morbidity of early

childhood asthma. *J Allergy Clin Immunol.* 2009;123(5):1055–1061.
30. Koponen P, Helminen M, Paassilta M, Luukkaala T, Korppi M. Preschool asthma after bronchiolitis in infancy. *Eur Respir J.* 2012;39(1):76–80.
31. Poorisrisak P, Halkjaer LB, Thomsen SF, et al. Causal direction between respiratory syncytial virus bronchiolitis and asthma studied in monozygotic twins. *Chest.* 2010;138(2):338–344.
32. Escobar GJ, Ragins A, Li SX, Prager L, Masaquel AS, Kipnis P. Recurrent wheezing in the third year of life among children born at 32 weeks' gestation or later: relationship to laboratory-confirmed, medically attended infection with respiratory syncytial virus during the first year of life. *Arch Pediatr Adolesc Med.* 2010;164(10):915–922.
33. Wu P, Dupont WD, Griffin MR, et al. Evidence of a causal role of winter virus infection during infancy in early childhood asthma. *Am J Respir Crit Care Med.* 2008;178(11):1123–1129.
34. Korppi M, Kuikka L, Reijonen T, Remes K, Juntunen-Backman K, Launiala K. Bronchial asthma and hyperreactivity after early childhood bronchiolitis or pneumonia: an 8-year follow-up study. *Arch Pediatr Adolesc Med.* 1994;148(10):1079–1084.
35. Stern DA, Morgan WJ, Halonen M, Wright AL, Martinez FD. Wheezing and bronchial hyper-responsiveness in early childhood as predictors of newly diagnosed asthma in early adulthood: a longitudinal birth-cohort study. *Lancet.* 2008;372(9643):1058–1064.
36. Korppi M, Piippo-Savolainen E, Korhonen K, Remes S. Respiratory morbidity 20 years after RSV infection in infancy. *Pediatr Pulmonol.* 2004;38(2):155–160.
37. Hall WJ, Hall CB, Speers DM. Respiratory syncytial virus infection in adults: clinical, virologic, and serial pulmonary function studies. *Ann Intern Med.* 1978;88(2):203–205.
38. Kusel MM, de Klerk NH, Kebadze T, et al. Early-life respiratory viral infections, atopic sensitization, and risk of subsequent development of persistent asthma. *J Allergy Clin Immunol.* 2007;119(5):1105–1110.
39. Jackson DJ, Gangnon RE, Evans MD, et al. Wheezing rhinovirus illnesses in early life predict asthma development in high risk children. *Am J Respir Crit Care Med.* 2008;178(7):667–672.
40. Duff AL, Pomeranz ES, Gelber LE, et al. Risk factors for acute wheezing in infants and children: viruses, passive smoke, and IgE antibodies to inhalant allergens. *Pediatrics.* 1993;92(4):535–540.
41. Gern JE, Rosenthal LA, Sorkness RL, Lemanske RF Jr. Effects of viral respiratory infections on lung development and childhood asthma. *J Allergy Clin Immunol.* 2005;115(4):668–674; quiz 675.
42. Stern DA, Morgan WJ, Wright AL, Guerra S, Martinez FD. Poor airway function in early infancy and lung function by age 22 years: a non-selective longitudinal cohort study. *Lancet.* 2007;370(9589):758–764.
43. Heymann PW, Carper HT, Murphy DD, et al. Viral infections in relation to age, atopy, and season of admission among children hospitalized for wheezing. *J Allergy Clin Immunol.* 2004;114(2):239–247.
44. Lemanske RF Jr, Jackson DJ, Gangnon RE, et al. Rhinovirus illnesses during infancy predict subsequent childhood wheezing. *J Allergy Clin Immunol.* 2005;116(3):571–577.
45. Rakes GP, Arruda E, Ingram JM, et al. Rhinovirus and respiratory syncytial virus in wheezing children requiring emergency care: IgE and eosinophil analyses. *Am J Respir Crit Care Med.* 1999;159(3):785–790.
46. Jackson DJ, Evans MD, Gangnon RE, et al. Evidence for a causal relationship between allergic sensitization and rhinovirus wheezing in early life. *Am J Respir Crit Care Med.* 2012;185(3):281–285.
47. Jartti T, Kuusipalo H, Vuorinen T, et al. Allergic sensitization is associated with rhinovirus-, but not other virus-, induced wheezing in children. *Pediatr Allergy Immunol.* 2010;21(7):1008–1014.
48. Illi S, von Mutius E, Lau S, Niggemann B, Gruber C, Wahn U. Perennial allergen sensitisation early in life and chronic asthma in children: a birth cohort study. *Lancet.* 2006;368(9537):763–770.
49. Kotaniemi-Syrjanen A, Vainionpaa R, Reijonen TM, Waris M, Korhonen K, Korppi M. Rhinovirus-induced wheezing in infancy: the first sign of childhood asthma? *J Allergy Clin Immunol.* 2003;111(1):66–71.
50. Hyvarinen MK, Kotaniemi-Syrjanen A, Reijonen TM, Korhonen K, Korppi MO. Teenage asthma after severe early childhood wheezing: an 11-year prospective follow-up. *Pediatr Pulmonol.* 2005;40(4):316–323.
51. Morgan WJ, Stern DA, Sherrill DL, et al. Outcome of asthma and wheezing in the first 6 years of life: follow-up through adolescence. *Am J Respir Crit Care Med.* 2005;172(10):1253–1258.
52. Piippo-Savolainen E, Korppi M. Wheezy babies—wheezy adults? Review on long-term outcome until adulthood after early childhood wheezing. *Acta Paediatr.* 2008;97(1):5–11.

53. Guilbert TW, Singh AM, Danov Z, et al. Decreased lung function after preschool wheezing rhinovirus illnesses in children at risk to develop asthma. *J Allergy Clin Immunol.* 2011;128(3):532–538, e510.
54. Kotaniemi-Syrjanen A, Reijonen TM, Korhonen K, Waris M, Vainionpaa R, Korppi M. Wheezing due to rhinovirus infection in infancy: bronchial hyperresponsiveness at school age. *Pediatr Int.* 2008;50(4):506–510.
55. Murray CS, Poletti G, Kebadze T, et al. Study of modifiable risk factors for asthma exacerbations: virus infection and allergen exposure increase the risk of asthma hospital admissions in children. *Thorax.* 2006;61(5):376–382.
56. Green RM, Custovic A, Sanderson G, Hunter J, Johnston SL, Woodcock A. Synergism between allergens and viruses and risk of hospital admission with asthma: case-control study. *BMJ.* 2002;324(7340):763.
57. Rosenstreich DL, Eggleston P, Kattan M, et al. The role of cockroach allergy and exposure to cockroach allergen in causing morbidity among inner-city children with asthma. *N Engl J Med.* 1997;336(19):1356–1363.
58. Stern DA, Guerra S, Halonen M, Wright AL, Martinez FD. Low IFN-gamma production in the first year of life as a predictor of wheeze during childhood. *J Allergy Clin Immunol.* 2007;120(4):835–841.
59. Subrata LS, Bizzintino J, Mamessier E, et al. Interactions between innate antiviral and atopic immunoinflammatory pathways precipitate and sustain asthma exacerbations in children. *J Immunol.* 2009;183(4):2793–2800.
60. Corne JM, Marshall C, Smith S, et al. Frequency, severity, and duration of rhinovirus infections in asthmatic and non-asthmatic individuals: a longitudinal cohort study. *Lancet.* 2002;359(9309):831–834.
61. DeMore JP, Weisshaar EH, Vrtis RF, et al. Similar colds in subjects with allergic asthma and nonatopic subjects after inoculation with rhinovirus-16. *J Allergy Clin Immunol.* 2009;124(2):245–252, e241–e243.
62. Isaacs D, Clarke JR, Tyrrell DA, Webster AD, Valman HB. Deficient production of leucocyte interferon (interferon-alpha) in vitro and in vivo in children with recurrent respiratory tract infections. *Lancet.* 1981;2(8253):950–952.
63. Parry DE, Busse WW, Sukow KA, Dick CR, Swenson C, Gern JE. Rhinovirus-induced PBMC responses and outcome of experimental infection in allergic subjects. *J Allergy Clin Immunol.* 2000;105(4):692–698.
64. Heaton T, Rowe J, Turner S, et al. An immunoepidemiological approach to asthma: identification of in-vitro T-cell response patterns associated with different wheezing phenotypes in children. *Lancet.* 2005;365(9454):142–149.
65. Holt PG, Upham JW, Sly PD. Contemporaneous maturation of immunologic and respiratory functions during early childhood: implications for development of asthma prevention strategies. *J Allergy Clin Immunol.* 2005;116(1):16–24; quiz 25.
66. Holgate ST, Roberts G, Arshad HS, Howarth PH, Davies DE. The role of the airway epithelium and its interaction with environmental factors in asthma pathogenesis. *Proc Am Thorac Soc.* 2009;6(8):655–659.
67. Bisgaard H, Hermansen MN, Bonnelykke K, et al. Association of bacteria and viruses with wheezy episodes in young children: prospective birth cohort study. *BMJ.* 2010;341:c4978.
68. Denlinger LC, Sorkness RL, Lee WM, et al. Lower airway rhinovirus burden and the seasonal risk of asthma exacerbation. *Am J Respir Crit Care Med.* 2011;184(9):1007–1014.
69. Strachan DP. Family size, infection and atopy: the first decade of the "hygiene hypothesis." *Thorax.* 2000;55(Suppl 1):S2–S10.
70. Gadomski AM, Brower M. Bronchodilators for bronchiolitis. *Cochrane Database Syst Rev.* 2010(12):CD001266.
71. Fernandes RM, Bialy LM, Vandermeer B, et al. Glucocorticoids for acute viral bronchiolitis in infants and young children. *Cochrane Database Syst Rev.* 2010(10):CD004878.
72. American Academy of Pediatrics Subcommittee on Diagnosis and Management of Bronchiolitis. Diagnosis and management of bronchiolitis. *Pediatrics.* 2006;118(4):1774–1793.
73. Simoes EA, Carbonell-Estrany X, Rieger CH, Mitchell I, Fredrick L, Groothuis JR. The effect of respiratory syncytial virus on subsequent recurrent wheezing in atopic and nonatopic children. *J Allergy Clin Immunol.* 2010;126(2):256–262.

10

GENETIC DISORDERS AND ASTHMA

COEXISTING AND DIFFERENTIAL DIAGNOSIS

Neetu Talreja and Ronald Dahl

KEY POINTS

- Primary ciliary dyskinesia (PCD) is a rare, inherited, usually autosomal recessive disorder with impaired ciliary function leading to unexplained neonatal respiratory distress, recurrent otitis media, chronic rhinosinusitis, bronchiectasis, and infertility.
- The diagnosis of PCD is made by identification of ciliary dysmotility and specific ciliary ultrastructural defects.
- Respiratory management of PCD consists of regular respiratory monitoring, airway clearance by means of chest physiotherapy, and early and aggressive antibiotic treatment.
- Cystic fibrosis (CF)[1] is characterized by mutations in the gene encoding the CF transmembrane conductance regulator (CFTR), with resultant abnormalities in airway epithelial ion transport, dysregulation of airway surface liquid, and abnormalities in airway host defense.
- The most common cause for the morbidity and mortality in patients with CF is severe lung disease and respiratory failure.
- α_1-Antitrypsin (AAT) deficiency is an autosomal codominant disease that increases the risk for emphysema in adults and causes chronic liver disease, cirrhosis, and hepatocellular carcinoma in children and adults.
- Treatment of AAT deficiency includes treatment of comorbid conditions and AAT augmentation therapy.

INTRODUCTION TO PRIMARY CILIARY DYSKINESIA

Primary ciliary dyskinesia (PCD) is a rare, inherited, usually autosomal recessive disorder with impaired ciliary function leading to unexplained neonatal respiratory distress, recurrent otitis media, chronic nasal drainage and sinusitis, chronic bronchitis leading to bronchiectasis, and, in approximately 50% of cases, situs inversus totalis or other laterality defect.[2] The incidence of PCD is about 1 in 15,000, although it is higher in populations in which consanguinity is common.[3] The diagnosis of PCD relies on the identification of ciliary dysmotility and specific ciliary ultrastructural defects in the outer dynein arms (ODAs), inner dynein arms (IDAs), or central apparatus. The diagnosis is often delayed or missed or is made incorrectly because these tests are not readily available or standardized. Access to early diagnosis and effective treatment is essential to reduce disease progression and to alleviate the burden of the disease.[4]

CLINICAL FEATURES

Upper and lower respiratory tract manifestations are cardinal features of PCD. They usually present in the first month of life; however, the diagnosis is delayed because features are similar to other pediatric disorders.[2] Upper respiratory tract features include chronic rhinosinusitis and chronic otitis media. Lower respiratory features include neonatal respiratory distress, chronic productive cough, chronic bronchitis, recurrent pneumonia, and bronchiectasis. Most patients have a history of neonatal respiratory distress with tachypnea, hypoxia, and occasionally respiratory failure requiring mechanical ventilation that is mistakenly attributed to transient tachypnea of the newborn or neonatal pneumonia.[4] So, too, a chronic productive cough often beginning in the first weeks of life is inappropriately attributed to recurrent viral infections, reflux, and aspiration or cough-variant asthma. Chronic bronchitis and recurrent pneumonia with radiographic features of air trapping and atelectasis are common in childhood PCD and lead to bronchiectasis typically involving the middle and lower lobes. It may occur in childhood and even in the first years of life.[5]

Laterality defects occur in about half of PCD patients. Indeed, the first reported patient in the early 1900s had situs inversus totalis, chronic sinusitis, and bronchiectasis, known as the Kartagener triad.[5] Almost all men with PCD are infertile from impaired sperm motility. Hydrocephalus, retinitis pigmentosa, polycystic kidney disease, liver cysts, and biliary atresia are reported rarely in PCD, suggesting that there may be an overlap of diseases associated with defects in motile and sensory cilia.[6]

DIAGNOSTIC STRATEGIES

The specialized techniques required for PCD diagnostic tests are not standardized or readily available; therefore, referral to research centers or tertiary diagnostic centers may be necessary.

Ciliary Ultrastructure

The cornerstone diagnostic test for PCD is examination of ciliary ultrastructure by transmission electron microscopy. Each normal cilium contains an array of longitudinal microtubules, consisting of nine doublets arranged in an outer circle around a central pair (9 + 2 pattern). Dynein arms are large protein complexes, including two to three heavy chains, two to four intermediate chains, and at least eight light chains, that are attached to the nine microtubule doublets as distinct inner and outer "arms" that are visualized on electron micrographs of ciliary cross sections (Figure 10.1). Dyneins generate the force for ciliary movement through microtubule sliding. The 9 + 2 array of microtubules is maintained by intertubular linkages and accessory proteins. Several ciliary ultrastructural defects are described, but the most frequent are absence or shortening of ODAs or IDAs, absence of radial spokes, or loss of the central pair of microtubules with transposition of a peripheral doublet to the center.[3] However, ultrastructural analysis alone does not identify all PCD cases, as described subsequently.

Ciliary Motility

Light microscopic examination of the ciliary beat was used as a screening test for PCD in the past. Although this approach may identify immotile or markedly dyskinetic cilia, the ciliary beat may appear normal in some cases of PCD. Digital high-speed

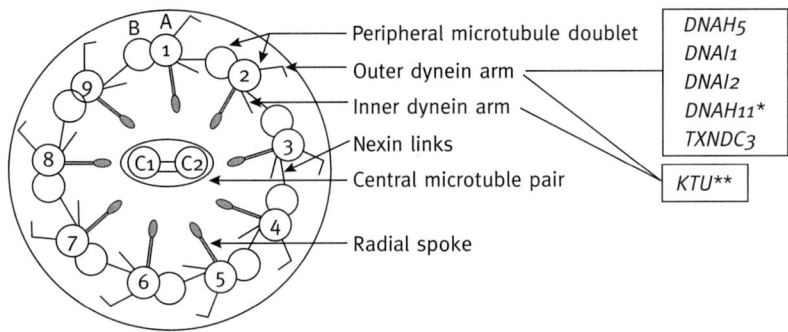

Peripheral microtubules are arranged in nine doublets (two microtubule components, A and B, are merged) with dynein arms arising from the A component. In the center is a pair of microtubules (C1 and C2). Genes mutated in human PCD are shown and linked with the corresponding axonemal structure that is involved. *Mutations seen in patient with normal dynein arms. **Encodes cytoplasmic protein that is required for ODA assembly, and mutations identified in patients with defects involving both outer and inner dynein arms. ODA, outer dynein arm; PCD, primary ciliary dyskinesia.

FIGURE 10.1 Schematic diagram showing 9 + 2 configuration in the cross section of an axoneme. (From Leigh MW, Zariwala MA, Knowles MR. Primary ciliary dyskinesia: improving the diagnostic approach. *Curr Opin Pediatr.* 2009;21:320–325. Reprinted with permission.)

videomicroscopy is used to detect more subtle abnormalities in the ciliary beat pattern and demonstrates that certain ciliary beat patterns are associated with specific ultrastructural defects; low-amplitude stiff beat for an isolated IDA or radial spoke defect; immotile or limited flickering for ODA defects; and circular, whiplike beat for central microtubular defects such as transposition.[7] This specialized technique is incorporated into the evaluation for this disease at some PCD diagnostic centers.

Nasal Nitric Oxide

Several studies have demonstrated that nasal nitric oxide (NNO) is extremely low (10% to 15% of normal) in PCD patients, suggesting that NNO measurement may be a useful screening test. Because low NNO levels also are reported in other disorders, sometimes with overlapping clinical features, such as cystic fibrosis (CF)[1] and panbronchiolitis and nasal polyposis, confirmatory ciliary ultrastructure analysis, genetic mutation analysis, or both are needed to make a firm diagnosis of PCD.[3] NNO measurements are used primarily for research in the United States, and cutoff values to delineate PCD from normal individuals range from 50 to 100 nL/minute depending on the technique used.[2]

Gene Mutation Analysis

Genetic diagnosis of PCD is challenging because of the extensive genetic heterogeneity and the large size of disease-causing genes. To date, six genes are linked with PCD (see Figure 10.1). Two dynein genes, encoding the ODA intermediate chain (DNAI1) and heavy chain (DNAH5), are mutated in approximately 30% to 38% of the families studied. Despite allelic heterogeneity, the presence of founder mutations and mutation clusters led to the development of the clinical molecular genetic test for PCD, which aids in the diagnosis in a subset of patients with the ODA defects. Mutations in other ODA genes (TXNDC3 and DNAI2) are noted in a small fraction (2%) of all patients but are not yet included in the clinical genetic panel.[6]

Genetic tests are very reliable because the presence of biallelic mutations is diagnostic, and the mutation identification techniques are more highly standardized and easier to perform than ciliary ultrastructural analysis. In summary, knowledge about the PCD disease-causing genes is still emerging.

Other Diagnostic Tests

Mucociliary clearance measurement, a noninvasive assessment of ciliary function in the upper and lower airways, is proposed as an adjunctive diagnostic test for PCD.[6]

DIAGNOSTIC APPROACH

The criteria to diagnose PCD include the presence of characteristic phenotypic features and supporting laboratory studies. Only a few phenotypic features are apparent at birth (e.g., neonatal respiratory distress and laterality defects), but some phenotypic features become more obvious during the first years of life; these include chronic sinusitis and recurrent respiratory infections. Others may not become apparent until adulthood (e.g., male infertility). Therefore, the minimum number of phenotypic features varies with age from at least three in early childhood to typically five or more in late childhood and adulthood. The diagnostic approach to PCD (outlined in Table 10.1) is subject to modification with further development and refinement of diagnostic tests for PCD and the better definition of phenotypic features. The availability of genetic testing has enhanced the ability to make a definitive diagnosis, even in individuals with normal ciliary ultrastructure. Further studies are necessary to provide more extensive genetic testing as well as to standardize other diagnostic testing. In the meantime, careful distinction between a definitive diagnosis of PCD and a probable or possible PCD diagnosis is important for clinical decision-making and research.

Criteria for a definitive diagnosis of PCD are the presence of at least three (typically five or more) phenotypic features and a genetic diagnosis, identification of two disease-causing mutations, or identification of ciliary ultrastructural defects that are specific for PCD with no overlap with secondary ciliary defects that occur following airway infections or exposure to airway irritants. Individuals who have ultrastructural defects that also may be seen in secondary ciliary dyskinesia warrant repeat biopsy to determine whether the defect resolves, as expected, after recovery. However, persistence of the defect does not exclude secondary dyskinesia from a chronic airway insult.[6]

ASTHMA AS COMORBIDITY

Asthma may coexist with PCD in some patients and should be recognized and treated. It has an estimated prevalence between 8% and 10% in the general population. Several cases are described in the literature of patients with PCD who have been misdiagnosed and treated for asthma.[8] Recurrent wheeze with chronic rhinosinusitis, chronic otitis media, and bronchiectasis may warrant detailed investigations for this disease. Similarly, any acute and chronic bronchial infection may be associated with a transient ciliary dysfunction and should not be mistaken for PCD. Alternatively, a study by Thomas and colleagues suggests that ciliary dysfunction and ultrastructural abnormalities are closely related to asthma severity.[9] Ciliary dysfunction was a feature of moderate to severe asthma, whereas profound ultrastructural abnormalities were restricted to severe disease. Hence, PCD and severe asthma both can present with ciliary dysfunction and ultrastructural abnormalities. The diagnostic approach mentioned previously, including NNO measurement, can be used for delineation in such complex patients.

PHARMACOLOGIC TREATMENT

Monitoring

PCD patients should be followed regularly at an expert center with a multidisciplinary team. Clinical follow-up is recommended to take place every 2 to 3 months for children and 6 to 12 months for adults. Relevant disciplines include pediatric and adult respiratory medicine; chest physiotherapy; ear, nose, and throat; genetic counseling; and fertility expertise.

Evaluation should consist of detailed symptom assessment (cough, sputum, exacerbations), spirometry, and pulse oximetry. Audiometry should be performed to detect loss of hearing. Regular cough swab cultures in young or nonexpectorating children or

Table 10.1. Diagnosis of Primary Ciliary Dyskinesia

Phenotypic clinical features (at least three, typically five or more)	Neonatal respiratory distress in a term infant Laterality defect (situs inversus totalis or heterotaxy) Chronic, year-round nasal congestion Chronic, year-round productive cough Recurrent lower respiratory tract infections Bronchiectasis Chronic otitis media (middle ear effusion of >6 months' duration) Chronic pansinusitis Male infertility due to impaired sperm motility History of PCD in the immediate family
Laboratory evidence for definitive PCD diagnosis (at least one)	Classic PCD ultrastructural ciliary defect Absence or shortening of outer dynein arms Absence or shortening of inner dynein arms Absence of radial spokes Absence of central pair of microtubules with transposition Genetic diagnosis based on two disease-causing mutations in: EAAH5, DNAI1 Other genes pending definition of disease-causing mutations
Laboratory evidence supporting diagnosis of "probable PCD" (if accompanied by at least three phenotypic clinical features)	Nasal nitric oxide levels in very row range (<100 nL/min)* Ultrastructural ciliary defects that may overlap with secondary ciliary dyskinesia Absence of central pair of microtubules (but no transposition) Absence of cilia on multiple biopsies (ciliary aplasia) Ciliary disorientation PCD genetic testing identifying only one disease-causing mutation Altered ciliary motility on high-speed video microscopy† Altered mucociliary clearance†

* Availability limited to research sites in the United States; more readily available outside United States.
† Specialized diagnostic centers are developing criteria to define specific characteristics that may be consistent with "probable PCD".
PCD, primary ciliary dyskinesia.
From Leigh MW, Zariwala MA, Knowles MR. Primary ciliary dyskinesia: improving the diagnostic approach. *Curr Opin Pediatr.* 2009;21:320–325. Reprinted with permission.

sputum cultures in productive patients are recommended. With exacerbations, regular cultures of sputum and bacterial composition and sensitivity to antibiotics are indicated. Fiberoptic bronchoscopy may be indicated in nonexpectorating patients who do not respond to conventional antibiotics or in patients with persistent atelectasis. Imaging with high-resolution computed tomography (HRCT) is used to detect and grade the occurrence of bronchiectasis.[10] HRCT can also be used to monitor the anatomic extent of lung injury every 4 to 5 years and before lung surgery. Lobectomy or segmentectomy in selected cases with severe, localized, and irreversible bronchiectasis may be necessary.[10]

Medical Interventions

MANAGEMENT OF OTOLOGIC AND SINUS DISEASE

In practice, all PCD patients have chronic otitis media with effusion. This is the reason that patients should be routinely screened for hearing deficits. Hearing aids should be provided to children and adults with conductive hearing impairment (deficit of >30 decibels). These can usually be discontinued at adolescence because chronic otitis media spontaneously becomes milder during puberty. Tympanostomy tubes are not recommended routinely because they can lead to chronic otorrhea, and evidence for benefit is conflicting. Aggressive use of antibiotics to manage otitis media may lead to resistant bacteria.

Like otitis media, chronic rhinitis and sinusitis affect almost all individuals with PCD. Chronic rhinosinusitis is managed symptomatically with nasal glucocorticoids, nasal and sinus lavage with saline, and intermittent courses of systemic antibiotics. Sometimes topical anticholinergics reduce nasal secretion. Sinus surgery may promote drainage and delivery of topical medications.

MUCUS CLEARANCE

Enhancing mucus clearance is the cornerstone of daily therapy in patients with PCD. Cough is the major route for mucus clearance, and instruction in cough techniques should be given and cough encouraged. Routine airway clearance using any of the available physiotherapy techniques such as positive expiratory pressure breathing and postural drainage should be done by all patients.

Mucolytics are of little benefit. Inhaled acetylcysteine is an irritant of the airway mucosa, whereas inhaled recombinant human deoxyribonuclease may be beneficial for purulent sputum in selected patients.[11] Inhaled mannitol is being explored for use in CF and chronic bronchitis patients.

Bronchial hyperresponsiveness may be observed in patients with chronic suppurative lung disease. The use of bronchodilators should be on an individual basis after the demonstration of a significant bronchodilator effect or a clinical trial to assess efficacy.

Maximal bronchodilation may improve the effectiveness of cough, and inhaled anticholinergics and β_2-agonists are regularly used for treatment. In addition, inhaled β_2-agonists may increase ciliary beat frequency.

ANTIBIOTICS

Common infecting organisms include *Haemophilus influenzae, Staphylococcus aureus,* and *Streptococcus pneumoniae.* Early therapeutic intervention results in better symptom control and slowing of lung function deterioration. Whenever possible, antibiotics should be selected on the basis of sputum or cough swab cultures and sensitivity. Occasionally, fiberoptic bronchoscopy with bronchoalveolar lavage[12] or bronchial washing may be necessary in nonexpectorating children to obtain adequate specimens. Antibiotic clearance is normal in patients with PCD. Multidrug-resistant bacteria, such as *Pseudomonas aeruginosa,* but also nontuberculous mycobacteria, may be isolated from adult patients. In these cases, treatment with intravenous and inhaled antibiotics is similar to that recommended in CF.[13]

There is no evidence to recommend prophylactic antibiotics. However, in children who require repeated courses of oral antibiotics, prophylaxis may be considered. An alternate regimen rotating three different classes of oral antibiotics may be instituted to avoid antibiotic resistance. High-dose antibiotics should be given at the first sign of worsening respiratory symptoms or deterioration of lung function.[10]

ANTI-INFLAMMATORY TREATMENT

Neutrophilic airway inflammation and elevated levels of interleukins are observed in children with PCD, but evidence for anti-inflammatory treatment is lacking. There is no rationale for prescribing inhaled corticosteroids, unless coincident asthma exists, in which case it should be treated based on the clinical or spirometric response.[10]

Adjunctive Measures

Patients with PCD should be appropriately immunized with the pneumococcal and yearly influenza vaccines. Contact with infected individuals should be avoided. Prophylaxis against respiratory syncytial virus by means of palivizumab during the first winter of life may be justified if the diagnosis is made in the first months of life. Any exposure to respiratory irritants, such as tobacco smoke, should be avoided. Any associated respiratory risk factor, such as malnutrition or gastroesophageal reflux, should be addressed. Surgical removal of localized irreversible bronchiectasis may be proposed in selected cases, but only after careful preparation using appropriate antibiotics and physiotherapy. Lung transplantation may be useful for the exceptional patients (usually adults) with end stage lung disease.[10]

Counseling

Patients should be informed as early as possible about infertility and referred to an appropriate specialist. Genetic counseling should be offered to patients to provide information about the risk for disease transmission to their children. Counseling also should be provided for the choice of education and work, ideally in an environment with less risk for infections and exposure to airborne irritants.

INTRODUCTION TO CYSTIC FIBROSIS

The name *cystic fibrosis* refers to the characteristic fibrosis and cyst formation in the pancreas, and the disorder is caused by a gene mutation for the protein called *cystic fibrosis transmembrane conductance regulator* (CFTR), required to regulate the components of sweat, digestive fluids, and mucus. CFTR regulates the movement of chloride and sodium ions across epithelial membranes in tubes, such as the bronchial and gastrointestinal epithelia, and all exocrine glands, such as those located in sweat glands and the pancreas. The excessive reabsorption of water and abnormal movement of chloride and sodium lead to blockage of the passages of affected organs with thickened secretions.

The presence of gram-negative bacteria, such as mucoid *P. aeruginosa,* leads to an inflammatory response, airway damage, bronchiectasis, and progressive obstructive airway disease. The morbidity and mortality in patients with CF is most commonly a result of severe lung disease and respiratory failure. Other organ systems involved in CF include the upper respiratory tract, hepatobiliary system, gastrointestinal tract and pancreas, endocrine system, and, less commonly, skin and joints.[12]

There are more than 1,900 known mutations that can lead to CF, and the most common, ΔF508-CFTR, is a deletion (Δ signifying deletion) of three nucleotides in the coding DNA that results in a loss of the amino acid phenylalanine (F) at the 508th position on the protein.[14] This mutation accounts for two-thirds of CF cases worldwide and 90% of the cases in the United States.[15] CF has the highest prevalence of 1 in 3,000 Caucasian children and 1 in 2,300 in the Ashkenazi Jewish population. Other ethnic and racial groups are less commonly affected, reflected in the prevalence of 1 in 10,000 in the Latino American population and 1 in 15,000 in African Americans. The disease is uncommon in Africa and Asia, with reported frequencies ranging from 1 in 35,000 to 1 in 350,000.

CLINICAL PRESENTATIONS BY AGE GROUP

Prenatal

HIGH-RISK PREGNANCIES

The prenatal diagnosis of CF is usually established in pregnancies known to be at increased risk based on the CF carrier status of the parents. In cases in which the genotype status of the parents is known, the diagnosis of CF can be confirmed or excluded with a high degree of certainty by direct mutation analysis performed on fetal cells obtained by chorionic villus sampling at 10 weeks or cultured amniotic fluid cells collected at 15 to 18 weeks. Prenatal testing should always be carried out in conjunction with an experienced geneticist. It is mandatory postnatally to carry out sweat testing in all cases in which the diagnosis of CF is made or excluded on the basis of prenatal DNA analysis.[16]

An alternative for at-risk couples is the use of preimplantation genetic diagnosis to screen embryos before implantation. After in vitro fertilization, a cleavage-stage biopsy is carried out on day 2 or 3, and one or two cells are removed for genetic analysis. Normal or carrier embryos are then transferred to establish pregnancy. This procedure can be followed by chorionic villus sampling or amniocentesis to confirm the original diagnosis.[17]

FETAL INTESTINAL OBSTRUCTION

The diagnosis is sometimes suggested by prenatal ultrasonographic findings, including a hyperechoic fetal bowel pattern and meconium peritonitis in pregnancies not known to be at increased risk for CF. Parental CF carrier testing with fetal mutation analysis in at-risk couples is considered in such cases.

Neonatal

Children with CF are often initially misdiagnosed as having food allergies, celiac disease, asthma, or bronchitis. The median age of clinical diagnosis on the basis of signs and symptoms other than meconium ileus is 14.5 months, compared with 0.2 months for meconium ileus and 0.5 months for newborn screening.[18]

MECONIUM ILEUS

Approximately 18% of patients with CF present with intestinal obstruction in the immediate postnatal period secondary to inspissation of tenacious meconium in the ileum. About 50% of cases are complicated by peritonitis, volvulus, atresia, necrosis, perforation, or pseudocyst formation of the bowel. Among full-term neonates with meconium ileus, CF is confirmed in approximately 98% of cases.[19] Patients presumptively should be treated for this diagnosis, and parents appropriately counseled, pending the results of sweat testing or mutation analysis.

MECONIUM PLUG SYNDROME

The meconium plug syndrome, in which there is transient distal colonic obstruction relieved by the passage of a meconium plug, may be the presenting manifestation of CF in the neonatal period. This syndrome also may occur in association with prematurity, hypotonia, hypermagnesemia, sepsis, hypothyroidism, or Hirschsprung's disease, but its presence should always alert one to the possibility of CF.[20]

JEJUNAL ATRESIA

Neonatal intestinal obstruction secondary to jejunal atresia, often in association with volvulus and meconium peritonitis, may be a presenting feature of CF.

LIVER DISEASE

Neonates with CF may present with prolonged obstructive jaundice, presumably secondary to obstruction of extrahepatic bile ducts by thick bile along with intrahepatic bile stasis. There may be associated hepatomegaly.[21]

PULMONARY MANIFESTATIONS

Respiratory symptoms may begin during the first month of life. Manifestations include cough, wheezing, chest retractions, and tachypnea. The chest radiograph may show hyperinflation. Segmental or lobar atelectasis, particularly involving the right upper lobe, is highly suggestive of CF.[22]

GROWTH FAILURE

Failure to regain birth weight by 2 weeks or inadequate weight gain at 4 to 6 weeks of age is common in neonates with CF. Growth failure often occurs despite normal or even increased caloric intake.

Infancy and Childhood

The diagnosis of CF in infants and young children is usually made based on respiratory tract symptoms or steatorrhea, along with some degree of failure to thrive.

UPPER RESPIRATORY TRACT

The upper respiratory tract is usually involved secondary to abnormal mucous gland secretions and hypertrophy and edema of the mucous membranes. Nasal polyps occur frequently and may be present at an early age. Their presence in a child is always an indication for a sweat test. Sweat testing should also be considered in a child with recurrent or chronic sinusitis refractory to antimicrobial therapy.[23]

LOWER RESPIRATORY TRACT

A CF diagnosis is first considered because of pulmonary symptoms in about 50% of patients. Lower respiratory manifestations may appear months or years after birth. CF should be considered in every patient with chronic or recurrent lower respiratory tract findings such as prolonged or recurrent pneumonia, bronchitis, bronchiectasis, atelectasis, refractory asthma, and empyema. The most consistent and prominent feature of pulmonary involvement is chronic cough. Cough is often initiated by an upper respiratory infection, after which it persists for weeks or may never resolve. Older patients may expectorate mucopurulent sputum, particularly in association with pulmonary exacerbations. Crackles, rhonchi, and wheezes can be auscultated in the presence of chest wall retractions and tachypnea. Air trapping occurs because of progressive airway obstruction, with an increase in the anterior-posterior diameter of the chest. Digital clubbing is almost universal in symptomatic patients older than 4 years of age. The presence of digital clubbing in a patient with chronic respiratory symptoms is always an indication for a sweat test.[19] Isolation of a mucoid variant of *P. aeruginosa* from the respiratory tract is almost uniquely associated with CF and again is an indication for a sweat test. However, organisms like *Burkholderia cepacia* and *S. aureus* in the sputum may suggest or support this diagnosis.[12]

GASTROINTESTINAL TRACT

Steatorrhea in infants and young children is strongly suggestive of CF. Clinical features include abdominal protuberance; crampy abdominal pain; flatulence; frequent, bulky, oily, malodorous stools; and poor weight gain. Associated rectal prolapse may occur. Other gastrointestinal manifestations of CF in infancy and childhood include intussusception, pancreatitis, gastroesophageal reflux, and mucoid impaction of the appendix.[24]

Adolescents and Adults

Approximately 8% of patients with CF have their diagnosis first made during adolescence and adulthood.[19] Many have a history of typical, somewhat mild respiratory tract and gastrointestinal features of CF with onset in childhood, often associated with a poor growth pattern. However, pulmonary symptoms may first become manifest after the age of 13 years in some patients. Chronic sinusitis, chronic cough, sputum production, wheezing, recurrent pneumonia, and chest imaging abnormalities are common presenting features. The diagnosis of CF should be considered in patients with hemoptysis, allergic bronchopulmonary aspergillosis (ABPA), and poorly controlled asthma, and in those in whom *P. aeruginosa* is recovered from the respiratory tract. All adolescents and adults with unexplained chronic lung disease, malabsorption, or both deserve a sweat test.[24]

Older patients may present with cirrhosis in the absence of pulmonary symptoms. CF should be considered in any patient with obscure liver disease. Other unusual presentations include pancreatitis, intussusception, night blindness, and intestinal obstruction.[24]

DIAGNOSIS OF CYSTIC FIBROSIS

The diagnosis of CF is based on the presence of one or more characteristic phenotypic features (Table 10.2), a history of CF in a sibling, or a positive newborn screening test, plus laboratory evidence of a CFTR abnormality as documented by elevated sweat chloride concentrations, identification of mutations in each CFTR gene known to cause CF, or in vivo demonstration of characteristic abnormalities in ion transport across the nasal epithelium.[25]

Table 10.2. Phenotypic Features Consistent with a Diagnosis of Cystic Fibrosis

1. Chronic sinopulmonary disease, manifested by:

   a. Persistent colonization/infection with typical CF pathogens, including *Staphylococcus aureus*, nontypeable *Haemophilus influenzae*, mucoid and nonmucoid *Pseudomonas aeruginosa*, *Stenotrophomonas maltophilia*, and *Burkholderia cepacia*
   b. Chronic cough and sputum production
   c. Persistent chest radiograph abnormalities (e.g., bronchiectasis, atelectasis, infiltrates, hyperinflation)
   d. Airway obstruction, manifested by wheezing and air trapping
   e. Nasal polyps; radiographic or CT abnormalities of the paranasal sinuses
   f. Digital clubbing

2. Gastrointestinal and nutritional abnormalities, including:

   a. Intestinal: meconium ileus, distal intestinal obstruction syndrome, rectal prolapse
   b. Pancreatic: pancreatic insufficiency, recurrent acute pancreatitis, chronic pancreatitis, pancreatic abnormalities on imaging
   c. Hepatic: prolonged neonatal jaundice, chronic hepatic disease manifested by clinical or histologic evidence of focal biliary cirrhosis or multilobular cirrhosis
   d. Nutritional: failure to thrive (protein-calorie malnutrition), hypoproteinemia and edema, complications secondary to fat-soluble vitamin deficiencies

3. Salt loss syndromes: acute salt depletion, chronic metabolic alkalosis
4. Genital abnormalities in males, resulting in obstructive azoospermia

From Farrell PM, Rosenstein BJ, White TB, et al. Guidelines for diagnosis of cystic fibrosis in newborns through older adults: Cystic Fibrosis Foundation consensus report. *J Pediatr.* 2008;153(2):S4–S14. Reprinted with permission.

Sweat Test

The sweat test remains the gold standard for the confirmation or exclusion of CF. During the first 24 hours after birth, sweat electrolyte values may be transiently elevated in normal infants. After the first 2 days of life, there is a rapid decline in sweat electrolyte concentrations, and an elevated value can be used to confirm the diagnosis of CF. The Cystic Fibrosis Foundation requires that sweat testing conducted at accredited CF care centers adhere to the standards recommended by a Cystic Fibrosis Foundation committee comprising CF center directors. The only acceptable procedure is the quantitative pilocarpine iontophoresis sweat test.[25,26]

Sweat test results should be interpreted in relation to the patient's clinical history and physical examination by a physician knowledgeable about the disease. The test results need to be consistent with the clinical picture; no single laboratory result is sufficient to establish or rule out the diagnosis of CF. The diagnosis should be made only if there is an elevated sweat chloride concentration on two separate occasions in a patient with one or more typical phenotypic features, a history of CF in a sibling, or a positive newborn screening test. In 0.1% to 1% of cases, the diagnosis of CF is established by way of nasal potential difference measurement, histopathology, and mutation analysis in patients with borderline or normal electrolyte concentrations.[26]

Mutation Analysis

The diagnosis can be confirmed in most patients with CF by a positive sweat test result; however, the cloning of the gene responsible for CF and the identification of disease-producing mutations raise the possibility that DNA testing may be a good substitute for the sweat test in certain circumstances. The presence of mutations known to cause CF in each CFTR gene predicts, with a high degree of certainty, that an individual has CF. To date, more than 1,900 putative CF mutations have been described.[14]

Alterations in the CFTR gene designated as CF-causing mutations should fulfill at least one of the following criteria: the mutation (1) causes a change in amino acid sequence that severely affects CFTR synthesis or function; (2) introduces a premature termination signal; (3) alters invariant nucleotides of intron splice sites; or (4) causes a novel amino acid sequence that does not occur in the normal CFTR genes from at least 100 carriers of CF mutations from the patient's ethnic group.[26]

Nasal Potential Difference Measurements

Abnormalities of ion transport in respiratory epithelia of patients with CF are associated with a different pattern of nasal PD compared with normal epithelia. Nasal PD can be measured in patients as young as a few hours of life; older children, ages 2 to 5 years, may require modest sedation.[25]

RECOMMENDED GENERAL PROCESS FOR DIAGNOSING CYSTIC FIBROSIS

In individuals presenting with symptoms of CF (see Table 10.2) or a positive family history, the following diagnostic process (Figure 10.2) is recommended:

1. A diagnosis of CF can be made if the sweat chloride value is at least 60 mmol/L. A second, confirmatory sweat chloride test is recommended unless mutation analysis identifies the presence of two CF-causing mutations.

2. A sweat chloride value of more than 39 mmol/L in individuals older than 6 months is not consistent with a diagnosis of CF. CF is unlikely in this group. However, two identified CF-causing mutations can occur in this group; these individuals have CF and should be followed in a CF care center.

3. Individuals with sweat chloride values in the intermediate range (30 to 59 mmol/L for infants younger than 6 months; 40 to 59 mmol/L for older individuals) should undergo extensive CFTR mutation analysis (i.e., expanded panel of CFTR mutations, evaluation for deletions, or gene sequencing).

   a. In the presence of two CF-causing mutations, a diagnosis of CF can be made.

   b. Individuals with no or one CF-causing mutation and clinical findings suggestive of CFTR dysfunction (i.e., obstructive azoospermia, bronchiectasis, or acute, recurrent, or chronic pancreatitis) may be diagnosed with a CFTR-related disorder, depending on their clinical picture or family history, and are at risk for CF. Sweat chloride testing should be repeated in infants by age 2 to 6 months and immediately in older individuals. If sweat chloride values remain in the intermediate range on repeat testing, then further assessment should be performed at a CF care center that can provide basic and ancillary testing to clarify the diagnosis, including:

- Clinical assessment
- Expanded genetic testing
- Exocrine pancreatic function tests
- Respiratory tract culture for CF-associated pathogens, especially *P. aeruginosa*

Depending on clinical presentation, assessment also may include ancillary tests, such as:

- Genital evaluation in males (i.e., genital examination, rectal ultrasound, semen analysis)
- Pancreatic imaging
- HRCT
- Bronchoalveolar lavage, including microbiology assessment
- Pulmonary function testing (not routinely recommended in infants)
- Nasal Potential difference (PD) testing
- Exclusionary testing for ciliary dyskinesia and immune deficiency

Significant clinical signs or symptoms of CF, laboratory indication of Pancreatic

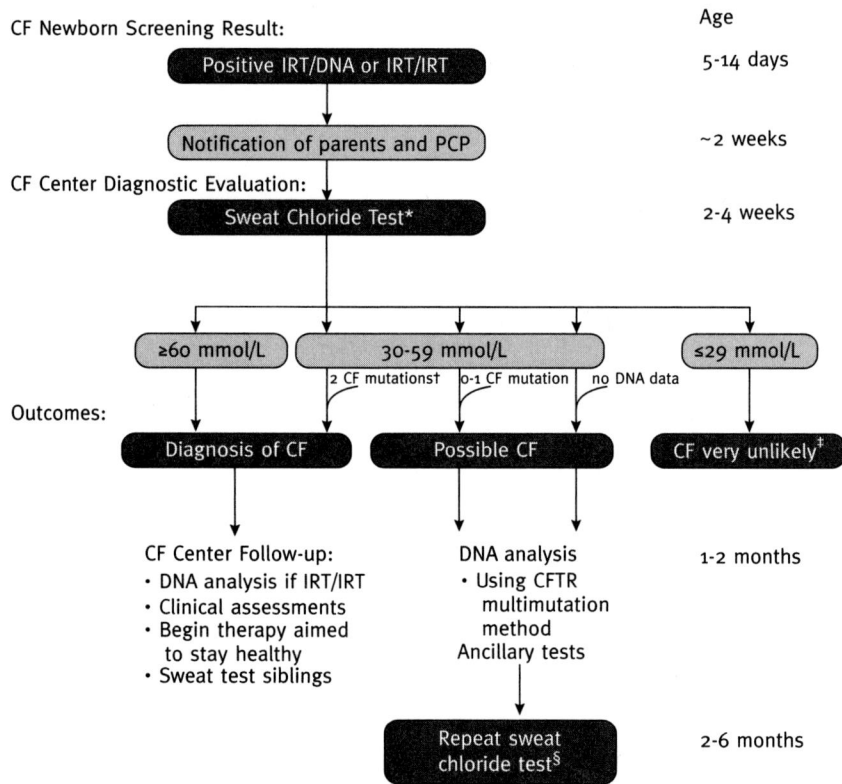

FIGURE 10.2 The cystic fibrosis diagnostic process for screened newborns. (From Farrell PM, Rosenstein BJ, White TB, et al. Guidelines for diagnosis of cystic fibrosis in newborns through older adults: Cystic Fibrosis Foundation consensus report. *J Pediatr.* 2008;153[2]:S4–S14. Reprinted with permission.)

insufficiency (PI), or a positive culture for a CF-associated pathogen (especially *P. aeruginosa*) should be considered strongly suggestive of CF. Individuals who have sweat chloride values in the intermediate range and exhibit no significant signs of CF should be monitored periodically for the appearance of symptoms until the diagnosis can be ruled in or out.[26]

ASTHMA AS COMORBIDITY

Cystic fibrosis and asthma are not always easily distinguishable. Wheeze, whether as in asthma or CF, involves airway mucosal edema, mechanical obstruction by accumulated secretions, airway smooth muscle contraction, and the dynamic collapse of airways. It occurs frequently in both diseases, and for this reason, it is difficult to determine which patients have concomitant asthma and which wheeze as a result of their underlying CF lung disease. There is, however, no consensus on how to define "CF asthma."[27] Acute airway obstruction reversed by bronchodilators, especially if seasonal or allergen induced, can be a valuable but not sensitive indicator. Similarly, laboratory data such as eosinophilia or high immunoglobulin E (IgE) levels are also of limited value.[28]

Standard spirometric tests, although useful to assess lung disease severity, are not reliable tools for diagnosing asthma in CF patients. The reason for the apparent ineffectiveness of lung function testing in patients suspected of having asthma is the degree of variability in lung function. Forced expiratory volume in 1 second (FEV_1) and forced vital capacity (FVC) can vary as much as 15% to 20%, even when testing on the same day. Likewise, the role of bronchodilator responsiveness in patients with CF is not well defined, and several studies report important limitations. CF patients often show a degree of bronchodilator responsiveness whether or not they have "CF asthma."[29]

Bronchial hyperresponsiveness (BHR) is a typical finding with asthma but not exclusive to this disease, and even though it is found in many CF patients, especially those with poorer lung function, the underlying mechanism is still debatable.[30] Even the hypothesized role of atopy in "CF asthma" needs clarification. According to some studies, a strong association exists between atopy and BHR.[31] However, other authors believe atopy may not be a significant risk factor for developing BHR in patients with CF.[32] BHR may be associated with colonization or infection with *P. aeruginosa* in patients with this disease, a risk factor that is probably more important than atopy.[32]

Asthma and CF differ not only clinically, but also in terms of immunopathology. CF is associated mainly with neutrophils in bronchoalveolar lavage (BAL), whereas asthma is primarily associated with eosinophils and lymphocytes in BAL; more severe forms of asthma, however, also are associated with neutrophils. A T_H2 immune response is characteristic of atopic asthma but, in general, CF does not fit this paradigm. However, CF patients with chronic *P. aeruginosa* infection and ABPA also develop predominantly a T_H2 type of response.[28] In summary, despite the similarities found in CF and asthma, the immunopathologic mechanisms are considerably different.

Some authors suggest a common genetic background linking asthma and CF, indicating that atopy in CF patients could result from the same genetic defect responsible for this disease.[33] Nevertheless, studies linking asthma and CFTR gene mutation heterozygosity have led to conflicting results. Dahl and colleagues, in a 15-year follow-up study from the Copenhagen (Denmark) City Heart Study, found that CF DF508 heterozygotes may be overrepresented among individuals with asthma and may have poorer lung function than noncarriers. Furthermore, DF508 heterozygosity, in the context of familial predisposition to asthma, may be associated with a greater annual FEV_1 decline.[34]

CF patients show several risk factors that might influence atopic progression, such as increased permeability of the bronchial mucosa, a defective secretory IgA system, and entrapment of antigens in infected areas of the lungs in association with ciliary dysfunction.[28] This could result in increased antigenic access through the tracheobronchial tree, favoring a constant stimulation of IgE production. The sensitization process occurs in genetically susceptible individuals and requires allergen processing by antigen-presenting cells, which then augment the T_H2 response within the bronchoalveolar lymphoid tissue.

Aspergillus fumigatus is the most prevalent mold allergen identified in CF patients. Colonization of the lower respiratory tract with this organism is common in patients with CF, with a reported incidence of 57% and a prevalence of 40%.[35] This organism is a widely distributed spore-bearing fungus and causes invasive pulmonary aspergillosis, aspergilloma, and different forms of hypersensitivity diseases in humans. Included are allergic asthma, hypersensitivity pneumonitis, and ABPA.

ABPA is a disease primarily occurring in patients with asthma (1% to 2% of asthma patients) or with CF (1% to 7.8% of CF patients).[36] The CFTR mutation is implicated in the etiology of ABPA, but no significant association with any particular CFTR genotype is documented.[37] Strong evidence exists that the atopic status may influence the appearance of comorbid conditions in patients with CF, such as "CF asthma," mold sensitization, and ABPA.

CF patients appear to be more prone to mold sensitization, in particular to *A. fumigatus*. Age, bacterial lung colonization, genetics, and the immunologic response of the host appear to be important factors for mold sensitization.[28]

PHARMACOLOGIC TREATMENT

The past and recently available treatment strategies for CF are summarized in Tables 10.3 and 10.4.[38]

Stem Cell and Gene Therapy Treatments

Since the gene for CFTR was identified in 1989, the CF research community has maintained great hope for a therapy that will correct the underlying defect through genetic manipulation. However, this has proved extremely challenging for a variety of reasons. The difficulty of gene therapy is reflected by the variable results of the 25 CF gene therapy trials performed to date.[14]

INTRODUCTION TO α_1-ANTITRYPSIN DEFICIENCY

α_1-Antitrypsin (AAT) deficiency is an autosomal codominant disease that increases the risk for emphysema in adults and causes chronic liver disease, cirrhosis, and hepatocellular carcinoma in children and adults.[39] It affects approximately 1 in 2,000 to 1 in 5,000 subjects and continues to be underdiagnosed.[40] AAT is a 52-kDa, single-chain glycoprotein with a 394–amino sequence that is synthesized primarily in the liver and functions as a serine protease inhibitor, providing essential protection to lung tissue against the actions of proteolytic enzymes, such as neutrophil elastase and proteinase 3.[41] More than 120 alleles for AAT deficiency are identified thus far. The M allele is the "normal" variant, and the most common deficiency variants are S and Z. The Z allele is usually responsible for severe deficiency and the disease state.[40]

EPIDEMIOLOGY

The SERPINA1 gene, located on the long arm of chromosome 14 (14q31–32.3), encodes the AAT protein.[41] Severe deficiency, classified by a serum AAT level below the protective threshold of 11 µM, has the PiZZ genotype. The highest prevalence of the Z variant is found in northern Europe, particularly southern Scandinavia.[42]

AAT deficiency is relatively common but underrecognized.[39] The combined results of the largest studies in the United States yield a frequency estimate of 1 in 4,455, suggesting that the number of PiZZ subjects in this country is approximately 70,000.[40] One example of underrecognition is that fewer than 10,000 AAT deficiency subjects are currently receiving augmentation therapy.[40]

PATHOPHYSIOLOGY

AAT is the prototypic member of the serine protease inhibitor (serpin) superfamily of proteins. Conformational instability of the β-sheet structure of serpins secondary to mutations and polymerization leads to serpinopathies. There may be a gain-of-toxic-function defect, that is, accumulation of the protein responsible for liver cirrhosis in AAT deficiency, or a loss-of-function defect responsible for emphysema. Hence, in PiZZ AAT deficiency, polymerization causes retention of AAT aggregates in hepatocytes causing liver cirrhosis. Similarly, loss of the anti-inflammatory effects of AAT and loss of protection of lung tissue against the actions of proteolytic enzymes, such as neutrophil elastase and proteinase 3, predisposes to emphysema.[43]

CLINICAL FEATURES

AAT deficiency can cause lung disease, emphysema, and bronchiectasis; liver disease, chronic hepatitis, cirrhosis, and hepatocellular carcinoma; skin disease; and panniculitis and is associated with vasculitis, especially anticytoplasmic antibody-positive vasculitis such as Wegener's granulomatosis.[40] In this chapter, the authors focus on the clinical manifestations of AAT deficiency in the lung.

Emphysema

The distinctive features of emphysema associated with AAT deficiency may include the

Table 10.3. Summary of Previous Recommendations

TREATMENT	RECOMMENDATION	CERTAINTY OF ESTIMATE OF: NET BENEFIT	NET BENEFIT	RECOM-MENDATION
Inhaled tobramycin—moderate to severe disease*	For individuals with CF ≥6 yr of age with moderate to severe lung disease and *Pseudomonas aeruginosa* persistently present in cultures of the airways, the CF Foundation strongly recommends the chronic use of inhaled tobramycin to improve lung function and quality of life and reduce exacerbations.	High	Substantial	A
Inhaled tobramycin—mild disease*	For individuals with CF ≥6 yr of age with mild lung disease and *P. aeruginosa* persistently present in cultures of the airways, the CF Foundation recommends the chronic use of inhaled tobramycin to reduce exacerbations.	Moderate	Moderate	B
Dornase alfa—moderate to severe disease*	For individuals with CF 6 years of age and older, with moderate to severe lung disease, the CF Foundation strongly recommends the chronic use of dornase alfa to improve lung function, improve the quality of life, and reduce exacerbations.	High	Substantial	A
Dornase alfa—mild disease*	For individuals with CF ≥6 yr of age with asymptomatic or mild lung disease, the CF Foundation recommends the chronic use of dornase alfa to improve lung function and reduce exacerbations.	High	Moderate	B
Inhaled hypertonic saline	For individuals with CF ≥6 yr of age, the CF Foundation recommends the chronic use of inhaled hypertonic saline to improve lung function and quality of life and reduce exacerbations.	Moderate	Moderate	B

(continued)

Table 10.3. (Continued)

TREATMENT	RECOMMENDATION	CERTAINTY OF ESTIMATE OF: NET BENEFIT	NET BENEFIT	RECOMMENDATION
Azithromycin with *P. aeruginosa*	For individuals with CF ≥6 yr with *P. aeruginosa* persistently present in cultures of the airways, the CF Foundation recommends the chronic use of azithromycin to improve lung function and reduce exacerbations.	High	Moderate	B
Oral anti-staphylococcal antibiotics, prophylactic	For individuals with CF the CF Foundation recommends against the prophylactic use of oral antistaphylococcal antibiotics to improve lung function and quality of life or reduce exacerbations.	Moderate	Negative	D
Inhaled corticosteroids	For individuals with CF ≥6 yr of age without asthma or allergic bronchopulmonary aspergillosis, the CF Foundation recommends against the routine use of inhaled corticosteroids to improve lung function or quality of life and reduce pulmonary exacerbations.	High	Zero	D
Oral corticosteroids	For individuals with CF ≥6 yr of age without asthma or allergic bronchopulmonary aspergillosis, the CF Foundation recommends against the chronic use of oral corticosteroids to improve lung function and quality of life or reduce exacerbations.	High	Negative	D
Other inhaled antibiotics	For individuals with CF ≥6 yr of age with *P. aeruginosa* persistently present in cultures of the airways, the CF Foundation concludes that the evidence is insufficient to recommend for or against the chronic use of other inhaled antibiotics (i.e., carbenicillin, ceftazidime, colistin, gentamicin) to improve lung function and quality of life or reduce exacerbations.	Low	—	I

(continued)

Table 10.3. (Continued)

TREATMENT	RECOMMENDATION	CERTAINTY OF ESTIMATE OF: NET BENEFIT	NET BENEFIT	RECOMMENDATION
Oral antipseudomonal antibiotics	For individuals with CF ≥6 yr of age with *P. aeruginosa* persistently present in cultures of the airways, the CF Foundation concludes that the evidence is insufficient to recommend for or against the routine use of chronic oral antipseudomonal antibiotics to improve lung function and quality of life or reduce exacerbations.	Low	—	I
Leukotriene modifiers	For individuals with CF ≥6 yr of age, the CF Foundation concludes that the evidence is insufficient to recommend for or against the routine chronic use of leukotriene modifiers to improve lung function and quality of life or reduce exacerbations.	Low	—	I
Inhaled or oral *N*-acetylcysteine or inhaled glutathione	For individuals with CF ≥6 yr of age the CF Foundation concludes that the evidence is insufficient to recommend for or against the chronic use of inhaled or oral *N*-acetylcysteine or inhaled glutathione to improve lung function and quality of life or reduce exacerbations.	Low	—	I
Inhaled anticholinergics	For individuals with CF ≥6 yr of age, the CF Foundation concludes that the evidence is insufficient to recommend for or against the chronic use of inhaled anticholinergic bronchodilators to improve lung function and quality of life or reduce exacerbations.	Low	—	I

*Severity of lung disease is defined by FEV1% predicted as follows: normal, >90% predicted; mildly impaired, 70%–89% predicted; moderately impaired, 40%–69% predicted; and severely impaired, <40% predicted.

CF, cystic fibrosis.

Reprinted with permission of the American Thoracic Society. Copyright © 2013 American Thoracic Society. Mogayzel PJ Jr, Naureckas ET, Robinson KA, et al. Cystic fibrosis pulmonary guidelines: chronic medications for maintenance of lung health. *Am J Respir Crit Care Med.* 2013;187:680–689.

Table 10.4. Summary of New and Modified Recommendations

TREATMENT	RECOMMENDATION	CERTAINTY OF NET BENEFIT	ESTIMATE OF NET BENEFIT	RECOMMENDATION
Ivacaftor*	For individuals with CF ≥6 yr of age with at least one G551D CFTR mutation, the Pulmonary Clinical Practice Guidelines Committee strongly recommends the chronic use of ivacaftor to improve lung function and quality of life and reduce exacerbations.	High	Substantial	A
Inhaled aztreonam—moderate to severe disease†	For individuals with CF ≥6 yr of age with moderate to severe lung disease and *Pseudomonas aeruginosa* persistently present in cultures of the airways, the CF Foundation strongly recommends the chronic use of inhaled aztreonam to improve lung function and quality of life.	High	Substantial	A
Inhaled aztreonam—mild disease†	For individuals with CF ≥6 yr of age with mild lung disease and *P. aeruginosa* persistently present in cultures of the airways, the CF Foundation recommends the chronic use of inhaled aztreonam to improve lung function and quality of life.	Moderate	Moderate	B
Chronic use of ibuprofen (age < 18 yr)	For individuals with CF 6–17 yr of age with an FEV_1 ≥ 60% predicted, the CF Foundation recommends the chronic use of oral ibuprofen, at a peak plasma concentration of 50–100 μg/mL, to slow the loss of lung function.	Moderate	Moderate	B

(continued)

Table 10.4. (Continued)

TREATMENT	RECOMMENDATION	CERTAINTY OF NET BENEFIT	ESTIMATE OF NET BENEFIT	RECOM-MENDATION
Chronic use of ibuprofen (age ≥ 18 yr)	For individuals with CF ≥18 yr of age, the CF Foundation concludes that the evidence is insufficient to recommend for or against the chronic use of oral ibuprofen to slow the loss of lung function or reduce exacerbations.	Low	—	I
Azithromycin without *P. aeruginosa*	For individuals with CF ≥6 yr of age without *P. aeruginosa* persistently present in cultures of the airways, the CF Foundation recommends the chronic use of azithromycin should be considered to reduce exacerbations.	Moderate	Small	C
Chronic inhaled β_2-adrenergic receptor agonists	For individuals with CF ≥6 yr of age, the CF Foundation concludes that the evidence is insufficient to recommend for or against chronic use of inhaled β_2-adrenergic receptor agonists to improve lung function and quality of life or reduce exacerbations.	Low	—	I
Oral antistaphylococcal antibiotics, chronic use	For individuals with CF ≥6 yr of age with *Staphylococcus aureus* persistently present in cultures of the airways, the CF Foundation concludes that the evidence is insufficient to recommend for or against the chronic use of oral antistaphylococcal antibiotics to improve lung function and quality of life or reduce exacerbations.	Low	—	I

* CF Foundation personnel did not participate in any activity related to ivacaftor.
† Severity of lung disease is defined by FEV_1% predicted as follows: normal, >90% predicted; mildly impaired, 70%–89% predicted; moderately impaired, 40%–69% predicted; and severely impaired, <40% predicted.

CF, cystic fibrosis.

Reprinted with permission of the American Thoracic Society. Copyright © 2013 American Thoracic Society. Mogayzel PJ Jr, Naureckas ET, Robinson KA, et al. Cystic fibrosis pulmonary guidelines: chronic medications for maintenance of lung health. *Am J Respir Crit Care Med.* 2013;187:680–689.

onset of emphysema in the fourth and fifth decades of life. The classic distribution of the disease is associated with lower lobe predominance; however, all zones of the lung can be affected. This is in contrast to the more apical distribution that occurs in cigarette-induced COPD.[44] However, underutilization of testing and atypical presentation of chest radiographs can result in underrecognition of this disease. Gishen and colleagues reported that 15% of the radiographs were normal and 20% demonstrated the typical pattern of lower lobe lung emphysematous changes in a series of 165 plain chest radiographs from PiZZ subjects.[44] Similarly, Parr and colleagues reported that 64% of PiZZ subjects with evidence of emphysema on CT had basal-prominent emphysema, whereas 36% had apical prominent emphysema.[45]

Bronchiectasis

The frequency of bronchiectasis with AAT deficiency is unclear. Cuvelier and colleagues reported no physiopathologic implications for the AAT genes in the development of bronchiectasis. They suggest that bronchiectasis is a consequence of emphysema in PiZZ subjects rather than a primary effect.[46] However, in a series of 74 PiZZ subjects, Parr and colleagues reported that bronchiectatic changes on chest CT were present in 95% of subjects, with severe, radiologic bronchiectasis in four or more bronchopulmonary segments, together with symptoms of regular sputum production, in 27% of subjects.[47] Current recommendations are to test for AAT deficiency when the cause of bronchiectasis remains unknown and after consideration of the usual etiologies, such as CF, hypogammaglobulinemia, and ciliary dysfunction.[48]

ASTHMA AS COMORBIDITY

Asthma is commonly misdiagnosed for AAT deficiency,[49] possibly secondary to the similar presenting symptoms of cough, sputum production, and wheezing.[50] Also, asthma has been associated with the AAT deficiency population.[51] A history of asthma was reported in 35% of patients, and reversible airflow obstruction, defined as a 12% and 200-mL increase in the FEV_1, was seen in 61% of participants over three serial post-bronchodilator spirometry tests in the National Heart, Lung and Blood Institute (NHLBI) Registry of AAT deficiency (N = 1,129).[52] Sixty-six percent of patients had wheezing, with a mean age at onset of 31 ± 16 years in the large cohort of 1,052 AAT deficiency subjects from the NHLBI Registry. A clinical diagnosis of asthma was present in 21% of the cohort as defined by reversible airflow obstruction, recurrent attacks of wheezing, and a reported diagnosis of asthma or allergy. Importantly, 12.5% of the subjects with a normal FEV_1 met the definition of asthma. An IgE level was elevated in 17% of the cohort and was associated with a history of allergy. The multivariable analysis showed that the bronchodilator response, but not asthma, age, and smoking, was a significant predictor of an FEV_1 decline.[53]

At a genomic level, studies on pathways that might modify the clinical course of AAT deficiency have identified interleukin-10 (IL-10) polymorphisms as being associated with a worse FEV_1 and FEV_1/FVC ratio.[54] Because IL-10 polymorphisms are associated with asthma severity, the finding is important in that asthma genes may play a role even in patients with AAT deficiency without clinical asthma. The difficulty in distinguishing asthma and COPD in patients with AAT deficiency is particularly challenging, and recognizing the overlap between the two conditions is important to ensure appropriate therapeutic strategies.

DIAGNOSIS

Screening

Recommendations for screening for AAT deficiency are available from the American Thoracic Society/European Respiratory Society (ATS/ERS) statement on diagnosis and management of this condition.[48] The four main benefits of early detection of AAT deficiency are as follows:

1. Smoking prevention or cessation
2. Minimization of hazards of occupational respiratory pollutants

3. Opportunities to receive augmentation therapy
4. Potential for family planning and guided genetic counseling and testing

Early diagnosis with screening programs allows this to be instigated while lung function is preserved. Symptomatic subjects may require lifelong therapy, and early detection may reduce the clinical and economic burdens of progressive lung deterioration. Screening with genotyping is recommended. AAT levels may be less expensive, but establishing the genotype gives more information about the likelihood of developing the clinical consequences of the disease.[39]

Lifestyle and Behavior Modification Strategies

Smoking cessation advice is effective in subjects with AAT deficiency. Follow-up of the original subjects from the 1970s AAT deficiency screening program in Sweden shows that smoking is less common than in control subjects.[39] Also, knowledge of how to diagnose AAT deficiency should aid affected subjects in their occupational choices, allowing them to avoid exposure to environmental pollutants, such as those associated with steel manufacturing.[39]

PHARMACOLOGIC TREATMENT

The treatment of COPD applies to AAT deficiency according to the Global Initiative for Diagnosis, Management, and Prevention of COPD guidelines. Most subjects with AAT deficiency and obstructive lung disease find symptomatic benefit from bronchodilators, even though objective bronchodilator responsiveness may be lacking. Those with proven bronchial hyperreactivity may be given an inhaled glucocorticosteroid with the presumption that a decrease in bronchial inflammation may reduce the loss in FEV_1 over time. Antibiotics are recommended for treatment of exacerbations triggered by bacterial infections. Portable oxygen is useful for those who desaturate with exercise, but otherwise long-term oxygen therapy is only recommended for those with respiratory insufficiency at rest. This should be prescribed in concordance with the ATS/ERS criteria. Oral glucocorticosteroids can be cautiously considered in subjects with a clear asthmatic component to their disease, and long-term use should be avoided when possible.

Comorbidities that accompany COPD outside the setting of AAT deficiency should always be borne in mind. These include depression, anxiety, and malnutrition. Pulmonary rehabilitation can offer benefit, improving endurance and reducing dyspnea and number of hospitalizations. Treatment specific to AAT deficiency is AAT augmentation therapy. Although definitive evidence from randomized controlled trials of augmentation therapy is lacking and therapy is expensive, the available evidence suggests that this approach is safe and can slow the decline of lung function and emphysema progression.[40] There are four potential treatment options: (1) intravenous human plasma-derived augmentation therapy, (2) augmentation therapy by inhalation, (3) recombinant AAT augmentation therapy, and (4) synthetic elastase inhibition.

Intravenous Human Plasma–Derived Augmentation Therapy

Since the early 1980s, intravenous administration of purified human AAT concentrate has been shown to increase lung levels of AAT in patients with AAT deficiency. In subjects receiving once-weekly[51] doses, the antineutrophil elastase capacity in lung epithelium lining fluid increased by 60% to 70%. A purified preparation shown to be biologically active led to its U.S. Food and Drug Administration approval in 1988. Randomized placebo-controlled trials evaluating the efficacy of intravenous AAT replacement therapy in attenuating the development of emphysema are lacking. Recommendations on the use of augmentation therapy are based on the ATS/ERS guidelines.[48] The decline in FEV_1 and mortality rates are lower in subjects treated with intravenous augmentation therapy than in untreated subjects.

Augmentation Therapy by Inhalation

Aerosol application of AAT in subjects with AAT deficiency increases AAT concentration and antielastase activity in the lower respiratory tract in a dose-dependent fashion. Preliminary data suggest that once- or twice-daily administration of aerosolized AAT may produce sustained antielastase protection of the lungs.

Recombinant Augmentation Therapy and Synthetic Elastase Inhibition

A number of recombinant forms of AAT, a recombinant secretory leukoprotease inhibitor, and several synthetic low-molecular-weight elastase inhibitors have been developed and are being evaluated, but their clinical efficacy and safety are not yet established.

Lung Transplantation

Lung transplantation is recommended for some subjects with end-stage lung disease. Because of limitations on available donor lungs, single-lung transplantation is more common despite the fact that outcomes are better for patients receiving a double-lung transplantation. Five-year survival rates after lung transplantation are about 50%, with bronchiolitis obliterans being the major cause of death after transplantation.

Lung Volume Reduction Surgery

Lung volume reduction surgery (LVRS) improves exercise capacity and relieves dyspnea in subjects with COPD, but its role is not yet established in AAT deficiency. One study shows benefit to bilateral LVRS in patients with AAT deficiency and emphysema, but functional measurements, except for the 6-minute walk test, returned to baseline after 6 to 12 months. LVRS is not recommended in the 2003 ATS/ERS guidelines for management of AAT deficiency.[48]

UNMET, FUTURE RESEARCH NEEDS

1. Optimizing and expanding access to the nongenetic diagnostic tests to ensure a timely and accurate diagnosis of PCD
2. Performing randomized controlled trials to study the benefit of anti-inflammatory agents and of mucoactive agents in patients with PCD and CF
3. Understanding the multitude of effects of CFTR on mucosal physiology and the susceptibility and progression of chronic lung disease and host immune responses that fail to adequately control lung infection
4. Determining the use of current therapies in the era of CFTR-modulation therapy
5. Performing large-scale genomic studies to define novel pathways to treat AAT deficiency
6. Determining the role of candidate modifier genes, anti-inflammatory proteins, and potential synthetic antiproteases in AAT deficiency
7. Developing a biomarker to diagnose PCD, CF, and AAT deficiency early in the course of disease

CONCLUSION

PCD, CF, and AAT deficiency are autosomal recessive hereditary diseases. These three diseases should always be considered in cases of asthma. The diagnosis and management of these diseases, particularly with asthma, is an important challenge for clinicians. However, the diagnosis of these chronic diseases is evolving with better definition of phenotypic features and expansion of diagnostic tests. Optimizing and expanding access to the nongenetic tests is critical to ensuring a timely and accurate diagnosis. Early diagnostic strategies, better understanding of the complex interactions underlying the pathophysiology of lung disease, and emerging treatments show great promise for the future. The discovery of genetic and biomarker studies that will predict individuals at risk for developing the clinical manifestations of these diseases can lead to more personalized treatment strategies and a better prognosis.

REFERENCES

1. Colombo C, Ellemunter H, Houwen R, et al. Guidelines for the diagnosis and management

of distal intestinal obstruction syndrome in cystic fibrosis patients. *J Cyst Fibros.* 2011;10(Suppl 2):S24–S28.
2. Leigh MW, O'Callaghan C, Knowles MR. The challenges of diagnosing primary ciliary dyskinesia. *Proc Am Thorac Soc.* 2011;8(5):434–437.
3. Noone PG, Leigh MW, Sannuti A, et al. Primary ciliary dyskinesia: diagnostic and phenotypic features. *Am J Respir Crit Care Med.* 2004;169(4):459–467.
4. Hogg C. Primary ciliary dyskinesia: when to suspect the diagnosis and how to confirm it. *Paediatr Respir Rev.* 2009;10(2):44–50.
5. Hossain T, Kappelman MD, Perez-Atayde AR, Young GJ, Huttner KM, Christou H. Primary ciliary dyskinesia as a cause of neonatal respiratory distress: implications for the neonatologist. *J Perinatol.* 2003;23(8):684–687.
6. Leigh MW, Zariwala MA, Knowles MR. Primary ciliary dyskinesia: improving the diagnostic approach. *Curr Opin Pediatr.* 2009;21(3):320–325.
7. Chilvers MA, Rutman A, O'Callaghan C. Ciliary beat pattern is associated with specific ultrastructural defects in primary ciliary dyskinesia. *J Allergy Clin Immunol.* 2003;112(3):518–524.
8. Hosoki K, Fujisawa T, Masuda S, et al. [A case of primary ciliary dyskinesia who had been treated as asthma]. *Arerugi.* 2010;59(7):847–854.
9. Thomas B, Rutman A, Hirst RA, et al. Ciliary dysfunction and ultrastructural abnormalities are features of severe asthma. *J Allergy Clin Immunol.* 2010;126(4):722–729, e2.
10. Fauroux B, Tamalet A, Clement A. Management of primary ciliary dyskinesia: the lower airways. *Paediatr Respir Rev.* 2009;10(2):55–57.
11. Lie H, Ferkol T. Primary ciliary dyskinesia: recent advances in pathogenesis, diagnosis and treatment. *Drugs.* 2007;67(13):1883–1892.
12. Lobo J, Rojas-Balcazar JM, Noone PG. Recent advances in cystic fibrosis. *Clin Chest Med.* 2012;33(2):307–328.
13. Amirav I, Cohen-Cymberknoh M, Shoseyov D, Kerem E. Primary ciliary dyskinesia: prospects for new therapies, building on the experience in cystic fibrosis. *Paediatr Respir Rev.* 2009;10(2):58–62.
14. Prickett M, Jain M. Gene therapy in cystic fibrosis. Translational research: the journal of laboratory and clinical medicine. 2013;161(4):255–264.
15. Boucher RC, Yankaskas JR. Cystic fibrosis. In: Mason RJ, Martin T, King T, et al., eds. *Murray and Nadel's Textbook of Respiratory Medicine.* 5th ed. Philadelphia: Saunders Elsevier; 2010: 985–1022.
16. Lemna WK, Feldman GL, Kerem B, et al. Mutation analysis for heterozygote detection and the prenatal diagnosis of cystic fibrosis. *N Engl J Med.* 1990;322(5):291–226.
17. Ao A, Ray P, Harper J, et al. Clinical experience with preimplantation genetic diagnosis of cystic fibrosis (delta F508). *Prenat Diagn.* 1996;16(2):137–142.
18. Comeau AM, Accurso FJ, White TB, et al. Guidelines for implementation of cystic fibrosis newborn screening programs: Cystic Fibrosis Foundation workshop report. *Pediatrics.* 2007;119(2):e495–e518.
19. FitzSimmons SC. The changing epidemiology of cystic fibrosis. *J Pediatr.* 1993;122(1):1–9.
20. Gaillard D, Bouvier R, Scheiner C, et al. Meconium ileus and intestinal atresia in fetuses and neonates. *Pediatr Pathol Lab Med.* 1996;16(1):25–40.
21. Valman HB, France NE, Wallis PG. Prolonged neonatal jaundice in cystic fibrosis. *Arch Dis Child.* 1971;46(250):805–809.
22. Lloyd-Still JD, Khaw KT, Shwachman H. Severe respiratory disease in infants with cystic fibrosis. *Pediatrics.* 1974;53(5):678–682.
23. Wiatrak BJ, Myer CM 3rd, Cotton RT. Cystic fibrosis presenting with sinus disease in children. *Am J Dis Child.* 1993;147(3): 258–260.
24. Rosenstein BJ. What is a cystic fibrosis diagnosis? *Clin Chest Med.* 1998;19(3):423–441, v.
25. Rosenstein BJ, Cutting GR. The diagnosis of cystic fibrosis: a consensus statement. Cystic Fibrosis Foundation Consensus Panel. *J Pediatr.* 1998;132(4):589–595.
26. Farrell PM, Rosenstein BJ, White TB, et al. Guidelines for diagnosis of cystic fibrosis in newborns through older adults: Cystic Fibrosis Foundation consensus report. *J Pediatr.* 2008;153(2):S4–S14.
27. Balfour-Lynn IM, Elborn JS. "CF asthma": what is it and what do we do about it? *Thorax.* 2002;57(8):742–748.
28. Antunes J, Fernandes A, Borrego LM, Leiria-Pinto P, Cavaco J. Cystic fibrosis, atopy, asthma and ABPA. *Allergol Immunopathol.* 2010;38(5):278–284.
29. Sanders DB, Rosenfeld M, Mayer-Hamblett N, Stamey D, Redding GJ. Reproducibility of spirometry during cystic fibrosis pulmonary exacerbations. *Pediatr Pulmonol.* 2008;43(11):1142–1146.
30. Weinberger M. Airways reactivity in patients with CF. *Clin Rev Allergy Immunol.* 2002;23(1):77–85.

31. Eggleston PA, Rosenstein BJ, Stackhouse CM, Alexander MF. Airway hyperreactivity in cystic fibrosis: clinical correlates and possible effects on the course of the disease. *Chest.* 1988;94(2):360–365.
32. Sanchez I, Powell RE, Pasterkamp H. Wheezing and airflow obstruction during methacholine challenge in children with cystic fibrosis and in normal children. *Am Rev Respir Dis.* 1993;147(3):705–709.
33. Warner JO, Norman AP, Soothill JF. Cystic fibrosis heterozygosity in the pathogenesis of allergy. *Lancet.* 1976;1(7967):990–991.
34. Dahl M, Nordestgaard BG, Lange P, Tybjaerg-Hansen A. Fifteen-year follow-up of pulmonary function in individuals heterozygous for the cystic fibrosis phenylalanine-508 deletion. *J Allergy Clin Immunol.* 2001;107(5):818–823.
35. Schonheyder H, Jensen T, Hoiby N, Andersen P, Koch C. Frequency of Aspergillus fumigatus isolates and antibodies to Aspergillus antigens in cystic fibrosis. *Acta Pathol Microbiol Immunol Scand B Microbiology.* 1985;93(2):105–112.
36. de Almeida MB, Bussamra MH, Rodrigues JC. Allergic bronchopulmonary aspergillosis in paediatric cystic fibrosis patients. *Paediatr Respir Rev.* 2006;7(1):67–72.
37. Kraemer R, Delosea N, Ballinari P, Gallati S, Crameri R. Effect of allergic bronchopulmonary aspergillosis on lung function in children with cystic fibrosis. *Am J Respir Crit Care Med.* 2006;174(11):1211–1220.
38. Mogayzel PJ Jr, Naureckas ET, Robinson KA, et al. Cystic fibrosis pulmonary guidelines: chronic medications for maintenance of lung health. *Am J Respir Crit Care Med.* 2013;187(7):680–689.
39. Kelly E, Greene CM, Carroll TP, McElvaney NG, O'Neill SJ. Alpha-1 antitrypsin deficiency. *Respir Med.* 2010;104(6):763–772.
40. Stoller JK, Aboussouan LS. A review of alpha1-antitrypsin deficiency. *Am J Respir Crit Care Med.* 2012;185(3):246–259.
41. Brantly M, Nukiwa T, Crystal RG. Molecular basis of alpha-1-antitrypsin deficiency. *Am J Med.* 1988;84(6A):13–31.
42. Hutchison DC. Alpha 1-antitrypsin deficiency in Europe: geographical distribution of Pi types S and Z. *Respir Med.* 1998;92(3):367–377.
43. Gooptu B, Ekeowa UI, Lomas DA. Mechanisms of emphysema in alpha1-antitrypsin deficiency: molecular and cellular insights. *Eur Respir J.* 2009;34(2):475–488.
44. Gishen P, Saunders AJ, Tobin MJ, Hutchison DC. Alpha 1-antitrypsin deficiency: the radiological features of pulmonary emphysema in subjects of Pi type Z and Pi type SZ. A survey by the British Thoracic Association. *Clin Radiol.* 1982;33(4):371–377.
45. Parr DG, Stoel BC, Stolk J, Stockley RA. Pattern of emphysema distribution in alpha1-antitrypsin deficiency influences lung function impairment. *Am J Respir Crit Care Med.* 2004;170(11):1172–1178.
46. Cuvelier A, Muir JF, Hellot MF, et al. Distribution of alpha(1)-antitrypsin alleles in patients with bronchiectasis. *Chest.* 2000;117(2):415–419.
47. Parr DG, Guest PG, Reynolds JH, Dowson LJ, Stockley RA. Prevalence and impact of bronchiectasis in alpha1-antitrypsin deficiency. *Am J Respir Crit Care Med.* 2007;176(12):1215–1221.
48. American Thoracic Society, European Respiratory Society. American Thoracic Society/European Respiratory Society statement: standards for the diagnosis and management of individuals with alpha-1 antitrypsin deficiency. *Am J Respir Crit Care Med.* 2003;168(7):818–900.
49. Stoller JK, Sandhaus RA, Turino G, Dickson R, Rodgers K, Strange C. Delay in diagnosis of alpha1-antitrypsin deficiency: a continuing problem. *Chest.* 2005;128(4):1989–1994.
50. Eden E, Strange C, Holladay B, Xie L. Asthma and allergy in alpha-1 antitrypsin deficiency. *Respir Med.* 2006;100(8):1384–1391.
51. Makino S, Chosy L, Valdivia E, Reed CE. Emphysema with hereditary alpha-1 antitrypsin deficiency masquerading as asthma. *J Allergy.* 1970;46(1):40–88.
52. McElvaney NG, Stoller JK, Buist AS, et al. Baseline characteristics of enrollees in the National Heart, Lung and Blood Institute Registry of alpha 1-antitrypsin deficiency. Alpha 1-Antitrypsin Deficiency Registry Study Group. *Chest.* 1997;111(2):394–403.
53. Eden E, Hammel J, Rouhani FN, et al. Asthma features in severe alpha1-antitrypsin deficiency: experience of the National Heart, Lung, and Blood Institute Registry. *Chest.* 2003;123(3):765–771.
54. Demeo DL, Campbell EJ, Barker AF, et al. IL10 polymorphisms are associated with airflow obstruction in severe alpha1-antitrypsin deficiency. *Am J Respir Cell Mol Biol.* 2008;38(1):114–120.

11

OTHER PULMONARY ABNORMALITIES

COMORBID, COEXISTING, AND DIFFERENTIAL DIAGNOSIS

Robert A. Wise and Emily P. Brigham

KEY POINTS

- Asthma may be mimicked by a number of conditions, including upper airway obstruction from tumors, foreign bodies, or diseases that cause intrinsic or extrinsic narrowing of the upper airway.
- Systemic diseases such as carcinoid or mastocytosis may cause wheezing that mimics asthma.
- Functional conditions such as sighing dyspnea or hyperventilation may also mimic asthma.
- Respiratory conditions that may coexist with asthma and that may worsen or obscure symptoms of asthma include congestive heart failure, interstitial lung disease, sarcoidosis, and lymphangioleiomyomatosis.
- Pneumothorax may occur in the setting of an acute asthma attack or may be a spontaneous event causing acute onset of dyspnea.

INTRODUCTION

The purpose of this chapter is to describe various disorders that are not described elsewhere in this text that may present as asthma, coexist with asthma, or be confused with asthma. The cardinal symptoms of asthma—cough, wheezing, and dyspnea—are associated with nearly all respiratory illnesses. Because asthma is a common disorder, it is a widespread practice to initially treat the syndrome of cough, wheeze, and dyspnea with bronchodilators or inhaled corticosteroids to determine whether it responds to treatment. When such treatment is unsuccessful or only partially effective, then further evaluation may be necessary, including lung imaging, comprehensive lung function testing, inhalation challenge testing with methacholine or mannitol, and more extensive examination of the upper airway.

UPPER AIRWAY OBSTRUCTION

Upper airway obstruction can present with episodic cough, dyspnea, and a history of wheezing (stridor). This condition is typically differentiated from asthma on physical examination. The high-pitched, musical wheezing sounds are both inspiratory and expiratory and tend to be monophonic in pitch rather than polyphonic, as in the wheeze of asthma. Moreover, the sounds are more prominent over the trachea and sternal notch than on the posterior chest. Flow-volume tracings are often diagnostic, demonstrating a fixed airway obstruction or a variable extrathoracic obstruction.

Both benign and malignant tumors may develop in the upper airway or mainstem bronchi and are usually detectable with chest and upper airway computed tomography (CT).[1] These tumors may be primary or secondary and include a broad differential diagnosis (Table 11.1). A definitive diagnosis usually requires bronchoscopy and biopsy, although care should be taken with forceps biopsy because of the risk for bleeding. Viral papillomatosis can be disseminated into the lungs by upper airway procedures. Accordingly, invasive procedures such as biopsy, debridement, or cryotherapy should be limited to those necessary to secure a patent upper airway. Adjuvant antiviral therapy or interferon-α may be used in cases in which there is extensive lower airway involvement, but the efficacy of these treatments is unclear.[2] Treatment of upper airway tumors depends on the type and extent of tumor and may range from local treatments with cryotherapy, laser resection, or electrocautery to surgical resections with tracheoplasty. Chemotherapy or radiation therapy may be necessary for disseminated or unresectable malignant lesions. Airway protection may require either a tracheotomy or bypass of the tumor with a T-tube. If a tracheal tumor causes a tracheoesophageal fistula, recurrent pneumonia and aspiration events may follow and require isolation of the airway and esophagus with a stent and gastrostomy.

Foreign bodies may also cause upper airway obstruction that can mimic asthma or worsen symptoms of preexisting asthma. These are particularly prevalent in children and may consist of food, small plastic toy parts, or household items.[3] Although imaging may be helpful, many such objects are not radiopaque. Direct visualization with laryngoscopy or bronchoscopy is necessary for diagnosis and removal. If the foreign object is present for a prolonged period, it can become obscured by granulation tissue, which may need to be excised to reveal the object.[4] Aspiration of foreign bodies is also reported in adults who have body piercings, especially in the tongue and lips, that have been aspirated into the lung. At times they require surgical removal.[5] Aspiration of peanuts is common in children, accounting for about one-third of foreign bodies in this age group.[6] Peanuts can be particularly problematic because of the local inflammatory response to the peanut oil. Aspirated teeth are another common foreign body that may go unrecognized and misdiagnosed for many years as recurrent asthma and pneumonias.[7]

Nonneoplastic processes also may cause airway obstruction that can coexist with asthma or mimic asthma.[8] A substernal goiter may compress the trachea and lead to wheezing and stridor. This can be diagnosed by CT; however, clinical examination alone will suggest the diagnosis if the stridor can be induced by having the patient raise the arms above the head, thereby narrowing the thoracic outlet. Vascular anomalies of the great vessels can cause wheezing and dyspnea and should be considered in the differential diagnosis, particularly when such symptoms are accompanied by dysphagia.[9]

Amyloidosis can involve the upper airway in about 1% of cases of systemic amyloidosis. In the diffuse submucosal form, it presents as concentric thickening of the airway wall with narrowing of the lumen. In the nodular form, amyloid may mimic other endobronchial tumors. In one series of benign tracheal lesions, amyloid accounted for 0.5% of cases. However, in a series of tracheal tumors that required laser resection, 23% of the cases were amyloid.[10,11] Moreover, amyloid may involve the lung either as single or multiple nodules or interstitial disease. When the interstitial disease is present, respiratory failure contributes to death in about 1 of 10 patients.

Table 11.1. Soft Tissue Tumors of the Trachea

EPITHELIAL TUMORS, BENIGN

Papillomas
Squamous cell papillomas, papillomatosis
Adenomas of salivary gland–type tumors
Mucous gland adenoma
Pleomorphic adenoma (benign mixed tumor)
Monomorphic adenoma, myoepithelioma
Oncocytoma

EPITHELIAL TUMORS, MALIGNANT

Endobronchial squamous cell carcinoma
Papillary variant of squamous cell carcinoma
Basaloid squamous cell carcinoma
Endobronchial adenocarcinoma, invasive adenocarcinoma
Carcinoid tumor—typical or atypical
Endobronchial small cell carcinoma
Large cell carcinoma, large cell neuroendocrine carcinoma
Adenoid cystic carcinoma
Mucoepidermoid carcinoma
Acinic cell carcinoma
Pleiotropic carcinomas with sarcomatoid elements, blastoma
Metastatic endobronchial carcinoma (e.g., breast, colon, renal cell, mesothelioma)
Fibroconnective tissue tumors (benign or malignant)
Chondroma, chondrosarcoma
Glomus tumor
Capillary hemangioma, hemangiosarcoma (Kaposi's sarcoma)
Granular cell tumor
Hamartoma
Leiomyoma, leiomyosarcoma, rhabdomyosarcoma
Lipoma, liposarcoma
Fibroma, fibrosarcoma
Neuroma, neurosarcoma
Osteosarcoma
Synovial sarcoma

MISCELLANEOUS TUMORS

Inflammatory pseudotumor
Malignant lymphoma of bronchial-associated lymphoid tissue
Primary pulmonary melanoma

Adapted from Litzky L. Epithelial and soft tissue tumors of the tracheobronchial tree. *Chest Surg Clin N Am.* 2003;13(1):1–40.

Diagnosis requires CT and biopsy. Optimal treatment of diffuse tracheal obstruction from amyloid is not established, but repeated rigid bronchoscopy with dilatation of the central airways is a temporizing measure.[12] If upper airway obstruction is the consequence of the nodular form, then laser or cryoresections may be used.

Iatrogenic stenosis of the trachea is the most common cause of tracheal stenosis and may result from prolonged airway intubation or occur at the site of a tracheotomy. This complication may go unrecognized in a patient with severe asthma who has had multiple episodes of mechanical ventilation. The use of low-pressure balloons in endotracheal tubes made this a relatively uncommon complication from intubation. However, one series suggests that mostly mild tracheal stenosis at the site of a tracheotomy may occur in as many as 30% of patients.[13]

Tracheomalacia and tracheobronchomalacia, which can be congenital or acquired through injury or inflammatory processes, can also lead to wheezing, dyspnea, cough, and airway compromise. Inspiratory and expiratory lung imaging may suggest this diagnosis when the posterior tracheal membrane invaginates or the trachea assumes a "saber sheath" profile. When conservative management fails, options include airway stenting and surgical repair.[14] Tracheomegaly (or Mounier-Kuhn syndrome) can also lead to impaired clearance of secretions and recurrent episodes of bronchitis, cough, and wheezing.

Rheumatic diseases may also cause upper airway obstruction that can be confused with asthma. Rheumatoid arthritis is commonly associated with *cricoarytenoid arthritis,* which can cause cough, hoarseness, and wheezing and may even be life threatening.[15] Wegener's granulomatosis can cause inflammation of the trachea that heals with fibrosis and narrowing or obstructive webs that may result in dyspnea.[16] Relapsing polychondritis is an uncommon autoimmune disorder that causes inflammation and necrosis of cartilage that can lead to upper airway obstruction. It is suggested radiographically by thickening of the anterior and lateral tracheal walls with the lack of involvement of the posterior tracheal membrane. Respiratory failure is one of the most common causes of disability and death from this condition.

Although uncommon, granulomatous diseases may also involve the larynx and trachea as a primary manifestation. Tracheal tuberculosis and sarcoidosis may cause primary mass-like lesions in the airway or may heal after treatment, with destruction of the airway wall leading to local fibrosis and narrowing.[17,18] Rhinoscleroma is a tropical disease caused by a chronic granulomatous infection with *Klebsiella rhinoscleromatis* that causes chronic obstruction of the airways due to inflammatory nodules that heal with scarring and stenosis.[19] *Aspergillus* species infection of the main airways can cause nodular narrowing in immune-compromised hosts.[20]

Granulomatous diseases of the lymph nodes may erode into the airway, leading to bronchial lithiasis and healing with airway narrowing. Tuberculosis and histoplasmosis are the infections most often associated with this condition, but *Nocardia* species and *actinomycosis* are also reported.[21] Anthracotic nodes are implicated in causing isolated major airway narrowing and black pigmentation, a condition known as *bronchial anthracofibrosis.*[22] An exuberant fibrotic process, *fibrosing mediastinitis,* may occur that envelops the major airways and central blood vessels, causing airway compromise, pulmonary hypertension, or superior vena cava syndrome in chronic granulomatous infections, particularly with histoplasmosis.[23] Less commonly, fibrosing mediastinitis can be caused by sarcoidosis.[24]

Vocal cord dysfunction and irritable larynx syndrome may coexist with asthma or may mimic severe asthma (see Chapter 22).

ACUTE INFECTIOUS DISEASES THAT CAN MIMIC ASTHMA

Acute stridor and wheezing, particularly in young children, can be caused by *acute epiglottitis.* In past years, this was mainly a disease of children caused by *Haemophilus influenzae* infection. However, since the widespread introduction of *H. influenzae* immunization in children, it presents predominantly as a streptococcal infection in adults.[25,26] Epiglottitis can progress to complete upper airway obstruction, and thus aggressive management is needed to prevent airway compromise. A lateral neck radiograph demonstrating the classic "thumbprint" sign or a neck CT examination is diagnostic when the condition is suspected.

Diphtheria and *pertussis*, although uncommon in children and young adults because of current immunization practices, can cause severe acute respiratory compromise in those who are unvaccinated.[27] Because of waning immunity of current vaccine preparations, pertussis outbreaks in preadolescents and adults who had received childhood immunization are now reported.[28,29]

OTHER CONDITIONS THAT MAY COMPLICATE OR MIMIC ASTHMA

Carcinoid syndrome is caused by secretion of neuropeptides from tumors derived from neuroendocrine cells. Serotonin is the signature neuropeptide of this syndrome, although several others are implicated in the disease. The syndrome manifests as episodic flushing, diarrhea, hypotension, and wheezing. When this occurs, it suggests that the tumor has metastasized from the intestinal tract to the liver, where the mediators can bypass the portal circulation and hepatic degradation. Octreotide, a somatostatin analog, suppresses the syndrome and may prevent progression of the disease. The clinical course of intestinal carcinoid is variable and can range from a chronic minimally symptomatic disease to one that is aggressive and fatal.[30]

Carcinoid tumors that arise in the airway do not typically cause carcinoid syndrome but instead lead to airway obstruction that results in chronic dyspnea, wheezing, and obstructive pneumonias (Figure 11.1). Multiple carcinoid tumorlets are associated with bronchiolitis obliterans with neuroendocrine cell hyperplasia that can lead to progressive airflow obstruction from small airway involvement.[31] This syndrome may also occur in infancy, presenting with respiratory distress.[32] Characteristic findings include a mosaic pattern on the expiratory CT scan in association with small interstitial nodules.

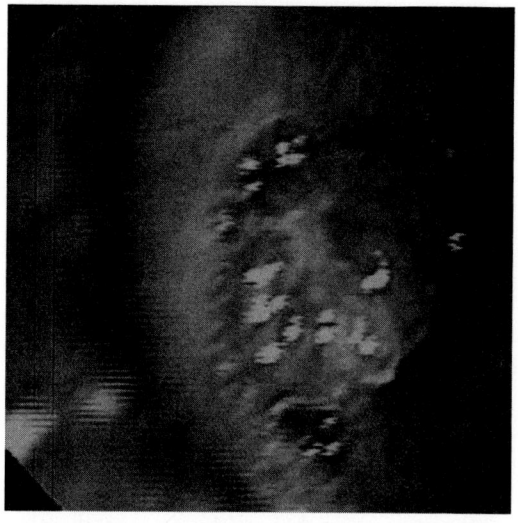

FIGURE 11.1 Bronchoscopic view of bronchial carcinoid tumor causing 90% obstruction of the left mainstem bronchus. The patient presented with dyspnea and unilateral wheezing and was initially treated with bronchodilators until the lesion was revealed on a chest computed tomogram. The lesion has a characteristic smooth, highly vascular appearance.

Systemic mastocytosis may overlap in its symptoms with carcinoid but usually does not cause wheezing as part of the mediator release syndrome. Most often, it results in abdominal pain, hypotension, and generalized flushing.[33] Abnormal accumulations of mast cells in tissues are responsible for this disease, which varies in presentation from benign with skin involvement only to malignant disease with bone marrow involvement.

Lymphangioleiomyomatosis is a chronic, progressive, obstructive airway disease that affects women of childbearing age. The disease is manifest by characteristic CT findings of cystic changes in the lung associated with increased interstitial markings (Figure 11.2). Evidence suggests that this is a proliferative disease related to mutations in the tuberous sclerosis gene complex and is benefitted by mTOR (mechanistic target of rapamycin) inhibitors such as sirolimus.[34] It usually presents with slowly progressive dyspnea or sudden-onset dyspnea from a pneumothorax or chronic chylothorax.[35]

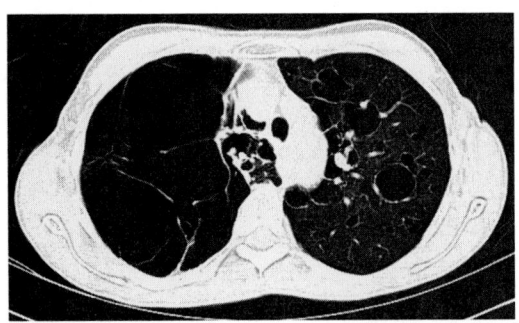

FIGURE 11.2 Computed tomogram (CT) appearance of lymphangioleiomyomatosis. The CT appearance of the left lung demonstrates round cystic lesions on a background of parenchyma with accentuated interstitial markings and ground glass opacities, typical for this disorder. The right lung shows more advanced disease with emphysematous changes that are not distinguishable from typical chronic obstructive pulmonary disease. This patient presented with exertional dyspnea and was treated with bronchodilators until the diagnosis was confirmed by a chest CT following a spontaneous pneumothorax.

Pulmonary thromboemboli are common causes of acute-onset dyspnea that are associated with wheezing in about 8% of patients.[36] The wheeze may result from serotonin release by platelets or be caused by pulmonary vascular congestion. In such patients, asthma may be considered in the differential diagnosis of acute dyspnea and wheezing. The diagnosis of pulmonary embolism may require CT angiography of the chest or a radionuclide ventilation-perfusion scan. Chronic or recurrent thromboembolic disease ought to be considered in patients with asthma who develop progressive dyspnea not associated with worsening airflow limitation.

Congestive heart failure and valvular heart disease may coexist with asthma or may mimic asthma with episodes of nocturnal dyspnea and wheezing. This is discussed in detail in Chapters 15 and 16.

Interstitial lung diseases are rarely difficult to distinguish from asthma because of a restrictive rather than obstructive ventilatory defect on pulmonary function testing and the characteristic CT scans. The diffusing capacity for carbon monoxide ($D_{L}CO$) is usually decreased in interstitial lung disease, whereas it is usually normal or increased in asthma.[37] Some interstitial diseases, however, are associated with involvement of airways that leads to a combined obstructive and restrictive defect. *Sarcoidosis* is a predominately peribronchial granulomatous disease that often leads to airflow obstruction. Sarcoidosis may also commonly coexist with asthma but can lead to increased airway reactivity and episodic wheezing in isolation. The estimated prevalence of methacholine reactivity varies widely, but it seems to be more common in those with more long-standing disease and airflow obstruction.[38,39] Follicular bronchiolitis is a low-grade lymphoproliferative disease that can be associated with rheumatoid arthritis or Sjögren's syndrome. More rarely, this condition is associated with common variable immunodeficiency or eosinophilic bronchiolitis of asthma.[40,41] The disorder may lead to progressive airflow limitation and air trapping but has a variable prognosis. The finding on CT of centrilobular nodules surrounding small airways in the context of an immune-mediated disease should suggest this diagnosis.

Idiopathic pulmonary fibrosis is a progressive interstitial inflammatory and fibrosing disease that mainly affects older men and has a predilection for those who have previously smoked. The disease has a progressive course that can be variable but often leads to disabling cough, dyspnea, and hypoxemia over a several-year timespan. The CT examination, which shows subpleural cystic changes and honeycombing in the lower and peripheral lung zones, is often diagnostic.[42] When the diagnosis is in doubt, an open lung biopsy may be required. There is no proven beneficial treatment for this disease, but a number of clinical trials are underway with promising agents. The histologic diagnosis of idiopathic pulmonary fibrosis is dictated by a pathologic diagnosis of *usual interstitial pneumonia*. Interstitial disease associated with collagen vascular diseases that may be responsive to immunosuppressive treatments more often have a histologic pattern of *nonspecific interstitial pneumonitis*, which is characterized by temporally homogeneous involvement of the lung and less end-stage honeycombing. Non-specific interstitial pneumonitis tends to occur in nonsmoking women and has a relatively good prognosis.[43] Mixed histologic patterns may coexist with a worse prognosis in those who show any evidence of usual interstitial pneumonia.[44]

Sighing dyspnea, or functional dyspnea, is a common disorder that is underrecognized in the medical literature. It has the typical presentation of an episodic sensation that the individual is unable to take a deep and satisfying breath. If this is described as a sensation of chest pressure, then a diagnosis of asthma may be made and bronchodilators prescribed.[45,46] A characteristic feature of this syndrome distinguishing it from asthma is that it is not associated with exertional dyspnea and does not waken individuals from sleep. In most cases, lung function testing and lung imaging are normal or show only mild impairment. The cause of this condition is not known, but it is hypothesized to result from impaired feedback from the chest wall mechanoreceptors indicating that a sufficiently deep inspiration has taken place. Typically, such individuals will adopt a pattern of sighing breathing during the episodes that may be evident on examination or by history from a family member. The disorder does not appear to be caused by stress or anxiety, although occasional individuals may have panic episodes in association with these spells. The course is benign, and usually the only necessary treatment is reassurance. Mild aerobic or isometric exercise is usually effective in diminishing symptoms if an episode becomes too uncomfortable.

Pneumothorax may occur spontaneously in healthy young adults, usually from rupture of a paraseptal emphysematous bleb. The presenting signs of sharp pleuritic chest pain and dyspnea are not usually confused with asthma. The diagnosis is confirmed by physical examination showing diminished breath sounds and hyperresonance to percussion on the affected hemithorax. The diagnosis is confirmed by chest imaging. When the pneumothorax is small, inspiratory and expiratory views are helpful to reveal air in the pleural space. However, in patients who are experiencing an acute asthma attack, pneumothorax or pneumomediastinum can be a serious or fatal complication.[47] Hyperinflation of the lung during an asthma attack increases the mechanical stresses on the alveoli and airways and can result in pneumothorax or pneumomediastinum. Thus, a "silent" chest during an asthma attack may reflect either severe bronchoconstriction and air trapping or pneumothorax, indicating urgent imaging of the chest. Pneumomediastinum is evidenced by a "crunching" sound in synchrony with the heart heard over the upper ribcage, often in association with subcutaneous emphysema. Although it may be benign in asymptomatic patients, it would be considered a portent of possible bilateral pneumothorax in patients experiencing acute asthma.[48] It may be necessary to perform emergency needle aspiration of the thorax as part of the resuscitation procedure in patients with severe asthma who suffer vascular collapse during an asthma attack. Definitive treatment of the pneumothorax with an asthma attack requires insertion of a chest tube or catheter drain to an underwater seal or suction. Maintenance of oxygenation with minimal airway pressures is the ideal approach to mechanically ventilate patients with severe asthma, regardless of hypercapnia—the so-called permissive hypercapnia strategy. This approach minimizes the prevalence of barotrauma and pneumothorax in severe asthma to about a 2.5% rate of pneumothorax of patients admitted to intensive care.[49]

UNMET, FUTURE RESEARCH NEEDS

1. Future research is needed to be able to unravel the role of comorbid conditions in asthma and how best to diagnose and treat them.

2. Both benign and malignant lesions of the upper airway may become amenable to tracheal reconstruction using tissue-engineering methods.

3. A better understanding of the role of neuropeptides and growth factors in the development of bronchiolitis obliterans may yield drug targets to address this devastating progressive disease.

4. More research is needed to understand the biochemical pathways and response of biomarkers in lymphangioleiomyomatosis, which show great promise in diagnosing and treating this previously fatal disease.

CONCLUSION

A number of conditions are reviewed in this chapter that may mimic asthma or coexist with asthma and exacerbate it. These include upper airway obstruction that may be either structural or functional and systemic diseases such as excess serotonin (carcinoid syndrome) or histamine (mastocytosis, anaphylaxis) that induce bronchospasm. Primary diseases of the lung, such as interstitial lung disease or sarcoidosis, may also be associated with episodic cough, wheezing, and dyspnea. Functional disorders such as sighing and dyspnea or hyperventilation may also mimic asthma. Pneumothorax can occur in the setting of asthma but also can present with acute symptoms that mimic asthma.

REFERENCES

1. Litzky L. Epithelial and soft tissue tumors of the tracheobronchial tree. *Chest Surg Clin N Am.* 2003;13(1):1–40.
2. Kimberlin DW. Current status of antiviral therapy for juvenile-onset recurrent respiratory papillomatosis. *Antiviral Res.* 2004;63(3):141–151.
3. Heim SW, Maughan KL. Foreign bodies in the ear, nose, and throat. *Am Fam Physician.* 2007;76(8):1185–1189.
4. Cutrone C, Pedruzzi B, Tava G, et al. The complimentary role of diagnostic and therapeutic endoscopy in foreign body aspiration in children. *Int J Pediatr Otorhinolaryngol.* 2011;75(12):1481–1485.
5. Holbrook J, Minocha J, Laumann A. Body piercing: complications and prevention of health risks. *Am J Clin Dermatol.* 2012;13(1):1–17.
6. Leong SC, Farook KS. Peanut aspiration in an adult. *Prim Care Respir J.* 2004;13(3):169–170.
7. Yurdakul AS, Kanbay A, Kurul C, Yorgancilar D, Demircan S, Ekim N. An occult foreign body aspiration with bronchial anomaly mimicking asthma and pneumonia. *Dent Traumatol.* 2007;23(6):368–370.
8. Grenier PA, Beigelman-Aubry C, Brillet PY. Nonneoplastic tracheal and bronchial stenoses. *Radiol Clin North Am.* 2009;47(2):243–260.
9. Phelan E, Ryan S, Rowley H. Vascular rings and slings: interesting vascular anomalies. *J Laryngol Otol.* 2011;125(11):1158–1163.
10. Berk JL, O'Regan A, Skinner M. Pulmonary and tracheobronchial amyloidosis. *Semin Respir Crit Care Med.* 2002;23(2):155–165.
11. Díaz-Jiménez J, Rodriguez A, Martinez-Ballarin J, Castro MJ, Argemi TM, Manresa F. Diffuse tracheobronchial amyloidosis. *J Bronchol.* 1999;6(1):13–17.
12. O'Regan A, Fenlon HM, Beamis JF Jr, Steele MP, Skinner M, Berk JL. Tracheobronchial amyloidosis: the Boston University experience from 1984 to 1999. *Medicine.* 2000;79(2):69–79.
13. Norwood S, Vallina VL, Short K, Saigusa M, Fernandez LG, McLarty JW. Incidence of tracheal stenosis and other late complications after percutaneous tracheostomy. *Ann Surg.* 2000;232(2):233–241.
14. Carden KA, Boiselle PM, Waltz DA, Ernst A. Tracheomalacia and tracheobronchomalacia in children and adults: an in-depth review. *Chest.* 2005;127(3):984–1005.
15. Blosser S, Wigley FM, Wise RA. Increase in translaryngeal resistance during phonation in rheumatoid arthritis. *Chest.* 1992;102(2):387–390.
16. Langford CA, Sneller MC, Hallahan CW, et al. Clinical features and therapeutic management of subglottic stenosis in patients with Wegener's granulomatosis. *Arthritis Rheum.* 1996;39(10):1754–1760.
17. Lenique F, Brauner MW, Grenier P, Battesti JP, Loiseau A, Valeyre D. CT assessment of bronchi in sarcoidosis: endoscopic and pathologic correlations. *Radiology.* 1995;194(2):419–423.
18. Lee JH, Park SS, Lee DH, Shin DH, Yang SC, Yoo BM. Endobronchial tuberculosis: clinical and bronchoscopic features in 121 cases. *Chest.* 1992;102(4):990–994. Erratum in: *Chest.* 1993;103(5):1640.
19. Yigla M, Ben-Izhak O, Oren I, Hashman N, Lejbkowicz F. Laryngotracheobronchial involvement in a patient with nonendemic rhinoscleroma. *Chest.* 2000;117(6):1795–1798.
20. Franquet T, Serrano F, Giménez A, Rodríguez-Arias JM, Puzo C. Necrotizing Aspergillosis of large airways: CT findings in eight patients. *J Comput Assist Tomogr.* 2002;26(3):342–345.
21. Kang EY. Large airway diseases. *J Thorac Imaging.* 2011;26(4):249–262.

22. Naccache JM, Monnet I, Nunes H, et al. Anthracofibrosis attributed to mixed mineral dust exposure: report of three cases. *Thorax.* 2008;63(7):655-657.
23. Devaraj A, Griffin N, Nicholson AG, Padley SP. Computed tomography findings in fibrosing mediastinitis. *Clin Radiol.* 2007;62(8):781-786.
24. Toonkel RL, Borczuk AC, Pearson GD, Horn EM, Thomashow BM. Sarcoidosis-associated fibrosing mediastinitis with resultant pulmonary hypertension: a case report and review of the literature. *Respiration.* 2010;79(4):341-345.
25. Bizaki AJ, Numminen J, Vasama JP, Laranne J, Rautiainen M. Acute supraglottitis in adults in Finland: review and analysis of 308 cases. *Laryngoscope.* 2011;121(10):2107-2113.
26. Wood N, Menzies R, McIntyre P. Epiglottitis in Sydney before and after the introduction of vaccination against Haemophilus influenzae type b disease. *Intern Med J.* 2005;35(9):530-535.
27. Bisgard KM, Rhodes P, Connelly BL, et al., for the Centers for Disease Control and Prevention. Pertussis vaccine effectiveness among children 6 to 59 months of age in the United States, 1998-2001. *Pediatrics.* 2005;116(2):e285-e294.
28. Centers for Disease Control and Prevention (CDC). Pertussis epidemic—Washington, 2012. *MMWR Morb Mortal Wkly Rep.* 2012;61(28):517-522.
29. Winter K, Harriman K, Zipprich J, et al. California pertussis epidemic, 2010. *J Pediatr.* 2012;161(6):1091-1096.
30. Chan JA, Kulke MH. New treatment options for patients with advanced neuroendocrine tumors. *Curr Treat Options Oncol.* 2011;12(2):136-148.
31. Miller RR, Müller NL. Neuroendocrine cell hyperplasia and obliterative bronchiolitis in patients with peripheral carcinoid tumors. *Am J Surg Pathol.* 1995;19(6):653-658.
32. Brody AS, Guillerman RP, Hay TC, et al. Neuroendocrine cell hyperplasia of infancy: diagnosis with high-resolution CT. *AJR Am J Roentgenol.* 2010;194(1):238-244.
33. Andersen CL, Kristensen TK, Severinsen MT, et al. Systemic mastocytosis: a systematic review. *Dan Med J.* 2012;59(3):A4397.
34. McCormack FX, Inoue Y, Moss J, et al., for the National Institutes of Health Rare Lung Diseases Consortium, MILES Trial Group. Efficacy and safety of sirolimus in lymphangioleiomyomatosis. *N Engl J Med.* 2011;364(17):1595-1606.
35. Harari S, Torre O, Moss J. Lymphangioleiomyomatosis: what do we know and what are we looking for? *Eur Respir Rev.* 2011;20(119):34-44.
36. Stein PD, Henry JW. Clinical characteristics of patients with acute pulmonary embolism stratified according to their presenting syndromes. *Chest.* 1997;112(4):974-979.
37. Keens TG, Mansell A, Krastins IR, et al. Evaluation of the single-breath diffusing capacity in asthma and cystic fibrosis. *Chest.* 1979;76(1):41-44.
38. Bechtel JJ, Starr T 3rd, Dantzker DR, Bower JS. Airway hyperreactivity in patients with sarcoidosis. *Am Rev Respir Dis.* 1981;124(6):759-761.
39. Olafsson M, Simonsson BG, Hansson SB. Bronchial reactivity in patients with recent pulmonary sarcoidosis. *Thorax.* 1985;40(1):51-53.
40. Shimizu K, Konno S, Nasuhara Y, Tanino M, Matsuno Y, Nishimura M. A case of follicular bronchiolitis associated with asthma, eosinophilia, and increased immunoglobulin E. *J Asthma.* 2010;47(10):1161-1164.
41. Aerni MR, Vassallo R, Myers JL, Lindell RM, Ryu JH. Follicular bronchiolitis in surgical lung biopsies: clinical implications in 12 patients. *Respir Med.* 2008;102(2):307-312.
42. Flaherty KR, Thwaite EL, Kazerooni EA, et al. Radiological versus histological diagnosis in UIP and NSIP: survival implications. *Thorax.* 2003;58(2):143-148.
43. Travis WD, Hunninghake G, King TE Jr, et al. Idiopathic nonspecific interstitial pneumonia: report of an American Thoracic Society project. *Am J Respir Crit Care Med.* 2008;177(12):1338-1347.
44. Flaherty KR, Travis WD, Colby TV, et al. Histopathologic variability in usual and nonspecific interstitial pneumonias. *Am J Respir Crit Care Med.* 2001;164(9):1722-1727.
45. Perin PV, Perin RJ, Rooklin AR. When a sigh is just a sigh...and not asthma. *Ann Allergy.* 1993;71(5):478-480.
46. Prys-Picard CO, Kellett F, Niven RM. Disproportionate breathlessness associated with deep sighing breathing in a patient presenting with difficult-to-treat asthma. *Chest.* 2006;130(6):1723-1725.
47. Sabin BR, Greenberger PA. Chapter 13: potentially (near) fatal asthma. *Allergy Asthma Proc.* 2012;33(Suppl 1):S44-S46.
48. Caceres M, Ali SZ, Braud R, Weiman D, Garrett HE Jr. Spontaneous pneumomediastinum: a comparative study and review of the literature. *Ann Thorac Surg.* 2008;86(3):962-966.
49. Peters JI, Stupka JE, Singh H, et al. Status asthmaticus in the medical intensive care unit: a 30-year experience. *Respir Med.* 2012;106(3):344-348.

12

PNEUMONIA

COMORBID AND COEXISTING

Chrysanthi L. Skevaki, Athanassios Tsakris, and Nikolaos G. Papadopoulos

KEY POINTS

- Community-acquired pneumonia (CAP) is a common worldwide health care concern with associated high morbidity and mortality rates.
- Common etiologic agents include *Streptococcus pneumoniae, Haemophilus influenzae, Legionella* species, atypical pathogens (*Mycoplasma pneumoniae* and *Chlamydophila pneumoniae*), and respiratory viruses (respiratory syncytial virus, human rhinovirus, influenza virus).
- Typical symptoms include cough, tachypnea, dyspnea, and fever, and there may be reduced or bronchial breath sounds, inspiratory crackles, and other auscultatory abnormalities on physical examination. Diagnosis can be confirmed by demonstration of an infiltrate on a chest radiograph or other imaging technique.
- Microbiologic diagnosis by means of culture, serology, antigen detection, or polymerase chain reaction should be considered for hospitalized patients and community patients not responding to initial empirical treatment.
- Amoxicillin in Europe and macrolide or doxycycline in the United States are the recommended first-choice antibiotics for community-treated patients based on empirical practice.
- Vaccination against pneumococcal disease and influenza and adherence to a healthy lifestyle, including proper nutritional support, can contribute to the prevention of CAP.
- Respiratory pathogens associated with pneumonia have been shown to have a role in the inception, exacerbation, and chronicity of asthma.
- Asthma can mimic other respiratory diseases and should be considered in the

differential diagnosis of pneumonia, especially in younger and older groups of patients, in whom presentation of pneumonia is often atypical.

INTRODUCTION

Pneumonia is defined as an acute infection of the lung caused by bacteria, viruses, fungi, or other microorganisms and is characterized by inflammation both within and around the alveolar tissues (consolidation). Three broader types of pneumonia are recognized based on the causative pathogens, the setting of infection, and the outcome. These are community-acquired pneumonia (CAP), which is the most common presentation, hospital-acquired (nosocomial) pneumonia, and pneumonia in the immunocompromised patient. CAP represents a challenge for physicians because of the large number and diversity of causative agents, the difficulty in reaching the appropriate clinical diagnosis, and the fact that a single antimicrobial regimen able to combat all possible etiologies is currently missing.

CAP stands as the seventh leading cause of death in the United States[1] and the fourth in Japan,[2] and despite considerable advances in antimicrobial therapy, pneumonia-associated mortality has not significantly decreased since the advent and broad use of penicillin in the 1950s.[1] The annual incidence of CAP diagnosed in the community is reported to be 5 to 11 per 1,000 adults based on studies from Europe and North America.[2] The incidence varies markedly with age and presents highest rates among elderly and very young people. Specifically, for European and North American children younger than 5 years, the annual incidence of pneumonia is 36 per 1,000, and the respective value is 10 times higher in the developing world, where childhood pneumonia accounts for more than 2 million deaths annually.[3]

The most common pathogens associated with CAP are presented in Table 12.1. *Streptococcus pneumoniae* (often referred to as pneumococcus) is one of the predominant causative organisms (Figure 12.1), yet an etiologic agent cannot be identified in 25% to 60% of patients, and the yield can be even lower

Table 12.1. Most Common Etiologic Agents of Community-Acquired Pneumonia According to Treatment Setting

NONHOSPITALIZED PATIENTS	HOSPITALIZED, NON-ICU PATIENTS	HOSPITALIZED, ICU PATIENTS
Streptococcus pneumoniae	*Streptococcus pneumoniae*	*Streptococcus pneumoniae*
Mycoplasma pneumoniae	*Mycoplasma pneumoniae*	*Mycoplasma pneumoniae*
Haemophilus influenzae	*Haemophilus influenzae*	*Haemophilus influenzae*
	Moraxella catarrhalis	
Chlamydophila pneumoniae	*Chlamydophila pneumoniae*	
Chlamydophila psittaci	*Chlamydophila psittaci*	*Chlamydophila psittaci*
	Staphylococcus aureus	*Staphylococcus aureus*
Respiratory viruses*	Respiratory viruses*	Respiratory viruses*
Legionella spp.	*Legionella* spp.	*Legionella* spp.
	Gram-negative enteric bacteria	Gram-negative enteric bacteria

*Respiratory viruses: influenza A, influenza B, parainfluenza virus, adenovirus, respiratory syncytial virus.
Modified from Mandell LA, Wunderink RG, Anzueto A, et al. Infectious Diseases Society of America/American Thoracic Society consensus guidelines on the management of community-acquired pneumonia in adults. *Clin Infect Dis*. 2007;44(Suppl 2):S27–S72.

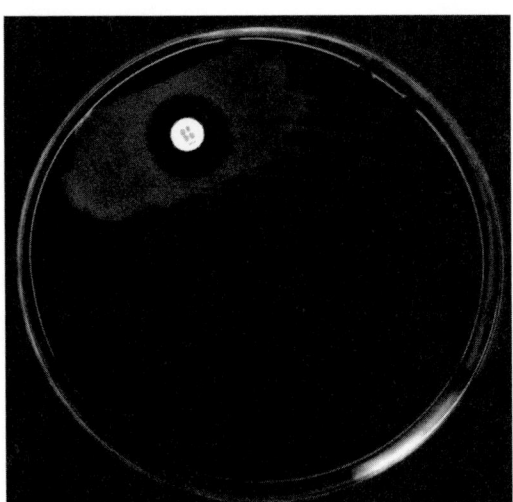

FIGURE 12.1 Culture of *Streptococcus pneumoniae* on blood agar with an inhibition zone around the optochin disk. (See Color Plate 4 in insert.)

in routine hospital practice.[2] Viruses also play an important role, particularly among infants and elderly people, but in school-aged children as well.[4] Bacteria, like *Haemophilus influenzae* and *Legionella* species, and atypical pathogens, such as *Mycoplasma pneumoniae* and *Chlamydophila pneumoniae*, play a distinct role in the etiology of CAP, causing about one in every five cases.[2] It is often assumed that a single pathogen is responsible for each CAP case, but the issue of mixed infections has received particular attention in recent years, largely because of improvements in virus diagnostic techniques.[4]

The purpose of this chapter is to provide a concise reference on pneumonia as a possible comorbid or coexisting condition with asthma. It provides basic information on pneumonia and its clinical features, mentions the main causative agents, and describes the diagnosis and treatment of the disorder. It also discusses lifestyle changes that could potentially reduce associated morbidity and argues on unmet needs in the area.

CLINICAL FEATURES

Symptoms of pneumonia include fever (>38°C), dyspnea, pleuritic chest pain, cough, production of sputum, and tachypnea. Physical examination of the chest may reveal dullness on percussion, crackles, bronchial breathing, or decreased chest expansion.[2]

Clinical features of the disease are also dependent on specific etiologic agents. *S. pneumoniae* is linked to increasing age, cardiovascular comorbidity, acute onset of symptoms, high fever, and pleuritic chest pain.

Bacteremia-associated pneumococcal pneumonia may be more likely in females or linked to the presence of a positive history for excessive alcohol consumption, diabetes mellitus, chronic obstructive pulmonary disease (COPD), and dry cough. *Legionella pneumophila* appears to be more common in men and young patients without comorbidities, in smokers, and in individuals who received antibiotic therapy. This microbe may cause neurologic and gastrointestinal symptoms, and the patient may be presenting a more severe infection in the absence of prominent upper respiratory tract symptoms, pleuritic pain, or purulent sputum. Pneumonia from infection with *M. pneumoniae* may occur in younger patients and in those with less multisystem involvement (compared with *Legionella*-caused pneumonia) and more frequent intake of antibiotics before hospital admission. *C. pneumoniae* is more commonly associated with headaches, usually infects older patients, and has a rather atypical clinical presentation that may lead to a longer duration of symptoms before hospital admission. CAP due to *Coxiella burnetii* is also associated with nonspecific clinical symptoms, but infection may be more common in younger men who present with high fever and dry cough. *Klebsiella pneumoniae* lower respiratory tract infection appears to be more common in men and in individuals with a history of alcohol abuse, and a complete blood count may demonstrate thrombocytopenia and leukopenia. Pneumonia caused by some less common respiratory pathogens, like *Acinetobacter* species, is observed more often in older patients with a history of alcoholism and is associated with a high mortality rate. CAP from other strains of *Streptococcus* such as *Streptococcus milleri* may originate from a dental or abdominal source of infection, whereas *Streptococcus viridans* is associated with aspiration.[2]

CAP in children commonly presents with fever, tachypnea, cough, chest pain, breathlessness or difficulty in breathing, and wheeze. Abdominal pain or vomiting, as well as headache, may also be present. Similar to adulthood pneumonia, clinical manifestations can be quite diverse, but classic presentation includes fever, cough, and tachypnea, preceded by upper respiratory symptoms and low-grade fever.[3] Tachypnea is a nonspecific clinical sign but is the most sensitive and most specific finding associated with pneumonia and indicates respiratory distress or hypoxemia.[5] Increased respiratory rate is present twice as often in children with radiographically proven pneumonia as in children without positive radiographs but with other symptoms of pneumonia.

The age of the child should always be considered during assessment for pneumonia because values for key criteria (e.g., respiratory rate or tachycardia) determining severity range are largely age dependent.[5,6] Clinical presentation of children with pneumonia can range from those who are acutely ill to those who look reasonably well, and this is partly dependent on the etiologic organism. In addition to the presence of persistent or repetitive fever (body temperature >38.5°C), together with chest recession and tachypnea, bacterial pneumonia can also be characterized by abdominal pain and mucus production. Atypical pneumonias, such as those caused by M. pneumoniae or C. pneumoniae, are often accompanied by less severe symptoms of a more gradual onset. Such symptoms may include headache, malaise, and low-grade fever.[7] Asthmatic children with deficient interleukin-18 (IL-18) response are reported to present with more severe forms of pneumonia caused by M. pneumoniae.[8]

Among elderly people, the clinical presentation of CAP is frequently described as more subtle. Nonspecific pneumonia symptoms, including fever, are often missing, whereas mental confusion of new onset may appear.[9]

Severity of CAP ranges from the mild, self-limited disease to severe and occasionally fatal disease, rendering the decision on site of care as the first and most vital in the management of CAP. A number of tools have been developed to assist the clinician in deciding whether a patient with pneumonia should be treated at home or requires either non–intensive care unit (ICU) or ICU hospitalization.[2] The Pneumonia Severity Index is a rather complex model involving 20 variables that performs well and is based on a 30-day mortality prognosis. Limitations include the requirement for sufficient support resources[10] and that it may underestimate pneumonia severity in younger patients.[10] A simpler, usually preferred index, CURB-65, evaluates the risk for mortality by means of a six-point score (one point for each of confusion, blood urea nitrogen level >7 mmol/L (20 mg/dL), Respiratory rate ≥30 breaths/minute, blood pressure [systolic <90 mmHg or diastolic ≤60 mmHg], and age ≥65 years). The even simpler severity assessment tool CRB-65 does not require blood urea nitrogen determination and is reported to be of similar value to CURB-65.[2]

DIAGNOSIS

The presence of pneumonia is supported by focal chest signs and a radiograph or other imaging techniques (e.g., computed tomography [CT]) indicating lung shadowing that is likely to be new. Commonly, CAP is diagnosed at the primary care level, where access to chest radiography is limited. In this setting, diagnosis is based on the history of the patient, clinical features, and physical examination.

Radiologic examination is perceived as the gold standard for the diagnosis of pneumonia. A chest radiograph will not necessarily provide a specific infiltrate pattern useful in identifying underlying etiology, although certain features may guide the physician. Pneumococcal pneumonias will present with lobar consolidation, cavitation, and large pleural effusions. The presence of a bilateral diffuse infiltrate is indicative of Pneumocystis, Legionella, or a primary viral pneumonia, whereas multiple nodular infiltrates throughout the lung point toward staphylococcal pneumonia. Pseudomonas and other gram-negative bacilli often yield lower lobe pneumonia. For Mycoplasma-caused pneumonia, an interstitial pattern in a peribronchial and perivascular distribution is present, cavitation is rare, and pleural effusions may exist occasionally. CT is particularly useful in cases of recurrent pneumonia and in pneumonia linked to tumors or other forms of immunosuppression, in which lung infection may be present in the absence of abnormal chest radiographs.

Although identification of the etiologic agent and its drug susceptibility would permit the confirmation and modification (if necessary) of the initial empirical choice of antimicrobials, microbiologic testing is not routinely recommended for patients managed in the community.[2] Pathogen-specific antimicrobial therapy is not any more effective than the empirical practice.[11] Specific microbial identification is, however, recommended in cases of severe pneumonia and ICU admission, failure of empirical antibiotic therapy, leukopenia, chronic liver disease, asplenia, pleural effusion, possibility of tuberculosis, and specific epidemiologic (e.g., alcohol abuse, intravenous illicit drug use, exposure to bird droppings or birds, travel to Southeast Asia or East Asia) and clinical (e.g., COPD, cystic fibrosis, HIV infection, chronic glucocorticosteroid treatment, lung abscess) conditions.[12] A positive result can be expected in about 60% of cases,[13] but this may require aggressive efforts and the use of most advanced techniques. Diagnostic yield is higher in severely ill patients, for whom the information obtained is most helpful.[13] A palette of diagnostic tests is available to identify microbial causes of pneumonia ranging from culture (e.g., of blood or sputum) to serology, antigen tests, and molecular techniques. In any case, microbiologic analyses should not delay the initiation of empirical treatment for acute pneumonia.

Blood Specimen

The presence of positive blood cultures is highly specific in pneumonia and can facilitate narrowing of antibiotic use, or it may identify the presence of unusual organisms that would not be adequately covered by routine empirical antibiotic coverage, thus helping patients who are not responsive to treatment. Blood culture yield (commonly *S. pneumoniae*) is reported to be 5% to 15% in an unselected hospitalized CAP population and higher in patients with severe CAP, chronic liver disease, asplenia, and leukopenia. Caution must be taken with contamination-related isolates of coagulase-negative staphylococci because misinterpretation can lead to longer hospital stay and overuse of vancomycin.[12] Strains of nonhemolytic *Streptococcus pyogenes* can also be difficult to recognize and isolate from blood culture. Given that β-hemolysis guides the preliminary identification of this species, the absence of hemolysis may be misleading to unimportant commensals. In this context, omission of further identification steps may be detrimental because such isolates appear to retain at least most of their pathogenicity.[14]

Serologic assays for influenza A and B virus antibody detection are often performed[2] and are simple, fast, and reliable tests with sensitivity ranging from 50% to 70% (depending on the type of test and sample and the time interval since the onset of symptoms).[15] However, an increased rate of false-negative results, especially 3 days after onset of symptoms, as well as false-positive results in association with adenovirus infections may occur.[1] Serum antibody assays are the gold standard for the conventional diagnosis of *M. pneumoniae* and are also used for the detection of *Chlamydophila* species because culture-based techniques for the aforementioned pathogens are usually not available in diagnostic laboratories. In this context, the serologic test most commonly applied is the complement fixation test (CFT). For *M. pneumoniae*, CFT titers normally take up to 10 to 14 days after infection to elevation, yet many patients already have elevated titers at the time of admission, because of the slow progression of symptoms.[2] Serology also has been used to diagnose infections caused by *Legionella* species and *C. burnetii*,[16] but their sensitivity and specificity are currently limiting their usefulness in rapid diagnosis.

Antigen detection tests, like enzyme immunoassays and microimmunofluorescence, are also available for blood samples and are routinely used for *M. pneumoniae* and *Chlamydophila* species identification. For the latter, enzyme immunoassays are considered more sensitive and specific than microimmunofluorescence.[17]

A variety of cytokines that are released into the circulation as a result of infection could serve as useful adjuncts in the diagnosis of pneumonia and prediction of disease severity. Procalcitonin, C-reactive protein, and soluble triggering receptor expressed on myeloid cells are the markers most often investigated in pneumonia, with procalcitonin being the earliest to appear during the course of the infection.[18]

Molecular approaches, mainly polymerase chain reaction, have been applied for the detection of *S. pneumoniae*[19] and of *Pneumocystis* species in patients with AIDS.[20]

Urine Specimen

Detection of the *S. pneumoniae* urinary antigen by an immunochromatographic technique provides satisfactory sensitivity (50% to 80%) and specificity (>90%),[21] is easy and rapid to perform (about 15 minutes), and is not affected by prior use of antibiotics. Nevertheless, it does not allow the isolation of the organism and thus does not provide information on drug susceptibility. False-positive results are possible in children colonized with *S. pneumoniae* and in subjects with a pneumococcal CAP episode within the previous 3 months.

Similarly, soluble *L. pneumophila* antigen can be detected in urine using a commercially available enzyme immunoassay (EIA). This test only detects *L. pneumophila* serogroup 1 (which is responsible for the majority of community-associated legionellosis), has an 80% to 95% sensitivity with an estimated 99% specificity, and is easy and rapid to perform.[22] It can provide a positive result from the first day of illness throughout weeks thereafter; however, it shares the same advantages and disadvantages with the pneumococcal urinary antigen test with respect to inability of organism isolation and persistence of antigenuria even after therapy completion.[22]

Sputum Specimen

The microscopic examination and culture of expectorated sputum are basic diagnostic techniques for pneumonia. Sputum samples should be taken from patients able to expectorate purulent samples who have not yet received antibiotic therapy. The specimen needs to be rapidly transported to the laboratory and promptly processed in order to reduce influence of the nasopharyngeal flora. Sputum should initially be observed for color, odor, and consistency. Given that pneumococci often constitute part of the nasopharyngeal flora among healthy adults and additionally colonize the lower airways of patients with chronic bronchitis, identification of the organism is not necessarily diagnostic. Anaerobic infection commonly presents organisms of mixed morphology, whereas Legionnaires' disease, mycoplasma, or viral pneumonias may be indicated by the presence of few bacteria. The sputum Gram stain is helpful to identify pneumococci, *H. influenzae*, and staphylococci, but special staining techniques must be employed for organisms like mycobacteria.

Antigen detection with direct fluorescent antibody assays is commonly used for *L. pneumophila* and *Pneumocystis jirovecii*. Although direct fluorescent tests have been used for *Chlamydophila trachomatis*, the assay has insufficient sensitivity for *C. pneumoniae*.[23]

Pleural Fluid

Early thoracocentesis is indicated for all patients with a parapneumonic effusion.[2] Microscopy and cultures are influenced by antibiotic therapy, and therefore, these investigations should ideally be initiated before treatment; nevertheless, several pathogens often involved in severe CAP (other than *S. pneumoniae*) may be unaffected by a single antibiotic dose.[1]

Other Respiratory Tract Specimens

Invasively collected specimens, like endotracheal aspirates, bronchoscopic or nonbronchoscopic bronchoalveolar lavage (BAL) fluid, protected specimen brushing, and transthoracic needle aspirates (TNAs), are more clinically significant than sputum. BAL can be considered for diagnosing pneumonia caused by *M. tuberculosis* because culture of this specimen has enhanced sensitivity even in the presence of negative sputum cultures. Additionally, BAL could be used for diagnosing atypical pneumonias caused by Legionella species and M. pneumoniae. TNA has been linked to high diagnostic yields,[23] but it should be applied only in specific cases of severe CAP because of potential complications. Endotracheal aspirates, which are safe to perform, are recommended for intubated patients, preferably soon after intubation to avoid tracheal colonization by nosocomial flora.[1]

Molecular techniques for the detection of pulmonary pathogens in respiratory tract samples are increasingly becoming available, but lack of standardization and high rates of false-negative results have withheld their wider application.

DIFFERENTIAL DIAGNOSIS

The clinician is challenged to differentiate pneumonia from other acute lower respiratory tract infections and alternative diagnoses. The key decisions are whether to administer an antibiotic, which antibiotic to use, and whether the patient should be hospitalized.[2]

A common disease interfering with the differential diagnosis of pneumonia is COPD, especially among adults with a history of tobacco use. Shadowing consistent with infection on a chest radiograph is suggestive of CAP.[2]

Chest signs on examination are not specific, and therefore consideration of other potential diagnoses, such as pulmonary edema, fibrosing alveolitis, pulmonary emboli, and bronchiectasis is needed. Chest radiographs are useful tools in reaching a definitive diagnosis of pneumonia,[24] although they cannot usually discriminate pulmonary tuberculosis. Clinicians should also be alert for the detection of an underlying malignancy, especially in heavy smokers presenting with CAP, even in the absence of obvious pointers to a neoplasm.[24]

Asthma and Pneumonia

The association between infectious agents and asthma is complex, and evidence implicates respiratory tract infection, including pneumonia, both at the inception and in exacerbations of preexisting asthma. The most common viruses identified during early-life wheezing illnesses are respiratory syncytial virus (RSV, the principal cause of pneumonia and bronchiolitis in infants), human rhinovirus (HRV, the most frequent cause of the common cold but also a potential cause of pneumonia and bronchiolitis), and multiple other respiratory viruses, such as parainfluenza, metapneumovirus, coronavirus, influenza virus, bocavirus, and adenovirus. RSV lower respiratory tract illnesses, particularly those severe enough to lead to hospitalization, are believed to be associated with an increased risk for asthma at school age[25]; however, several studies argue against a causal role of RSV in asthma inception. However, wheezing illnesses caused by HRV are a more robust predictor of asthma development than RSV episodes.[26]

Regarding atypical pathogens, there is convincing evidence linking infection caused by M. pneumoniae and C. pneumoniae with exacerbations and chronicity of asthma. M. pneumoniae has been detected significantly more often in adult patients with chronic stable asthma and children with acute episodes of wheezing compared with healthy subjects.[27,28] An association between M. pneumoniae infection and the pathogenesis of atopic asthma in children has been suggested, but more studies are required to demonstrate causality.[29] Additionally, subjects with refractory asthma appeared to be chronically infected with M. pneumoniae, without, however, an accompanying increase in immunoglobulin G or the ability to eradicate the infectious agent with macrolides.[30]

Typical bacteria, like S. pneumoniae, H. influenzae, Moraxella catarrhalis, and Staphylococcus aureus, seem to have no role in asthma pathogenesis in children, unlike their atypical counterparts.[31] However, asthma is an important risk factor for severe pneumococcal infections, even more so when the underlying disease is not well controlled and necessitates frequent oral use of corticosteroids.[32] Individuals with severe asthma have been found to present a history of pneumonia at 63%, compared with 35% to 36% in individuals with nonsevere asthma.[33]

Table 12.2. Comparison of Asthma and Pneumonia in Children

CLINICAL FEATURES	PNEUMONIA	ASTHMA
History	Commonly acute onset of a single episode	Chronic or recurrent with acute exacerbations
Symptoms and signs	Cough, tachypnea, dyspnea, fever, chest retraction, nasal flaring, chest pain, reduced or bronchial breath sounds, inspiratory crackles, lethargy, cyanosis, inability to feed in severe cases	Cough, dyspnea, wheezing, tachypnea, fever (if viral infection acts as a trigger for asthma exacerbation), chest retraction, nasal flaring, chest pain, prolonged expiration, lethargy, cyanosis, inability to feed in severe cases
Causative agents	Bacteria, viruses, and other	Viruses (commonly respiratory syncytial virus, human rhinovirus), allergens
Laboratory tests	Nonspecific	Nonspecific
Chest radiograph	Lobar consolidation ± cavitation and pleural effusion, bilateral diffuse, multiple nodular infiltrates, interstitial perihilar changes, atelectasis	Hyperinflation, airway wall thickening, perihilar changes, atelectasis

Modified from Ostergaard MS, Nantanda R, Tumwine JK, Aabenhus R. Childhood asthma in low income countries: an invisible killer? *Prim Care Respir J.* 2012;21(2):214–219; and Brand PL, Hoving MF, de Groot EP. Evaluating the child with recurrent lower respiratory tract infections. *Paediatr Respir Rev.* 2012;13(3):135–138.

Pneumonia and asthma in children can represent a differential diagnostic challenge because they have a number of similarities (Table 12.2). Indeed, a large proportion of infants and children with asthma are mistakenly referred for recurrent pneumonia (or other respiratory tract infections).[34]

Asthma is commonly reported as an underlying cause for recurrent pneumonia, but this notion was challenged based on results failing to indicate a causality between these two conditions.[35] In the differential workup of an asthma exacerbation, wheezing is a supporting feature,[24] and chest radiography can help further: a pneumonia-indicative radiograph would present with the typical appearance of lobar consolidation, which is strongly associated with bacterial pneumonia, whereas the presence of mild perihilar changes would point toward viral infections or asthma.[36]

Certain disorders can cause both pneumonia and asthma, like extrinsic allergic alveolitis, allergic bronchopulmonary aspergillosis, or both allergic angiitis and granulomatosis (Churg-Strauss syndrome). The clinician will be prompted to consider such conditions when generalized wheezing or other signs of bronchospasm are present during physical examination in the absence of underlying lung disease.

LIFESTYLE AND BEHAVIOR MODIFICATION STRATEGIES

Prevention of pneumonia heavily relies on vaccination; based on existing recommendations, all elderly adults (>65 years of age) are advised to receive vaccination against pneumococcal disease and influenza. Immunization is also recommended for patients affected by chronic diseases such as heart and kidney disorders, asthma, COPD, diabetes mellitus, hepatic cirrhosis, functional or anatomic asplenia, and alcoholism, and in the case of immunocompromised hosts, including HIV infection, cancer chemotherapy, and hematologic malignancies.[32]

A number of risk factors significantly predispose to the occurrence of pneumococcal pneumonia, including lifestyle factors. Smoking is linked to increased susceptibility to CAP in several epidemiologic studies, so smoking cessation is advisable. Daily hygiene may offer protection from pneumonia because hand washing (even with a nonmedicated soap) is known to be an effective means of preventing bacterial transmission.[37] Hand washing with an antimicrobial agent may prove even more effective, and proper hygiene of the nasal and oropharyngeal cavities is also important because the primary step in the pathogenesis of pneumococcal invasive infections is nasopharyngeal colonization.[38]

Sufficient hours of sleep and an enhanced social role of elderly women are associated with a reduced mortality from pneumonia and other age-related diseases.[39] Excessive weight gain is a risk factor for CAP among men and women in the United States, whereas physical activity is inversely associated with the risk for development of CAP among women.[40]

Malnutrition is a key contributor to the development of pneumonia among ICU patients, probably by impairing host defense. Along these lines, the use of immune-enhancing feeds enriched with a variety of nutrients including the amino acids arginine and glutamine, as well as nucleotides, is associated with fewer nosocomial infections, such as pneumonia.[41] Still, further studies are needed to precisely establish the blend of nutrients able to provide the most beneficial effects. Nutritional studies suggest that higher intakes of α-linolenic and linoleic acids and possibly of fish may significantly reduce the risk for pneumonia.[37]

In children, a wide range of environmental factors is thought to potentially have a positive impact on health, including proper nutrition (proteins, vitamins, antioxidants), lifestyle and behavior choices (abstinence from tobacco and alcohol use), good parental health, socioeconomic status, choice of living environment (urban versus rural), and parent-sibling behavior.[42]

PHARMACOLOGIC TREATMENT

The principal treatment of pneumonia relies on addressing the underlying etiology. At presentation, clinical and laboratory features do not allow prediction of microbial cause; thus, knowledge of likely causative pathogens based on local epidemiology and consideration of possible antibiotic resistance spread are important to direct appropriate treatment. Prompt initiation of empirical antibiotic therapy is paramount for a favorable outcome, although this is not always achieved. Common reasons for delaying antibiotic therapy are administrative issues; incorrect diagnosis; and insufficient knowledge, experience, or confidence on the part of the physician, often leading to a delay in obtaining results of microbial testing. Administration of an antimicrobial effective for isolated or suspected pathogens within the first hour of documented hypotension has been associated with a survival rate of 79.9%, whereas each hour of delay over the next 6 hours was related to an average decrease in survival of 7.6%.[43]

Recommendations for initial empirically reasoned antibiotic therapy in CAP are based on prediction of the most likely pathogen, after consideration of both the regional patterns of resistance and the individual patient toxicity risk associated with selected antibiotics. Available guidelines also evaluate the need for and feasibility of more aggressive treatment and the setting of the individual patient because this pragmatically reflects disease severity and mortality risk. For home-treated patients, U.S. recommendations indicate the use of macrolides or doxycycline (if the former is not tolerated), whereas European guidelines advocate administration of amoxicillin, which, although ineffective for atypical pathogens, may successfully treat the often macrolide-resistant S. pneumoniae strains circulating in Europe.[2,12] For non-ICU hospitalized patients, both European[2] and U.S.[1] guidelines advise the use of a respiratory fluoroquinolone alone or a β-lactam and macrolide combination. For patients hospitalized in the ICU because of severe CAP, institution of therapy targeting S. pneumoniae, Legionella species, and most of the clinically relevant

Enterobacteriaceae family is warranted,[1,2] thus directing the use of a potent antipneumococcal β-lactam in combination with either a macrolide or a fluoroquinolone.

Asthma and lower respiratory tract infections such as pneumonia can be significant causes of chest pain. Analgesic medications can improve chest pain associated with pulmonary pathologies, but the mainstay of therapy is to treat the underlying etiology. The chest pain generally resolves with the resolution of other respiratory symptoms.

Considerations for Patients with Asthma

Antibiotics prescribed for pneumonia do not currently play a major role in the treatment of chronic asthma in stable patients. Nevertheless, emerging evidence depicts improvement of the symptoms and markers of airway inflammation in patients who have atypical bacterial infection as a cofactor in their asthma and are treated with macrolide antibiotics.[44]

Inhaled corticosteroids (ICSs) are the mainstay of asthma treatment, but the effect of such inhaled agents on CAP is unclear. Studies in COPD reported increased rates of pneumonia associated with ICS intake,[45] and there are concerns about an increased pneumonia risk in patients with asthma under ICS treatment. A study illustrated that there was no increased risk for pneumonia acquisition among patients with asthma receiving budesonide.[46] In contrast, according to a Japanese report, there may be a greater risk for nontuberculous *Mycobacterium* infection in asthmatic patients who are older, have more severe airflow limitation, and receive higher doses of ICS therapy.[47]

Inhaled anticholinergics also are associated with an increased risk for development of CAP among asthmatic patients.[48] Although it is difficult to differentiate between the effect of inhaled therapy and the impact of asthma severity on the risk for CAP, this relationship, even if not causal, could call attention to inhaled therapy in COPD and asthma patients.[48]

An earlier report describes the development of *Pneumocystis carinii* pneumonia as a consequence of asthma treatment with methotrexate. Investigation of new infiltrates in a patient with asthma receiving methotrexate treatment should be thoroughly performed to determine the cause and to differentiate from drug-induced pneumonitis.[49]

UNMET, FUTURE RESEARCH NEEDS

1. There is a need to improve clinical outcomes in hospitalized patients with bacterial CAP because 6% to 15% of such patients and up to 40% of those initially admitted to the ICU fail to respond to original antibiotic therapy.[1]

2. There are limitations to identifying the etiologic agent of CAP in more than 50% of cases,[11] a fact that dictates the necessity of faster and more specific diagnostic methods.

3. There is a documented emergence of drug-resistant strains of *S. pneumoniae* (DRSP) and community-acquired methicillin-resistant *S. aureus* (CA-MRSA), often associated with necrotizing pneumonia, shock, respiratory failure, and formation of abscesses and empyemas.[2] Still, the clinical relevance of DRSP remains uncertain, with current levels of β-lactam resistance not resulting in treatment failures in patients with CAP, as long as appropriate dosages and compounds are used. However, macrolide-resistant *S. pneumoniae* strains may lead to clinical failure.[50] Drug-resistance levels in DRSP and CA-MRSA are highly location specific, as are penicillin-, macrolide-, or dual-resistance rates of *S. pneumoniae*.[50] The European Antimicrobial Resistance Surveillance Network project (http://www.ecdc.europa.eu/en/activities/surveillance/EARS-Net/Pages/index.aspx) regularly provides data on the resistance of *S. pneumoniae* across many European countries; nevertheless, related data must soon become available for the widest range of countries possible. Improvement in both the identification rate of the causative agent and the acquisition of data on resistance patterns will substantially aid advances toward prescribing narrow-spectrum and effective antibiotics for the management of bacterial CAP.

4. Future research efforts also should contribute to unraveling the complex relationship between causative agents of pneumonia and asthma. Viruses are the most common triggers of wheezing attacks; however, the mechanism by which they contribute to disease onset or progression remains elusive. Even less is known about the role of bacterial pathogens related to CAP (including the atypical pathogens) in the pathogenesis of asthma. Moreover, the microbial flora colonizing the airway may also influence asthma onset or progression. Serologic evidence of an immune response to *S. pneumoniae, H. influenzae,* and *M. catarrhalis* can be found in 20% of wheezing children,[7] whereas *M. pneumoniae* and *C. pneumoniae* have been identified in 5% to 25% of children with asthma exacerbations.[8]

5. Finally, in regard to cost-related aspects of pneumonia, national health systems should consider increasing support to infection control programs in order to ultimately avert or reduce preventable community and nosocomial infections and their associated expenditures, which in the case of pneumonia are exceptionally high.

CONCLUSION

Pneumonia is an acute lower respiratory tract infection with significant worldwide morbidity and mortality, especially in underdeveloped nations. The clinical presentation of pneumonia is quite diverse with a range of symptoms, of which fever, cough, and tachypnea are most common. Diagnosis of pneumonia is supported by a chest radiograph displaying new shadowing, but most often, diagnosis is performed at the primary care level, in the absence of an imaging technique, and based only on symptoms and physical examination. Pneumonia is caused by a broad spectrum of microorganisms, whose identification can be difficult and time consuming and may often require invasive techniques and procedures of uncertain diagnostic success. Therefore, antimicrobial treatment is provided empirically and before any diagnostic test because prompt initiation of treatment is imperative and decisive for patient outcome.

Viral and bacterial causative agents of CAP are implicated in asthma pathogenesis. Early-life RSV and HRV lower respiratory tract infections are linked to an increased asthma risk at school age, whereas pneumonia caused by *Mycoplasma* or *Chlamydia* is associated with the inception, exacerbation, and chronicity of asthma. Moreover, asthma presents an important risk factor for the acquisition of severe pneumococcal infections. Macrolide antibiotics are found to benefit asthma patients with an atypical bacterial pulmonary infection.

Vaccination against pneumococci and influenza virus may significantly contribute to pneumonia prevention. A proactive lifestyle including refraining from smoking, avoidance of increased weight, physical activity, and proper nutrition can also significantly reduce the risk for pneumonia.

Future research should include efforts toward a better understanding of the epidemiology of pneumonia and related microorganisms and development of improved and more rapid diagnostics. Another scientific area requiring particular attention is in relation to the clinical relevance of the continuously increasing appearance of drug-resistant strains. Finally, research efforts should also decipher the interactions between asthma pathogenesis and lower respiratory tract infections.

REFERENCES

1. Mandell LA, Wunderink RG, Anzueto A, et al. Infectious Diseases Society of America/American Thoracic Society consensus guidelines on the management of community-acquired pneumonia in adults. *Clin Infect Dis.* 2007;44(Suppl 2):S27–S72.
2. Lim WS, Baudouin SV, George RC, et al. BTS guidelines for the management of community acquired pneumonia in adults: update 2009. *Thorax.* 2009;64(Suppl 3):iii1–55.
3. Hale KA, Isaacs D. Antibiotics in childhood pneumonia. *Paediatr Respir Rev.* 2006;7(2):145–151.
4. Tsolia MN, Psarras S, Bossios A, et al. Etiology of community-acquired pneumonia in hospitalized school-age children: evidence for high prevalence of viral infections. *Clin Infect Dis.* 2004;39(5):681–686.

5. Bradley JS, Byington CL, Shah SS, et al. The management of community-acquired pneumonia in infants and children older than 3 months of age: clinical practice guidelines by the Pediatric Infectious Diseases Society and the Infectious Diseases Society of America. *Clin Infect Dis.* 2011;53(7):e25–e76.
6. Harris M, Clark J, Coote N, et al. British Thoracic Society guidelines for the management of community acquired pneumonia in children: update 2011. *Thorax.* 2011;66(Suppl 2):ii1–23.
7. Durbin WJ, Stille C. Pneumonia. *Pediatr Rev.* 2008;29(5):147–158; quiz 159–160.
8. Chung HL, Shin JY, Ju M, Kim WT, Kim SG. Decreased interleukin-18 response in asthmatic children with severe *Mycoplasma pneumoniae* pneumonia. *Cytokine.* 2011;54(2):218–221.
9. Loeb M. Pneumonia in older persons. *Clin Infect Dis.* 2003;37(10):1335–1339.
10. Dean NC, Suchyta MR, Bateman KA, Aronsky D, Hadlock CJ. Implementation of admission decision support for community-acquired pneumonia. *Chest.* 2000;117(5):1368–1377.
11. van der Eerden MM, Vlaspolder F, de Graaff CS, et al. Comparison between pathogen directed antibiotic treatment and empirical broad spectrum antibiotic treatment in patients with community acquired pneumonia: a prospective randomised study. *Thorax.* 2005;60(8):672–678.
12. Carbonara S, Stano F, Scotto G, Monno L, Angarano G. The correct approach to community-acquired pneumonia in immunocompetent adults: review of current guidelines. *New Microbiol.* 2008;31(1):1–18.
13. Hohenthal U, Vainionpaa R, Meurman O, et al. Aetiological diagnosis of community acquired pneumonia: utility of rapid microbiological methods with respect to disease severity. *Scand J Infect Dis.* 2008;40(2):131–138.
14. Taylor MB, Barkham T. Fatal case of pneumonia caused by a nonhemolytic strain of Streptococcus pyogenes. *J Clin Microbiol.* 2002;40(6):2311–2312.
15. Bellei N, Benfica D, Perosa AH, Carlucci R, Barros M, Granato C. Evaluation of a rapid test (QuickVue) compared with the shell vial assay for detection of influenza virus clearance after antiviral treatment. *J Virol Methods.* 2003;109(1):85–88.
16. Campbell JF, Spika JS. The serodiagnosis of nonpneumococcal bacterial pneumonia. *Semin Respir Infect.* 1988;3(2):123–130.
17. Miyashita N, Ouchi K, Kawasaki K, et al. Comparison of serological tests for detection of immunoglobulin M antibodies to *Chlamydophila pneumoniae*. *Respirology.* 2008;13(3):427–431.
18. Jensen JU, Heslet L, Jensen TH, Espersen K, Steffensen P, Tvede M. Procalcitonin increase in early identification of critically ill patients at high risk of mortality. *Crit Care Med.* 2006;34(10):2596–2602.
19. Kee C, Palladino S, Kay I, et al. Feasibility of real-time polymerase chain reaction in whole blood to identify *Streptococcus pneumoniae* in patients with community-acquired pneumonia. *Diagn Microbiol Infect Dis.* 2008;61(1):72–75.
20. Schluger N, Godwin T, Sepkowitz K, et al. Application of DNA amplification to pneumocystosis: presence of serum *Pneumocystis carinii* DNA during human and experimentally induced *Pneumocystis carinii* pneumonia. *J Exp Med.* 1992;176(5):1327–1333.
21. Dominguez J, Gali N, Blanco S, et al. Detection of *Streptococcus pneumoniae* antigen by a rapid immunochromatographic assay in urine samples. *Chest.* 2001;119(1):243–249.
22. Ruf B, Schurmann D, Horbach I, Fehrenbach FJ, Pohle HD. Prevalence and diagnosis of Legionella pneumonia: a 3-year prospective study with emphasis on application of urinary antigen detection. *J Infect Dis.* 1990;162(6):1341–1348.
23. Skerrett SJ. Diagnostic testing for community-acquired pneumonia. *Clin Chest Med.* 1999;20(3):531–548.
24. Hoare Z, Lim WS. Pneumonia: update on diagnosis and management. *BMJ.* 2006;332(7549):1077–1079.
25. Sigurs N, Bjarnason R, Sigurbergsson F, Kjellman B. Respiratory syncytial virus bronchiolitis in infancy is an important risk factor for asthma and allergy at age 7. *Am J Respir Crit Care Med.* 2000;161(5):1501–1507.
26. Jackson DJ, Gangnon RE, Evans MD, et al. Wheezing rhinovirus illnesses in early life predict asthma development in high-risk children. *Am J Respir Crit Care Med.* 2008;178(7):667–672.
27. Esposito S, Blasi F, Arosio C, et al. Importance of acute *Mycoplasma pneumoniae* and *Chlamydia pneumoniae* infections in children with wheezing. *Eur Respir J.* 2000;16(6):1142–1146.
28. Kraft M, Cassell GH, Henson JE, et al. Detection of *Mycoplasma pneumoniae* in the airways of adults with chronic asthma. *Am J Respir Crit Care Med.* 1998;158(3):998–1001.
29. Jeong YC, Yeo MS, Kim JH, Lee HB, Oh JW. *Mycoplasma pneumoniae* infection affects the serum levels of vascular endothelial growth

factor and interleukin-5 in atopic children. *Allergy Asthma Immunol Res.* 2012;4(2):92–97.
30. Peters J, Singh H, Brooks EG, et al. Persistence of community-acquired respiratory distress syndrome toxin-producing *Mycoplasma pneumoniae* in refractory asthma. *Chest.* 2011;140(2): 401–407.
31. Korppi M. Bacterial infections and pediatric asthma. *Immunol Allergy Clin N Am.* 2010;30(4):565–574, vii.
32. Obert J, Burgel PR. Pneumococcal infections: association with asthma and COPD. *Med Mal Infect.* 2012;42(5):188–192.
33. Moore WC, Bleecker ER, Curran-Everett D, et al. Characterization of the severe asthma phenotype by the National Heart, Lung, and Blood Institute's Severe Asthma Research Program. *J Allergy Clin Immunol.* 2007;119(2):405–413.
34. Ostergaard MS, Nantanda R, Tumwine JK, Aabenhus R. Childhood asthma in low income countries: an invisible killer? *Prim Care Respir J.* 2012;21(2):214–219.
35. Brand PL, Hoving MF, de Groot EP. Evaluating the child with recurrent lower respiratory tract infections. *Paediatr Respir Rev.* 2012;13(3):135–138.
36. Greenberg D, Leibovitz E. Community-acquired pneumonia in children: from diagnosis to treatment. *Chang Gung Med J.* 2005;28(11):746–752.
37. Vincent JL. Prevention of nosocomial bacterial pneumonia. *Thorax.* 1999;54(6):544–549.
38. Oliveira TF, Gomes Filho IS, Passos Jde S, et al. Factors associated with nosocomial pneumonia in hospitalized individuals. *Rev Assoc Med Bras.* 2011;57(6):630–636.
39. Goto A, Yasumura S, Nishise Y, Sakihara S. Association of health behavior and social role with total mortality among Japanese elders in Okinawa, Japan. *Aging Clin Exp Res.* 2003;15(6): 443–450.
40. Baik I, Curhan GC, Rimm EB, Bendich A, Willett WC, Fawzi WW. A prospective study of age and lifestyle factors in relation to community-acquired pneumonia in US men and women. *Arch Intern Med.* 2000;160(20):3082–3088.
41. Merchant AT, Curhan GC, Rimm EB, Willett WC, Fawzi WW. Intake of n-6 and n-3 fatty acids and fish and risk of community-acquired pneumonia in US men. *Am J Clin Nutr.* 2005;82(3):668–674.
42. Pallapies D. Trends in childhood disease. *Mutat Res.* 2006;608(2):100–111.
43. Rello J. Demographics, guidelines, and clinical experience in severe community-acquired pneumonia. *Crit Care.* 2008;12(Suppl 6):S2.
44. Kraft M, Cassell GH, Pak J, Martin RJ. Mycoplasma pneumoniae and *Chlamydia pneumoniae* in asthma: effect of clarithromycin. *Chest.* 2002;121(6):1782–1788.
45. Drummond MB, Dasenbrook EC, Pitz MW, Murphy DJ, Fan E. Inhaled corticosteroids in patients with stable chronic obstructive pulmonary disease: a systematic review and meta-analysis. *JAMA.* 2008;300(20):2407–2416.
46. O'Byrne PM, Pedersen S, Carlsson LG, et al. Risks of pneumonia in patients with asthma taking inhaled corticosteroids. *Am J Respir Crit Care Med.* 2011;183(5):589–595.
47. Hojo M, Iikura M, Hirano S, et al. Increased risk of nontuberculous mycobacterial infection in asthmatic patients using long-term inhaled corticosteroid therapy. *Respirology.* 2012;17(1):185–190.
48. Almirall J, Bolibar I, Serra-Prat M, et al. Inhaled drugs as risk factors for community-acquired pneumonia. *Eur Respir J.* 2010;36(5): 1080–1087.
49. Kuitert LM, Harrison AC. *Pneumocystis carinii* pneumonia as a complication of methotrexate treatment of asthma. *Thorax.* 1991;46(12): 936–937.
50. Woodhead M, Blasi F, Ewig S, et al. Guidelines for the management of adult lower respiratory tract infections—full version. *Clin Microbiol Infect.* 2011;17(Suppl 6):E1–E59.

13

COUGH

COMORBID, COEXISTING, AND DIFFERENTIAL DIAGNOSIS

Pramod Kelkar, Alan Goldsobel, and Riccardo Polosa

KEY POINTS

- Cough is a common symptom in adults and children.
- Cough reflex sensitivity and airway hyperreactivity are separate physiologic processes. Either or both can be upregulated in a given patient.
- Cough-asthma syndrome includes asthma per se, cough-variant asthma, nonasthmatic eosinophilic bronchitis, and atopic cough.
- Cough in an asthmatic person does not always represent worsening asthma and can be associated with other coexisting or comorbid diseases.
- Other common causes of cough include upper airway cough syndrome and gastroesophageal reflux disease in a nonasthmatic adult with chronic cough and normal chest x-ray.
- Pediatric chronic cough, particularly in children younger than 6 to 8 years, may have different etiologies, such as protracted bacterial bronchitis.

MECHANISMS, EPIDEMIOLOGY, AND COUGH MEASUREMENT

Cough results from forced expulsion, usually against a closed glottis, creating a characteristic sound. It is a natural reflex and defense mechanism, helping the body clear excessive secretions, and it prevents foreign material from entering the respiratory tract. At times, cough can become excessive, nonproductive, disturbing to the patient, and potentially harmful.[1]

Cough is the most common symptom for which adult patients seek outpatient medical care. It is also one of the main symptoms associated with asthma with or without wheeze, dyspnea, and chest tightness. Cough allegedly is the most troublesome presenting symptom in adults with asthma,[2] and they are willing to trade higher levels of other symptoms for a reduction in this symptom. In children, cough is the most frequent symptom predicting subsequent wheezing and an asthma exacerbation.[3,4]

Cough can be predictive of poorer outcomes in asthma. In a 9-year study in adults, worsening cough had the highest predictive value for increasing asthma severity.[5] Methods to measure cough in asthma as well as in other conditions are important because subjective patient reporting of frequency does not correlate well with objective measurements in asthma. Objective ambulatory cough counts in asthmatic patients do not correlate with airway hyperresponsiveness, pulmonary function, or exhaled nitric oxide (NO) levels. However, objective cough frequency in patients with asthma is related to asthma control.[6] Objective cough rates also correlate with cough-related quality of life.[7] The presence of cough does not always imply worsening asthma, and other causes need to be considered in the differential diagnosis.

CLINICAL FEATURES: ASTHMA SYNDROME AND CHRONIC COUGH

Chronic cough in adults is defined as persisting for more than 8 weeks.[1] Multiple prospective studies show that asthma is one of the more common causes of chronic cough in nonsmoking adults with a normal chest x-ray (CXR).[8] In asthma, cough is usually associated with wheeze and dyspnea, but in some patients, it can be the sole symptom. This presentation is termed *cough-variant asthma*, first described by Glauser in 1972[9] and subsequently named by Corrao and colleagues.[10] In classic asthma and cough-variant asthma, airway inflammation (typically eosinophilic), bronchial hyperresponsiveness, and variable airflow obstruction are present. Cough-variant asthma is thought to be not a "forme fruste" of asthma but rather a clinical manifestation of asthma with similar pathologic changes in the airways.[11]

Two other cough-predominant eosinophilic airway disorders are described: nonasthmatic eosinophilic bronchitis (NAEB) and atopic cough (AC). These eosinophilic airway conditions can be linked to asthma by thinking of them as being part of the "asthma syndrome." NAEB and AC have been described in nonwheezing adults with chronic cough who demonstrate eosinophilic airway inflammation without airway hyperresponsiveness, variable airflow obstruction, or bronchodilator responsiveness. A striking pathophysiologic difference between asthma and NAEB is the absence of mast cell infiltration in smooth muscle bundles in NAEB.[12] NAEB accounts for about 10% to 30% of cases of chronic cough referred to a tertiary care center. Its etiology is uncertain but can be associated with exposure to occupational sensitizing agents or inhaled allergens.[13] Its natural history is somewhat unclear; long-term follow-up data of 32 patients suggest that although a minority (16%) of patients developed fixed airway obstruction, 66% of patients had persistent symptoms or inflammation.[14] Some studies have observed that up to 40% of patients with chronic obstructive pulmonary disease (COPD) without a history of asthma and no bronchodilator reversibility have sputum evidence of an airway eosinophilia. This observation provides one possible explanation for the presence of eosinophilic airway inflammation in some patients with COPD without apparent preexisting asthma, implying that NAEB may in some circumstances be a prelude to COPD.[15,16]

Fujimura and colleagues proposed the new cough category of AC, a bronchodilator-resistant, nonproductive chronic cough associated with atopy. They described the pathologic characteristics of AC as eosinophilic tracheobronchitis with bronchoalveolar lavage eosinophilia and the physiologic characteristics as cough hypersensitivity without bronchial hyperresponsiveness.[17] Affected patients did not have a higher incidence of developing asthma. AC has only been described in Japan. Other cough researchers believe that AC is merely a collection of atopic individuals with cough-variant asthma and its existence as a separate entity is debatable.[18] See Table 13.1 for a complete list of cough-asthma syndromes.

Table 13.1. Cough-Asthma Syndromes

	CLASSIC ASTHMA	COUGH-VARIANT ASTHMA	ATOPIC COUGH	NONASTHMATIC EOSINOPHILIC BRONCHITIS
Symptoms	Cough, dyspnea, wheeze, chest tightness	Cough only	Nonproductive cough only	Cough, possibly upper airway symptoms
Atopy	Common	Common	Very common	Same as general population
Variable airflow obstruction	Present	May be present	Absent	Absent
Airway hyperresponsiveness	Present	Present	Absent	Absent
Bronchodilator response	Present	Present	Absent	Absent
Progression to classic asthma	NA	30%	Rare	10%
Sputum eosinophilia >3%	Frequent	Frequent	Frequent	Always
Mast cells in airway smooth muscle bundles	Yes	Possibly increased	Unknown	No
Exhaled NO	Increased	Increased	Not increased	Increased
Cough reflex hypersensitivity	Normal or increased	Normal or increased	Increased	Increased
Steroid-responsive (inhaled and oral)	Yes	Yes	Yes	Yes
Bronchial biopsy eosinophilia	Common	Common	Common	Very common

Modified from Magni C, Chellini E, Zanasi A. Cough variant asthma and atopic cough. *Multidiscip Respir Med.* 2010; 5:99–103.

OTHER CAUSES OF NONASTHMATIC CHRONIC COUGH: DIFFERENTIAL DIAGNOSIS

In adults with a normal CXR, the most common causes of chronic cough other than asthma include gastroesophageal reflux disease (GERD) and upper airway cough syndrome (UACS). Other, less common causes include angiotensin-converting enzyme inhibitor (ACEI) therapy, COPD, bronchiectasis, and interstitial lung disease. Chronic cough has also been associated with obstructive sleep apnea.[19] Lung cancer has been found to be the cause in less than 2% of adults with chronic cough.[1] Some studies of chronic cough in adults find that up to 40% of cases have no definable cause after extensive investigation and treatment and are labeled idiopathic cough (Table 13.2). A more detailed list of the possible causes of chronic cough can be found in the American College of Chest Physicians (ACCP) guidelines on cough.[1] Some of the more common causes include the following:

A. *Gastroesophageal reflux disease.* GERD is a common medical problem with an estimated prevalence of 10% to 20%. It frequently results in gastrointestinal symptoms such as heartburn but may be asymptomatic or result in other symptoms, which include cough, hoarseness, and chest pain. A variety of pathophysiologic mechanisms are proposed, including (1) micro-aspiration of gastric contents into the laryngopharyngeal region, creating an inflammatory response; (2) esophageal distention and distal esophageal acid exposure, which trigger vagal reflexes; (3) esophageal acidification, triggering local axonal reflexes and leading to an inflammatory response in the airways[20]; and (4) higher cough sensitivity from acidic or weakly acidic refluxate or nonacid gastric contents. One mechanism for nonacid or weakly acid reflux is transient lower esophageal sphincter relaxation.[21,22] Reflux can cause cough, but cough can also cause or worsen reflux through increased intraabdominal pressure causing gastric contents to be pushed into the esophagus and macro- or micro-aspiration into the larynx causing laryngopharyngeal reflux.[23] In the early stages of reflux-induced cough, structural changes may not be apparent on indirect laryngoscopy or esophagogastroduodenoscopy, and thus such studies can be completely normal in some patients.

B. *Rhinitis and rhinosinusitis (UACS–postnasal drip syndrome)*. UACS is a common cause of chronic cough. There are no pathognomonic features to prove its existence, and the diagnosis is principally based on the patient's description of symptoms, the physical and radiologic findings (CXR or computed tomography scan of sinuses), and response to therapy. All forms of allergic and nonallergic rhinosinusitis can be associated with cough. The mechanism of cough is thought to be stimulation of the afferent pharyngeal branch of the vagus nerve. There is either mechanical or chemical irritation of receptors located in the nasopharynx or larynx or, rarely, actual aspiration of secretions into the lower airways. The secretions

Table 13.2. Common Causes of Chronic Cough in Adult Patients Investigated in Specialist Clinics

STUDY	PATIENT'S MEAN AGE (YR)	ASTHMA SYNDROME	GERD	RHINITIS	MOST COMMON OTHER CAUSES
Irwin et al., 1981[60]	50.3 (17–88)	25	10	29	Chronic bronchitis (12)
Poe et al., 1982[61]	? (15–89)	36	0	8	Postinfectious (27)
Poe et al., 1989[62]	44.8 (19–79)	35	5	26	Idiopathic (12)
Irwin et al., 1990[8]	51 (6–83)	24	21	41	Chronic bronchitis (5)
Hoffstein, 1994[63]	47	25	24	26	Postinfectious (21)
O'Connell et al., 1994[64]	49 (19–83)	6	10	13	Idiopathic (22)
Smyrnios et al., 1995[65] (G)	58 (18–86)	24	15	40	Chronic bronchitis (11)
Mello et al., 1996[66]	53.1 (15–83)	14	40	38	Bronchiectasis (4)
Marchesani et al., 1998[67]	51	14	5	56	Chronic bronchitis (16)
McGarvey et al., 1998[68]	47.5 (18–77)	23	19	21	Idiopathic (18)
Palombini et al., 1999[69]	57 (15–81)	59	41	58	Bronchiectasis (18)
Brightling et al., 1999[70]	No figures given	31	8	24	Postviral (13)

Adapted from Morice AH. Epidemiology of cough. In: F. Chung, J. Widdicombe, and H. Boushey, eds. *Cough: Causes, Mechanisms and Theory.* Oxford, UK: Blackwell; 2003:11–16.

originate from the nose or sinuses and drip into the hypopharynx. Treatment is individualized and directed at the specific cause. Further details can be found in specific chapters on rhinitis and sinusitis.

C. *Unexplained or idiopathic cough.* The diagnosis of unexplained or idiopathic cough is one of exclusion. In some studies of patients with chronic cough, up to 40% are not found to have a definable underlying etiology and are labeled as having idiopathic cough.[24] Chronic cough hypersensitivity syndrome is used to describe this type of cough.[25] Its features include female predominance, minimal or no sputum production, one or more sensory cough reflex triggers (i.e., cold air, speech, odors), urge to cough caused by a tickle or itch localized to the oropharynx and larynx (laryngeal hypersensitivity), and significant adverse impact of cough on the quality of life.

There are overlapping possible mechanisms for chronic cough hypersensitivity syndrome, all of which suggest laryngeal hypersensitivity:

1. Postviral vagal neuropathy is a laryngeal sensory neuropathy following an antecedent viral illness of undetermined time. Motor and sensory nerve branches can be involved, leading to cough or laryngospasm, vocal cord paresis, globus sensation, or odynophonia. Medical treatments tried with varied success include gabapentin, pregabalin, amitriptyline, and botulinum toxin type A.

2. Laryngeal dysfunction with chronic cough and throat clearing can be associated with chronic laryngeal irritation in which inflammatory and irritant stimuli result in laryngeal hypersensitivity to external stimuli. This triggers paradoxical vocal cord dysfunction during inspiration and leads to shortness of breath, often clinically mistaken for asthma. It can present with cough as a protective mechanism, attempting to open the glottic constriction that occurs during vocal cord dysfunction. Behavioral therapy or speech pathology may be helpful in treating this condition. Medical therapy with neuromodulator medication can also be tried.

3. Irritable larynx syndrome is defined as paradoxical vocal cord adduction as determined by a decrease in inspiratory flow rate (laryngeal hyperreactivity) measured through histamine inhalation challenge. Laryngeal hyperreactivity is proposed as a marker of upper airway involvement irrespective of the trigger of chronic cough and can be followed as an objective tool to evaluate response to therapy of the underlying triggers.

D. *Psychological factors and habit or psychogenic cough.* Habit or psychogenic cough can be challenging to diagnose and treat. It may be preceded by a routine viral upper respiratory infection with a characteristic persistent nonproductive, paroxysmal cough. It should be considered a diagnosis of exclusion, and underlying organic causes should be eliminated. Patients may complain of a tickle sensation in the throat leading to coughing fits. It is more common in children and adolescents, who frequently display the affect of showing no distress over the severity and frequency of a cough ("la belle indifference") that is frequently disruptive to normal activities and disturbing to parents and others around the patient. The cough characteristically diminishes with vigorous physical exertion and pleasurable activities and usually ceases during sleep. It can be difficult to differentiate this type of cough from Tourette's syndrome or other tic disorders. In children, males and females are equally affected, and severe underlying psychopathology is not typically seen. In adults, females are more affected, and it is more likely associated with a somatoform disorder. Using the term *unexplained cough* rather than *psychogenic cough* will minimize stigmatizing patients with a wrong diagnosis and implying that they are the cause of their own cough. Nevertheless, cough may rarely present as a form of somatization. In such cases, problems such as anxiety, depression, domestic violence, and child abuse or neglect that are often associated with somatization disorders should be evaluated.[26] Treatment modalities include forms of biofeedback, clinical hypnosis, suggestion therapy, and psychotherapy when indicated.

PEDIATRIC COUGH

Cough is a common symptom in healthy school-aged children, who could experience 10 to 11 cough episodes per day in a general survey.[27] Postviral cough (also called postinfectious cough) due to heightened chronic rhinosinusitis (CRS) is also common in children and typically lasts less than 4 weeks in nonasthmatic children.[1] Chronic cough in children is defined as lasting longer than 4 to 8 weeks and is associated with significant quality-of-life issues for the patient and family members, teachers, and other caregivers. Age seems to play a role in the etiology of chronic cough in children because older children and teens have similar problems as adults, in whom the evaluation and treatment are similar. Younger children, particularly those younger than 6 years, may have asthma, GERD, or upper airway diseases causing cough, but they frequently have a chronic "wet cough" caused by protracted bacterial bronchitis (PBB).[28] PBB is increasingly recognized in young children and associated with neutrophilic airway inflammation and infection with *Streptococcus pneumoniae*, *Haemophilus influenzae*, and *Moraxella catarrhalis*. CXR may be normal or show central airway prominence. Specific infiltrates are not seen. Antibiotic treatment for 2 to 4 weeks usually resolves this problem, although it may recur. Airway malacia abnormalities were observed in 30% to 74% of the subjects in published series[29] and may be associated with nonacid reflux or weakly acid reflux.[30] Most children with PBB are not immunodeficient, but specific antibody deficiency with abnormal response to pneumococcal vaccination has been described in some PBB patients.[31] Habit cough, a functional respiratory disorder, is more commonly seen in children and adolescents.

LIFESTYLE MODIFICATIONS

Lifestyle modifications that may help cough are directed toward managing the underlying cause. It is important to control or avoid environmental irritant and allergic triggers such as dust mites, indoor pets, and cigarette smoke, all of which exacerbate asthma and can trigger cough. Dietary modifications, such as avoiding alcohol, soda and other carbonated beverages, fried foods, and caffeine; avoiding postprandial recumbency; elevating the head of the bed; weight reduction; and stress reduction are important to treat GERD. Avoiding smoking is critical in all patients with cough.

MANAGEMENT

In patients with chronic cough, the management approach should focus on the detection of one or more underlying causes and therapeutic trials individualized based on each patient's unique history and physical examination. In up to 25% of adults with chronic cough, more than one underlying cause may be operative, requiring concurrent therapy. CXR and spirometry should be obtained in all patients with chronic cough. ACEI therapy should be discontinued in all patients with chronic cough. This cough can persist for up to 4 weeks. UACS, asthma, and GERD can all manifest with cough as the sole symptom. The character or timing of cough and the presence or absence of sputum are helpful in thinking about specific causes (e.g., cough after meals, GERD, barking or honking cough in children, habit cough, wet-sounding cough, protracted bacterial bronchitis) but should not be used as the sole criterion to rule in or rule out specific causes.

In UACS, treatment is directed toward the cause. Allergic rhinitis can be treated with antihistamines, intranasal corticosteroid sprays, and allergen immunotherapy. Nonallergic rhinitis responds to water-salt sinus rinses, intranasal antihistamine and corticosteroid sprays, and intranasal anticholinergic sprays. Sinusitis is treated with antibiotics, corticosteroids, and also surgery if medical management fails. Further details on therapy of these entities are provided in the chapter on rhinitis. When a specific cause of UACS is not apparent, the ACCP guidelines recommend empirical therapy with a first-generation antihistamine-decongestant combination before embarking on a workup.

Asthmatic cough typically responds to standard asthma therapy. NAEB and AC respond to inhaled corticosteroid therapy. Rarely, systemic steroids are needed. Other antiasthmatic medications like leukotriene receptor antagonists have not been studied for this condition. In patients with severe or refractory cough due to asthma, the ACCP guidelines recommend giving a short course (1 to 2 weeks) of systemic (oral) corticosteroids followed by inhaled corticosteroids.

The ACCP guidelines recommend doing therapeutic trials in lieu of testing in patients who fit the clinical profile for GERD-induced cough. GERD-induced cough usually responds to an empirical trial of medical antireflux therapy. This typically involves (1) lifestyle modifications, (2) acid-suppression (proton pump inhibitors and histamine-2 blockers), (3) the addition of prokinetic therapy, and (4) detection and treatment of comorbid conditions like sleep apnea. The response should be assessed in 1 to 3 months. If the therapeutic trial fails, further systematic evaluation to rule out GERD can be undertaken. This involves 24-hour pH probe monitoring and barium esophagogram. The performance of 24-hour pH probe tests is recommended with antireflux therapy to gauge whether the therapy needs to be intensified or whether the medical therapy has failed. A normal esophagoscopy finding does not rule out GERD as the cause of cough. Prior history of antireflux surgery does not rule out GERD as the cause of cough because in some patients a revision surgery is necessary. In some uncontrolled studies, antireflux surgery shows potential benefit.[32]

The management of unexplained or idiopathic cough is based on empirical, time-limited therapeutic trials and focuses on eliminating all causes of cough in a sequential stepwise manner. Because multiple etiologies of cough exist, therapy should be additive on a case-by-case basis. Laryngeal dysfunction can be present in unexplained or chronic cough from other causes. Symptoms of laryngeal dysfunction include voice hoarseness, dyspnea, wheeze, and cough. Extrathoracic airway hyperresponsiveness is another manifestation of laryngeal dysfunction and has been reported in several conditions in which cough is prominent, such as rhinosinusitis, ACEI-induced cough, GERD, and patients with asthma-like symptoms.[33] Speech therapy can be a valuable adjunct in cases of chronic refractory cough through a behavioral approach to cough suppression or improved vocal hygiene, thereby leading to reduced laryngeal irritation, which further results in decreased cough sensitivity, decreased urge to cough, and an increased cough threshold. This was shown by a study by Ryan and colleagues[34] in which primary outcome measures were capsaicin cough reflex sensitivity, automated cough frequency detection, and cough-related quality of life.

COUGH SUPPRESSION AND FUTURE THERAPIES

When diagnostic and treatment trials have failed to resolve the cough, a different approach is necessary: cough suppression with or without normalization of the cough reflex. A number of medications can be used to suppress cough, and others are in clinical development. Cough suppressants are divided into centrally acting and peripherally acting antitussives.

1. *Centrally acting antitussives.* Morphine, an opiate, is an excellent cough suppressor through its action on the κ receptor, which also mediates its sedative side effects. A randomized controlled study of low-dose modified-release morphine sulfate (5 mg twice daily) in refractory cough showed significant improvement in subjective measurements of cough (Leicester Cough Questionnaire and daily cough diary), but no improvement in evoked cough challenge.[35] Codeine, also an opiate, showed little benefit for cough suppression in experimental models of cough and in clinical trials.[36-38] However, large intersubject variability of codeine's effect was reported. Dextromethorphan is a synthetic opioid that has been shown to attenuate cough count in experimental cough challenge in normal volunteers.[39] The only study showing a clinical reduction in cough with dextromethorphan is a meta-analysis using cough-counting methodology in which the drug was significantly beneficial over placebo in attenuating naturally occurring cough after viral respiratory infection.[40] Gabapentin is a gamma-aminobutyric acid (GABA) analog and a centrally acting neuroleptic agent. It is superior to placebo in

both subjective and objective measurements of cough in patients with cough hypersensitivity, but the effect is small. Gabapentin and pregabalin (a precursor to gabapentin with a better pharmacologic profile) subjectively ameliorate cough secondary to laryngeal sensory neuropathy.[41,42] Amitriptyline is another centrally acting neuroleptic agent that causes subjective improvements in postviral vagal neuropathy and idiopathic chronic cough.[43,44]

2. *Peripherally acting antitussives.* There are also antitussive agents known to act peripherally. These include the GABA-B agonist lesogaberan as well as the TRPV1 and TRPA1 antagonists. They are all being investigated for clinical development. In phase II studies, lesogaberan is superior to placebo in reducing transient lower esophageal sphincter relaxation, acid reflux episodes, and lower esophageal sphincter pressure.[45,46] In a large randomized controlled study of lesogaberan versus placebo in subjects on proton pump inhibitors with persisting GERD symptoms, lesogaberan improved significantly their heartburn and regurgitation symptoms and was well tolerated.[47] Moreover, days with a cough were recorded as a secondary endpoint, and more patients reported improvement in daytime cough in treatment versus placebo with active treatment. TRPV1 and TRPA1 are cation channels coexpressed in primary sensory neurons that can be activated by a number of exogenous and endogenous irritants.[48,49] Increased cough hypersensitivity to heat and low pH may be mediated by both cation channels, and for that reason antagonists to TRPV1 and TRPA1 are currently in development for the treatment of intractable cough. Clinical studies are now in progress to evaluate the efficacy and safety of TRPV1 and TRPA1 antagonists.[50]

3. *Other mechanisms.* Other agents are under investigation for clinical development that exert antitussive function by alternative mechanisms. Macrolides may attenuate mucous hypersecretion, modulate systemic and pulmonary cytokine profiles, and exert an inhibitory effect on the innate immune response.[51] With the premise that chronic cough may be linked with neutrophilic airway inflammation, a randomized placebo-controlled study of low-dose erythromycin was conducted in patients with unexplained cough.[52] Although a reduction in induced sputum neutrophil count after 12 weeks of treatment was reported, there was no change in cough frequency or severity in the patients. In an observational assessment of azithromycin in patients undergoing lung transplantation, there were significant improvements in total number of reflux events (acid and nonacid) and proximal extent of the refluxate, implying that this medication may attenuate GERD and bile acid aspiration possibly by enhancing prokinetic effects on esophageal and gastric motility.[53] These notions may have practical implications for refractory cough in general, and specifically for difficult-to-treat asthmatic patients. Theobromine and theophylline are nonspecific PDE inhibitors used as bronchodilators. However, there is now evidence that these drugs are efficacious in ameliorating the citric acid–induced cough in ovalbumin-sensitized animal models.[54,55] Moreover, in a phase 1 randomized controlled trial of 10 healthy subjects, theobromine suppressed capsaicin-induced cough with no adverse events.[56] To improve their adverse effect profile, more specific phosphodiesterase (PDE) inhibitors have been recently developed. PDE3 (cilostazol) and PDE4 (citalopram) inhibitors have been shown to have antitussive activity in citric acid and capsaicin challenges in guinea pigs.[57-59]

UNMET, FUTURE RESEARCH NEEDS

1. More research is necessary to better delineate the characteristics of cough in patients who have asthma, in particular, cough variant asthma.

2. Better cough suppressive pharmacotherapy is necessary.

3. Chronic cough is a debilitating symptom and is socially unacceptable.

4. When the etiology of cough is uncertain, specialized care is necessary.

5. More research is necessary, in particular, for post-viral induced cough. Its etiology and treatment remain to be better elucidated.

CONCLUSION

Cough is a complex symptom and often requires a multidisciplinary approach to ascertain its cause and effective treatment. Evaluation should be guided by a thorough history and physical examination, and testing should be individualized for cost effectiveness. In children, particular attention needs to be paid to postviral cough because children can get three to five virus infections per year, mostly concentrated in the winter months. Also, parental anxiety can magnify the importance of this symptom, and the clinician has to be discerning in order to avoid overmedicating a child. Habit cough and unexplained cough are diagnoses of exclusion, and any tendency to underdiagnose or overdiagnose these conditions should be avoided. Most over-the-counter cough suppressants are not as effective as previously thought, and their use in routine practice should be minimized. Future research should be conducted to elucidate the mechanisms of cough production and to develop cough-suppressive pharmacotherapy. Allergists, as experts in the management of upper and lower airway disorders, should play a central role in the diagnosis and management of cough.

REFERENCES

1. Irwin RS, Boulet LP, Cloutier MM, et al. Managing cough as a defense mechanism and as a symptom: a consensus panel report of the American College of Chest Physicians. Chest. 1998;114:133S-181S.
2. Osman LM, McKenzie L, Cairns J, et al. Patient weighting of importance of asthma symptoms. Thorax. 2001;56(2):138-142.
3. Rivera-Spoljaric K, Chinchilli VM, Camera LJ, et al., for the Childhood Asthma Research and Education (CARE) Network. Signs and symptoms that precede wheezing in children with a pattern of moderate-to-severe intermittent wheezing. J Pediatr. 2009;154(6):877-881.e4.
4. Skytt N, Bønnelykke K, Bisgaard H. "To wheeze or not to wheeze": that is not the question. J Allergy Clin Immunol. 2012;130(2):403-407.e5.
5. de Marco R, Marcon A, Jarvis D, et al., for the European Community Respiratory Health Survey Therapy Group. Prognostic factors of asthma severity: a 9-year international prospective cohort study. J Allergy Clin Immunol. 2006;117(6):1249-1256.
6. Marsden PA, Smith JA, Kelsall AA, et al. A comparison of objective and subjective measures of cough in asthma. J Allergy Clin Immunol. 2008;122(5):903-907.
7. Sunger K, Powley W, Kelsall A, Sumner H, Murdoch R, Smith JA. Objective measurement of cough in otherwise healthy volunteers with acute cough. Eur Respir J. 2013;41(2):277-284.
8. Irwin RS, Curley FJ, French CL. Chronic cough: the spectrum and frequency of causes, key components of the diagnostic evaluation, and outcome of specific therapy. Am Rev Respir Dis. 1990;141(3):640-647.
9. Glauser FL. Variant asthma. Ann Allergy. 1972;30(8):457-459.
10. Corrao WM, Braman SS, Irwin RS. Chronic cough as the sole presenting manifestation of bronchial asthma. N Engl J Med. 1979;300(12):633-637.
11. Niimi A, Matsumoto H, Minakuchi M, Kitaichi M, Amitani R. Airway remodeling in cough-variant asthma. Med J Aust. 2000;356(9229):564-565.
12. Brightling CE, Woltmann G, Wardlaw AJ, et al. Development of irreversible airflow obstruction in a patient with eosinophilic bronchitis without asthma. Eur Respir J. 1999;14:1228-1230.
13. Lemiere C, Efthimiadis A, Hargreave FE. Occupational eosinophilic bronchitis without asthma: an unknown occupational airway disease. J Allergy Clin Immunol. 1997;100:852-853.
14. Berry MA, Hargadon B, McKenna S, et al. Observational study of the natural history of eosinophilic bronchitis. Clin Exp Allergy. 2005;35:598-601.
15. Pizzichini E, Pizzichini MM, Gibson P, et al. Sputum eosinophilia predicts benefit from prednisone in smokers with chronic obstructive bronchitis. Am J Respir Crit Care Med. 1998;158:1511-1517.
16. Brightling CE, Monteiro W, Ward R, et al. Sputum eosinophilia and short-term response to prednisolone in chronic obstructive pulmonary disease: a randomized controlled trial. Lancet. 2000;356:1480-1485.
17. Fujimura M, Ogawa H, Nishizawa Y, Nishi K. Comparison of atopic cough with cough variant asthma: is atopic cough a precursor of asthma? Thorax. 2003;58:14-18.
18. McGarvey L, Morice AH. Atopic cough: little evidence to support a new clinical entity. Thorax. 2003;58:736-738.
19. Chan KK, Ing AJ, Laks L, Cossa G, Rogers P, Birring SS. Chronic cough in patients with

sleep-disordered breathing. *Eur Respir J.* 2010;35:368–372.
20. Patterson RN, Johnston BT, Ardill JE, Heaney LG, McGarvey LP. Increased tachykinin levels in induced sputum from asthmatic and cough patients with acidic reflux. *Thorax.* 2007;62(6):491–495.
21. Javorkova N, Varechova S, Pecova R, et al. Acidification of the esophagus acutely increases the cough sensitivity in patients with gastro-esophageal reflux and chronic cough. *Neurogastroenterol Motil.* 2008;20(2):119–124.
22. Sifrim D, Dupont L, Blondeau K, Zhang X, Tack J, Janssens J. Weakly acidic reflux in patients with chronic unexplained cough during 24-hour pressure, pH, and impedance monitoring. *Gut.* 2005;54(4):449–454.
23. Blondeau K, Dupont L, Mertens V, et al. Gastro-esophageal reflux and aspiration of gastric contents in adult patients with cystic fibrosis. *Gut.* 2008;57(8):1049–1055.
24. McGarvey LP. Does idiopathic cough exist? *Lung.* 2008;186(Suppl 1):S78–S81.
25. Chung KF. Chronic "cough hypersensitivity syndrome": a more precise label for chronic cough. *Pulm Pharmacol Ther.* 2011;24(3):267–271.
26. Bhatia MS, Chandra R, Vaid L. Psychogenic cough: a profile of 32 cases. *Int J Psychiatry Med.* 2002;32:353–360.
27. Hay AD, Wilson A, Fahey T, Peters TJ. The duration of acute cough in preschool children presenting to primary care: a prospective cohort study. *Fam Pract.* 2003;20:696–705.
28. Marchant J, Masters IB, Taylor SM, Cox NC, Seymour GJ, Chang AB. Evaluation and outcome of young children with chronic cough. *Chest.* 2006;129(1 Suppl):1132S–1141S.
29. Kompare M, Weinberger M. Protracted bacterial bronchitis in young children: association with airway malacia. *J Pediatr.* 2012;160(1):88–92.
30. Rosen R, Nurko S. The importance of multichannel intraluminal impedance in the evaluation of children with persistent respiratory symptoms. *Am J Gastroenterol.* 2004;99:2452–2458.
31. Lim MT, Jeyarajah K, Jones P, et al. Specific antibody deficiency in children with chronic wet cough. *Arch Dis Child.* 2012;97(5):478–480.
32. Mainie I, Tutuian R, Agrawal A, et al. Fundoplication eliminates chronic cough due to non-acid reflux identified by impedance pH monitoring. *Thorax.* 2005;60(6):521–523.
33. Bucca C, Rolla G, Scappaticci E, Baldi S, Caria E, Oliva A. Histamine hyperresponsiveness of the extrathoracic airway in patients with asthmatic symptoms. *Allergy.* 1991;46:147–153.
34. Ryan NM, Vertigan AE, Bone S, Gibson PG. Cough reflex sensitivity improves with speech language pathology management of refractory chronic cough. *Cough.* 2010;6:5.
35. Morice AH, Menon MS, Mulrennan SA, et al. Opiate therapy in chronic cough. *Am J Respir Crit Care Med.* 2007;175(4):312–315.
36. Davenport PW, Bolser DC, Vickroy T, et al. The effect of codeine on the urge-to-cough response to inhaled capsaicin. *Pulm Pharmacol Ther.* 2007;20(4):338–346.
37. Eccles R, Morris S, Jawad M, et al. Lack of effect of codeine in the treatment of cough associated with acute upper respiratory tract infection. *J Clin Pharm Ther.* 1992;17(3):175–180.
38. Smith J, Owen E, Earis J, Woodcock A. Effect of codeine on objective measurement of cough in chronic obstructive pulmonary disease. *J Allergy Clin Immunol.* 2006;117(4):831–835.
39. Grattan TJ, Marshall AE, Higgins KS, Morice AH. The effect of inhaled and oral dextromethorphan on citric acid induced cough in man. *Br J Clin Pharmacol.* 1995;39(3):261–263.
40. Pavesi L, Subburaj S, Porter-Shaw K. Application and validation of a computerized cough acquisition system for objective monitoring of acute cough: a meta-analysis. *Chest.* 2001;120(4):1121–1128.
41. Lee B, Woo P. Chronic cough as a sign of laryngeal sensory neuropathy: diagnosis and treatment. *Ann Otol Rhinol Laryngol.* 2005;114(4):253–257.
42. Halum SL, Sycamore DL, McRae BR. A new treatment option for laryngeal sensory neuropathy. *Laryngoscope.* 2009;119(9): 1844–1847.
43. Jeyakumar A, Brickman TM, Hayben M. Effectiveness of amitriptyline versus cough suppressants in the treatment of chronic cough resulting from postviral vagal neuropathy. *Laryngoscope.* 2006;116(12):2108–2112.
44. Bastian RW, Vaidua AM, Delsupehe KG. Sensory neuropathic cough: a common and treatable cause of chronic cough. *Otolaryngol Head Neck Surg.* 2006;135(1):17–21.
45. Boeckxstaens GE, Rydholm H, Lei A, Adler J, Ruth M. Effect of lesogaberan, a novel GABA(B)-receptor agonist, on transient lower oesophageal sphincter relaxations in male subjects. *Aliment Pharmacol Ther.* 2010;31(11):1208–1217.
46. Boeckxstaens GE, Beaumont H, Mertens V, et al. Effects of lesogaberan on reflux and lower esophageal sphincter function in patients with gastroesophageal reflux disease. *Gastroenterology.* 2010;139(2):409–417.

47. Boeckxstaens GE, Beaumont H, Hatlebakk JG, et al. A novel reflux inhibitor lesogaberan (AZD3355) as add-on treatment in patients with GORD with persistent reflux symptoms despite proton pump inhibitor therapy: a randomised placebo-controlled trial. *Gut.* 2011;60(9):1182–1188.
48. Andre E, Campi B, Materazzi S, et al. Cigarette smoke-induced neurogenic inflammation is mediated by alpha, beta-unsaturated aldehydes and the TRPA1 receptor in rodents. *J Clin Invest.* 2008;118(7):2574–2582.
49. Birrell MA, Belvisi MG, Grace M, et al. TRPA1 agonists evoke coughing in guinea pig and human volunteers. *Am J Respir Crit Care Med.* 2009;180(11):1042–1047.
50. Krarup AL, Ny L, Astrand M, et al. Randomised clinical trial: the efficacy of a transient receptor potential vanilloid 1 antagonist AZD1386 in human oesophageal pain. *Aliment Pharmacol Ther.* 2011;33(10):1113–1122.
51. Rubin BK, Henke MO. Immunomodulatory activity and effectiveness of macrolides in chronic airway disease. *Chest.* 2004;125(2 Suppl):70S–78S.
52. Yousaf N, Monteiro W, Parker D, et al. Long-term low-dose erythromycin in patients with unexplained chronic cough: a double-blind placebo controlled trial. *Thorax.* 2010;65(12):1107–1110.
53. Mertens V, Blondeau K, Pauwels A, et al. Azithromycin reduces gastroesophageal reflux and aspiration in lung transplant recipients. *Dig Dis Sci.* 2009;54(5):972–979.
54. Usmani OS, Belvisi MG, Patel HJ, et al. Theobromine inhibits sensory nerve activation and cough. *FASEB J.* 2005;19(2):231–233.
55. Mokry J, Nosalova G. The influence of the PDE inhibitors on cough reflex in guinea pigs. *Bratisl Lek Listy.* 2011;112(3):131–135.
56. Usmani OS, Belvisi MG, Patel HJ, et al. Theobromine inhibits sensory nerve activation and cough. *FASEB J.* 2005;19(2):231–233.
57. Mokry J, Nosalova G. The influence of the PDE inhibitors on cough reflex in guinea pigs. *Bratisl Lek Listy.* 2011;112(3):131–135.
58. Mokry J, Mokra D, Nosalova G, et al. Influence of selective inhibitors of phosphodiesterase 3 and 4 on cough and airway reactivity. *J Physiol Pharmacol.* 2008;59(Suppl 6):473–482.
59. Fujimura M, Liu Q. Selective inhibitors for phosphodiesterase 3 and 4 in antigen induced increase of cough reflex sensitivity in guinea pigs. *Pulm Pharmacol Ther.* 2007;20(5):543–548.
60. Irwin RS, Corrao WM, Pratter MR. Chronic persistent cough in the adult: the spectrum and frequency of causes and successful outcome of specific therapy. *Am Rev Respir Dis.* 1981;123(4 Pt 1):413–417.
61. Poe RH, Israel RH, Utell MJ, Hall WJ. Chronic cough: bronchoscopy or pulmonary function testing. *Am Rev Respir Dis.* 1982;126(1):160–162.
62. Poe RH, Harder RV, Israel RH, Kallay MC. Chronic persistent cough: experience in diagnosis and outcome using an anatomic diagnostic protocol. *Chest.* 1989;95(4):723–728.
63. Hoffstein V. Persistent cough in nonsmoker. *Can Respir J.* 1994;1:40–47.
64. O'Connell F, Thomas VE, Pride NB, Fuller RW. Capsaicin cough sensitivity decreases with successful treatment of chronic cough. *Am J Respir Crit Care Med.* 1994;150:374–380.
65. Smyrnios NA, Irwin RS, Curley FJ. Chronic cough with a history of excessive sputum production. *Chest.* 1995;108(4):991–997.
66. Mello CJ, Irwin RS, Curley FJ. Predictive values of the character, timing and complications of chronic cough in diagnosing its cause. *Arch Intern Med.* 1996;156(9):997–1003.
67. Marchesani F, Cecarini L, Pla R, Sanguinetti CM. Causes of chronic persistent cough in adult patients: the results of a systematic management protocol. *Monaldi Arch Chest Dis.* 1998;53(5):510–514.
68. McGarvey LP, Heaney LG, Lawson JT, et al. Evaluation and outcome of patients with chronic nonproductive cough using a comprehensive diagnostic protocol. *Thorax.* 1998;53(9):738–743.
69. Palombini BC, Villanova CA, Araujo E, et al. A pathogenic triad in chronic cough: asthma, postnasal drip syndrome, and gastroesophageal reflux disease. *Chest.* 1999;116(2):279–284.
70. Brightling CE, Ward R, Goh KL, Wardlaw AJ, Pavord ID. Eosinophilic bronchitis is an important cause of chronic cough. *Am J Respir Crit Care Med.* 1999;160(2):406–410.

14

OCCUPATIONAL ASTHMA

COMORBID AND DIFFERENTIAL DIAGNOSIS

Manon Labrecque, Roberto Castaño, Grégory Moullec, Ignacio Ansottegui, and Denyse Gautrin

KEY POINTS

- Work-related asthma can be divided into two major entities: work-exacerbated asthma and occupational asthma.
- Adult-onset asthma is attributable to occupational exposures in 15% to 20% of cases.
- Medical history (type of symptoms and timing) is not sufficient to diagnose occupational asthma. The diagnosis requires an objective confirmation of asthma and of work-related functional changes.
- Chronic exposure to relatively low concentrations of irritant gases, fumes, or aerosols has been reported to cause low-dose irritant asthma (or low-dose reactive airways dysfunction syndrome).
- Occupational rhinitis and occupational asthma often coexist, wherein symptoms of rhinitis appear to develop before asthma symptoms.
- Psychological distress, health-related quality-of-life impairment, and comorbid psychiatric disorder are frequent in patients with work-related asthma or work-related asthma symptoms and have to be considered in the evaluation and treatment of the patient.

INTRODUCTION

In 2008, the American College of Chest Physicians published their updated state-of-the-art consensus statement, "Diagnosis and Management of Work-Related Asthma."[1] *Work-related asthma* (WRA) can be divided into two major entities, shown in Figure 14.1[2]: work-exacerbated asthma (WEA) and occupational asthma (OA). The term encompasses all cases of workers who develop new respiratory symptoms and obstructive airway physiology consistent with the diagnosis of asthma, and the cause can be directly attributed to an exposure in the workplace.

The key element is that OA is asthma caused by exposure to an organic protein, chemical, or other compound that is unique to the workplace. OA is further split into two subtypes—sensitizer-induced occupational asthma (>90% of the cases) and irritant-induced asthma (IIA), which includes reactive airways dysfunction syndrome (RADS).[3]

WEA, also called *work-aggravated asthma*, refers to previously diagnosed asthma that is worsened, but not caused, by agents found in the workplace. The distinction between these two entities is not superfluous because it affects treatment strategies and medicolegal decisions.

More recently, Sabin and Grammer proposed a slightly different approach for classification. They included OA under the term of *occupational immunologic lung disease* (OILD).[4] This entity is characterized by an immunologic response in the lung to an airborne agent inhaled in the work environment and can be subdivided into immunologically mediated occupational asthma and hypersensitivity pneumonitis (HP). The authors have separated into a different category the following: irritant-induced occupational asthma (IIOA), which is defined like a nonimmunologic entity, can be caused by chronic exposure to inhaled irritants or RADS and generally occurs abruptly after a single exposure to a high concentration of an irritating industrial agent. The authors also insist that OILD must be differentiated from WEA in which preexisting or concurrent asthma is worsened by workplace conditions such as cold air or dust exposure rather than caused by an immune response to a workplace sensitizer.

Occupational exposures may account for a significant proportion of adult-onset asthma cases.[5] Recent data indicate that the range of incidence of OA is estimated between 12 and 300 cases per 1 million workers per year.[6]

Registries and surveillance schemes of occupational respiratory diseases including OA have been created in several countries (e.g., Finland, United Kingdom, South Africa, France, United States, and Germany)[7] to observe trends in the occurrence of OA and identify workplaces at risk; as such, they provide estimates of the incidence rates of OA. These vary among countries from 13 new cases of OA with confirmed clinical diagnosis to more than 70 per 1 million employed individuals per year as published between 2000 and 2011. The large variations are to be interpreted with caution because they are possibly due to country-specific factors, including but not limited to case identification, reporting system, occupational health care system, and type of industrial activities. Several occupations are considered at risk for OA, and these include traditionally identified jobs such as spray-painters, bakers, farmers, food processors, hospital workers, hairdressers, animal technicians, and woodworkers. Other occupations have been recently identified: nurses, cleaners, and construction workers.[8]

More than 350 substances have been identified as causal factors[9]; among the high-risk substances are some of high molecular weight (HMW) (e.g., flour, latex, and animal epithelia) and some of low molecular weight (LMW) (e.g., isocyanates, anhydrides, and sensitizing drugs), and mixed work environments with single or multiple exposures (e.g., metalworking fluids, welding fumes, disinfectants, irritant gases or fumes, damp and moldy workplaces).[6,10–16]

The evidence of the importance of occupational exposures in the etiology of asthma also comes from large epidemiologic population-based studies. Interestingly, it was in population-based studies in Europe and the United States that an increased risk for asthma was first found to be also associated with exposure to irritants at work such as dusts, gases, fumes, welding fumes, and disinfectants in occupations not traditionally associated with OA (Table 14.1).[6]

In Finland, data from national registers of clinically well-established persistent asthma were combined at an individual level with population census data; all employed Finns without preexisting asthma were followed for the incidence of asthma over 5 years. Among 49,575 incident cases of asthma, 2,464 were cases of recognized OA; in that study, it was estimated that the proportion of adult-onset asthma attributable to exposures at work, expressed

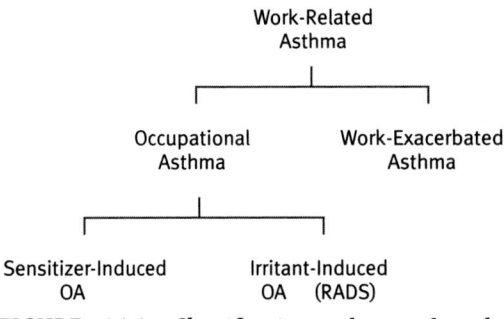

FIGURE 14.1 Classification scheme for the major types of asthma in the workplace. This scheme is based on the American College of Chest Physicians 2008 guidelines and is adapted from Tarlo et al.[1] RADS, reactive airways dysfunction syndrome.

(From Kenyon N, Morrissey B, Schivo M, Albertson T. Occupational asthma. *Clin Rev Allergy Immunol.* 2012;43[1–2]:3–13.)

as the population attributable risk (PAR), was 29% (95% confidence interval [CI], 25% to 33%) for men and 17% (95% CI, 15% to 19%) for women.[17] In the United States, a prospective investigation among a large population of adults, members of a health maintenance organization in Massachusetts, identified 906 cases of asthma, either incident cases or reactivated cases, with a confirmed clinical diagnosis; these individuals were invited to answer a structured questionnaire on work-related symptoms and work history. The study estimated that 29% (95% CI, 25% to 34%) of adult-onset asthma was attributable to workplace exposures, whether to occupational sensitizers or irritants.[18] Another example comes from the large international prospective population-based European Community Respiratory Health Survey. The PAR for adult asthma due to exposures at work ranged between 11% (95% CI, 1% to 20%) and 26% (95% CI, 2% to 44%); the variation was due to differences in the definition of asthma, with risks being highest when asthma was defined by bronchial hyperactivity in addition to symptoms and when exposure was defined as having a high-risk occupation (vs. exposure to high-risk substances).[10]

Toren and Blanc performed a synthesis from 26 studies (longitudinal, case-control, cross-sectional), including the three aforementioned studies, to estimate the PAR for asthma due to occupational exposures.[19] Overall the median value for the PAR was 17.6%, and the authors estimated that the likely range for the burden of asthma attributable to occupational exposures was between 15% and 20%. PAR is high in industrialized countries and developing countries characterized by rapid industrialization, but the lower figures in other developing countries (i.e., 6%) may be due to underrecognition of the disease.[20]

CLINICAL FEATURES

The clinical history can be suggestive of OA when asthmatic symptoms (dyspnea,

Table 14.1. Common Agents and Jobs Related to Occupational Asthma

SOURCE AGENT OR JOB

Most commonly reported agents causing occupational asthma: isocyanates, flour and grain dust, colophony and fluxes, latex, animals, aldehydes, adhesives, metals, resins, and wood dust

Workers most commonly reported to surveillance schemes of occupational asthma: animal handlers, bakers and pastry makers, chemical workers, food processing workers, hairdressers, paint sprayers, nurses and other health professionals, timber workers, and welders

Workers reported from population studies to be at increased risk for developing asthma: bakers, chemical workers, cleaners, cooks, electrical and electronic production workers, farm workers, food processors, forestry workers, health care workers, laboratory technicians, mechanics, metalworkers, painters, plastics and rubber workers, storage workers, textile workers, waiters, welders, and woodworkers wheezing, cough, and tightness in the chest) appear in conjunction with work, that is, are worse at work or after a shift at work and improve during weekends and holidays.

All the information in Appendix 14.1[21] was reported to be important in the clinical assessment of OA and includes information related to (1) the type of job, work shift, and agents that the workers identified as potential causes of symptoms; (2) the nature of symptoms during working periods, including chest symptoms (cough, sputum, chest tightness, wheezing, shortness of breath at rest or on exertion, change in voice), general symptoms (fever, chills, muscle or joint pain), nasal symptoms (blocked nose, runny nose, sneezing, nasal or throat itching), eye symptoms (itching, runny eyes, redness of the eyes), and skin symptoms (rash, eczema); and (3) timing of the onset of symptoms in relation to the beginning of the occupation and the interval between the last occupational exposure and the questionnaire. The relationship between work and respiratory, nasal, conjunctival, or skin symptoms has also been addressed by asking whether symptoms differed on days at work and away from work, whether there was a specific product causing the onset of symptoms, and whether there was an improvement in or disappearance of symptoms on weekends and on vacation. The temporal pattern of asthmatic symptoms has also been addressed, including time interval necessary to develop symptoms after starting work, persistence of symptoms after the work shift, and presence of symptoms only on return from work.

However, we have to insist on the fact that symptoms alone (type and timing) did not provide a satisfactory differentiation between those subjects with and those without occupational asthma. The predictive value of a suggestive history to a final diagnosis of OA confirmed by objective tests like a specific-inhalation challenge (SIC) is only 63%.[22]

Concerning the IIOA subclass, when asthma follows a single short-term accidental massive exposure to a respiratory irritant and symptoms appear within 24 hours without a latency period, the designation of RADS is employed. The classic features of RADS are presented in Table 14.2.[23] IIOA was later extended from multiple, somewhat lower, exposure incidents with a less sudden onset.[23-25] Furthermore, there is evidence that a susceptible subgroup of subjects with mainly atopic symptoms and nonspecific bronchial hyperresponsiveness or asthma in remission can be susceptible to IIOA. Chronic exposure to relatively low concentrations of irritant gases, fumes, or aerosols has been reported to cause this disorder, which has been called *low-dose irritant asthma* or *low-dose RADS*. Demonstrably causative concentrations of particular irritants are often below their occupational exposure limits or permissible exposure limits. An extensive review of IIOA and its causes has recently been published.[26]

Table 14.2. Cardinal Diagnostic Features of Reactive Airways Dysfunction Syndrome

Identification of date, time, frequency, and extent of exposure: the latter may be a single high exposure or multiple somewhat high exposures (higher than TLV or PEL concentrations)
Symptoms appear within 24 hours
No latency period between exposure and symptoms
Symptoms less likely to improve away from work
Objective pulmonary function tests demonstrate airway obstruction
Presence and persistence of BHR (as measured by methacholine or histamine challenge tests)

BHR, bronchial hyperresponsiveness; PEL, permissible exposure level; TLV, threshold limit value.
From Gautrin D, Bernstein I, Brooks S, Henneberger P. Reactive airways dysfunction syndrome and irritant-induced asthma. In: Bernstein IL, Chan-Yeung M, Malo JL, Bernstein DI, eds. *Asthma in the Workplace*. 3rd ed. New York: Taylor and Francis, 2006:579–627.

In this paper, all the following causative irritants are listed: wine confinement facilities, exposures to cleaning agents, solvents, ozone, endotoxin, formaldehyde, quaternary ammonium compounds, chlorine, bisulfite and SO_2, acid mist, diesel exhaust, fumigant residues, and dusts in the textile paper, mineral fiber, or construction industries or in mines, as well as a proportion of cases of pot-room asthma and meat-wrapper asthma.

DIAGNOSIS

Approaches to the diagnosis of WRA are based on a recent update of the consensus statement on the diagnosis and management of WRA by the American College of Chest Physicians[1] and on the updated standards of care for OA by the British Thoracic Society.[6] The approach varies according to the form of WRA, that is, whether it is irritant-induced WRA or sensitizer-induced OA.

More than 350 substances have been identified that may cause sensitizer-induced OA.[1] Patients with sensitizer-induced OA should avoid further exposure to the causal agent; indeed, early diagnosis and avoidance of exposure have been shown to be associated with a better outcome. Removal from work will inevitably have socioeconomic consequences,[27] and thus an objective diagnosis of OA is especially important. The diagnosis requires objective confirmation of asthma and of work-related functional changes, along with a history and exposure to an agent known to cause OA.[28] The most commonly used tool for investigating the possibility of OA is a questionnaire. Key elements have been suggested by Bernstein and colleagues[29] and include employment history and job description and a list of all processes and substances used in the employee's environment and prior jobs. The symptoms are described in terms of their nature, time of onset, duration, and temporal pattern and their relationship to the workplace. Recent evidence supports the importance of nasal symptoms; rhinoconjunctivitis may precede or appear concurrently with asthma symptoms. It is known that a history consistent with OA has good sensitivity but poor specificity for this diagnosis; a variety of differential diagnoses such as adult-onset asthma coincidental to the workplace, unrelated asthma aggravated by exposure to irritants at work, chronic bronchitis, and rhinitis should be considered.

Immunologic assessment, including skin-prick testing and measures of serum-specific immunoglobulin E (IgE) antibodies to HMW allergens, are useful to detect specific IgE response to HMW allergens. They are safe and quick to administer, but their value is limited by the lack of commercially available and standardized extracts of most allergens.[30] Immunologic tests in the diagnosis of OA due to LMW agents are limited to the assessment of specific serum antibodies by radioallergosorbent tests and enzyme-linked immunosorbent assays.

An important step is to objectively confirm or reject a diagnosis of asthma with lung function tests before and after administration of a bronchodilator and preferably with methacholine or histamine challenge tests according to a standard protocol.[31,32] Because of the high sensitivity and specificity of these tests for identifying subjects with asthma, a negative test can be used to exclude asthma and OA if the worker is symptomatic and remains exposed. Indeed, OA cannot be excluded if an individual has a negative methacholine test when he has been away from exposure for some time.[28]

In individuals with suspected sensitizer-induced asthma who are currently working at the job associated with the development of symptoms, it is recommended to record serial measurements of peak expiratory flow (PEF) as an additional step in the diagnostic procedure. The patient should optimally record PEF rates four times per day for 2 weeks at work and for 2 weeks off work.[8] Medication should be stable during the period of recording. Although the sensitivity and specificity of serial PEF are high in compliant patients, this method has well-documented limitations; for example, it relies on compliance of the patients and is not always useful in identifying the causative agent.[3,7] Although high-quality recordings can be obtained with appropriate training, the guidelines still recommend, concurrently with PEF measurements, assessing nonspecific bronchial hyperresponsiveness through methacholine challenge or a comparable method during a working period and at least 2 weeks from the work exposure to identify work-related changes. If there is disagreement between results from the PEF measurements and nonspecific bronchial challenges, or if the nature of the causative agent is equivocal, further tests may be necessary.

SIC should be performed only in specialized (tertiary) centers with medical supervision throughout the testing or in a closely supervised workplace. With an SIC, the clinical and functional status of the patient can be monitored during and after exposure to the suspected causative agent. A positive SIC identifies the causal agent, but a negative SIC does not necessarily exclude OA because the suspected agent used for the challenge may not reproduce exposure at work. Under such circumstances, workplace challenge is considered. SICs are considered as the reference standard for the diagnosis of OA.[3]

New noninvasive measures for assessing airway inflammation are being introduced in the investigation of OA. These include sputum induction and sampling of exhaled breath.[8] There is evidence that the sputum cell count may add useful information to the diagnosis of OA. Presently, there is only limited evidence that the use of exhaled nitric oxide level may have additional value in the diagnostic process; further research is needed to determine the value of this test.[8]

Physicians and other health care professionals who suspect a worker of having OA should refer the patient to a specialized physician without delay.[9]

DIFFERENTIAL DIAGNOSIS

When faced with a patient with WRA-like symptoms, the physician must first confirm or exclude asthma by objective measures (see "Diagnosis"). When asthma has been proved, the physician then must establish the distinction between WEA and OA. Some clinical signs (Table 14.3) may provide insight in differentiating these two conditions, but none is exclusive to either diagnosis.

Lemière and colleagues recently published a prospective cohort study comparing the clinical, functional, and inflammatory characteristics of workers with objectively confirmed diagnoses of WEA and OA.[33] This cohort included 154 subjects: 53 with WEA, 68 with OA, and 33 control asthmatic subjects (non-WRA). WEA was associated with more frequent prescriptions of inhaled corticosteroids (odds ratio, 4.4; 95% CI, 1.4 to 13.6; $P = .009$), a noneosinophilic phenotype (odds ratio, 0.3; 95% CI, 0.1 to 0.9; $P = .04$), a trend toward a lower FEV_1 (odds ratio, 0.9; 95% CI, 0.9 to 1.0; $P = .06$), and a higher proportion of smokers (odds ratio, 2.5; 95%, CI, 0.96 to 9.7; $P = .06$) compared with the OA group. The health care use of the WRA group and related costs were 10 times higher than those of the control subjects with non-WRA.

When there are asthma-like symptoms at work but no asthma, the diagnosis is still broad.[34] To help the clinician and simplify the list, we tried to regroup the differential diagnosis into five categories (Table 14.4): WRA; other OILDs (e.g., hypersensitivity pneumonitis and eosinophilic bronchitis); nonasthmatic obstructive diseases (e.g., chronic obstructive pulmonary disease [COPD], obliterative bronchiolitis); work-related rhinitis (including occupational rhinitis [OR] and others); and dysfunctional breathing, which includes work-related laryngeal dysfunction (WRLD), vocal cord dysfunction (VCD), hyperventilation syndrome, panic disorder, and multiple chemical sensitivity syndrome.

In the subsections that follow, we highlight the most important conditions for each nonasthmatic category.

Occupational Immunologic Lung Disease

OILD is characterized by an immunologic response in the lung to an airborne agent inhaled in the work environment and can be subdivided into immunologically mediated OA and HP. Even if we are unaware of the pathophysiologic mechanism of eosinophilic bronchitis, we have included this condition in the category labeled *immunologic disease of the lung*.

Table 14.3. Distinguish Work-Exacerbated Asthma from Occupational Asthma

CONDITIONS	WORK-EXACERBATED ASTHMA	OCCUPATIONAL ASTHMA
Sex	Men > women	Men >>> women
Atopy	Often present	More frequent with high-molecular-weight agents
Preexisting asthma	Present	Usually absent
Sensitizing agent at work	Can be present, but it is not the cause of asthma	Usually present and is the cause of asthma
Latency period	Usually no latency period	Always present
Asthma triggers	Various work-related factors; aeroallergens, irritants, or exercise	Exposure to the specific agent
Symptoms of rhinitis at work	Frequent	Frequent (more pronounced with high-molecular-weight agents)
Peak expiratory flow or FEV_1 decrease at work	Yes	Yes
Improving PC_{20} after a period away from work	No	Yes
Specific inhalation challenge	Negative	Positive
Eosinophilic phenotype	Less frequent	More frequent

Table 14.4. Asthma-like Symptoms at Work: Differential Diagnosis

GROUP	WORK-RELATED ASTHMA (WRA)	OCCUPATIONAL IMMUNOLOGIC LUNG DISEASE (OILD)	NONASTHMATIC OBSTRUCTIVE DISEASE	WORK-RELATED RHINITIS	DYSFUNCTIONAL BREATHING GROUP
Specific conditions	Work-exacerbated asthma	Hypersensitivity pneumonitis	Chronic obstructive pulmonary disease	Occupational rhinitis Irritant-induced occupational rhinitis	Work-related laryngeal dysfunction Vocal cord dysfunction
	Occupational asthma Reactive airways dysfunction syndrome Irritant-induced occupational asthma	Eosinophilic bronchitis	Obliterative bronchiolitis	Work-exacerbated rhinitis	Hyperventilation syndrome Panic disorder Multiple chemical sensitivity syndrome

Hypersensitivity Pneumonitis

Occupational HP results from occupational dust derived from fungal spores or bacteria such as moldy hay and avian dust or from chemicals such as isocyanates. HP can present in acute, chronic, or subacute form. Classically, the bronchoalveolar lavage shows a CD4/CD8 ratio of less than 1. Later in the course of the disease, there may be a skewing toward helper T-cell type 2 lymphocytes and interleukin-4 production. The acute form results from short-term, high-level exposure to a workplace antigen. Symptoms occur 4 to 8 hours after inhalation exposure and include fever, chills, nonproductive cough, dyspnea, and myalgias. The chronic form results from persistent low-level exposure to an antigen. Patients present with cough, dyspnea, weight loss, and fatigue. In the subacute form, patients usually have an insidious onset of symptoms after several days to weeks of exposure. Symptoms in the subacute form include exertional dyspnea, productive cough, and malaise. All three forms can progress to irreversible lung disease with severe pulmonary fibrosis. Early recognition of HP and avoidance of further exposure to the causative antigen are instrumental in preventing the progression to an irreversible disease.

Eosinophilic Bronchitis

Eosinophilic bronchitis causes chronic cough with phlegm, dyspnea, and, on rare occasions, wheezing. It is characterized by increased eosinophils in sputum (>3%) in the absence of increased nonallergic bronchial responsiveness.[4] The syndrome is considered a variant of OA when it develops as a consequence of occupational exposure, and hence it should be considered in the spectrum of work-related airway diseases. Occupational eosinophilic bronchitis is characterized by the presence of isolated chronic cough (lasting more than 3 weeks) that worsens at work; sputum eosinophilia (>3% in sputum); increase in sputum eosinophils related to exposure to the offending agent (either at work or after SIC); normal spirometric parameters that are not significantly affected by exposure to the offending agent; and absence of bronchial hyperresponsiveness to methacholine both at work and away from work, when other causes of chronic cough are ruled out.[35-37] This entity reinforces the importance of examining induced sputum as part of the diagnostic algorithm for individuals who complain of asthma-like symptoms in the workplace.[38] Bakers are at high risk for developing occupational respiratory disorders, and three cases of occupational NAEB have been described with exposure to flour.[39,40] Other occupational sensitizers, such as natural rubber latex, mushroom spores, acrylates, and an epoxy resin hardener, have also been reported to cause eosinophilic bronchitis without asthma.

Nonasthmatic Obstructive Diseases

CHRONIC OBSTRUCTIVE PULMONARY DISEASE

COPD should be considered in patients experiencing dyspnea at work. A history of smoking, chronic cough and phlegm, and irreversible airway obstruction will help to make the diagnosis. Tobacco smoking is the most important risk factor for COPD, but other environmental factors such as occupational exposures are likely to contribute in some patients.[41,42] In 2010, the American Thoracic Society[43] estimated that more than 20% of COPD cases are attributable to occupational exposure. General population-based studies or community-based cohorts of patients with COPD found an increased risk for COPD in subjects exposed to vapors, dust, gas, or fumes or working in agricultural, paper, cleaning, wood, and food-processing industries.

BRONCHIOLITIS

Obliterate bronchiolitis (OB) (formerly termed *bronchiolitis obliterans*) is a rare fibrotic disorder involving terminal and respiratory bronchioles.[44] The term *constrictive bronchiolitis* is synonymous with OB. Clinically, OB is characterized by a progressive (often fatal) airflow obstruction, the absence of parenchymal infiltrates on chest radiographs, a mosaic pattern of perfusion on high-resolution computed tomography, poor responsiveness to therapy, and high mortality rates. Currently, most cases of OB occur in lung transplant recipients with chronic allograft rejection or hematopoietic stem cell transplant recipients with graft versus host disease. Other causes of OB include connective tissue diseases (particularly rheumatoid arthritis); lower respiratory tract infections; inhalation injury; and occupational exposure to or inhalation of toxic fumes, metals, and dusts. One publication reported subjects who had developed persistent airflow obstruction (reduced FEV_1/FVC ratio and FEV_1 at 25% to 44% of predicted) after 1 to 3 years of exposure to diacetyl,[45] without the use of personal protective equipment, at a cookie factory. The high-resolution computed tomography findings were indicative of bronchiolitis. In one patient, the surgical lung biopsy revealed bronchiolitis obliterans accompanied by giant cells. OB in fiberglass workers[46] and after occupational ammonia poisoning has been reported recently,[47] and a recent interesting review has been published.[48]

Work-Related Rhinitis

Work-related rhinitis (WRR) is two to four times more frequent than OA[49,50] and includes OR and work-exacerbated rhinitis. OR has recently been classified as allergic or nonallergic.[51,52] Allergic OR is caused by immunologically mediated hypersensitivity reactions characterized by a latency period, which may be IgE mediated or not. If IgE mediated, it is usually due to HMW and some LMW agents. If not IgE mediated, it is due to LMW chemicals for which the allergic mechanism has not yet been characterized.

Nonallergic, irritant-induced OR is caused by an irritant, nonimmunologic mechanism. An extensive review was recently published on the epidemiology of non–IgE-mediated and irritant-induced OR.[53] The authors reviewed all cross-sectional studies done in all working groups in 2011 and 2012. Several irritants and LMW agents have been described in epidemiologic, surveillance, and experimental studies, case reports, and reviews. Among new agents are drugs, wood dust, chemicals, metals, and biocides, and among activities causing nonallergic irritant-induced OR, health care, antibiotic manufacturing, and cleaning were more frequently reported.

Cross-sectional studies in working groups published in the past 2 years estimated the prevalence of nasal symptoms (e.g., stuffy, runny, or blocked nose; sneezing; rhinorrhea; bleeding; and nasal congestion) in 3% to 74% of workers in different settings and exposed to LMW and irritant agents.[48]

Work-exacerbated rhinitis has not been specifically investigated, and few data are available on the subject. Moreover, there is some evidence that WRR symptoms are frequently associated with WEA. At least one work-related nasal symptom was reported by 83% of patients with WEA, and work-related ocular-nasal symptoms were a strong predictor of WEA (odds ratio, 6.7; 95% CI, 2.4 to 19.1).

Dysfunctional Breathing Group

The term "dysfunctional breathing" (DB) has been introduced here to describe patients who display divergent breathing patterns and have breathing problems that cannot be attributed to a specific medical diagnosis. Patients with DB are often misdiagnosed as having asthma. We include in this group patients with WRLD. WRLD is a larger spectrum of clinical features that includes a more defined condition: VCD. We also include in the DB group hyperventilation syndrome, panic disorder, and multiple chemical sensitivity syndrome.

WORK-RELATED LARYNGEAL DYSFUNCTION

Workplace exposures have been reported as precipitants for the development of nonorganic laryngeal dysfunction and also as triggers for recurrent symptoms. Laryngeal dysfunction may be difficult to clinically differentiate from asthma; it is important to consider this diagnosis as a cause of work-related respiratory symptoms. Unfortunately, there is a lack of consensus regarding clinical features and terminology of laryngeal dysfunction, but a recent review tried to clarify the spectrum of this disease.[53]

VCD is likely to be the most well-appreciated manifestation of nonorganic dysfunctional laryngeal behavior. It is characterized by inappropriate laryngeal closure by involuntary adduction of the vocal cords (folds) during respiration, resulting in variable upper airway obstruction and the most typical symptoms of VCD. Symptoms of intermittent dyspnea, wheeze, and cough are common to both asthma and VCD. Features that suggest VCD include a sensation of aspiratory limitation, rather than expiratory limitation as is usual in asthma, and tightness in throat rather than chest. During an acute episode, the wheeze may be loudest over the neck and upper thorax but is transmitted to the chest wall. Hyperventilation during an episode may lead to symptoms such as tingling of the perioral area and digits, dizziness, and lightheadedness. Frequently, episodes have a rapid onset and resolution. Exposure of the upper respiratory tract to an irritant at the workplace, such as caused by an accidental spill of a water-soluble agent, may be associated with the onset of symptoms. The event may have been psychologically traumatic and required emergency medical treatment. Perkner and colleagues[55] described a variable latency between occupational irritant exposure and the onset of VCD symptoms, ranging from 1 hour or less to 24 hours; they described the condition of "irritant-associated VCD" as with the following criteria:

a. Documented absence of preceding VCD or laryngeal disease
b. Onset of symptoms after a single specific exposure or accident
c. Exposure to an irritating gas, smoke, fume, vapor, mist, or dust
d. Onset of symptoms within 24 hours after exposure
e. Symptoms of wheezing, stridor, dyspnea, cough, or throat tightness
f. Abnormal direct laryngoscopy for vocal cord dysfunction in the asymptomatic state, during symptoms, or with a provocative study
g. Exclusion of other types of significant vocal cord disease

Concerning the epidemiology of this syndrome, the available literature suggests a female-to-male ratio of 2:1 or 3:1. The prevalence of VCD in association with asthma and WRA exists, but no known studies have addressed its exact prevalence. The association of both diseases could make the differential diagnosis of work-related symptoms difficult.[54]

Psychopathology has commonly been proposed as the etiologic basis of VCD; however, more recent theories have placed emphasis on organic causes, such as altered neurologic control of laryngeal reflexes and the role of olfaction.[55]

Chronic postnasal drip, laryngopharyngeal reflux, and gastroesophageal reflux may contribute to laryngeal hyperresponsiveness.[56] The diagnosis of VCD may be difficult because a physical examination and spirometry may be normal between episodes. During symptomatic episodes, spirometry typically reveals variable extrathoracic airway obstruction (truncated inspiratory flow volume loop). The gold standard for identifying VCD is flexible fiberoptic rhinolaryngoscopy. Management of VCD includes identification and treatment of underlying disorders (e.g., chronic postnasal drip, laryngopharyngeal reflux, gastroesophageal reflux, anxiety, depression) and a multidisciplinary approach including highly trained speech therapists. Speech therapy and biofeedback play a critical role in teaching techniques to override various dysfunctional breathing habits. When postnasal drip, laryngopharyngeal reflux, or gastroesophageal coexists, the disorder should be aggressively treated.

Hyperventilation Syndrome and Panic Disorder

Hyperventilation syndrome and DB are often synonymous.[57,58] They are both defined by chronic or recurrent changes in breathing patterns that cannot be attributed to a specific medical diagnosis, causing respiratory and nonrespiratory complaints such as anxiety, lightheadedness, and fatigue.

Symptoms of hyperventilation syndrome, or DB, include dyspnea with normal lung function, chest tightness, chest pain, deep sighing, exercise-induced breathlessness, frequent yawning, and hyperventilation. There is no gold standard for the diagnosis of hyperventilation syndrome beyond the clinical description.

The Nijmegen Questionnaire can be used to discriminate adult dysfunctional breathers from normal breathers.[59] In moderate to severe asthma, a positive Nijmegen score might overestimate the presence of DB, and confirmation using progressive exercise testing has been suggested.[60]

Several breathing therapies are used to manage DB. The most popular ones are the Buteyko breathing method, pursed-lip breathing, and traditional Hatha yoga. All breathing therapies focus on strengthening the diaphragmatic breathing during breath work; some also address lifestyle changes and have strict criteria for success or progress (Hatha yoga and Buteyko method).

Many symptoms overlap between acute hyperventilation and panic disorder. Patients with panic disorder suffer from chronic episodes of hyperventilation, in which they shift toward hypocapnic alkalosis as a consequence of stress-induced acute hyperventilation, generating panic attacks. Diagnoses of panic disorder must be consistent with the *Diagnostic and Statistical Manual of Mental Disorders* (DSM-IV) criteria. Generally, panic disorders are diagnosed when the subject has recurrent unexpected panic attacks and at least one of these attacks has been followed by persistent concern about having additional attacks, worry about the implications of the attack or its consequences, or a significant change in behavior related to the attacks.

COMORBID, COEXISTING DISEASE

Psychiatric Comorbidity

Given the sudden or often unexpected onset of OA in otherwise previously healthy individuals and the magnitude of its health and socioeconomic impacts for the affected worker, OA should have similar, if not greater, psychological impacts than non-OA. As stated in a recent review by Lavoie and colleagues,[61] there is a paucity of knowledge concerning the psychological characteristics, including psychological distress and health-related quality-of-life impairment, in patients with WRA. For the purpose of the current chapter, *psychological distress* is defined as the experience of negative emotions such as sadness/depression or fear/anxiety. The experience of psychological distress may be acute and transient (e.g., feeling anxious about an upcoming medical examination) or more severe and chronic (e.g., feeling so depressed that one cannot get out of bed in the morning). When psychological distress is severe and chronic, it may reach clinical levels and become a psychiatric disorder, which is a clinical diagnosis based on established diagnostic DSM-IV-R criteria.[62] To be diagnosed with a psychiatric disorder (e.g., a mood or anxiety disorder), one must meet established symptom criteria, which must have persisted for a minimum duration (often 2 consecutive weeks to several months) and caused significant functional impairment (i.e., interfered with an individual's ability to work or engage in social relationships).

To our knowledge, only two original studies have so far specifically assessed the level of psychological distress in patients with OA.[27,63] Yacoub and colleagues[63] assessed psychological distress levels using two self-report instruments—the Psychiatric Symptom Index (PSI) and the Millon Clinical Multiaxial Inventory (MCMI)—in 40 patients with OA 2 years after cessation of exposure to the sensitization agent determined to have caused OA. According to the PSI, levels of depression, anxiety, and cognitive dysfunction were all in the clinical range based on the established cut-off score, indicating that psychological distress in patients with OA not only is severe but also may affect a range of psychological factors.[27,63] In the same study, Yacoub and colleagues[63] also assessed clinical levels of psychological distress—for example, the prevalence of psychiatric disorders—using the MCMI. Although diagnoses of psychiatric disorders may only be strictly made using structured psychiatric interviews such as the PRIME-MD, this study used a validated, 175-item self-report questionnaire that yields probable diagnoses using algorithms that are based on DSM-IV criteria. The results indicated that certain psychiatric disorders were common in patients with OA, with anxiety disorders and dysthymia affecting about 35% and 23% of patients, respectively. In the same way, a recent Quebec follow-up study of 60 subjects compensated for OA has shown, using the PRIME-MD, that 15% and 32% of them suffered from anxiety and mood disorders, respectively, associated with moderate impairment in health-related quality of life, 2 years after diagnosis.[27]

Although additional evidence is needed, these results suggest that patients with OA are highly anxious and that many are chronically depressed, which is consistent with previous studies conducted in non-OA patients.[64] However, the overall rates of depressive and anxiety disorders in the studies by Yacoub and colleagues[63] and Miedinger and colleagues[27] were generally higher (25% to 40%) than those observed in a previous study with non-OA patients (20% to 25%),[65] suggesting that the psychological burden of OA may exceed that of non-OA. The paucity of original data on the association of psychological distress and OA represents an important gap in the clinical literature.

The fact that OA is a chronic, debilitating illness that is caused by the workplace may place an additional psychological burden on the affected worker in a number of ways. First, given that workers' symptoms are related to their workplace, a diagnosis of OA frequently involves complete removal from the workplace,[66,67] threatening their ability to earn a living. This may be a source of significant psychological distress because OA often affects individuals working in occupations or regions where alternative job opportunities are either limited or nonexistent (e.g., fish and shellfish occupations), leading to fears of unemployment and financial loss. These fears appear to be well founded. Although removing the worker from the workplace has been linked to better medical outcomes (e.g., improved lung function and reduced asthma severity),[68,69] it has been linked to worse socioeconomic outcomes, including loss of income, professional downgrading, and unemployment.[68,70,71]

Ameille and colleagues[70] have estimated that the mean loss of annual income in OA patients is higher than 40%, which represents a significant and potentially life-changing drop in earnings for affected workers.[70]

These findings highlight the potential personal financial burden of receiving a diagnosis of OA and how a confirmed diagnosis of OA (even in cases in which compensation claims are accepted, as in Quebec[72]) may be a source of significant psychological distress in those affected. Workers need not have a confirmed diagnosis of OA to experience the psychological burden of this disease. Simply experiencing symptoms suggestive of OA may elicit anxiety about the consequences of an eventual diagnosis. Just the thought of receiving a diagnosis of OA may elicit fears about being removed from the only work environment and culture the worker has ever known, one that often forms a large part of the worker's identity. In fact, there is evidence to suggest that workers' fears about the negative consequences of disclosing WRA symptoms, submitting a claim to a workers' compensation board, or both are associated with nondisclosure of symptoms to colleagues and management as well as failing to file claims with a board.[73-75] Workers may even continue to expose themselves to the causative workplace environment when they are aware of the risks, just to avoid the negative socioeconomic consequences of a diagnosis.[76] This suggests that many workers may put their health at risk in order to protect their livelihood, a situation that undoubtedly places considerable stress on the affected worker.

Occupational Rhinitis and Asthma Comorbidity

OA is the most common form of occupational lung disease, but there is increasing interest in OR, which may be regarded as an early stage of OA.[77] A diagnosis of OR could easily be missed in patients with OA because they focus all their attention on asthma symptoms, which often generate more morbidity and affect quality of life to a greater extent than rhinitis symptoms. Thus, OR appears to be underdiagnosed, and there are no standardized criteria for diagnosing this disease.[78]

Evidence from epidemiologic studies indicates that OR and OA often coexist, with OR occurring two to three times more frequently than OA.[78] Symptoms of OR appear to develop before OA symptoms. For example, rhinitis symptoms were reported by 92% of subjects with a confirmed diagnosis of OA and were more often reported as appearing before OA in the case of HMW agents.[79] Also, work-related rhinitis symptoms have been reported to appear before asthma in bakers, apprentice bakers, and hairdressers.[80]

There is evidence that OR may be a risk factor for the development of OA. A register-based study showed that patients with OA were older than patients with OR, suggesting that OR precedes OA.[81] Another study showed an increased risk for asthma (risk ratio, 4.8; 95% CI, 4.3 to 5.4) among subjects with OR compared with subjects with other occupational diseases, with the higher risk being observed among farmers, animal handlers, and woodworkers.[12] Also, it has been shown that nasal symptoms less frequently precede asthma symptoms in subjects with WEA (17%) than in those with OA (43%).[82] Other recent studies have observed a high frequency of rhinitis symptoms among subjects referred to specialized clinics for investigation of WRA-like symptoms.[82-84] A multicenter study of 212 subjects referred to four tertiary care clinics for investigation of OA showed that nasal itching was a satisfactory predictor of OA objectively confirmed by SIC, particularly in subjects exposed to HMW agents.[21]

There also appears to be a pathophysiologic link between OR and OA. Clinical challenge testing studies have examined the association between OR and OA. SIC performed in subjects with probable OR showed a concomitant clinically significant nasal and bronchial reaction indicative of OR and OA in the same patient in 13% of the challenge investigations.[85] A similar study evaluated 43 subjects with histories suggestive of OA and, at the same time, complaining of work-related rhinitis symptoms.[86] An isolated clinically significant nasal response was observed in 25 SICs (58%), an isolated significant bronchoconstriction in 17 SICs (39.5%), and a parallel positive nasal and bronchial response in 13 SICs (30.2%), with OR occurring in 76.4% of confirmed cases of OA. The observed association between positive nasal and bronchial responses was significant (risk ratio, 1.7; 95% CI, 1.0 to 2.4; $P = .04$) and more frequent in subjects undergoing challenge with HMW agents.[86]

The emerging evidence supporting the relationship between OR and OA is growing, but this area of research is in its early stages. The management of OR and OA is similar with regard to exposure preventive measures. It is yet to be determined whether interventions aiming to reduce the incidence of OR will alter the natural history of OA. In the meantime, an integrated diagnostic and management approach for patients suffering from work-related rhinitis and asthma may result in improved care and better treatment outcomes.[87]

UNMET, FUTURE RESEARCH NEEDS

Many aspects of WRA are not well understood and need to be explained.

1. Mechanisms of sensitization remain unknown for many LMW sensitizers, such as diisocyanates.
2. Further understanding may lead to better immunologic testing that could be relevant to exposure assessment, diagnosis, and disease management.
3. The role of irritants in asthma causation and exacerbation, acting alone or as adjuvant factors or cofactors, also requires more research.

CONCLUSION

WRA can be divided in two major entities: WER and OA. OA is further split into two subtypes—sensitizer-induced occupational asthma (>90% of the cases) and IIA, which includes RADS.

Adult-onset asthma is attributable to occupational exposures in 15% to 20% of cases. Symptoms alone (type and timing) did not provide a satisfactory differentiation between subjects with and those without OA. The predictive value of a suggestive history to a final diagnosis of OA confirmed by objective tests like an SIC is only 63%. The differential diagnosis of asthma-like symptoms at work is large and relatively complex. OR and OA often coexist, with OR occurring two to three times more frequently than OA, and symptoms of OR appear to develop before OA symptoms.

Psychological distress, health-related quality-of-life impairment, and comorbid psychiatric disorder are frequent in patients with WRA or WRA symptoms and have to be considered in the evaluation and treatment of patients.

Many areas of research are still needed to understand the complexity of WRAs.

REFERENCES

1. Tarlo SM, Balmes J, Balkissoon R, et al. Diagnosis and management of work-related asthma. *Chest.* 2008;134(3 Suppl):1S–41S.
2. Kenyon N, Morrissey B, Schivo M, Albertson T. Occupational asthma. *Clin Rev Allergy Immunol.* 2012;43(1–2):3–13.
3. Gautrin D, Bernstein I, Brooks S, Henneberger P. Reactive airways dysfunction syndrome and irritant-induced asthma. In: Bernstein IL, Chan-Yeung M, Malo JL, Bernstein DI, eds. *Asthma in the Workplace.* 3rd ed. New York: Taylor and Francis, 2006:579–627.
4. Sabin BR, Grammer LC. Occupational immunologic lung disease. *Allergy Asthma Proc.* 2012;33:S58–S60.
5. Chan-Yeung M, Malo JL. Occupational asthma. *N Engl J Med.* 1995;333(2):107–112.
6. Fishwick D, Barber CM, Bradshaw LM, et al. Standards of care for occupational asthma: an update. *Thorax.* 2012;67(3):278–280.
7. Becklake M, Malo J, Chan-Yeung M. Epidemiological approaches in occupational asthma. In: Bernstein IL, Chan-Yeung M, Malo JL, Bernstein DI, eds. *Asthma in the Workplace.* 3rd ed. New York: Taylor and Francis; 2006:37–86.
8. Bernstein IL, Chan-Yeung M, Malo JL, Bernstein DI, eds. *Asthma in the Workplace.* 3rd ed. New York: Taylor and Francis; 2006.
9. Szram J, Cullinan P. Occupational asthma. *Semin Respir Crit Care Med.* 2012;33(6):653–665.
10. Kogevinas M, Zock JP, Jarvis D, et al. Exposure to substances in the workplace and new-onset asthma: an international prospective population-based study (ECRHS-II). *Lancet.* 2007;370(9584):336–441.
11. Karjalainen A, Kurppa K, Martikainen R, Karjalainen J, Klaukka T. Exploration of asthma risk by occupation—extended analysis of an incidence study of the Finnish population. *Scand J Work Environ Health.* 2002;28(1):49–57.
12. Karjalainen A, Martikainen R, Oksa P, Saarinen K, Uitti J. Incidence of asthma among Finnish construction workers. *J Occup Environ Med.* 2002;44(8):752–757.
13. Jaakkola JJ, Piipari R, Jaakkola MS. Occupation and asthma: a population-based incident case-control study. *Am J Epidemiol.* 2003;158(10):981–987.
14. Jaakkola MS, Nordman H, Piipari R, et al. Indoor dampness and molds and development of adult-onset asthma: a population-based incident case-control study. *Environ Health Perspect.* 2002;110(5):543–547.
15. Karvala K, Toskala E, Luukkonen R, Uitti J, Lappalainen S, Nordman H. Prolonged exposure to damp and moldy workplaces and new-onset asthma. *Int Arch Occup Environ Health.* 2011;84(7):713–721.
16. Zock JP, Cavalle N, Kromhout H, et al. Evaluation of specific occupational asthma risks in a community-based study with special reference to single and multiple exposures. *J Expo Anal Environ Epidemiol.* 2004;14(5):397–403.
17. Karjalainen A, Kurppa K, Martikainen R, Klaukka T, Karjalainen J. Work is related to a substantial portion of adult-onset asthma incidence in the Finnish population. *Am J Respir Crit Care Med.* 2001;164(4):565–568.
18. Sama SR, Milton DK, Hunt PR, Houseman EA, Henneberger PK, Rosiello RA. Case-by-case assessment of adult-onset asthma attributable to occupational exposures among members of a health maintenance organization. *J Occup Environ Med.* 2006;48(4):400–407.
19. Toren K, Blanc PD. Asthma caused by occupational exposures is common: a systematic analysis of estimates of the population-attributable fraction. *BMC Pulm Med.* 2009;9:7.
20. Jeebhay MF, Quirce S. Occupational asthma in the developing and industrialised world: a review. *Int J Tubercl Lung Dis.* 2007;11(2):122–133.
21. Vandenplas O, Ghezzo H, Munoz X, et al. What are the questionnaire items most useful in identifying subjects with occupational asthma? *Eur Respir J.* 2005;26(6):1056–1063.
22. Malo JL, Ghezzo H, L'Archevêque J, Lagier F, Perrin C, Cartier A. History in diagnosing occupational asthma. *Am Rev Respir Dis.* 1991;143:528–532.
23. Gautrin et al. Reactive airways dysfunction syndrome and irritant-induced asthma.

In: Bernstein IL, Chan-Yeung M, Malo JL, Bernstein DI, eds. *Asthma in the Workplace*. 3rd ed. New York: Taylor and Francis; 2006:581–625.

24. Brooks SM, Hammad Y, Richards I, Giovinco-Barbas J, Jenkins K. The spectrum of irritant-induced asthma. *Chest*. 1998;113(1):42–49.

25. Burge SP, Moore VC, Robertson AS. Sensitization and irritant-induced occupational asthma with latency are clinically indistinguishable. *Occup Med*. 2012;62(2):129–133.

26. Baur X, Bakehe P, Vellguth H. Bronchial asthma and COPD due to irritants in the workplace: an evidence-based approach. *J Occup Med Toxicol*. 2012;7:19.

27. Miedinger D, Lavoie KL, L'Archeveque J, et al. Quality-of-life, psychological, and cost outcomes 2 years after diagnosis of occupational asthma. *J Occup Environ Med*. 2011;53(3):231–238.

28. Moscato G, Malo JL, Bernstein D. Diagnosing occupational asthma: how, how much, how far? *Eur Respir J*. 2003;21(5):879–885.

29. Bernstein DI, Campo P, Baur X. Clinical assessment and management of occupational asthma. In: Bernstein IL, Chan-Yeung M, Malo JL, Bernstein DI, eds. *Asthma in the Workplace*. 3rd ed. New York: Taylor and Francis; 2006:161–178.

30. Malo JL, Chan-Yeung M. Occupational asthma. *J Allergy Clin Immunol*. 2001;108(3):317–328.

31. Society AT. Guidelines for methacholine and exercise challenge testing—1999. *Am J Respir Crit Care Med*. 2000;161:309–329.

32. Tarlo SM, Liss GM. Occupational asthma: an approach to diagnosis and management. *CMAJ*. 2003;168(7):867–871.

33. Lemière C, Boulet LP, Chaboillez S, et al. Work-exacerbated asthma and occupational asthma: do they really differ? *J Allergy Clin Immunol*. 2013;131(3);704–710.

34. Cartier A, Sastre J. Clinical assessment of occupational asthma and its differential diagnosis. *Immunol Allergy Clin N Am*. 2011;31(4):717–728.

35. Quirce S. Eosinophilic bronchitis in the workplace. *Curr Opin Allergy Clin Immunol*. 2004;4:87–91.

36. Quirce S, Fernández-Nieto M, de Miguel J, Sastre J. Chronic cough due to latex-induced eosinophilic bronchitis. *J Allergy Clin Immunol*. 2001;108:143.

37. Brihtling CE. Chronic cough due to non-asthmatic eosinophilic bronchitis: ACCP evidence-based clinical practice guidelines. *Chest*. 2006;129(Suppl 1):116S–121S.

38. Quirce S, Lemiere C, De BF, et al. Noninvasive methods for assessment of airway inflammation in occupational settings. *Allergy*. 2010;65(4):445–458.

39. Barranco P, Fernández-Nieto M, del Pozo V, Sastre B, Larco JI, Quirce S. Nonasthmatic eosinophilic bronchitis in a baker caused by fungal alpha-amylase and wheat flour. *J Invest Allergol Clin Immunol*. 2008;18(6):494–495.

40. Di Stefano F, Di Giampaolo L, Verna N, Di Gioacchino M. Occupational eosinophilic bronchitis in a foundry worker exposed to isocyanate and a baker exposed to flour. *Thorax*. 2007;62(4):368–370.

41. Blanc PD, Eisner MD, Trupin L, Yelin EH, Katz PP, Balmes JR. The association between occupational factors and adverse health outcomes in chronic obstructive pulmonary disease. *Occup Environ Med*. 2004;61(8):661–667.

42. Blanc PD, Iribarren C, Trupin L, et al. Occupational exposures and the risk of COPD: dusty trades revisited. *Thorax*. 2009;64(1):6–12.

43. Eisner MD, Anthonisen N, Coultas D, et al. An official American Thoracic Society public policy statement: novel risk factors and the global burden of chronic obstructive pulmonary disease. *Am J Respir Crit Care Med*. 2010;182(5):693–718.

44. Ryu JH, Myers JL, Swensen SJ. Bronchiolar disorders. *Am J Respir Crit Care*. 2003;168(11):1277–1292.

45. Kreiss K, Gomaa A, Kullman G, et al. Clinical bronchiolitis obliterans in workers at a microwave-popcorn plant. *N Engl J Med*. 2002;347(5):330–338.

46. Cullinan P, McGavin CR, Kreiss K, et al. Obliterative bronchiolitis in fiberglass workers: a new occupational disease? *Occup Environ Med*. 2013;70(5):357–359.

47. Mao WJ, Xia W, Chen JY. [Lung transplantation for bronchiolitis obliterans after occupational ammonia poisoning: report of one case]. *Zhonghua Lao Dong Wei Sheng Zhi Ye Bing ZaZhi*. 2012;30(9):703–704.

48. Lynch JP 3rd, Weigt SS, DerHovanessian A, Fishbein MC, Gutierrez A, Belperio JA. Obliterative (constrictive) bronchiolitis. *Semin Respir Crit Care Med*. 2012;33(5):509–532.

49. Siracusa A, Desrosiers M, Marabini A. Epidemiology of occupational rhinitis: prevalence, aetiology and determinants. *Clin Exp Allergy*. 2000;30:1519–1534.

50. Ruoppi P, Koistinen T, Susitaival P, Honkanen J, Soininen H. Frequency of allergic rhinitis

50. to laboratory animals in university employees as confirmed by chamber challenges. *Allergy.* 2004;59:295–301.
51. Moscato G, Vandenplas O, Gerth Van Wijk R, et al. EAACI Task Force on Occupational Rhinitis. *Allergy.* 2008;63:969–980.
52. Moscato G, Siracusa A. Rhinitis guidelines and implications for occupational rhinitis. *Curr Opin Allergy Clin Immunol.* 2009;9:110–115.
53. Siracusa A, Follettia I, Moscato G. Non-IgE-mediated and irritant-induced work-related rhinitis. *Curr Opin Allergy Clin Immunol.* 2013;13(2):159–166.
54. Hoy R. Work-related laryngeal syndromes. *Curr Opin Allergy Clin Immunol.* 2012;12(2):95–101.
55. Perkner JJ, Fennelly K, Balkissoon R, et al. Irritant-associated vocal cord dysfunction. *J Occup Environ Med.* 1998;40:136–143.
56. Ayres JG, Gabbott PLA. Vocal cord dysfunction and laryngeal hyperresponsiveness: a function of altered autonomic balance? *Thorax.* 2002;57:284–285.
57. Balkissoon R, Kenn K. Asthma: vocal cord dysfunction (VCD) and other dysfunctional breathing disorders. *Semin Respir Crit Care Med.* 2012;33(6):595–605.
58. Agache I, Ciobanu C, Pauland G, Rogozea L. Dysfunctional breathing phenotype in adults with asthma: incidence and risk factors. *Clin Transl Allergy.* 2012;2:18.
59. van Dixhoorn DJ, Duivenvoorden HJ. Efficacy of Nijmegen Questionnaire in recognition of the hyperventilation syndrome. *J Psychosom Res.* 1985;29:199–206.
60. Stanton AE, Vaughn P, Carter R, Bucknall CE. An observational investigation of dysfunctional breathing and breathing control therapy in a problem asthma clinic. *J Asthma.* 2008;45:75.
61. Lavoie KL, Joseph M, Bacon SL. Psychological distress and occupational asthma. *Curr Opin Allergy Clin Immunol.* 2009;9(2):103–109.
62. American Psychiatric Association. *Diagnostic and Statistical Manual of Mental Disorders, Text Revision (DSM-IV-TR).* 4th ed. Washington, DC: American Psychiatric Association; 2000.
63. Yacoub MR, Lavoie K, Lacoste G, et al. Assessment of impairment/disability due to occupational asthma through a multidimensional approach. *Eur Respir J.* 2007;29(5):889–896.
64. Goodwin RD, Jacobi F, Thefeld W. Mental disorders and asthma in the community. *Arch Gen Psychiatry.* 2003;60(11):1125–1130.
65. Lavoie KL, Bacon SL, Barone S, Cartier A, Ditto B, Labrecque M. What's worse for asthma control and quality of life: mood disorders, anxiety disorders, or both? *Chest.* 2006;130(4):1039–1047.
66. American Thoracic Society. Guidelines for assessing and managing asthma risk at work, school, and recreation. *Am J Respir Crit Care Med.* 2004;169(7):873–881.
67. Mapp CE, Boschetto P, Maestrelli P, Fabbri LM. Occupational asthma. *Am J Respir Crit Care Med.* 2005;172(3):280–305.
68. Moscato G, Dellabianca A, Perfetti L, et al. Occupational asthma: a longitudinal study on the clinical and socioeconomic outcome after diagnosis. *Chest.* 1999;115(1):249–256.
69. Gannon PF, Weir DC, Robertson AS, Burge PS. Health, employment, and financial outcomes in workers with occupational asthma. *Br J Ind Med.* 1993;50(6):491–496.
70. Ameille J, Pairon JC, Bayeux MC, et al. Consequences of occupational asthma on employment and financial status: a follow-up study. *Eur Respir J.* 1997;10(1):55–58.
71. Cannon J, Cullinan P, Newman Taylor A. Consequences of occupational asthma. *BMJ.* 1995;311(7005):602–603.
72. Dewitte JD, Chan-Yeung M, Malo JL. Medicolegal and compensation aspects of occupational asthma. *Eur Respir J.* 1994;7(5):969–980.
73. Bradshaw LM, Barber CM, Davies J, Curran AD, Fishwick D. Work-related asthma symptoms and attitudes to the workplace. *Occup Med.* 2007;57(1):30–35.
74. Munir F, Leka S, Griffiths A. Dealing with self-management of chronic illness at work: predictors for self-disclosure. *Soc Sci Med.* 2005;60(6):1397–1407.
75. Howse D, Gautrin D, Neis B, et al. Gender and snow crab occupational asthma in Newfoundland and Labrador, Canada. *Environ Res.* 2006;101(2):163–174.
76. Slater T, Erkinjuntti-Pekkanen R, Fishwick D, et al. Changes in work practice after a respiratory health survey among welders in New Zealand. *N Z Med J.* 2000;113(1114):305–308.
77. Gautrin D, Desrosiers M, Castano R. Occupational rhinitis. *Curr Opin Allergy Clin Immunol.* 2006;6:77–84.
78. Moscato G, Vandenplas O, Gerth Van WR, et al. Occupational rhinitis. *Allergy.* 2008;63:969–980.
79. Malo JL, Lemiere C, Desjardins A, Cartier A. Prevalence and intensity of rhinoconjunctivitis in subjects with occupational asthma. *Eur Respir J.* 1997;10:1513–1515.
80. Moscato G, Vandenplas O, Van Wijk RG, et al. EAACI position paper on occupational rhinitis. *Respir Res.* 2009;10:16.

81. Hytonen M, Kanerva L, Malmberg H, Martikainen R, Mutanen P, Toikkanen J. The risk of occupational rhinitis. *Int Arch Occup Environ Health*. 1997;69:487–490.
82. Vandenplas O, Van BP, D'Alpaos V, Wattiez M, Jamart J, Thimpont J. Rhinitis in subjects with work-exacerbated asthma. *Respir Med*. 2010;104:497–503.
83. Miedinger D, Gautrin D, Castano R. Upper airway symptoms among workers with work-related respiratory complaints. *Occup Med*. 2012;62:427–434.
84. Chiry S, Boulet LP, Lepage J, et al. Frequency of work-related respiratory symptoms in workers without asthma. *Am J Ind Med*. 2009;52:447–454.
85. Airaksinen LK, Tuomi TO, Tuppurainen MO, Lauerma AI, Toskala EM. Inhalation challenge test in the diagnosis of occupational rhinitis. *Am J Rhinol*. 2008;22:38–46.
86. Castano R, Gautrin D, Theriault G, Trudeau C, Ghezzo H, Malo JL. Occupational rhinitis in workers investigated for occupational asthma. *Thorax*. 2009;64:50–54.
87. Castano R, Malo JL. Toward a "united" management of "united airways disease": the role of otorhinolaryngologists and pneumologists. *Allergy*. 2007;62:708.

APPENDIX 14.1

INFORMATION COLLECTED FROM THE QUESTIONNAIRE

1. OCCUPATIONAL DATA

Job title
Duration of work under the same job title
Products made by the company
Work shift
Products causing symptoms

2. NATURE OF SYMPTOMS

2.1. Respiratory

Cough
Sputum
Chest tightness
Wheezing
Shortness of breath at rest
Shortness of breath on exercise
Loss of voice

2.2. Systemic

Fever
Chills
Muscle or joint aches

2.3. Rhinitis

Nasal obstruction
Runny nose
Sneezing
Nasal/pharyngeal itching

2.4. Conjunctivitis

Ocular itching
Watery eyes
Redness of the eyes

2.5. Skin symptoms

Rash/urticaria
Eczema

3. TIMING OF SYMPTOMS IN RELATION TO WORK

Interval between onset of exposure at work and onset of symptoms
Interval between onset of symptoms and current questionnaire

Interval between last occupational exposure and current questionnaire

4. RELATIONSHIP OF WORK AND RESPIRATORY SYMPTOMS

4.1. Status of respiratory symptoms on working days compared with days away from work

Better, worse, same
If better or worse:

1. Every day
2. Progressively over the week
3. As a function of working conditions; if yes,

On physical exertion
On exposure to mist, hot or cold temperature
On exposure to dust, fumes, gas

4.2. Possibility of identifying a process or a product that is responsible for respiratory symptoms

Yes, No
If yes, identify the process or product
If yes, is this exposure regular or intermittent?

4.3. Status of respiratory symptoms on weekends

They disappear
They improve
No change

4.4. Status of respiratory symptoms on vacations (more than 1 week)

They disappear
They improve
No change
If they disappear or improve, after how many days?

4.5. Timing of respiratory symptoms in relation to work

Interval between onset of work and onset of symptoms
Persistence or reappearance of symptoms on return to home
Onset of symptoms only upon returning home
Change of timing of symptoms over time

5. RELATIONSHIP OF WORK AND NASAL, CONJUNCTIVAL, OR SKIN SYMPTOMS

5.1. Status of symptoms on working days compared with days away from work

Better, worse, same
If better or worse:

1. Every day
2. Progressively over the week
3. As a function of working conditions; if yes,

On physical exertion
On exposure to mist, hot or cold temperature
On exposure to dust, fumes, gas

6. OTHER INFORMATION

6.1. Smoking habits: smoker, nonsmoker, ex-smoker; number of pack-years

6.2. Presence of chronic bronchitis

6.3. Asthma before starting work that causes symptoms

6.4. Respiratory drugs at the time of investigation

From Vandenplas O, Ghezzo H, Munoz X, et al. What are the questionnaire items most useful in identifying subjects with occupational asthma? *Eur Respir J.* 2005;26(6):1056–1063.

SECTION THREE

CARDIAC AND CARDIOVASCULAR

15

ADULT CARDIAC CONDITIONS

COEXISTING AND DIFFERENTIAL DIAGNOSIS

Paola Rogliani, Andrea Segreti, and Mario Cazzola

KEY POINTS

- Asthma is not a risk factor for coronary heart disease in middle-aged adults.
- There is no difference in gender risk for various kinds of cardiovascular diseases in different age groups with asthma, except for women, in whom there is a higher risk for angina and coronary artery disease.
- Age does not seem to influence the association between asthma and cardiovascular and hypertensive diseases.
- Adult-onset asthma is associated with increased carotid atherosclerosis in women.
- Contrary to what is observed in patients with chronic obstructive pulmonary disease, asthma is only weakly associated with cardiovascular and hypertensive diseases.
- Cardiac asthma, which shares common symptoms and signs with asthma such as wheezing, cough, and dyspnea, must be accurately differentiated from asthma.

INTRODUCTION

Asthma is a chronic inflammatory disease of the airways characterized by bronchospasm and airflow obstruction. It affects an estimated 300 million people worldwide. Comorbidities of asthma may share a common pathophysiologic mechanism, influencing asthma control and its phenotypes and response to treatment.[1] Different studies show that the prevalence of cardiovascular disease (CVD) is increased in asthma.[2-8] In this chapter, the relationship between asthma and its cardiovascular comorbidities will be reviewed.

CLINICAL FEATURES OF ASTHMA

Asthma is a serious global health care problem—people of all ages throughout the world are affected by this chronic airway disorder that can place severe limits on daily life, and it is sometimes fatal. It is a major cause of chronic airflow obstruction, but its pathogenesis and pathology are different from those of chronic obstructive pulmonary disease (COPD).[9] The pathophysiology of asthma is complex and heterogeneous, involving airway inflammation, intermittent airflow obstruction, and bronchial hyperresponsiveness. The inflammation in asthma may be acute, subacute, or chronic, and the presence of airway edema and mucus secretion may also contribute to airflow obstruction. Varying degrees of cellular infiltration, mucus hypersecretion, desquamation of the epithelium, smooth muscle hypertrophy and hyperplasia, and airway remodeling are present.[10] In fact, asthma is a heterogeneous disease with different phenotypes. Inflammation can be predominantly eosinophilic or neutrophilic and involve other cell types.[11]

Both clinical and basic scientific studies indicate that inflammation plays a vital role in the initiation and progression of several comorbidities.[12] For example, Togias[13] suggests that although the initial manifestations of a mucosal allergic reaction are localized (i.e., in the lung), a systemic component also develops that perpetuates the reaction in the respiratory tract as well as leads to inflammatory reactions in other organ systems.

RISK FOR CARDIOVASCULAR DISEASE

Many studies have examined the association of impaired lung function and CVD[14,15]; however, there are relatively few about asthma. These studies support the association between these two diseases, most frequently in females and in late-onset asthma.[16,17]

Asthma seems not to be a risk factor for coronary heart disease in middle-aged adults[6]; nevertheless, some reports suggest that subjects with severe asthma, especially females, are at significant risk for ischemic heart disease.[4] Also, adult-onset asthma, particularly in females, may be a significant risk factor for coronary heart disease.[16] Asthma, contrary to what is observed in patients with COPD, appeared to be only weakly associated with cardiovascular and hypertensive diseases in one large population-based cross-sectional study. There is no difference in gender risk for various kinds of CVDs in different age groups with asthma, except for women, in whom there is a higher risk for angina and coronary artery disease. In males, asthma is not associated with hypertensive disease.[3]

In both genders, asthma is not associated with acute or a past myocardial infarction. Moreover, age does not seem to influence the association between asthma and cardiovascular and hypertensive diseases.[18]

Local inflammation in the lung may spill over into the circulation,[19] inducing low-grade systemic inflammation, which is believed to be a key pathogenetic mechanism underlying most of the systemic manifestations of this disease.[12] Proposed hypotheses to explain the link between asthma and cardiovascular comorbidities are included in Table 15.1.

ASTHMA, CHRONIC OBSTRUCTIVE PULMONARY DISEASE, AND CONGESTIVE HEART FAILURE

Airflow limitation in asthma is usually reversible either spontaneously or after treatment. However, long-standing asthma can lead to

Table 15.1. Asthma and Cardiovascular Comorbidities: Proposed Hypotheses

PATHOPHYSIOLOGIC FEATURES	REFERENCES
Systemic inflammation	12, 13, 19, 50, 62
Asthma medications	8, 42, 44, 45, 46, 56
Transitory and/or chronic hypoxia (pulmonary hypertension)	31

airflow limitation that is not fully reversible.[20] A history of asthma and a higher degree of reversibility of airflow obstruction by an inhaled β_2-agonist are helpful to clinically differentiate asthma from COPD, although clinical overlap between these diseases occurs, in particular in asthmatic patients who smoke. In many cases, it is difficult to differentiate between these two chronic pulmonary diseases.

The most frequent clinical manifestations of asthma include cough, wheezing, chest tightness, and dyspnea. However, these signs and symptoms are not specific for this disease because they also occur in other diseases, such as COPD and CVD. Therefore, the differential diagnosis between asthma and a CVD can be a difficult diagnostic problem, in particular when these two conditions can coexist.

When congestive heart failure (CHF) presents with wheezing, cough, and orthopnea, it referred to as *cardiac asthma*, a condition that must be differentiated from bronchial asthma. Orthopnea also can be a clinical manifestation of asthma and COPD, and paroxysmal nocturnal dyspnea associated with CHF can be mistaken for nocturnal asthma.[21] Furthermore, inhaled bronchodilators, which reduce bronchospasm, may improve the dyspnea associated with pulmonary edema and therefore not help differentiate CHF from asthma. A smoking history may also confuse the picture by producing cough, dyspnea, and wheezing with diminished lung function (and COPD), complicating the differential diagnosis.[22]

Asthma symptoms are usually worse in the early morning and are triggered by cigarette smoke, perfumes, cold air, exercise, laughter, exposure to various allergens, infections, and occupational substances.[23] Other features include variability in symptoms, with periods of disease stability and exacerbations characterized by dyspnea, cough, and chest tightness. The disease can be confirmed either by appropriate pulmonary function studies and the response to a bronchodilator or by a pulmonary challenge study with methacholine or mannitol. However, a bronchial provocation test, although useful to diagnose asthma, thanks to its high predictive value, is not specific for asthma; airway hyperresponsiveness also occurs with other respiratory diseases, such as cystic fibrosis, COPD, and CHF.[24]

Orthopnea associated with CHF often occurs during the night and is referred to as *paroxysmal nocturnal dyspnea*. The airway obstruction associated with CHF is postulated to be due to vascular congestion of the bronchial circulation, dilatation of the pulmonary circulation, and interstitial pulmonary edema, with compression of the airways, squamous metaplasia of bronchial epithelial cells, and smooth muscle cell hypertrophy and subepithelial fibrosis.[25]

The physical examination, in addition to wheezing, may show tachypnea, jugular venous distension, dependent edema, basilar rales (in acute cases), a split or accentuated second heart sound, or a gallop sound.[22] The patient's symptoms may be due to either left- or right-sided failure, or both. Left heart failure is manifested by pulmonary edema and characterized by degrees of dyspnea, orthopnea, paroxysmal nocturnal dyspnea, and wheezing. Right heart failure manifests primarily as peripheral edema, hepatomegaly, and a pulsatile liver with or without ascites, jugular vein distension, and hepatojugular reflux. Decreased cardiac output may occur in either right or left heart failure. Lung hyperinflation may displace the liver and mimic hepatomegaly, particularly in patients with COPD.[26]

Paroxysmal nocturnal dyspnea is caused by interstitial pulmonary edema and sometimes by intraalveolar edema, most commonly as a consequence of left ventricular failure. It is often ameliorated by sitting up, in particular by sitting on the side of the bed or getting out of the bed. Relief is not instantaneous. The dyspnea usually precedes cough. In contrast, nocturnal dyspnea associated with pulmonary disease (i.e., asthma, COPD) is often relieved by coughing up secretions rather than assuming a sitting or upright position.[27]

An electrocardiogram, echocardiogram, and serum B-type natriuretic peptide, a cardiac neurohormone that is increased in CHF, can help differentiate cardiac from respiratory dyspnea. The electrocardiogram may show evidence of left- or right-sided hypertrophy, ischemic heart disease, cardiomyopathy, arrhythmias, and conduction abnormalities. The echocardiogram may confirm the diagnosis. The chest x-ray may show cardiomegaly and signs of pulmonary venous congestion, as occurs with interlobular (Kerley B lines) and peribronchial interstitial thickening, pleural effusion, apical vascular redistribution, dilatation of the azygos vein, and, in cases of alveolar edema, pulmonary consolidations.

Levels of plasma B-type natriuretic peptide, together with other clinical manifestations, permit the diagnosis of this disease in patients with acute dyspnea.[28] It also can help distinguish new-onset CHF in patients with COPD or asthma who present to the emergency department with dyspnea.[29]

Other useful tests to confirm CHF include a Holter electrocardiographic monitor, 6-minute walk test (6MWT), cycle ergometer or treadmill exercise test, and cardiac catheterization.

Management of CHF depends on its etiology and is based on both nonpharmacologic and pharmacologic treatments. Nonpharmacologic treatment includes smoking cessation and sodium restriction. Pharmacologic treatment includes the use of angiotensin-converting enzyme inhibitors, β-blockers, aldosterone antagonists, angiotensin receptor blockers, hydralazine and isosorbide dinitrate, digoxin, and diuretics. The acute management may include use of oxygen, diuretics, opiates, vasodilators, inotropes, vasopressors, and mechanical ventilation.[30] Table 15.2 illustrates the major differences between bronchial and cardiac asthma.

PULMONARY HYPERTENSION

Another problem to consider is the occurrence of complications secondary to transitory or chronic hypoxia, such as occurs with pulmonary hypertension. Eighteen percent of patients with mild to moderate asthma have pulmonary hypertension as demonstrated by Doppler echocardiography. These patients are older, have later onset of disease, and have lower $FEF_{25\%-75\%}$ (forced expiratory flow between 25% and 75% of the forced expiratory capacity), PaO_2, basal SpO_2, and SpO_2 at 6MWT.[31] The 6MWT is a submaximal exercise test in which the patient is asked to walk as quickly as possible on a flat surface for 6 minutes to assess the submaximal level of functional capacity.[32]

Symptoms in patients affected by all forms of pulmonary hypertension are nonspecific, such as dyspnea on exertion and fatigue. In more advanced forms, signs of right ventricular failure, such as peripheral edema, elevated jugular venous pressure, a loud pulmonary component of the second heart sound, and/or a holosystolic murmur of tricuspid insufficiency, are present.[33]

β-BLOCKERS

It is important to assess the treatment for patients with asthma who have concomitant CVD. For example, even though β-blocker therapy is efficacious in reducing the mortality after a myocardial infarction,[34] noncardioselective β-blockers should be avoided in patients with asthma because they may induce acute bronchospasm.[35] In contrast, a meta-analysis indicates that cardioselective β-blockers ($β_1$-blockers) do not significantly adversely affect patients with mild to moderate asthma. The minimal decrease in forced expiratory volume in 1 second (FEV_1) observed after a single dose tends to attenuate after a few days to weeks of use. Moreover, continued treatment improves response to $β_2$-agonists versus placebo, as a result of upregulation or sensitization of $β_2$-adrenergic receptors. Therefore, in patients with asthma who have concomitant cardiovascular pathologies, cardioselective β-blockers are safe and should not be withheld.[36,37]

The benefit of using low-dose $β_1$-blockers following a myocardial infarction outweighs the risk in patients with well-controlled, mild intermittent or persistent asthma, but when possible these drugs should be avoided in moderate to severe persistent asthma, in which they have been associated with fatal or life-threatening asthma.[38] Evidence suggests that β-blockers should not be withheld in patients with mild to moderate well-controlled asthma and, if used carefully, may even improve symptoms in patients with both cardiovascular and obstructive airways disease.[39] Although a single administration of β-blockers

Table 15.2. Differential Diagnosis between Bronchial Asthma and Cardiac Asthma

	BRONCHIAL ASTHMA	CARDIAC ASTHMA
Clinical manifestations	Dyspnea Wheezing Cough Viscous sputum Chest tightness Nocturnal awakenings associated with sputum production	Dyspnea Wheezing Cough Frothy or bloody sputum Orthopnea Paroxysmal nocturnal dyspnea
Thoracic auscultation	Diminished vesicular breath sound Expiratory wheezes	Diminished vesicular breath sound Inspiratory crackles (dependent on gravity) Expiratory wheezes
Electrocardiogram and echocardiogram	Normal in stable asthma Alterations due to chronic hypoxemia and pulmonary arterial hypertension in case of severe asthma and/or exacerbations	Alterations depend on the etiology
Chest x-ray	Bronchial thickening Hyperinflation	Cardiomegaly Interlobular and peribronchial interstitial thickening Pleural effusion Redistribution of pulmonary veins toward apical fields Dilatation of azygos vein Pulmonary consolidations (alveolar edema)
Laboratory tests	Eosinophilia Total serum immunoglobulin E levels increased Positive in vivo (skin allergy test) or in vitro allergy test	B-type natriuretic peptide levels increased
Inhaled bronchodilators	In most cases improve the clinical manifestations	May improve the clinical manifestations

may be accompanied by acute bronchoconstriction, their chronic use may attenuate airway hyperresponsiveness and be beneficial in treating asthma. In fact, chronic exposure to β_2-agonists causes β_2-adrenergic downregulation, whereas chronic administration of β-blockers causes receptor upregulation.[40]

ASTHMA TREATMENT AND CARDIOVASCULAR DISEASE

Cardiovascular complications have been attributed to asthma treatment.[17,41] However, it is possible that the initial presentation of symptoms that suggest asthma, presumably including dyspnea, is in some cases ischemic heart disease.[42] The risk for a myocardial infarction is similar with inhaled corticosteroids, long-acting β-agonists, and short-acting β-agonists, with the highest risks in first-time users and long-term heavy users of these asthma medications.[43]

A review of randomized controlled trials shows that the use of $β_2$-agonists to treat asthma and COPD is statistically associated with a significant risk for increased heart rate and decreased serum potassium. Consequently, risk for adverse cardiovascular events is higher than with placebo.[44]

Patients with asthma, relative to subjects with no history of the disease, seem to have an increased risk for coronary heart disease, cerebrovascular disease, and heart failure, and these risks are correlated with the use of asthma medications. In particular, patients not taking asthma medications are at reduced risk for CVD, although they are at increased risk for all-cause mortality. Those taking one or more asthma medications are at enhanced risk for both CVD and all-cause mortality.[45] These observations indicate that the increased prevalence of CVDs in asthmatic patients may be associated with the medications that patients use to treat the disease. In this case, the presence of cardiovascular comorbidities could represent side effects of anti-asthmatic treatment. Table 15.3 illustrates the cardiovascular side effects associated with medications used to treat asthma.

Cardiac arrest with asthma is usually caused by hypoxemia, which can be of sudden onset. Cardiovascular arrest, secondary to asthma, can be caused by severe asthma associated with hypoxia, medication use, electrolyte abnormalities, hyperinflation of the lungs with reduction in blood pressure, and unilateral or bilateral tension pneumothorax.[46]

ASTHMA AND MARKERS OF SYSTEMIC INFLAMMATION

The connection between asthma and CVDs is not completely understood. Markers of systemic

Table 15.3. Cardiovascular Side Effects of Asthma Medications

MEDICATION	CARDIOVASCULAR SIDE EFFECTS
$β_2$-Agonist	Arrhythmias
	Cardiac ischemia
	Hyperglycemia
	Hypopotassemia
	Increase of plasma free fatty acid
	Tachycardia
Corticosteroids	Arterial hypertension
	Hypernatremia
	Hypopotassemia
	Increase of plasma free fatty acids
Anticholinergics	Arrhythmias
	Tachycardia
Theophyllines	Arrhythmias
	Arterial hypotension
	Tachycardia
	Hypopotassemia
	Hyperglycemia
	Hypercalcemia

inflammation, a risk factor for CVDs, are elevated in patients with asthma.[19] For example, adults with asthma or asthmatic symptoms have higher levels of high-sensitivity C-reactive protein (Hs-CRP),[47] a known inflammatory marker and risk factor for CVD. In corticosteroid-naïve asthmatic patients, serum levels of Hs-CRP are increased and correlated with sputum eosinophils and decreased pulmonary function.[48] Likewise, concentrations of serum tumor necrosis factor-α, interleukin-6 (IL-6), and tissue inhibitor of metalloproteinases-1 are significantly higher in patients with stable COPD and those with asthma than in control subjects. Also, serum $α_1$-antitrypsin levels are higher in COPD patients than in asthma and control patients, and transforming growth factor-β1 levels are higher in patients with asthma versus COPD.[49]

Adipocyte dysfunction could be the link between asthma and COPD and associated comorbidities.[12] Airway inflammation in asthma is heterogeneous and may involve an allergen-specific acquired immune response with IL-5–mediated eosinophilic inflammation or a dysregulation of the innate immune responses involving IL-8–induced neutrophilic airway inflammation.[50] Systemic inflammation is increased in asthmatic patients with neutrophilic airway inflammation and is associated with worse clinical outcomes.[51] However, the possibility that comorbidities of asthma are the result of systemic inflammation is not well established.

ASTHMA AND VASCULAR COMPLICATIONS

A significant association of asthma with cardiac and vascular complications is demonstrated in several epidemiologic studies.[3,8] Schanen and colleagues[6] report an increased risk for stroke, but not coronary heart disease, associated with asthma. Adult-onset asthma is associated with increased carotid atherosclerosis in women,[7] and subjects who have bronchial hyperresponsiveness to methacholine demonstrate increased carotid intima-media thickness.[52]

Asthma and atherosclerosis are both associated with systemic inflammation. Animal studies show increased myocardial vulnerability in rabbits with systemic allergy and asthma.[53] An intriguing report reveals that the induction of allergic pulmonary inflammation in mice depresses endothelium-dependent and -independent vascular relaxation, which can contribute to cardiovascular complications associated with allergic inflammation.[54]

The prevalence of asthma is increased in patients affected by the long QT syndrome, indicating a possible genetic link. The presence of asthma as a comorbidity of this syndrome is independently associated with an increased risk for cardiac events, and the risk is reduced by β-blocker therapy.[55] Tachycardia and premature ventricular contractions are more prevalent in subjects with asthma versus those without and more pronounced in patients who receive $β_2$-agonists.[56]

LIFESTYLE AND BEHAVIOR MODIFICATION STRATEGIES

Asthmatic patients should avoid factors that can trigger an asthma exacerbation and properly take their medications as prescribed. There is some evidence to suggest that dietary sodium intake, a recognized risk factor for CVD, is involved in the increased prevalence of asthma and that asthmatic patients should reduce their salt intake. For example, reduced dietary salt intake improves pulmonary function and decreases bronchoconstriction in response to exercise in individuals with asthma.[57] Adoption of a low-sodium diet improves lung function and decreases bronchial reactivity and exercise-induced bronchoconstriction in asthmatic subjects.[58] There was a relationship between low sodium intake and improvement of asthma and bronchial reactivity to methacholine in a randomized controlled trial.[59] Reduction of salt intake has multiple beneficial health effects, and thus it can be considered as a therapeutic option for asthmatic patients, regardless of the presence or absence of hypertension and other cardiovascular problems.

Although the reasons that the Mediterranean diet is beneficial in reducing CVD are under review, its likely beneficial effects are probably secondary to its anti-inflammatory properties. A high intake of fruits, vegetables, legumes, nuts, whole grains, and olive oil; moderately high intake of oily fish; moderate intake of dairy products (mainly cheese and yogurt); and low intake of meat, poultry, and ω-6 fatty acids, the latter being essential fatty acids that improve health, characterize the Mediterranean diet. Asthma is an inflammatory disease, and the Mediterranean diet is associated with reduced asthma risk in epidemiologic studies. Small but consistent improvements were seen in quality of life and spirometric parameters among adults in a randomized controlled trial. Regardless, the Mediterranean diet is a healthy diet that also could produce clinical improvements in asthma.[60]

PHARMACOLOGIC TREATMENT

Inhaled and systemic glucocorticosteroids are the most effective anti-inflammatory medications used to treat persistent asthma. Short- and long-acting β_2-agonist bronchodilators can be added to improve asthma control. In a large population-based cohort of asthma patients, the use of inhaled corticosteroids reduced the risk for myocardial infarction, particularly among those with more severe disease. This effect was attributable to improved asthma control, with a consequent reduction in episodes of hypoxemia and various types of tachycardia. Another variable suggests that asthmatic patients who take inhaled corticosteroids regularly are more compliant and therefore maintain a healthier lifestyle than patients who do not regularly take their medications. One other possibility is that inhaled corticosteroids may exert anti-inflammatory effects on coronary plaques.[61]

However, possible cardiovascular side events may result from the use of medications commonly administered for the treatment of asthma, in particular β_2-agonists. The risk for myocardial infarction was highly associated with the Framingham myocardial infarction risk score in patients prescribed asthma medications. These findings imply that the initial presentation with symptoms suggesting asthma (presumably dyspnea) is, in some cases, the presentation of ischemic heart disease.[42]

It is not yet established whether controlling asthma will actually reduce comorbidities or whether treatment of comorbid conditions improves asthma control, or even whether treatment of asthma is altered by the presence of a concomitant comorbid disease. Nevertheless, there is the suggestive documentation that escalating doses of β_2-adrenoceptor inverse agonists reduce airway hyperresponsiveness in patients with asthma. β_2-adrenergic receptor inverse agonists are medications that act at the same receptor as the agonists but produce an opposite effect; such a medication is nadolol, one of the first options to treat CHF. Furthermore, the simultaneous administration of nadolol and a corticosteroid is more effective in reducing indexes of airway inflammation than either drug given alone, at least in an asthma model. Moreover, emerging evidence suggests beneficial effects of statins in asthma management.[62]

UNMET, FUTURE RESEARCH NEEDS

1. The presence of CVD may affect asthma control or modulate treatment response.
2. Asthma may be responsible for inducing other comorbidities such as CVD.
3. Better control of asthma may reduce such comorbidities.
4. Systemic inflammation occurs with asthma; it is unclear whether treating systemic inflammation will prevent comorbidities such as CVD.
5. More data are needed to determine whether local inflammation in the lung spills over into systemic inflammation.
6. Another question is whether or not asthma treatment causes cardiovascular complications.
7. It is possible that inhaled corticosteroids decrease the formation of coronary plaques via their anti-inflammatory effects.
8. More emphasis is needed on making sure that the presenting signs and symptoms of asthma, in some cases, are associated with ischemic heart disease.
9. Information is also necessary on lifestyle and behavior modification strategies such as

the use of a low-sodium or Mediterranean diet to help control asthma.

CONCLUSION

Asthma is frequently associated with different types of CVD. Although various hypotheses have been advanced to explain this association, the exact mechanisms are not understood. What is clear is that the identification of these comorbidities must become an integral part of the core management of asthma. Likewise, a physician should know how to differentiate between asthma, COPD, and cardiac asthma (CHF), often a difficult proposition. A systematic evaluation, not only of the presence of comorbid conditions, is necessary to ensure that such comorbidities are adequately treated and controlled so that the effect on asthma is minimized.

REFERENCES

1. Boulet LP, Boulay MÈ. Asthma-related comorbidities. *Expert Rev Respir Med*. 2011;5(3):377–393.
2. Boulet LP. Influence of comorbid conditions on asthma. *Eur Respir J*. 2009;33(4):897–906.
3. Cazzola M, Calzetta L, Bettoncelli G, et al. Cardiovascular disease in asthma and COPD: a population-based retrospective cross-sectional study. *Respir Med*. 2012;106(2):249–256.
4. Toren K, Lindholm NB. Do patients with severe asthma run an increased risk from ischaemic heart disease? *Int J Epidemiol*. 1996;25(3):617–620.
5. Knoflach M, Kiechl S, Mayr A, Willeit J, Poewe W, Wick G. Allergic rhinitis, asthma, and atherosclerosis in the Bruneck and ARMY studies. *Arch Intern Med*. 2005;165(21):2521–2526.
6. Schanen J, Iribarren C, Shahar E, et al. Asthma and incident cardiovascular disease: the Atherosclerosis Risk in Communities Study. *Thorax*. 2005;60(8):633–638.
7. Onufrak S, Abramson J, Vaccarino V. Adult-onset asthma is associated with increased carotid atherosclerosis among women in the Atherosclerosis Risk in Communities (ARIC) study. *Atherosclerosis*. 2007;195(1):129–137.
8. Appleton SL, Ruffin RE, Wilson DH, Taylor AW, Adams RJ. Cardiovascular disease risk associated with asthma and respiratory morbidity might be mediated by short-acting beta2-agonists. North West Adelaide Cohort Health Study Team. *J Allergy Clin Immunol*. 2009;123(1):124–130.
9. Fabbri LM, Romagnoli M, Corbetta L, et al. Differences in airway inflammation in patients with fixed airflow obstruction due to asthma or chronic obstructive pulmonary disease. *Am J Respir Crit Care Med*. 2003;167(3):418–424.
10. Horwitz RJ, Busse WW. Inflammation and asthma. *Clin Chest Med*. 1995;16(4):583–602.
11. The ENFUMOSA cross-sectional European multicentre study of the clinical phenotype of chronic severe asthma. European Network for Understanding Mechanisms of Severe Asthma. *Eur Respir J*. 2003;22(3):470–477.
12. Wouters EF, Reynaert NL, Dentener MA, Vernooy JH. Systemic and local inflammation in asthma and chronic obstructive pulmonary disease: is there a connection? *Proc Am Thorac Soc*. 2009;6(8):638–647.
13. Togias A. Systemic effects of local allergic disease. *J Allergy Clin Immunol*. 2004;113(1 Suppl):S8–S14.
14. Kannel WB, Hubert H, Lew EA. Vital capacity as a predictor of cardiovascular disease: the Framingham study. *Am Heart J*. 1983;105(2):311–315.
15. Lange P, Nyboe J, Appleyard M, Jensen G, Schnohr P. Spirometric findings and mortality in never-smokers. *J Clin Epidemiol*. 1990;43(9):867–873.
16. Onufrak SJ, Abramson JL, Austin HD, Holguin F, McClellan WM, Vaccarino LV. Relation of adult-onset asthma to coronary heart disease and stroke. *Am J Cardiol*. 2008;101(9):1247–1252.
17. Appleton SL, Ruffin RE, Wilson DH, Taylor AW, Adams RJ, for the North West Adelaide Cohort Health Study Team. Cardiovascular disease risk associated with asthma and respiratory morbidity might be mediated by short-acting b2-agonists. *J Allergy Clin Immunol*. 2009;123(1):124–130.
18. Cazzola M, Calzetta L, Bettoncelli G, Novelli L, Cricelli C, Rogliani P. Asthma and comorbid medical illness. *Eur Respir J*. 2011;38(1):42–49.
19. Magnussen H, Watz H. Systemic inflammation in chronic obstructive pulmonary disease and asthma: relation with comorbidities. *Proc Am Thorac Soc*. 2009;6(8):648–651.
20. Lange P, Parner J, Vestbo J, Schnohr P, Jensen G. A 15-year follow up study of ventilatory function in adults with asthma. *N Engl J Med*. 1998;339(17):1194–1200.

21. Kasper DL, Braunwald E, Fauci AS, Hauser SL, Longo DL, Jameson JL. *Harrison's Principles of Internal Medicine*. 16th ed. New York: McGraw-Hill Medical; 2005.
22. Slaughter MC. Not quite asthma: differential diagnosis of dyspnea, cough, and wheezing. *Allergy Asthma Proc*. 2007;28(3):271–281.
23. Hopkin JM. The diagnosis of asthma, a clinical syndrome. *Thorax*. 2012;67(7):660–662.
24. Fishman AP, Elias JA, Fishman JA, Grippi MA, Senior RM, Pack AI. *Fishman's Pulmonary Diseases and Disorders*. 4th ed. New York: McGraw-Hill Professional; 2008.
25. Tanabe T, Rozycki HJ, Kanoh S, Rubin BK. Cardiac asthma: new insights into an old disease. *Expert Rev Respir Med*. 2012;6(6):705–714.
26. Buckner K. Cardiac asthma. *Immunol Allergy Clin North Am*. 2013;33(1):35–44.
27. Zipes DP, Libby P, Bonow RO, Braunwald E. *Braunwald's Heart Disease, A Textbook of Cardiovascular Medicine*. 7th ed. Philadelphia: W.B. Saunders; 2005.
28. Maisel AS, Krishnaswamy P, Nowak RM, et al., for the Breathing Not Properly Multinational Study Investigators. Rapid measurement of B-type natriuretic peptide in the emergency diagnosis of heart failure. *N Engl J Med*. 2002;347(3):161–167.
29. McCullough PA, Hollander JE, Nowak RM, et al., for the Breathing Not Properly Multinational Study Investigators. Uncovering heart failure in patients with a history of pulmonary disease: rationale for the early use of B-type natriuretic peptide in the emergency department. *Acad Emerg Med*. 2003;10(3):198–204.
30. McMurray JJ, Adamopoulos S, Anker SD, et al., for the Task Force for the Diagnosis and Treatment of Acute and Chronic Heart Failure 2012 of the European Society of Cardiology, Committee for Practice Guidelines. ESC guidelines for the diagnosis and treatment of acute and chronic heart failure 2012: The Task Force for the Diagnosis and Treatment of Acute and Chronic Heart Failure 2012 of the European Society of Cardiology. Developed in collaboration with the Heart Failure Association (HFA) of the ESC. *Eur J Heart Fail*. 2012;14(8):803–869.
31. Gunen H, Hacievliyagil SS, Kosar F, Gulbas G, Kizkin O, Sahin I. The role of arterial blood gases, exercise testing, and cardiac examination in asthma. *Allergy Asthma Proc*. 2006;27(1):45–52.
32. ATS Committee on Proficiency Standards for Clinical Pulmonary Function Laboratories. ATS statement: guidelines for the six-minute walk test. *Am J Respir Crit Care Med*. 2002;166(1):111–117.
33. Preston IR. Properly diagnosing pulmonary arterial hypertension. *Am J Cardiol*. 2013;111 (8 Suppl):2C–9C.
34. Gottlieb SS, McCarter RJ, Vogel RA. Effect of beta-blockade on mortality among high-risk and low-risk patients after myocardial infarction. *N Engl J Med*. 1998;339(8):489–497.
35. Covar RA, Macomber BA, Szefler SJ. Medications as asthma triggers. *Immunol Allergy Clin North Am*. 2005;25(1):169–190.
36. Salpeter SR, Ormiston TM, Salpeter EE. Cardioselective beta-blockers in patients with reactive airway disease: a meta-analysis. *Ann Intern Med*. 2002;137(9):715–725.
37. Salpeter S, Ormiston T, Salpeter E. Cardioselective beta-blockers for reversible airway disease. *Cochrane Database Syst Rev*. 2002;4:CD002992.
38. Chafin CC, Soberman JE, Demirkan K, Self T. Beta-blockers after myocardial infarction: do benefits ever outweigh risks in asthma? *Cardiology*. 1999;92(2):99–105.
39. Ashrafian H, Violaris AG. Beta-blocker therapy of cardiovascular diseases in patients with bronchial asthma or COPD: the pro viewpoint. *Prim Care Respir J*. 2005;14(5):236–241.
40. Lipworth BJ, Williamson PA. Think the impossible: beta-blockers for treating asthma. *Clin Sci*. 2009;118(2):115–120.
41. Varas-Lorenzo C, Rodriguez LA, Maguire A, Castellsague J, Perez-Gutthann S. Use of oral corticosteroids and the risk of acute myocardial infarction. *Atherosclerosis*. 2007;192(2):376–383.
42. Squire I. Shortness of breath, prescription of bronchodilators and the risk of myocardial infarction. *J Hypertens*. 2009;27(7): 1358–1359.
43. Zhang B, de Vries F, Setakis E, van Staa TP. The pattern of risk of myocardial infarction in patients taking asthma medication: a study with the General Practice Research Database. *J Hypertens*. 2009;27(7):1485–1492.
44. Salpeter SR, Ormiston TM, Salpeter EE. Cardiovascular effects of beta-agonists in patients with asthma and COPD: a meta-analysis. *Chest*. 2004;125(6):2309–2321.
45. Iribarren C, Tolstykh IV, Miller MK, Sobel E, Eisner MD. Adult asthma and risk of coronary heart disease, cerebrovascular disease, and heart failure: a prospective study of 2 matched cohorts. *Am J Epidemiol*. 2012;176(11):1014–1024.

46. Soar J, Perkins GD, Abbas G, et al. European Resuscitation Council Guidelines for Resuscitation; 2010, Section 8. Cardiac arrest in special circumstances: electrolyte abnormalities, poisoning, drowning, accidental hypothermia, hyperthermia, asthma, anaphylaxis, cardiac surgery, trauma, pregnancy, electrocution. *Resuscitation*. 2010;81(10):1400–1433.
47. Arif AA, Delclos GL, Colmer-Hamood J. Association between asthma, asthma symptoms and C-reactive protein in US adults: data from the National Health and Nutrition Examination Survey, 1999–2002. *Respirology*. 2007;12(5):675–682.
48. Takemura M, Matsumoto H, Niimi A, et al. High sensitivity C-reactive protein in asthma. *Eur Respir J*. 2006;27(5):908–912.
49. Higashimoto Y, Yamagata Y, Taya S, et al. Systemic inflammation in chronic obstructive pulmonary disease and asthma: similarities and differences. *Respirology*. 2008;13(1):128–133.
50. Wood LG, Baines KJ, Fu J, Scott HA, Gibson PG. The neutrophilic inflammatory phenotype is associated with systemic inflammation in asthma. *Chest*. 2012;142(1):86–93.
51. Sexton P, Black P, Metcalf P, et al. Influence of Mediterranean diet on asthma symptoms, lung function, and systemic inflammation: a randomized controlled trial. *J Asthma*. 2013;50(1):75–81.
52. Zureik M, Kony S, Neukirch C, et al. Bronchial hyperresponsiveness to methacholine is associated with increased common carotid intima-media thickness in men. *Arterioscler Thromb Vasc Biol*. 2004;24(6):1098–1103.
53. Hazarika S, Van Scott MR, Lust RM. Myocardial ischemia-reperfusion injury is enhanced in a model of systemic allergy and asthma. *Am J Physiol Heart Circ Physiol*. 2004;286(5):H1720–H1725.
54. Hazarika S, Van Scott MR, Lust RM, Wingard CJ. Pulmonary allergic reactions impair systemic vascular relaxation in ragweed sensitive mice. *Vascul Pharmacol*. 2010;53(5-6):258–263.
55. Rosero SZ, Zareba W, Moss AJ, et al. Asthma and the risk of cardiac events in the Long QT syndrome. Long QT Syndrome Investigative Group. *Am J Cardiol*. 1999;84(12):1406–1411.
56. Warnier MJ, Rutten FH, Kors JA, et al. Cardiac arrhythmias in adult patients with asthma. *J Asthma*. 2012;49(9):942–946.
57. McKeever TM, Britton J. Diet and asthma. *Am J Respir Crit Care Med*. 2004;170(7):725–729.
58. Mickleborough TD. Salt intake, asthma, and exercise-induced bronchoconstriction: a review. *Phys Sportsmed*. 2010;38(1):118–131.
59. Pogson ZE, Antoniak MD, Pacey SJ, Lewis SA, Britton JR, Fogarty AW. Does a low sodium diet improve asthma control? A randomized controlled trial. *Am J Respir Crit Care Med*. 2008;178(2):132–138.
60. Sexton P, Black P, Metcalf P, et al. Influence of Mediterranean diet on asthma symptoms, lung function, and systemic inflammation: a randomized controlled trial. *J Asthma*. 2013;50(1):75–81.
61. Suissa S, Assimes T, Brassard P, Ernst P. Inhaled corticosteroid use in asthma and the prevention of myocardial infarction. *Am J Med*. 2003;115(5):377–381.
62. Cazzola M, Segreti A, Calzetta L, Rogliani P. Comorbidities of asthma: current knowledge and future research needs. *Curr Opin Pulm Med*. 2013;19(1):36–41.

16

PEDIATRIC CARDIAC CONDITIONS

COEXISTING AND DIFFERENTIAL DIAGNOSIS

Louis I. Bezold

KEY POINTS

- Asthma is one of the most common associated conditions in children with congenital heart disease.
- Respiratory distress or frank wheezing may be caused by a number of congenital or acquired heart diseases seen in children.
- Chronic asthma is associated with several cardiac comorbid conditions, including subclinical cardiac dysfunction, obesity, and tamponade physiology (in status asthmaticus).
- Pharmacologic treatment of asthma may have negative cardiac effects.

INTRODUCTION

The relationship between asthma and pediatric cardiac conditions is complex. A number of cardiac conditions in children result in physiology either associated with or actually causing wheezing and/or respiratory distress and hence should be considered in the differential diagnosis of bronchial asthma (Table 16.1).

The converse is also true: asthma is one of the most common associated conditions in children with congenital heart disease (2.4% in one study of 1,058 children with congenital heart disease, trailing only developmental issues in frequency).[1] Chronic asthma is also associated with several cardiac comorbid conditions, including subclinical cardiac dysfunction and obesity, and certain intravenous therapies for status asthmaticus may have negative cardiac effects, including transient cardiac ischemia.

Table 16.1. Pediatric Cardiac Anatomy and Physiology Associated with Wheezing

Bronchial compression and/or bronchomalacia
- Congenital heart disease with pulmonary artery dilatation
- Congenital heart disease with aortopulmonary collaterals
- Vascular rings, pulmonary sling
- Aortic aneurysm

Congestive heart failure
- Congenital heart disease with pulmonary overcirculation
- Left ventricular dysfunction or ischemia (congenital or acquired)

Pulmonary venous or left atrial hypertension
- Congenital heart disease
- Postoperative congenital heart disease
- Left ventricular dysfunction, congestive heart failure

Palliated single ventricle (Fontan) with plastic bronchitis

PEDIATRIC CARDIAC CONDITIONS MIMICKING ASTHMA (DIFFERENTIAL DIAGNOSIS)

Congenital Heart Disease Associated with Bronchial Compression or Bronchomalacia

Congenital cardiac defects that result in compression of the airways due to aortopulmonary malformations can mimic asthma.[2,3] Although the severity of symptoms varies widely, common features include chronic airway issues such as tachypnea, retractions, wheezing, and poor tolerance of pulmonary infections, particularly in infancy.

Tetralogy of Fallot with Absent Pulmonary Valve Syndrome

Tetralogy of Fallot is a fairly common form of cyanotic congenital heart disease consisting of a ventricular septal defect, overriding aorta, significant right ventricular outflow tract obstruction, and secondary right ventricular hypertrophy. There may be associated pulmonary valve and pulmonary artery hypoplasia.

Tetralogy of Fallot with absent pulmonary valve (also known as *absent pulmonary valve syndrome*) is an uncommon variant (about 3% of patients with tetralogy of Fallot) characterized by severe pulmonary regurgitation due to very dysplastic and rudimentary pulmonary valve leaflets, often in association with congenital absence of the ductus arteriosus. The right ventricular outflow tract obstruction is often relatively mild in this syndrome. In conjunction with the pulmonary regurgitation, there is aneurysmal dilatation of the main and branch pulmonary arteries (often to a massive degree; Figure 16.1) that extends to more distal pulmonary branches.[4] Bronchial and bronchiolar compression and malacia are common, leading to symptoms of wheezing, stridor, and respiratory distress.

The diagnosis of absent pulmonary valve syndrome is generally made in infancy by echocardiography in patients with symptoms of respiratory distress and possible cyanosis and with the classic "to-and-fro" murmur of pulmonary stenosis and regurgitation. Surgical repair of the congenital heart lesions is typically performed in the first year or so of life and may include pulmonary arterioplasty in an attempt to relieve airway compromise. Respiratory symptoms often persist after repair, although improvement can occur with age and somatic growth.[5-7] This disease may actually represent a true pulmonary arteriopathy in conjunction with the congenital heart disease.[4]

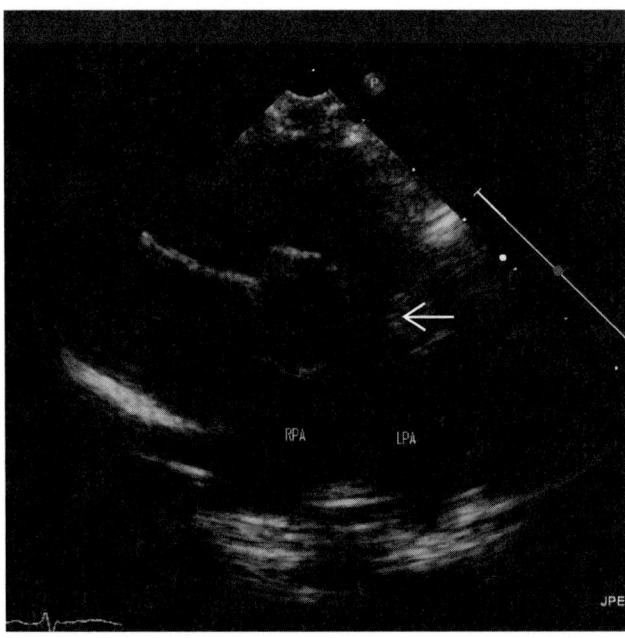

FIGURE 16.1 Transthoracic echocardiographic image (parasternal short-axis view) demonstrating massive enlargement of the branch pulmonary arteries in an infant with absent pulmonary valve syndrome after repair. The branch pulmonary arteries both measure between 1.5 and 2 cm and contributed to significant airway compression and respiratory symptoms in this patient. The arrow points out the main pulmonary artery. LPA, left pulmonary artery; RPA, right pulmonary artery; P, echo machine left-right indicator.

Pulmonary Atresia with Ventricular Septal Defect and Aortopulmonary Collaterals

Other types of complex congenital heart disease that include pulmonary atresia as part of the diagnosis may have associated major aortopulmonary collateral arteries (MAPCAs) that develop as an alternative means of providing pulmonary blood flow. The classic cardiac lesion with MAPCAs is pulmonary atresia with ventricular septal defect, which arguably may be thought of as the most severe manifestation of tetralogy of Fallot.[8-11] MAPCAs are usually multiple and bilateral and may be relatively large vessels. They arise most commonly from the thoracic aorta but can also originate from major aortic branches such as the subclavian or internal mammary arteries, the abdominal aorta, or, rarely, the coronary arteries. MAPCAs are often very tortuous, with areas of stenosis. Depending on their specific course and relationship to the bronchi and smaller airways, they can result in airway compression or malacia, similar to the absent pulmonary valve syndrome described previously.

Patients with pulmonary atresia are obviously cyanotic and come to attention early after birth because of their heart disease. Although respiratory symptoms are typically much less severe in this disease compared with absent pulmonary valve syndrome, they can complicate diagnosing true asthma, if present, in these patients. Multiple surgical and transcatheter procedures are needed to palliate the congenital heart disease and deal with the MAPCAs in these cases.[8,10]

Other Cardiac or Vascular Anomalies

Vascular rings are relatively uncommon congenital anomalies (<1% of congenital heart defects) that involve anomalous configuration of the aortic arch or branch vessels, resulting in an encircling of the trachea or esophagus and trachea. Rings may be complete or incomplete. By far, the most common types are double aortic arch and right aortic arch with a left ductus or ligamentum arteriosum (>85% to 90% of cases). Other variations are much less common. Timing and specifics of clinical presentation also vary depending on the severity of airway or esophageal compression. Most patients present early in life (infancy or early childhood) with stridor, respiratory distress, wheezing, apnea, or a characteristic cough. Older patients may have a previous diagnosis of asthma, dysphagia, or history of recurrent lower tract respiratory infections. Some patients present much later in adulthood or even remain asymptomatic.[12-15]

Chest radiography may demonstrate pulmonary hyperinflation, sometimes mistaken for asthma. Radiography can also suggest the presence of a right arch, which should be specifically looked for in patients with airway difficulties. Most cases can be definitively diagnosed using barium esophagram. Echocardiography can also help to define the anatomy and exclude other cardiac structural anomalies. Computed tomography and magnetic resonance imaging can provide additional anatomic definition in unclear cases but are not routinely necessary to diagnose the typical vascular ring. Treatment is by surgical division and is indicated in all symptomatic patients.

Pulmonary artery sling (anomalous origin of the left pulmonary artery from the right pulmonary artery) makes up about 10% of vascular rings and can also cause tracheomalacia. In this condition, the left pulmonary artery courses over the right mainstem bronchus and between the esophagus and trachea. There may be other associated congenital heart disease (10% to 15% of patients) or other congenital anomalies, including gastrointestinal (biliary atresia, Hirschsprung's disease) or airway anomalies (complete tracheal rings). Most patients present within the first few weeks of life. Although the history and physical examination may be more consistent with upper airway issues (i.e., stridor), associated pulmonary parenchymal anomalies also occur and may generate signs or symptoms that may be mistaken for asthma, similar to the other types of vascular rings.[16,17]

Although extremely rare in childhood, an aortic aneurysm or pseudoaneurysm may cause bronchial compression and wheezing mimicking asthma. These vascular anomalies are most commonly caused by infection or trauma.[18]

Bronchodilator therapy is frequently used in patients with respiratory issues related to the congenital heart lesions mentioned previously; however, their effectiveness is questionable at best, unless there is concomitant bronchial asthma.

CONGESTIVE HEART FAILURE

Congestive heart failure in children is quite different than in adults with respect to potential causes and clinical findings. Two basic physiologies can lead to pediatric heart failure: (1) left-to-right cardiac shunts of sufficient magnitude to cause symptomatic pulmonary overcirculation (perhaps a more appropriate term than "heart failure"); and (2) left ventricular dysfunction (due to multiple potential etiologies), which is physiologically similar to adult heart failure, but clinically distinct. Both types of physiology can lead to symptoms of shortness of air, respiratory distress, and wheezing on examination ("cardiac asthma"), thus potentially being mistaken for true bronchial asthma.

Left-to-Right Shunts

Left-to-right shunts are typically due to congenital heart disease with intracardiac septal defects or aortopulmonary connections. The most common defects include ventricular septal defect, atrial septal defect, and patent ductus arteriosus. Physiologically, large defects result in a significant shunting of blood from the left heart to the right heart (assuming relatively normal pulmonary vascular resistance), leading to increased pulmonary blood flow. A significant increase in pulmonary blood flow causes pulmonary vascular engorgement, which in severe cases can result in wheezing or "cardiac asthma." Associated cardiomegaly (primarily due to left atrial and ventricular enlargement) may also contribute to airway compression and respiratory symptoms that can be confused with asthma.[19-21]

Wheezing due to this physiology is usually a finding restricted to severe, untreated pulmonary overcirculation because of very large left-to-right shunts. As a result, it would be unusual to find cardiac wheezing as an isolated finding in these patients, who typically exhibit a multitude of symptoms and physical findings; in fact, wheezing without any other typical cardiac findings should prompt evaluation for other etiologies. Infants may demonstrate tachypnea, tachycardia, diaphoresis, poor feeding, failure to thrive, murmurs, a gallop rhythm, and hepatomegaly on examination. The rare older child who has not been repaired in infancy may have similar physical examination findings and also exercise intolerance. Notably, children typically do not exhibit pulmonary crackles, nor do they have peripheral edema like adults with heart failure. These children are also more likely to have difficulties with respiratory illnesses of childhood, including developing wheezing more readily and suffering a more severe or protracted course.

Palliative treatment involves anticongestive measures, including diuretics and in some cases digoxin or angiotensin-converting enzyme inhibitors. Definitive therapy generally involves closure of the defect either surgically or by a transcatheter approach, depending on the lesion.

Left Ventricular Dysfunction

Other types of congenital or acquired heart disease can result in left ventricular dysfunction (failure) in children. Anomalous left coronary artery from the pulmonary artery (ALCAPA) results in left ventricular myocardial ischemia similar to adult myocardial infarction. The electrocardiogram (ECG) in ALCAPA classically shows a myocardial ischemia or infarction pattern in left-sided leads (I and aVL). Other coronary artery anomalies with the potential to cause myocardial ischemia and left ventricular failure include congenital coronary stenosis and acquired coronary thrombosis or stenosis associated with Kawasaki disease.

Pediatric left ventricular failure may also be caused by dilated cardiomyopathy or myocarditis. Children with myocarditis often present with symptoms suggesting other illnesses, including asthma.[22,23] In one pediatric emergency department study, 32% of patients with myocarditis presented with primarily respiratory symptoms, and 57% were originally diagnosed with either asthma or pneumonia before being ultimately found to have myocarditis. Chest radiography was found to be fairly nonspecific in these patients; ECG had a much higher diagnostic sensitivity for myocarditis.[24] Echocardiography (including focused ultrasonography in the emergency department with pediatric cardiology oversight) may detect myocarditis, cardiomyopathy, or pericardial effusion and should be considered in patients with wheezing that does not respond to usual treatment measures.[25]

Physiologically, left ventricular failure results in left atrial congestion and hypertension with concomitant pulmonary venous hypertension and vascular congestion. The resulting pulmonary vascular engorgement and cardiomegaly may manifest as cardiac wheezing, like in adult patients with heart failure. Patients with left ventricular failure exhibit signs and symptoms similar to patients with large intracardiac shunts in childhood. Murmurs specific to the type of problem include a mitral regurgitation murmur in ALCAPA, other ischemic heart disease, and possibly myocarditis. Cardiac rhythm disturbances can also occur in these patients. Chest radiography will demonstrate cardiomegaly with pulmonary edema in severe cases. ECG findings vary according to the underlying diagnosis but are often helpful in making a diagnosis. Echocardiography is usually confirmatory of the diagnosis.

Treatment of these patients is similar to that of children with left-to-right shunts, including anticongestive measures (including β-blockers) and aspirin. Interventional therapy depends on the diagnosis and clinical status of the patient.

PULMONARY VENOUS HYPERTENSION

Another cardiac physiologic abnormality that can result in so-called cardiac wheezing is left atrial hypertension or pulmonary venous obstruction. The classic scenario of pulmonary venous obstruction is in the postoperative total anomalous pulmonary venous return repair patient, but it can also arise de novo through fibromuscular intimal hypertrophy or sclerosis of the pulmonary veins, following other intracardiac surgery, or after radiofrequency ablation of tachycardia.[26]

Left atrial hypertension can mimic pulmonary venous hypertension. Causes include congenital or acquired (i.e., rheumatic or postoperative) mitral stenosis or (less commonly) mitral regurgitation. From a functional standpoint, mitral regurgitation secondary to cardiomyopathy or other causes of left ventricular pump dysfunction results in markedly increased left ventricular diastolic pressures and therefore left atrial pressure results in similar physiology. With this physiology, wheezing mimicking asthma is not typically seen, except in severe cases, in children.

POSTOPERATIVE SINGLE VENTRICLE PATIENTS

Patients with single ventricle anatomy and physiology of varying types most often proceed down a similar interventional palliative pathway resulting in so-called Fontan physiology. Anatomically, this involves connection of the superior and inferior venae cavae directly to the branch pulmonary arteries; physiologically, systemic venous blood flows directly into the pulmonary vessels without the benefit of the right ventricle as a pump. The driving pressure for pulmonary blood flow is therefore the central venous pressure, which typically is at least mildly elevated and determined largely by the pulmonary vascular resistance. Increased pulmonary pressures may be exacerbated by concomitant single-ventricle systolic or diastolic dysfunction. One of the mid- to late-term complications seen in a subgroup of Fontan patients is plastic bronchitis.[27] Patients with plastic bronchitis suffer from exudation of proteinaceous material into the airways, resulting in respiratory symptoms and in some cases obstruction due to castlike formations in the airways. Wheezing may be seen in patients with plastic bronchitis; therefore, in post-Fontan patients with new onset of wheezing, this diagnosis should be considered in the differential diagnosis.

Table 16.2 summarizes several features that may assist in distinguishing potential cardiac causes for respiratory symptoms from asthma.

Table 16.2. Clinical Features Suggesting Possible Cardiac Disease in a Wheezing Child

- History of poor feeding, failure to thrive, excessive diaphoresis, or exercise intolerance (CHD with pulmonary overcirculation, CHF)
- History of syncope with exertion
- Presence of other congenital anomalies or syndromes associated with CHD
- Cyanosis minimally or not responsive to oxygen administration (cyanotic CHD)
- Stridor and/or dysphagia in addition to wheezing (vascular rings)
- Cardiac murmurs (CHD, CHF)
- Hepatomegaly (CHF)
- Pulsus paradoxus (pericardial effusion with tamponade)
- Cardiomegaly and/or increased pulmonary vascular markings on CXR (CHD, CHF)
- Right aortic arch on CXR (vascular rings)
- Abnormal ECG

CHD, congenital heart disease; CHF, congestive heart failure; CXR, chest x-ray; ECG, electrocardiogram.

PEDIATRIC CARDIAC SYMPTOMS OR CONDITIONS COEXISTING WITH ASTHMA

Chest Pain

One of the most common reasons for referral of children for pediatric cardiac evaluation is chest pain. This is the case despite multiple studies demonstrating a very low incidence (<1% to 5%) of cardiac causes for pediatric chest pain.[28,29] Most cases of cardiac chest pain can be diagnosed with a thorough history (including family history) and physical examination, with selected testing (i.e., chest x-ray, ECG, and, rarely, echocardiography). Referral to a pediatric cardiologist should be considered for patients with hypertension, dizziness, pain only with exertion, or exertional syncope. Important cardiac causes to exclude include coronary anomalies, myocarditis, pericarditis, cardiomyopathy (especially hypertrophic cardiomyopathy with left ventricular outflow obstruction), and arrhythmias. A much more common reason for chest pain in childhood, including pain associated with physical exertion, is asthma.[30] Generally, a detailed history and physical examination assist in making this diagnosis as well, particularly the finding of associated shortness of breath or cough with exercise. In unclear cases, an exercise treadmill with pulmonary function testing (including at least peak flow measurements before and after exercise) can help to rule out cardiac ischemia as a cause and may help to confirm reversible exercise-induced bronchospasm.[30]

Cardiac Tamponade

Cardiac tamponade results from an accumulation of pericardial fluid resulting in increased intrapericardial pressure leading to decreased ventricular diastolic filling, which, if severe enough, causes low cardiac output. Status asthmaticus can also result in tamponade physiology and thus can mimic symptomatic, hemodynamically significant pericardial effusion.

Pulsus paradoxus (or paradoxical pulse), an exaggerated decline in systolic arterial pressure with inspiration of greater than 12 mmHg or 9%, was actually initially described in severe asthma and is considered an index of acute disease severity.[31,32] It is also a diagnostically important finding in pericarditis and large pericardial effusions with tamponade physiology. The paradox is that the pulse may be weak or nonpalpable during inspiration, although the heart sounds are still present on auscultation. Physiologically, asthma results in decreased left ventricular filling by right ventricular dilation competing with the left ventricle for limited pericardial space in diastole, as well as impedance to right ventricular ejection.[33]

In addition to asthma, the differential diagnosis of pulsus paradoxus includes cardiac conditions such as tricuspid atresia, constrictive pericarditis, restrictive cardiomyopathy, and acute right ventricular failure. Pulmonary differential diagnoses include obstructive pulmonary disease, pulmonary embolism, respiratory distress, and large pleural effusions. Tension pneumothorax or pneumopericardium, which may be associated with asthma (or its treatment), can also cause tamponade physiology.

CARDIAC DYSFUNCTION ASSOCIATED WITH ASTHMA

Asthma is increasingly recognized to have effects on numerous other organ systems. Children with chronic asthma often have somewhat limited physical endurance and engage in less physical activity, at least in part because of poor lung capacity and reduced aerobic exercise capacity. Despite this, exercise capacity in patients with asthma may improve with regular exercise.[34,35] There are emerging data on cardiac functional changes in children with asthma.[36-38] Data from a study using treadmill stress testing and conventional echocardiography suggest measurable cardiac changes in children with chronic moderate to severe asthma, including lower aerobic capacity, decreased systolic function, and lower left ventricular mass than healthy children. Diastolic cardiac function as measured by echocardiography was not affected in this study.[34] Another study using tissue

Doppler imaging (TDI), an echocardiographic technique to assess both systolic and diastolic function of either ventricle, demonstrated significant left and right ventricular dysfunction in children with moderate chronic asthma compared with healthy children.[38] When broken down into specific asthma phenotypes (shortness of breath versus wheezing), children in the shortness of breath group had significant biventricular diastolic dysfunction compared with the wheezing asthmatic group. The shortness of breath group also demonstrated worse global myocardial performance as measured by the TDI-derived myocardial performance index (MPI), a reproducible Doppler-derived measure of global myocardial performance, compared with the wheezing group. TDI and MPI may be more sensitive indicators than conventional echocardiography. As in the prior study, these findings are subclinical but highlight the need for further investigation, particularly in specific asthma phenotypes.[38]

The right ventricular findings noted in studies to date have been thought to possibly be secondary to pulmonary hypertension associated with multiple asthma exacerbations. The cardiac findings, particularly in patients with the shortness of breath phenotype, may be linked to various mediators of airway inflammation (i.e., interleukins and tumor necrosis factor-α) that have potent negative effects on cardiac contractility and which have differential expression in different asthma phenotypes.[38,39] Another study using TDI found similar results.[40] These findings typically are subclinical and do not require medical therapy, but they suggest that increased vigilance for cardiac functional anomalies in chronic asthma patients is reasonable. More studies are needed to evaluate cardiac functional changes, the specific etiologies for these changes, the effect of asthma severity, and the differences accounted for by the various asthma phenotypes.

Obesity

Another comorbidity of asthma with potential cardiac implications is obesity (see Chapter 24). Prevalence rates of overweight have increased markedly over the past several decades, resulting in a major public health issue. Several studies have shown an association of higher rates of asthma in overweight children (particularly girls), although controversy remains regarding the veracity of this association.[41-43] Possible mechanisms for this association have been proposed, including reduced lung volumes, low-grade inflammation, hormonal changes due to obesity (including diabetes), dyslipidemia, gastroesophageal reflux, and systemic hypertension.[44] However, exercise limitations due to asthma may also contribute to inactivity and weight gain. Whether causal or not, long-term obesity, hypertension, diabetes, and dyslipidemia are known to increase cardiac morbidity and mortality. Lifestyle modifications, including proper diet, regular aerobic exercise (which emphasizes the importance of optimal control of asthma to allow reasonable levels of physical activity), and avoidance of tobacco products, are important in all children, but especially in asthma sufferers. More research is needed to evaluate the association of asthma and obesity and to evaluate treatment options.

CARDIAC EFFECTS OF PHARMACOLOGIC TREATMENT OF ASTHMA

Several medications used in the treatment of asthma have real or potential cardiac effects or toxicity. β-Agonists are a mainstay of asthma therapy, but they can also trigger pathologic tachycardia in patients with an underlying substrate for supraventricular tachycardia; conversely, β-blockers used to manage tachycardia can exacerbate bronchospasm and therefore may be contraindicated in some asthma patients. Medications used to treat status asthmaticus can have negative cardiac effects, particularly intravenous infusions of β-agonists. Intravenous isoproterenol has been shown to cause myocardial ischemia, which is typically transient and reversible with cessation of the infusion.[45] Albuterol and terbutaline have relative $β_2$ selectivity and, in theory, potentially less cardiac effects. However, terbutaline still has significant cardiac side effects, including tachycardia, prolongation of the QT interval, and hypokalemia. Some studies demonstrate subclinical myocardial ischemia even with these drugs, including elevated cardiac troponin I in up to 50% of patients treated with intravenous terbutaline for status asthmaticus.[46-48] There does not appear to be an association between asthma severity and likelihood of ischemia with β-agonist infusion. Clearly, intravenous β-agonists have the potential for significant toxicity and should be used with appropriate caution and patient monitoring. Research and development of new, less cardiotoxic agents to treat asthma are needed.

UNMET, FUTURE RESEARCH NEEDS

1. Further evaluation of the etiology of asthma-induced cardiac systolic and diastolic dysfunction, including the effect of asthma severity and phenotypic differences

2. Further evaluation of the potential association of asthma and obesity, including optimal treatment options

3. Research and development of new, less cardiotoxic agents to treat asthma, especially in severe disease

CONCLUSION

When it comes to the complex relationship between asthma and pediatric cardiac disease, whether congenital or acquired, the old adage that "all that wheezes is not asthma" is certainly true. Many cardiac conditions presenting in childhood belong on the differential diagnosis list of bronchial asthma, and vice versa. Asthma, through either direct disease action or undesired side effects of therapy, is associated with subclinical cardiac dysfunction and ischemia. Obesity, a tremendous public health issue, shares a common association with both cardiac disease and asthma. Considering these facts, close collaboration between pediatric subspecialists and physicians and other health care practitioners is absolutely necessary to effectively manage children with the multiple comorbidities associated with asthma. Finally, more research is needed to optimize asthma therapies while reducing complications, with the goal of the best possible outcomes for all children struggling with these medical issues.

REFERENCES

1. Massin M, Astadicko I, Dessy H. Noncardiac comorbidities of congenital heart disease in children. *Acta Paediatr.* 2007;96:753–755.
2. Austin J, Ali T. Tracheomalacia and bronchomalacia in children: pathophysiology, assessment, treatment and anaesthesia management. *Paediatr Anaesth.* 2003;13(1):3–11.
3. Bandla HP, Hopkins RL, Beckerman RC, Gozal D. Pulmonary risk factors compromising postoperative recovery after surgical repair for congenital heart disease. *Chest.* 1999;116(3):740–747.
4. Rabinovitch M, Grady S, David I, et al. Compression of intrapulmonary bronchi by abnormally branching pulmonary arteries associated with absent pulmonary valves. *Am J Cardiol.* 1982;50(4):804–813.
5. Alsoufi B, Williams WG, Hua Z, et al. Surgical outcomes in the treatment of patients with tetralogy of Fallot and absent pulmonary valve. *Eur J Cardiothorac Surg.* 2007;31(3):354–359.
6. Moon-Grady AJ, Tacy TA, Brook MM, Hanley FL, Silverman NH. Value of clinical and echocardiographic features in predicting outcome in the fetus, infant, and child with tetralogy of Fallot with absent pulmonary valve complex. *Am J Cardiol.* 2002;89(11):1280–1285.
7. Galindo A, Gutierrez-Larraya F, Martinez JM, et al. Prenatal diagnosis and outcome for fetuses with congenital absence of the pulmonary valve. *Ultrasound Obstet Gynecol.* 2006;28(1):32–39.
8. d'Udekem Y, Alphonso N, Norgaard MA, et al. Pulmonary atresia with ventricular septal defects and major aortopulmonary collateral arteries: unifocalization brings no long-term benefits. *J Thorac Cardiovasc Surg.* 2005;130(6):1496–1502.
9. Faletra F, Giardina A, Petroni R, et al. Evaluation of pulmonary atresia with 64-slice multidetector computed tomography (MDCT). *Echocardiography.* 2007;24(9):998–999.
10. Reddy VM, McElhinney DB, Amin Z, et al. Early and intermediate outcomes after repair of pulmonary atresia with ventricular septal defect and major aortopulmonary collateral arteries: experience with 85 patients. *Circulation.* 2000;101(15):1826–1832.

11. Schulze-Neick I, Ho SY, Bush A, et al. Severe airflow limitation after the unifocalization procedure: clinical and morphological correlates. *Circulation.* 2000;102(19 Suppl 3):III142–III147.
12. Tehrai M, Saidi B, Goudarzi M. Multi-detector computed tomography demonstration of double-lumen aortic arch—persistent fifth arch—as an isolated anomaly in an adult. *Cardiol Young.* 2012;22(3):353–355.
13. Humphrey C, Duncan K, Fletcher S. Decade of experience with vascular rings at a single institution. *Pediatrics.* 2006;117(5):e903–e908.
14. Dillman JR, Attili AK, Agarwal PP, Dorfman AL, Hernandez RJ, Strouse PJ. Common and uncommon vascular rings and slings: a multi-modality review. *Pediatr Radiol.* 2011;41(11):1440–1454.
15. Castaneda AR, Jonas RA, Mayer JE. Vascular rings, slings, and tracheal anomalies. In: *Cardiac Surgery of the Neonate and Infant.* Philadelphia: WB Saunders; 1994:397–408.
16. Morrow R, Huhta J. Aortic arch and pulmonary artery anomalies. In: Garson A, Bricker TJ, Fisher DJ, Neish SR, eds. *The Science and Practice of Pediatric Cardiology.* Baltimore: William and Wilkins; 1998:1347–1381.
17. Newman B, Cho YA. Left pulmonary artery sling-anatomy and imaging. *Semin Ultrasound CT MR.* 2010;31(2):158–170.
18. Gaspar L, Mariano A, Caetano S, Mendes P, Neves JP, Anjos R. "Asthma" cured after cardiac surgery. *Arch Dis Child.* 2012;97(5):433–435.
19. Buchhorn R, Hammersen A, Bartmus D, Bursch J. The pathogenesis of heart failure in infants with congenital heart disease. *Cardiol Young.* 2001;11(5):498–504.
20. Talner NS. The physiology of congenital heart disease. In: Garson A, Bricker TJ, Fisher DJ, Neish SR, eds. *The Science and Practice of Pediatric Cardiology.* Baltimore: William and Wilkins; 1998:1107–1118.
21. Yau KI, Fang LJ, Wu MH. Lung mechanics in infants with left-to-right shunt congenital heart disease. *Pediatr Pulmonol.* 1996;21(1):42–47.
22. Levi D, Alejos J. Diagnosis and treatment of pediatric viral myocarditis. *Curr Opin Cardiol.* 2001;16(2):77–83.
23. Bohn D, Benson L. Diagnosis and management of pediatric myocarditis. *Paediatr Drugs.* 2002;4(3):171–181.
24. Freedman SB, Haladyn JK, Floh A, Kirsh JA, Taylor G, Thull-Freedman J. Pediatric myocarditis: emergency department clinical findings and diagnostic evaluation. *Pediatrics.* 2007;120(6):1278–1285.
25. Pershad J, Chin T. Early detection of cardiac disease masquerading as acute bronchospasm: the role of bedside limited echocardiography by the emergency physician. *Pediatr Emerg Care.* 2003;19(2):E1–E3.
26. Lee ML, Wang JK, Lue HC. Visualization of pulmonary vein obstruction by pulmonary artery wedge injection and documentation by pressure tracings: report of one case with persistent wheezing following correction of total anomalous pulmonary venous connection. *Int J Cardiol.* 1995;49(2):167–172.
27. Costello JM, Steinhorn D, McColley S, Gerber ME, Kumar SP. Treatment of plastic bronchitis in a Fontan patient with tissue plasminogen activator: a case report and review of the literature. *Pediatrics.* 2002;109(4):e67.
28. Hambrook JT, Kimball TR, Khoury P, Cnota J. Disparities exist in the emergency department evaluation of pediatric chest pain. *Congenit Heart Dis.* 2010;5(3):285–291.
29. Drossner DM, Hirsh DA, Sturm JJ, et al. Cardiac disease in pediatric patients presenting to a pediatric ED with chest pain. *Am J Emerg Med.* 2011;29(6):632–638.
30. Singh AM, McGregor RS. Differential diagnosis of chest symptoms in the athlete. *Clin Rev Allergy and Immunol.* 2005;29(2):87–96.
31. Rebuck AS, Pengelly LD. Development of pulsus paradoxus in the presence of airways obstruction. *N Engl J Med.* 1973;288(2):66–69.
32. Knowles GK, Clark TJ. Pulsus paradoxus as a valuable sign indicating severity of asthma. *Lancet.* 1973;2:1356–1359.
33. Jardin F, Farcot JC, Boisante L, Prost JF, Gueret P, Bourdarias JP. Mechanism of paradoxic pulse in bronchial asthma. *Circulation.* 1982;66(4):887–894.
34. Alioglu B, Ertugrul T, Unal M. Cardiopulmonary response of asthmatic children to exercise: analysis of systolic and diastolic cardiac function. *Pediatr Pulmonol.* 2007;42(3):283–289.
35. Hallstrand TS, Bates PW, Schoene RB. Aerobic conditioning in mild asthma decreases the hyperpnea of exercise and improves exercise and ventilatory capacity. *Chest.* 2000;118(5):1460–1469.
36. Zeybek C, Yalcin Y, Erdem A, et al. Tissue Doppler echocardiographic assessment of cardiac function in children with bronchial asthma. *Pediatr Int.* 2007;49(6):911–917.
37. Shedeed SA. Right ventricular function in children with bronchial asthma: a tissue Doppler image echocardiography study. *Pediatr Cardiol.* 2010;31(7):1008–1015.

38. Zedan M, Alsawah GA, El-Assmy MM, Hasaneen B, Zedan MM, Nasef NA. Clinical asthma phenotypes: is there an impact on myocardial performance? *Echocardiography*. 2012;29(5):528–534.
39. Uyan AP, Uyan C, Ozyurek H. Assessment of right ventricular diastolic filling parameters by Doppler echocardiography. *Pediatr Int*. 2003;45(3):263–267.
40. Ozdemir O, Ceylan Y, Razi CH, Ceylan O, Andiran N. Assessment of ventricular functions by tissue Doppler echocardiography in children with asthma. *Pediatr Cardiol*. 2013;34(3):553–559.
41. Schaub B, von Mutius E. Obesity and asthma, what are the links? *Curr Opin Allergy Clin Immunol*. 2005;5(2):185–193.
42. De Groot EP, Duiverman EJ, Brand PL. Comorbidities of asthma during childhood: possibly important, yet poorly studied. *Eur Respir J*. 2010;36(3):671–678.
43. Story RE. Asthma and obesity in children. *Curr Opin Pediatr*. 2007;19(6):680–684.
44. Shore SA. Obesity and asthma: possible mechanisms. *J Allergy Clin Immunol*. 2008;121(5):1087–1093.
45. Maguire JF, O'Rourke PP, Colan SD, Geha RS, Crone R. Cardiotoxicity during treatment of severe childhood asthma. *Pediatrics*. 1991;88(6):1180–1186.
46. Kalyanaraman M, Bhalala U, Leoncio M. Serial cardiac troponin concentrations as marker of cardiac toxicity in children with status asthmaticus treated with intravenous terbutaline. *Pediatr Emerg Care*. 2011;27(10):933–936.
47. Fisher AA, Davis MW, McGill DA. Acute myocardial infarction associated with albuterol. *Ann Pharmacother*. 2004;38(12):2045–2049.
48. Chiang VW, Burns JP, Rifai N, Lipshultz SE, Adams MJ, Weiner DL. Cardiac toxicity of intravenous terbutaline for the treatment of severe asthma in children: a prospective assessment. *J Pediatr*. 2000;137(1):73–77.

17

PULMONARY HYPERTENSION

COEXISTING AND DIFFERENTIAL DIAGNOSIS

Aaron B. Waxman and Kerri Akaya Smith

KEY POINTS

- Pulmonary hypertension (PH), defined as an elevation in pulmonary arterial pressures, is often misdiagnosed as asthma.
- A delay in the diagnosis of PH results in the lack of initiation of appropriate treatment and a poorer prognosis.
- A high index of suspicion is necessary to make the diagnosis of PH for the symptoms are often non-specific and variable. Most patients present with dyspnea, fatigue, or both whereas edema, chest pain, presyncope and actual syncope are less common and are associated with more severe disease.
- The current classification system of the Fourth World Symposium on Pulmonary Hypertension recognizes five categories of PH, including pulmonary arterial hypertension, PH due to left heart disease, PH due to chronic lung disease, PH associated with chronic thromboemboli, and finally a group of miscellaneous diseases that only rarely cause PH.
- Interstitial lung disease is the second most common cause of PH.
- Improved medications to treat PAH include prostacyclin analogs, phosphodiesterase-5 inhibitors and endothelin receptor agonists that have dramatically improved the outlook of this disease.

INTRODUCTION

Pulmonary hypertension (PH) is a spectrum of diseases involving the pulmonary vascular circuit and is defined as an elevation in pulmonary arterial pressures. Pulmonary arterial hypertension (PAH) is a relatively rare form of PH and is characterized by symptoms of dyspnea, chest pain, and syncope. If left untreated, the disease carries a high mortality rate, with the most common cause of death being decompensated right heart failure. There have been significant advances in this field in regard to understanding the pathogenesis, diagnosis, and classification of PAH. Despite these significant advances, there is still a substantial delay in diagnosis of up to 2 years. Many patients whose primary complaint is dyspnea on exertion are misdiagnosed with more common diseases such as asthma. The availability of newer drugs has resulted in a radical change in the management of PAH, with significant improvement in both quality of life and mortality. A delay in diagnosis results in an obvious delay in the initiation of appropriate treatment. Increasing data from clinical trials suggest that delay in treatment negatively affects long-term outcomes. Timely diagnosis remains an important challenge. Clinicians should be able to recognize the signs and symptoms of PH and to complete a systematic workup in patients suspected of having it. In this way, early diagnosis, prompt treatment, and improved outcomes for patients become possible. This process is best illustrated by reviewing a case that presented to our pulmonary vascular clinic. We will also discuss the usual approach to evaluating a patient with dyspnea and suspected PH.

CLINICAL FEATURES OF PULMONARY HYPERTENSION

The patient is a 33-year-old woman, Gravida 2, Para 1, Sab 1, with a 5-year-old son who was the product of an uncomplicated pregnancy. She began complaining of shortness of breath about three years before her presentation to the clinic. During the preceding 6 months, she was increasingly limited, having difficulty going up a flight of stairs, carrying things on a flat surface, and keeping up with her son. She was diagnosed with asthma and treated over a 2-year period with multiple inhalers, including a combination long-acting β-agonist and inhaled corticosteroid. She reported that she never had any benefit using the inhalers. Likewise, she had been treated with multiple glucocorticosteroid tapers that also never provided any benefit. Her past medical history was notable only for Raynaud's disease. She had no family history of medical problems, and no history of tobacco, alcohol, or illicit drug use. She was referred to the pulmonary vascular clinic after an incidental finding of enlarged pulmonary arteries on a chest radiograph (Figure 17.1). The chest radiograph was done because she had complained of dyspnea as part of a preoperative evaluation for gynecologic surgery.

On presentation, her physical examination was notable for a heart rate of 113 beats/minute, a respiratory rate of 18 breaths/minute, a systemic blood pressure of 112/78 mm Hg, and a resting oxygen saturation of 93% on room air. The physical examination was notable for jugular venous distension to 7 cm, clear lungs, and a regular cardiac rhythm with a variably splitting second heart sound (S_2) and a prominent pulmonic sound (P_2). There were no murmurs or gallops. She had mild pedal edema. At no time previously had she had pulmonary function testing performed.

As part of the evaluation performed in the pulmonary vascular clinic, as part of

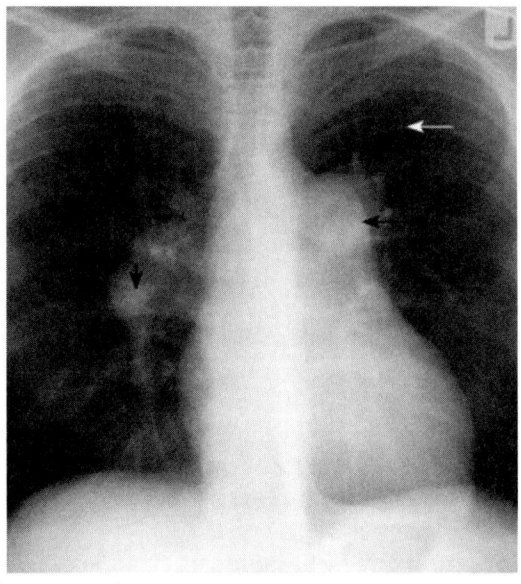

FIGURE 17.1 Posteroanterior chest radiograph showing enlarged pulmonary arteries (*black arrows*) and pruning of the distal pulmonary vasculature (*white arrow*) commonly seen with advanced pulmonary arterial hypertension.

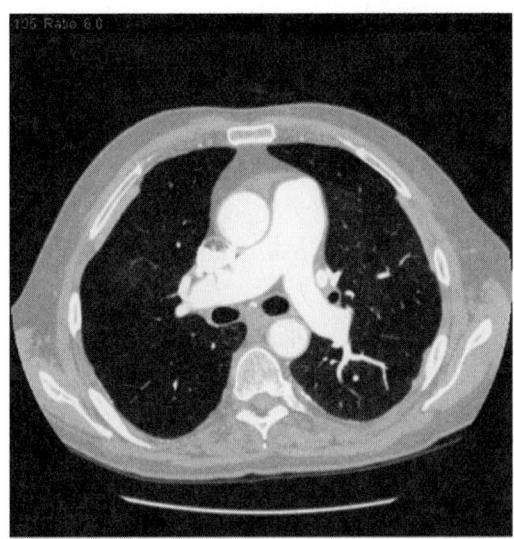

FIGURE 17.2 Representative computed tomography scan of the chest demonstrating enlarged main pulmonary arteries. There is a mosaic pattern evident both lungs.

the evaluation for a patient with dyspnea, she did have pulmonary function testing that was consistent with mild restriction and a decreased diffusing capacity for carbon monoxide (D_{LCO}/alveolar ventilation 53% of predicted). There was no reversibility after the administration of inhaled albuterol. Chest computed tomography (CT) showed no evidence of parenchymal lung disease. The main pulmonary arteries were enlarged, and there was a mosaic pattern evident on the lung windows (Figure 17.2).

The ventilation-perfusion (V/Q) study showed no evidence of pulmonary embolism. It was not read as normal because of a moth-eaten appearance that is typical in patients with PH. The electrocardiogram showed sinus tachycardia with a rate of 112 beats/minute and right atrial enlargement, right-axis deviation, and an incomplete right bundle branch block. The screening echocardiogram demonstrated marked right atrial enlargement, right ventricular dilatation and dysfunction, and an estimated right ventricular systolic pressure of 75 mm Hg. The left atrium was compressed by the enlarged right atrium (Figure 17.3), and left ventricular function was normal. The patient was referred for right heart catheterization that was significant for pulmonary arterial hypertension (Table 17.1). Based on the mean pulmonary artery pressure, the patient was diagnosed with severe PAH. Based on her subjective description of her functional limitation, she was designated as World Health Organization (WHO) functional class 3. On the baseline 6-minute walk test (6MWT), she walked 318 meters and had a Borg dyspnea index of 5 on a scale of 1 to 10, which is consistent with a significant exercise limitation. Importantly, she also desaturated to 89% on room air.

A number of features of this patient's presentation were not consistent with obstructive lung disease including asthma. A comprehensive history obtained from the

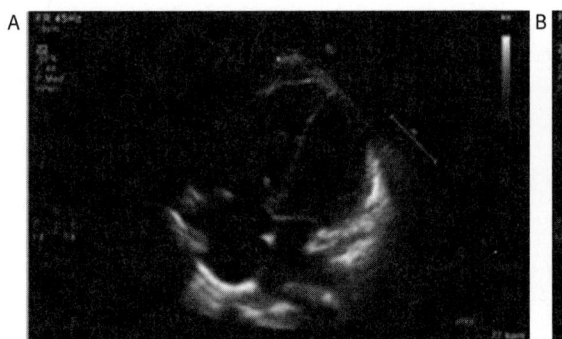
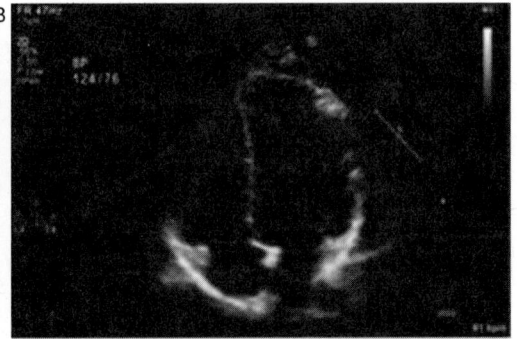

FIGURE 17.3 **A,** A representative echocardiogram showing the apical four-chamber view in a patient with pulmonary hypertension demonstrating an enlarged right atrium and ventricle with some compression of the left side of the heart. **B,** The same echocardiographic view showing a normal echocardiogram.

Table 17.1. Right Heart Catherterization Data for Pulmonary Arterial Hypertension

RIGHT HEART CATHETERIZATION	PATIENT DATA	NORMAL
Right atrial pressure	25 mm Hg	≤12 mm Hg
Right ventricular pressure	89/12	25/0–8
Right ventricular end diastolic pressure	22 mm Hg	≤12 mm Hg
Pulmonary artery pressure	89/36	
Mean pulmonary artery pressure	54 mm Hg	<25 mm Hg
Pulmonary capillary wedge pressure	14 mm Hg	<15 mm Hg
Cardiac output	4.6 L/min	4–5 L/min
Pulmonary vascular resistance	710 dynes · sec/cm^5	<240 dynes · sec/cm^5
Systemic vascular resistance	871 dynes · sec/cm^5	

patient with unexplained dyspnea is often instructive and can be helpful in narrowing a differential diagnosis. The patient had a history that was notable for progressive dyspnea rather than episodes of worsening or acute exacerbations. Likewise, there were no apparent triggers for her shortness of breath. The earliest symptoms in patients with PH are often apparent only with exercise or significant exertion. PH typically has a slow progressive course. As the disease advances, patients may develop right ventricular failure, with lower extremity edema and limiting dyspnea, as well as angina. As the cardiac output decreases, patients may have episodes of near syncope or syncope.

Our patient's physical findings of a resting sinus tachycardia in combination with a relatively low blood pressure and chronic dyspnea would suggest a systemic disorder affecting her cardiac output. Most important, the low normal oxygen saturation in an otherwise healthy person should be a sign that something is wrong. Asthmatic patients typically have normal oxygen saturations unless they are in the throes of a serious exacerbation. It is also concerning that she was "diagnosed" with and treated for asthma while never having had pulmonary function testing. The case presentation is regrettably fairly common among patients with PH, such that the average time to diagnosis for patients with PH is about a year and a half.[1]

HOW TO ACCURATELY DIAGNOSE PULMONARY HYPERTENSION

The diagnosis of PH can be missed without a reasonable index of suspicion. Dyspnea is the most common presenting symptom, but this complaint is far from specific for the diagnosis of PH. PH symptoms are insidious and overlap considerably with many common conditions, including asthma and other lung disease and cardiac disease. The symptoms of PH are often nonspecific and variable. Most patients will present with dyspnea, fatigue, or both, whereas edema, chest pain, presyncope, and actual syncope are less common and associated with more advanced disease. On examination, there may be evidence of right ventricular failure with elevated jugular venous pressure, lower extremity edema, and ascites. Additionally, the cardiovascular examination may reveal an accentuated P_2 component of the second heart sound, a right-sided S_3 or S_4, and a holosystolic tricuspid regurgitant murmur. It is also important to look for markers of the diseases that are often concurrent with PH; clubbing may be seen in some chronic lung diseases, sclerodactyly and telangiectasia may signify scleroderma, and crackles and systemic hypertension may be clues to left-sided systolic or diastolic heart failure.

After clinical suspicion is raised, a systematic approach to diagnosis and assessment is essential. An echocardiogram with bubble study is the most important initial screening test. Echocardiography not only is important for the diagnosis of PH but also is often essential in determining the cause. All forms of PH may demonstrate a hypertrophied and dilated right ventricle with elevated estimated pulmonary artery systolic pressure. Important additional information can be gleaned about specific etiologies of PH, such as valvular disease, left ventricular systolic and diastolic function, intracardiac shunts, and other cardiac diseases.

Although the accuracy of Doppler echocardiography is often debated, Becker and colleagues reported that systematic overestimation of pulmonary artery systolic pressure may occur in low-risk populations.[2] More recently, Fischer and colleagues evaluated 65 patients who underwent Doppler echocardiography within 1 hour of right heart catheterization and found that in 48% of cases, the echocardiogram differed from the invasive measurement by more than 10%, overestimating the pressures as often as underestimating them.[3] These findings suggest that, although a high-quality echocardiogram that is absolutely normal may obviate the need for further evaluation for PH, an echocardiogram is a screening test, whereas invasive hemodynamic monitoring is the gold standard for diagnosis and assessment of disease severity.

This need for invasive hemodynamic measurements to accurately diagnose PH poses an additional problem when evaluating older patients. Physicians are understandably more reluctant to refer older patients for invasive procedures. However, the diagnosis of PH is increasing in the older population, at least in part because of an increased awareness of this disease in elderly people and increased use of screening echocardiograms. Further, the increased availability of oral and less toxic therapeutic options has encouraged the referral of older patients for evaluation and treatment.

With a normal echocardiogram, there may still be some concern for PH. This is particularly true if there is unexplained dyspnea or hypoxemia. In this setting, it is reasonable to proceed to right heart catheterization for definitive diagnosis. Alternatively, if the patient has a reasonable functional capacity, a cardiopulmonary exercise test may help to identify a true physiologic limitation as well as differentiate between cardiac and pulmonary causes of dyspnea.[4,5] If this is normal, there is no indication for a right heart catheterization. If a cardiovascular limitation to exercise is found, a right heart catheterization should be pursued.

If the echocardiogram or cardiopulmonary exercise test suggests PH and this is confirmed by catheterization, a reasonable effort must be made to establish the etiology, because this will largely determine the therapeutic approach. A stepwise approach to evaluation is outlined later.

Chest imaging and lung function tests are essential because lung disease is an important cause of PH. Signs of PH that may be evident on chest x-ray include enlargement of the central pulmonary arteries associated with "vascular pruning," a relative paucity of peripheral vessels. Cardiomegaly, with specific evidence of right atrial and ventricular enlargement, can often be observed. The chest x-ray may also demonstrate significant interstitial lung disease or suggest hyperinflation from obstructive lung disease, which may be the underlying cause of or contributor to the development of PH. High-resolution computed tomography (HRCT) may provide additional useful information. Classic findings of PH on HRCT include those found on chest x-ray: enlarged pulmonary arteries, peripheral pruning of the small vessels, and enlarged right ventricle and atrium. However, HRCT may also reveal signs of venous congestion, including centrilobular ground-glass infiltrate and thickened septal lines. In the absence of left heart disease, these findings suggest pulmonary-venous disease, a rare cause of PAH that can be quite challenging to diagnose.

CT angiograms are commonly used to evaluate acute thromboembolic disease and have demonstrated excellent sensitivity and specificity for that purpose.[6,7] Even for acute emboli, however, early studies suggested that CT angiograms may be less sensitive for detecting segmental and subsegmental pulmonary emboli, with a 7% false-negative rate compared with pulmonary angiography.[8] V/Q scanning has traditionally been used for screening because of its high sensitivity and its role in qualifying patients for surgical intervention.[9] The role of CT angiograms in the diagnosis of chronic thromboembolic pulmonary hypertension (CTEPH) remains controversial, even with the advent of spiral CT. A study reported the high sensitivity of V/Q scans at 97.4%, whereas the sensitivity of spiral CT may be as low as 51% for CTEPH.[10] Thus, although a negative V/Q virtually rules out CTEPH, many cases may be missed through the use of CT angiograms.

Pulmonary function tests are an important component of the evaluation. Although an isolated reduction in D_{LCO} is the classic finding in PAH, results of pulmonary function tests may also suggest restrictive or obstructive lung diseases as the cause of dyspnea or PH. The 6MWT is also important to evaluate the degree of exertional hypoxemia and limitation and to monitor progression and response to therapy.

Sleep-disordered breathing is another important cause of PH, but a sleep study is generally necessary only when indicated by the patient's history. Nocturnal desaturation is a common finding in PH, even in the absence of sleep-disordered breathing.[11] Thus, all patients should undergo nocturnal oximetry screening, regardless of whether classic symptoms of obstructive sleep apnea or obesity hypoventilation syndrome are observed. The finding of nocturnal desaturation should prompt a full sleep study.

Laboratory tests that are important for screening include an HIV test. In addition, all patients should have their blood tested for antinuclear antibodies, rheumatoid factor, and scl-70 antibodies to screen for the most common rheumatologic causes of PH. Liver function and hepatitis serology tests are important to screen for underlying liver disease. Finally, there is an increasing role for brain natriuretic peptide (BNP) testing in the diagnosis and management of PH. Levels of these peptides, which are released from the atria and ventricles in response to stretch, are assessed to monitor left ventricular dysfunction. BNP and the N-terminus of its pro-peptide also appear to correlate with right ventricular function, hemodynamic severity, and functional status in PAH; this testing may also be useful in non-PAH forms of PH.

PULMONARY HYPERTENSION AS A COMORBID DISEASE

PAH is but one of a number of disease classifications that affect the pulmonary vascular bed. PH was previously classified as primary or secondary, but as understanding of the various contributing diseases has increased, classification systems have attempted to group these diseases by clinical features to aid in diagnosis. The current classification system, last revised in 2008 during the Fourth World Symposium on Pulmonary Hypertension held in Dana Point, California, recognizes five categories of PH, including PAH, PH due to left heart disease, PH due to chronic lung disease, PH associated with chronic thromboemboli, and finally a group of miscellaneous diseases that only rarely cause PH.

Pulmonary Arterial Hypertension

Classified as WHO group I PH, PAH is a relatively rare cause of PH, with an estimated annual incidence of 2 cases per 1 million.[12-14] PAH includes a group of diseases that result in pulmonary arterial precapillary remodeling marked by intimal fibrosis, increased medial thickness, pulmonary arteriolar occlusion, and classic plexiform lesions. PAH is defined as a sustained elevation in resting mean pulmonary arterial pressure (mPAP) of 25 mm Hg or more, pulmonary vascular resistance (PVR) of more than 240 dynes · sec/cm^5, and pulmonary capillary wedge pressure (PCWP) or left ventricle end diastolic pressure of 15 mm Hg or less based on a right heart catheterization.[12] With a normal PCWP and an elevated mPAP, these diseases demonstrate an increased transpulmonary gradient (mPAP − PCWP); in addition, the PVR is elevated.

Idiopathic pulmonary arterial hypertension (IPAH) is a progressive disease that leads to right heart failure and death. It is typically seen in young women. The National Institutes of Health registry, the first large registry of patients with PAH, reported that the average age at diagnosis was 36 years, with only 9% of patients with IPAH older than 60 years. However, the more current clinical studies suggest that the patient demographics are changing. The Pulmonary Hypertension Connection registry found that the average age of diagnosis for IPAH was 45 years, with 8.5% of patients older than 70 years at diagnosis.[15] This finding is supported by data from the Registry to Evaluate Early and Long-term PAH Disease Management (REVEAL), the largest cohort of PAH to date, which reported that the average age of diagnosis with IPAH was 44.9 ± 0.6 years.[14] The reasons for this older age at diagnosis likely reflect the increased use of screening echocardiograms in the general population and increased referral of older patients for evaluation.

Other forms of PAH that deserve specific consideration in patients are those associated with HIV, connective tissue disease, and portal hypertension. Although HIV is a rare cause of PAH, this form of PAH is indistinguishable from IPAH and is an important cause of mortality in the HIV-infected population.[16,17] Importantly, there is no correlation between the stage of HIV infection and the development of PAH.

Among connective tissue diseases, the prevalence of PAH has been established only for systemic sclerosis. Two catheter-based studies found that the prevalence was 7% to 12%; however, echocardiographic studies report a much higher prevalence.[18,19] Although the average age of scleroderma onset is 30 to 50 years old, patients who eventually develop scleroderma-associated PAH tend to be older at the time of scleroderma diagnosis, with an average age of 65 to 66 years.[18,19] Several studies demonstrate that outcomes of scleroderma are closely linked to the development of PAH, as diagnosed by echocardiogram or catheterization.[18,20,21] In addition, of all forms of PAH, scleroderma-related PAH is associated with the poorest prognosis, despite advances in treatment.[22,23] For a given increase in PVR, there is a greater impairment in right ventricular function in patients with scleroderma than in patients with nonscleroderma PAH.[24] Although this poor right ventricular adaptation may be partially explained by the older age of this population, scleroderma appears to cause right ventricular dysfunction even in the absence of PAH.[25] Nonetheless, modern therapies have improved outcomes, with 1-year survival rates estimated at 80% to 85%, which is considerably higher than a previously reported 1-year survival rate of 50%.[21,26,27]

Portopulmonary hypertension occurs in 2% to 10% of patients with established portal hypertension and is most commonly observed in advanced disease.[28,29] Its occurrence appears to be independent of the cause of liver disease and is observed in patients with nonhepatic causes of portal hypertension.[28,29] A hyperdynamic circulatory state is common, as in most patients with advanced liver disease; however, the same pulmonary vascular remodeling observed in other forms of PAH is seen in the pulmonary vascular bed in portopulmonary hypertension. It is important to distinguish this process from hepatopulmonary syndrome, which can also manifest with dyspnea and hypoxemia but is pathophysiologically distinct from portopulmonary hypertension in that abnormal vasodilation of the pulmonary vasculature effectively leads to intrapulmonary shunting. Although the prognosis in hepatopulmonary syndrome is also quite poor, it is not a form of PH.

Pulmonary Hypertension Associated with Left Heart Disease

WHO group II PH includes patients with left heart systolic failure, aortic and mitral valvulopathies, and heart failure with preserved ejection fraction (HFpEF). PH can develop as a result of all of these conditions. The hallmark of group II PH (i.e., PH due to left heart disease) is elevated left atrial pressure with resultant pulmonary-venous hypertension. In general, the transpulmonary gradient and pulmonary vascular resistance remain normal. Although this phenomenon is well described in both left-sided valvular disease and left-sided systolic heart failure, studies suggest that HFpEF may carry a higher overall risk. The prevalence of PH in HFpEF may be as high as 52.5% to 83%.[30-32]

Whatever the cause of elevated left atrial pressure (i.e., systolic or diastolic heart failure or valvular disease), this increased pulmonary venous pressure indirectly leads to a rise in pulmonary arterial pressure. The presence of PH portends a poor prognosis in all forms of heart failure.[31] In particular, chronic pulmonary venous hypertension may lead to a reactive pulmonary arterial vasculopathy, seen as an elevated transpulmonary gradient (>12 mm Hg) and elevated pulmonary vascular resistance (>3 Wood units). Pathologically, this process is marked by pulmonary arteriolar remodeling with intimal fibrosis and medial hyperplasia akin to that seen in PAH.[33]

Pulmonary Hypertension Associated with Lung Disease

Intrinsic lung disease is the second most common cause of PH, although its actual prevalence is hard to ascertain. PH has been observed in both chronic obstructive lung disease and interstitial lung disease and appears to be particularly important in diseases with mixed obstructive-restrictive physiology: bronchiectasis, cystic fibrosis, mixed obstructive-restrictive disease marked by fibrosis in the lower lung zones, and emphysema predominantly in the upper lung zones.[34] As in patients with left heart disease, PH associated with chronic lung disease is usually modest. However, some of these patients appear to have PH "out of proportion" to their parenchymal lung disease, suggesting intrinsic pulmonary arterial disease.[35]

Since the 1970s, studies have demonstrated that even mild PH has prognostic implications in chronic obstructive pulmonary disease (COPD). In a 7-year longitudinal study, Burrows and colleagues[36] found that survival in COPD was inversely proportional to PVR, and in a 15-year follow-up of 200 patients with COPD, PH was one of the strongest predictors of mortality. Most studies suggest a prevalence of PH of 30% to 70% in COPD; however, in most patients, COPD causes relatively modest PH, and severe PH is uncommon in this population.[35,37-39] Many studies, however, identify a subset of patients with COPD (1% to 5%) who have severe PH "out of proportion" to their underlying lung disease.[35,40] These patients typically have severe PH, with results of pulmonary function tests demonstrating a very low D_{LCO} associated with only moderate airflow obstruction. Causes for PH other than COPD, such as pulmonary emboli and sleep-disordered breathing, are frequently observed in this population.[35,41] The 5-year survival rate of these patients (10%) appears to be much lower than that of patients with less severe PH (nearly 60%) and patients without PH (almost 90%).[35,42]

Although PH is described in most forms of interstitial lung disease, it has been most extensively studied in idiopathic pulmonary fibrosis; however, the individual studies have been small. Early echocardiographic data suggested that the prevalence of PH in interstitial lung diseases was as high as 84%,[43-45] but more current studies using invasive hemodynamic monitoring suggest that the incidence is considerably lower.[46-48] PH portends poor outcome in pulmonary fibrosis.[44,48] Indeed, a small prospective trial by Hamada and colleagues detected a resting mPAP greater than 25 mm Hg in only 8.1% of patients but demonstrated that mPAP greater than 17 mm Hg was predictive of mortality despite being below the diagnostic threshold for PH.[48]

Also included in group III PH is sleep-disordered breathing. Sleep apnea has long been associated with PH, with early studies suggesting a prevalence of PH as high as 15% to 20% in this population.[49,50] However, PH associated with sleep-disordered breathing is generally mild. It is not clear whether sleep-disordered breathing is sufficient to cause PH; many studies suggest that coexisting daytime hypoxemia must also be present.[50-52]

Pulmonary Hypertension Associated with Chronic Thromboembolic Disease

The development of PH after chronic obstruction of the pulmonary arteries is well described, but its incidence is not known. Most studies suggest that the incidence of PH after a single pulmonary embolic event is quite low (0.5% to 1.5%).[9,53,54] Others have suggested the incidence may be as high as 3.8% to 8% after the first episode and 13.4% following recurrent embolism.[55,56] The risk factors for developing CTEPH are also unclear, but several studies have suggested that larger perfusion defects at presentation and a history of multiple emboli are risk factors.[55,57] Up to 40% of patients have no history of clinical venous thromboembolism.[58,59] A history of malignancy has also been implicated as a risk factor.[59] It is important to note that although venous thromboembolism or pulmonary embolism occurs more often in older patients, CTEPH is more common in younger patients.[60]

The pathogenesis of CTEPH is poorly understood. Obstruction of the proximal pulmonary vasculature is important and often the dominant factor; however, studies suggest that additional pulmonary vascular remodeling occurs. About 10% to 15% of patients will develop a disease very similar clinically and pathologically to PAH after resection of the proximal thrombus.[61]

PHARMACOLOGIC TREATMENT OF PULMONARY ARTERIAL HYPERTENSION

PH was a consistently fatal condition with no effective medical treatment options before 1996; however, since then there has been an upsurge in the development of novel therapeutic agents for PAH. There are several approved agents for PAH, including prostacyclin and prostacyclin analogs, phosphodiesterase-5 inhibitors, and endothelin receptor antagonists, that have improved the outlook dramatically. Although there is no cure for PAH, current pharmacologic therapies improve morbidity and, in some cases, mortality.

PROSTANOIDS

In PAH, endothelial dysfunction and platelet activation cause an imbalance of arachidonic acid metabolites with reduced prostacyclin levels and increased thromboxane A_2 production. Prostacyclin (prostaglandin I_2, or PGI_2) activates cyclic adenosine monophosphate–dependent pathways that mediate vasodilation. PGI_2 also has antiproliferative effects on vascular smooth muscle and inhibits platelet aggregation. Protein levels of prostacyclin synthase are decreased in pulmonary arteries of patients with PAH.[58] This imbalance of mediators is addressed by the exogenous administration of prostanoids as therapy in advanced PAH.

Epoprostenol was the first prostanoid available for the management of PAH. Epoprostenol delivered as a continuous intravenous infusion improves functional capacity and survival in PAH.[62-64] The efficacy of epoprostenol in WHO class 3 and 4 PAH patients was demonstrated in a randomized clinical trial that showed improved quality of life, mPAP, PVR, 6MWT, and mortality compared with placebo.[65]

Continuous subcutaneous and intravenous administration of treprostinil has been shown to improve pulmonary hemodynamics, symptoms, exercise capacity, and possibly survival in PAH.[66-68] Inhaled treprostinil has been approved for patients with class III and IV PAH. Studies comparing inhaled treprostinil to iloprost suggest that inhaled treprostinil has a comparable and more sustained PVR decrease with fewer systemic side effects. The main advantage of treprostinil is less frequent administration.

Inhaled iloprost has the advantage of targeting the lung vasculature and does not require intravenous administration. However, the main disadvantage is the need for very frequent administration. A large trial investigating the use of inhaled iloprost in class III and IV PAH patients over 12 weeks demonstrated improved WHO functional class and increased 6MWT compared with placebo.[69] The addition of phosphodiesterase-5 (PDE-5) inhibitor augments the pulmonary hemodynamic and functional capacity benefits of prostanoids in PAH.[70]

ENDOTHELIN RECEPTOR ANTAGONISTS

Endothelin receptor antagonists (ERAs) target endothelin-1 (ET-1), a potent endogenous vasoconstrictor and vascular smooth muscle mitogen. Stewart and colleagues first reported elevated ET-1 levels in PAH patients.[71] There is a positive correlation between ET-1 and PVR and mean PAP, and a strong negative correlation between cardiac output (CO) and 6MWT.[72]

ERAs block the binding of ET-1 to either endothelin receptor A (ET-A) or endothelin receptor B (ET-B). ET-A receptors found on pulmonary artery smooth muscle cells mediate vasoconstriction. In normal pulmonary vasculature, ET-B receptors are found on endothelial cells and mediate vasodilation through production of prostacyclin and nitric oxide as well as ET-1 clearance. However, in PAH, ET-B mediates vasoconstriction through a separate population of receptors that are upregulated in vascular smooth muscle cells.[73] The two ERAs approved for use in the United States are bosentan, a nonselective receptor antagonist, and ambrisentan, a selective ET-A receptor antagonist.

Studies have shown that bosentan improves hemodynamics and exercise capacity and delays clinical worsening. The placebo-controlled, phase 3 trial Bosentan Randomized Trial of Endothelin Antagonist Therapy (BREATHE)-1, comparing bosentan and placebo, demonstrated improved symptoms, 6MWT, and WHO functional class.[74] The Endothelin Antagonist Trial in Mildly Symptomatic Pulmonary Arterial Hypertension Patients (EARLY) study comparing bosentan with placebo demonstrated improved PVR and 6MWT.[75]

Several studies, including the phase 3 placebo-controlled Ambrisentan in Pulmonary Arterial Hypertension (ARIES)-1 trial, suggest that ambrisentan improves exercise tolerance, WHO functional class, hemodynamics, and quality of life in patients with PAH.[76,77] There are no trial data to evaluate whether selective ET-A receptor antagonism of ambrisentan has any advantaged over nonselective ET receptor antagonism of bosentan. There are also no data comparing the efficacy of ERAs and PDE-5 inhibitors. However, results of a 2-year follow-up study of ambrisentan reveal sustained improvement in mean 6MWT, 72% freedom from clinical worsening, and 88% survival at 2 years.[77]

PHOSPHODIESTERASE-5 INHIBITORS

Nitric oxide derived from endothelial cells activate guanylyl cyclase, which in turn dephosphorylates guanyl triphosphate to cyclic guanyl monophosphate (cGMP) in vascular smooth muscle cells. cGMP is a second messenger that induces vasodilation through relaxation of the arterial smooth muscle cells. PDE-5 enzymes metabolize cGMP. Therefore, cGMP PDE-5 inhibitors prolong the vasodilatory effect of nitric oxide, especially within the pulmonary arterial bed, where high concentrations of cGMP are found. There are currently two PDE-5 inhibitors used for the treatment of PAH: sildenafil[78] and tadalafil.[79] Both agents have been shown to improve hemodynamics and 6MWT.

UNMET, FUTURE RESEARCH NEEDS IN PULMONARY HYPERTENSION

1. Presently there are only three classes of therapy for patients with PAH, and even with therapy, the median survival for a person with PAH is only 5 to 6 years.

2. Although there are five subtypes of PH, current approved therapies only address one subtype. Not only do we need to expand the treatment options for patients with PAH, but we also need to develop effective therapies for all patients with PH.

3. Limited survival is, in part, a result of delay in diagnosis. Improved awareness among clinicians and patients could lead to more timely diagnosis that will affect response to therapy and survival. PH needs to be diagnosed in a timely manner so that patients can be started on therapy as soon as possible.

4. Patients should also have the option of referral to a specialty center that focuses on treatment of patients with pulmonary vascular disease, which will ensure them access to state-of-the-art care and a multidisciplinary approach to care.

5. Finally, there needs to be continued efforts at developing new therapies that target the increasingly complex and overlapping pathways involved in the various forms of PH.

CONCLUSION

In summary, PH is an uncommon disorder that presents with nonspecific complaints. There remains a significant delay in the diagnosis of PH and initiation of appropriate therapy because often patients are misdiagnosed with more common causes of dyspnea, such as obstructive lung diseases like asthma. The diagnosis of PH should be considered in patients who do not fit the usual profile of patients presenting with dyspnea and asthma, especially if they do not respond to therapy. The finding of PH foreshadows a poor outcome if not discovered early and treated aggressively. Patients found to have PH should be referred to a physician experienced in its evaluation and treatment.

REFERENCES

1. Brown LM, Chen H, Halpern S, et al. Delay in recognition of pulmonary arterial hypertension: factors identified from the REVEAL Registry. *Chest.* 2011;140(1):19–26.
2. Brecker SJ, Gibbs JS, Fox KM, Yacoub MH, Gibson DG. Comparison of Doppler derived haemodynamic variables and simultaneous high fidelity pressure measurements in severe pulmonary hypertension. *Br Heart J.* 1994;72(4):384–389.
3. Fisher MR, Forfia PR, Chamera E, et al. Accuracy of Doppler echocardiography in the hemodynamic assessment of pulmonary hypertension. *Am J Respir Crit Care Med.* 2009;179(7):615–621.
4. Tolle JJ, Waxman AB, Van Horn TL, Pappagianopoulos PP, Systrom DM. Exercise-induced pulmonary arterial hypertension. *Circulation.* 2008;118(21):2183–2189.
5. Oudiz RJ, Barst RJ, Hansen JE, et al. Cardiopulmonary exercise testing and six-minute walk correlations in pulmonary arterial hypertension. *Am J Cardiol.* 2006;97(1):123–126.
6. van Belle A, Buller HR, Huisman MV, et al. Effectiveness of managing suspected pulmonary embolism using an algorithm combining clinical probability, D-dimer testing, and computed tomography. *JAMA.* 2006;295(2):172–179.
7. Stein PD, Woodard PK, Weg JG, et al. Diagnostic pathways in acute pulmonary embolism: recommendations of the PIOPED II Investigators. *Radiology.* 2007;242(1):15–21.
8. Bergin CJ, Rios G, King MA, Belezzuoli E, Luna J, Auger WR. Accuracy of high-resolution CT in identifying chronic pulmonary thromboembolic disease. *AJR Am J Roentgenol.* 1996;166(6):1371–1377.
9. Fedullo PF, Auger WR, Kerr KM, Rubin LJ. Chronic thromboembolic pulmonary hypertension. *N Engl J Med.* 2001;345(20):1465–1472.
10. Tunariu N, Gibbs SJ, Win Z, et al. Ventilation-perfusion scintigraphy is more sensitive than multidetector CTPA in detecting chronic thromboembolic pulmonary disease as a treatable cause of pulmonary hypertension. *J Nucl Med.* 2007;48(5):680–684.
11. Rafanan AL, Golish JA, Dinner DS, Hague LK, Arroliga AC. Nocturnal hypoxemia is common in primary pulmonary hypertension. *Chest.* 2001;120(3):894–899.
12. Gaine SP, Rubin LJ. Primary pulmonary hypertension. *Lancet.* 1998;352(9129):719–725.
13. Humbert M, Sitbon O, Chaouat A, et al. Pulmonary arterial hypertension in France: results from a national registry. *Am J Respir Crit Care Med.* 2006;173(9):1023–1030.
14. Frost AE, Badesch DB, Barst RJ, et al. The changing picture of pulmonary arterial hypertension (PAH) patients in the United States: how the REVEAL Registry differs from historic and non-US contemporary registries. *Chest.* 2011;139(1):128–137.
15. Thenappan T, Shah SJ, Rich S, Gomberg-Maitland M. A USA-based registry for pulmonary arterial hypertension: 1982–2006. *Eur Respir J.* 2007;30(6):1103–1110.
16. Janda S, Quon BS, Swiston J. HIV and pulmonary arterial hypertension: a systematic review. *HIV Med.* 2010;11(10):620–634.
17. Nunes H, Humbert M, Capron F, et al. Pulmonary hypertension associated with sarcoidosis: mechanisms, haemodynamics and prognosis. *Thorax.* 2006;61(1):68–74.
18. Mukerjee D, St George D, Coleiro B, et al. Prevalence and outcome in systemic sclerosis associated pulmonary arterial hypertension: application of a registry approach. *Ann Rheum Dis.* 2003;62(11):1088–1093.
19. Hachulla E, Gressin V, Guillevin L, et al. Early detection of pulmonary arterial hypertension in systemic sclerosis: a French nationwide prospective multicenter study. *Arthritis Rheum.* 2005;52(12):3792–3800.
20. Tyndall AJ, Bannert B, Vonk M, et al. Causes and risk factors for death in systemic sclerosis: a study from the EULAR Scleroderma Trials

and Research (EUSTAR) database. *Ann Rheum Dis.* 2010;69(10):1809-1815.
21. Williams MH, Das C, Handler CE, et al. Systemic sclerosis associated pulmonary hypertension: improved survival in the current era. *Heart.* 2006;92(7):926-932.
22. Condliffe R, Kiely DG, Peacock AJ, et al. Connective tissue disease-associated pulmonary arterial hypertension in the modern treatment era. *Am J Respir Crit Care Med.* 2009;179(2):151-157.
23. Fisher MR, Mathai SC, Champion HC, et al. Clinical differences between idiopathic and scleroderma-related pulmonary hypertension. *Arthritis Rheum.* 2006;54(9):3043-3050.
24. Kawut SM, Al-Naamani N, Agerstrand C, et al. Determinants of right ventricular ejection fraction in pulmonary arterial hypertension. *Chest.* 2009;135(3):752-759.
25. Bezante GP, Rollando D, Sessarego M, et al. Cardiac magnetic resonance imaging detects subclinical right ventricular impairment in systemic sclerosis. *J Rheumatol.* 2007;34(12):2431-2437.
26. Stupi AM, Steen VD, Owens GR, Barnes EL, Rodnan GP, Medsger TA Jr. Pulmonary hypertension in the CREST syndrome variant of systemic sclerosis. *Arthritis Rheum.* 1986;29(4):515-524.
27. Campo A, Mathai SC, Le Pavec J, et al. Hemodynamic predictors of survival in scleroderma-related pulmonary arterial hypertension. *Am J Respir Crit Care Med.* 2010;182(2):252-260.
28. Hoeper MM, Krowka MJ, Strassburg CP. Portopulmonary hypertension and hepatopulmonary syndrome. *Lancet.* 2004;363(9419):1461-1468.
29. Porres-Aguilar M, Zuckerman MJ, Figueroa-Casas JB, Krowka MJ. Portopulmonary hypertension: state of the art. *Ann Hepatol.* 2008;7(4):321-330.
30. Hoeper MM, Barberà JA, Channick RN, et al. Diagnosis, assessment, and treatment of non-pulmonary arterial hypertension pulmonary hypertension. *J Am Coll Cardiol.* 2009;54(1):S85-S96.
31. Grigioni F, Potena L, Galie N, et al. Prognostic implications of serial assessments of pulmonary hypertension in severe chronic heart failure. *J Heart Lung Transplant.* 2006;25(10):1241-1246.
32. Leung CC, Moondra V, Catherwood E, Andrus BW. Prevalence and risk factors of pulmonary hypertension in patients with elevated pulmonary venous pressure and preserved ejection fraction. *Am J Cardiol.* 2010;106(2):284-286.
33. Delgado JF, Conde E, Sanchez V, et al. Pulmonary vascular remodeling in pulmonary hypertension due to chronic heart failure. *Eur J Heart Fail.* 2005;7(6):1011-1016.
34. Simonneau G, Robbins IM, Beghetti M, et al. Updated clinical classification of pulmonary hypertension. *J Am Coll Cardiol.* 2009;54(1):S43-S54.
35. Chaouat A, Bugnet AS, Kadaoui N, et al. Severe pulmonary hypertension and chronic obstructive pulmonary disease. *Am J Respir Crit Care Med.* 2005;172(2):189-194.
36. Burrows B, Bloom JW, Traver GA, Cline MG. The course and prognosis of different forms of chronic airways obstruction in a sample from the general population. *N Engl J Med.* 1987;317(21):1309-1314.
37. Thabut G, Dauriat G, Stern JB, et al. Pulmonary hemodynamics in advanced COPD candidates for lung volume reduction surgery or lung transplantation. *Chest.* 2005;127(5):1531-1536.
38. Scharf SM, Iqbal M, Keller C, Criner G, Lee S, Fessler HE. Hemodynamic characterization of patients with severe emphysema. *Am J Respir Crit Care Med.* 2002;166(3):314-322.
39. Minai OA, Chaouat A, Adnot S. Pulmonary hypertension in COPD: epidemiology, significance, and management. Pulmonary vascular disease: the global perspective. *Chest.* 2010;137(6 Suppl):39S-51S.
40. Weitzenblum E, Chaouat A, Canuet M, Kessler R. Pulmonary hypertension in chronic obstructive pulmonary disease and interstitial lung diseases. *Semin Respir Crit Care Med.* 2009;30(4):458-470.
41. Marin JM, Soriano JB, Carrizo SJ, Boldova A, Celli BR. Outcomes in patients with chronic obstructive pulmonary disease and obstructive sleep apnea: the overlap syndrome. *Am J Respir Crit Care Med.* 2010;182(3):325-331.
42. Hoeper MM. Treating pulmonary hypertension in COPD: where do we start? *Eur Respir J.* 2008;32(3):541-542.
43. Vizza CD, Lynch JP, Ochoa LL, Richardson G, Trulock EP. Right and left ventricular dysfunction in patients with severe pulmonary disease. *Chest.* 1998;113(3):576-583.
44. Nadrous HF, Pellikka PA, Krowka MJ, et al. Pulmonary hypertension in patients with idiopathic pulmonary fibrosis. *Chest.* 2005;128(4):2393-2399.
45. Nathan SD, Shlobin OA, Ahmad S, et al. Serial development of pulmonary hypertension in patients with idiopathic pulmonary fibrosis. *Respiration.* 2008;76(3):288-294.
46. Lettieri CJ, Nathan SD, Barnett SD, Ahmad S, Shorr AF. Prevalence and outcomes of

46. [continued] pulmonary arterial hypertension in advanced idiopathic pulmonary fibrosis. *Chest.* 2006;129(3): 746–752.
47. Shorr AF, Wainright JL, Cors CS, Lettieri CJ, Nathan SD. Pulmonary hypertension in patients with pulmonary fibrosis awaiting lung transplant. *Eur Respir J.* 2007;30(4):715–721.
48. Hamada K, Nagai S, Tanaka S, et al. Significance of pulmonary arterial pressure and diffusion capacity of the lung as prognosticator in patients with idiopathic pulmonary fibrosis. *Chest.* 2007;131(3):650–656.
49. Kessler R, Chaouat A, Weitzenblum E, et al. Pulmonary hypertension in the obstructive sleep apnoea syndrome: prevalence, causes and therapeutic consequences. *Eur Respir J.* 1996;9(4):787–794.
50. Minai OA, Ricaurte B, Kaw R, et al. Frequency and impact of pulmonary hypertension in patients with obstructive sleep apnea syndrome. *Am J Cardiol.* 2009;104(9): 1300–1306.
51. Sajkov D, Cowie RJ, Thornton AT, Espinoza HA, McEvoy RD. Pulmonary hypertension and hypoxemia in obstructive sleep apnea syndrome. *Am J Respir Crit Care Med.* 1994;149(2 Pt 1): 416–422.
52. Bady E, Achkar A, Pascal S, Orvoen-Frija E, Laaban JP. Pulmonary arterial hypertension in patients with sleep apnoea syndrome. *Thorax.* 2000;55(11):934–939.
53. Becattini C, Agnelli G, Pesavento R, et al. Incidence of chronic thromboembolic pulmonary hypertension after a first episode of pulmonary embolism. *Chest.* 2006;130(1):172–175.
54. Miniati M, Monti S, Bottai M, et al. Survival and restoration of pulmonary perfusion in a long-term follow-up of patients after acute pulmonary embolism. *Medicine.* 2006;85(5):253–262.
55. Pengo V, Lensing AW, Prins MH, et al. Incidence of chronic thromboembolic pulmonary hypertension after pulmonary embolism. *N Engl J Med.* 2004;350(22):2257–2264.
56. Dentali F, Donadini M, Gianni M, et al. Incidence of chronic pulmonary hypertension in patients with previous pulmonary embolism. *Thromb Res.* 2009;124(3):256–258.
57. Lang I, Kerr K. Risk factors for chronic thromboembolic pulmonary hypertension. *Proc Am Thorac Soc.* 2006;3(7):568–570.
58. Tuder RM, Abman SH, Braun T, et al. Development and pathology of pulmonary hypertension. *J Am Coll Cardiol.* 2009;54(1):S3–S9.
59. Bonderman D, Wilkens H, Wakounig S, et al. Risk factors for chronic thromboembolic pulmonary hypertension. *Eur Respir J.* 2009;33(2):325–331.
60. Tapson VF, Humbert M. Incidence and prevalence of chronic thromboembolic pulmonary hypertension: from acute to chronic pulmonary embolism. *Proc Am Thorac Soc.* 2006;3(7):564–567.
61. Moser KM, Bloor CM. Pulmonary vascular lesions occurring in patients with chronic major vessel thromboembolic pulmonary hypertension. *Chest.* 1993;103(3):685–692.
62. Barst RJ, Rubin LJ, McGoon MD, Caldwell EJ, Long WA, Levy PS. Survival in primary pulmonary hypertension with long-term continuous intravenous prostacyclin. *Ann Intern Med.* 1994;121(6):409–415.
63. Rubin LJ, Mendoza J, Hood M, et al. Treatment of primary pulmonary hypertension with continuous intravenous prostacyclin (epoprostenol): results of a randomized trial. *Ann Intern Med.* 1990;112(7):485–491.
64. Shapiro SM, Oudiz RJ, Cao T, et al. Primary pulmonary hypertension: improved long-term effects and survival with continuous intravenous epoprostenol infusion. *J Am Coll Cardiol.* 1997;30(2):343–349.
65. Barst RJ, Rubin LJ, Long WA, et al. A comparison of continuous intravenous epoprostenol (prostacyclin) with conventional therapy for primary pulmonary hypertension. *N Engl J Med.* 1996;334(5):296–301.
66. Barst RJ, Galie N, Naeije R, et al. Long-term outcome in pulmonary arterial hypertension patients treated with subcutaneous treprostinil. *Eur Respir J.* 2006;28(6):1195–1203.
67. Tapson VF, Gomberg-Maitland M, McLaughlin VV, et al. Safety and efficacy of IV treprostinil for pulmonary arterial hypertension: a prospective, multicenter, open-label, 12-week trial. *Chest.* 2006;129(3):683–688.
68. Benza RL, Rayburn BK, Tallaj JA, Pamboukian SV, Bourge RC. Treprostinil-based therapy in the treatment of moderate-to-severe pulmonary arterial hypertension: long-term efficacy and combination with bosentan. *Chest.* 2008;134(1):139–145.
69. Olschewski H, Simonneau G, Galie N, et al. Inhaled iloprost for severe pulmonary hypertension. *N Engl J Med.* 2002;347(5):322–329.
70. Simonneau G, Rubin LJ, Galie N, et al. Addition of sildenafil to long-term intravenous epoprostenol therapy in patients with pulmonary arterial hypertension: a randomized trial. *Ann Intern Med.* 2008;149(8):521–530.
71. Stewart DJ, Levy RD, Cernacek P, Langleben D. Increased plasma endothelin-1 in pulmonary hypertension: marker or mediator of disease? *Ann Intern Med.* 1991;114(6):464–469.

72. Rubens C, Ewert R, Halank M, et al. Big endothelin-1 and endothelin-1 plasma levels are correlated with the severity of primary pulmonary hypertension. *Chest.* 2001;120(5):1562–1569.
73. Hirata Y, Emori T, Eguchi S, et al. Endothelin receptor subtype B mediates synthesis of nitric oxide by cultured bovine endothelial cells. *J Clin Invest.* 1993;91(4):1367–1373.
74. Rubin LJ, Badesch DB, Barst RJ, et al. Bosentan therapy for pulmonary arterial hypertension. *N Engl J Med.* 2002;346(12):896–903.
75. Galie N, Rubin L, Hoeper M, et al. Treatment of patients with mildly symptomatic pulmonary arterial hypertension with bosentan (EARLY study): a double-blind, randomised controlled trial. *Lancet.* 2008;371(9630):2093–2100.
76. Galie N, Olschewski H, Oudiz RJ, et al. Ambrisentan for the treatment of pulmonary arterial hypertension: results of the ambrisentan in pulmonary arterial hypertension, randomized, double-blind, placebo-controlled, multicenter, efficacy (ARIES) study 1 and 2. *Circulation.* 2008;117(23):3010–3019.
77. Oudiz RJ, Galie N, Olschewski H, et al. Long-term ambrisentan therapy for the treatment of pulmonary arterial hypertension. *J Am Coll Cardiol.* 2009;54(21):1971–1981.
78. Galie N, Ghofrani HA, Torbicki A, et al. Sildenafil citrate therapy for pulmonary arterial hypertension. *N Engl J Med.* 2005;353(20):2148–2157.
79. Galie N, Brundage BH, Ghofrani HA, et al. Tadalafil therapy for pulmonary arterial hypertension. *Circulation.* 2009;119(22):2894–2903.

SECTION FOUR

UPPER/EXTRATHORACIC AIRWAY

18

ALLERGIC RHINITIS

COMORBID

Robert M. Naclerio and Ruby Pawankar

KEY POINTS

- Allergic rhinitis is an inflammatory disease that profoundly affects quality of life.
- Treatments exist to treat allergic rhinitis, but there is still a need for more efficacious therapy.
- Allergic rhinitis is associated with multiple comorbidities.
- How allergic rhinitis affects comorbidities is an important question.

INTRODUCTION

Allergic rhinitis (AR) is the most common atopic disease, with an increasing prevalence worldwide. It is an immunoglobulin E (IgE)-mediated inflammatory disease of the nasal mucosa, characterized by symptoms of nasal itching, sneezing, runny nose, and stuffy nose. The stuffy nose is the most burdensome symptom to patients, but the itch and sneeze are the most characteristic.[1] Although it is not a fatal disease, AR has a negative impact on the patient's quality of life (QOL), which is detected not only on disease-specific QOL measures but also on general QOL measures such as the SF36. Sleep, presenteeism, mood and cognition, and participation in sports and leisure activities are all affected, causing a great physical and financial burden on the patient.

Allergic rhinitis is traditionally classified into seasonal and perennial allergic types, which remain the classification used by the U.S. Food and Drug Administration (FDA) for approval of treatments for AR. This classification works best as an attempt to identify the allergens causing the disease, particularly in certain parts of the world where there are distinct seasons. It provides an excellent model for the study and diagnosis of AR. To provide a classification that is useful for the clinician who treats the disease, the Allergic Rhinitis and Its Impact on Asthma (ARIA) guidelines classified AR along two axes: mild versus moderate/severe and intermittent versus persistent. The ARIA guidelines emphasize asthma as a significant comorbidity of AR and indicate that AR is a risk factor for asthma.[2]

DIAGNOSIS

The prevalence of AR in the United States ranges between 10% and 30%. This prevalence varies according to the definition used and whether it is based on physician diagnosis or physician diagnosis and allergy testing. Because more than 50% of Americans are skin test positive for common allergens, skin testing does not always accurately confirm a diagnosis of AR in the absence of a definitive history.[3] Some false-positive skin tests are easy to recognize because the timing of symptoms and the seasonality of the allergen do not match. Another quandary is presented by nasal symptoms with a false-positive skin test. Further confusing the issue is the recognition of local IgE production in the nose, leading to symptoms on exposure to an antigen, but in the presence of negative skin tests. The diagnosis of AR is usually made by a history that correlates a positive allergy test with a positive nasal examination showing signs of AR or a negative examination showing the absence of another disease that could explain the symptoms.

A negative physical examination can eliminate serious diseases that mimic perennial AR. Unilateral otitis media with effusion can signal a mass in the nasopharynx and is an indication for nasopharyngoscopy. A unilateral nasal polyp is more suspicious for a noninflammatory process. Facial numbness raises concern about a sinus malignancy. Facial swelling or interference with ocular movements portends a complication of sinusitis. Fever and enlarged neck lymph nodes are not associated with AR. Although most sinusitis is rhinogenic in nature, dental infections can initiate sinusitis. Purulent-appearing postnasal discharge is a strong sign of a sinus infection. Lack of response to a 2-week course of intranasal glucocorticoid (INS) justifies nasal endoscopy in the effort to try to identify structural or more subtle forms of pathology. Imaging studies, primarily computed tomography (CT) scans, are useful after medical therapy fails or when the diagnosis is not apparent.

Other diseases in the differential diagnosis of AR include non-AR, immotile cilia syndrome, hormonal rhinitis, drug-induced rhinitis, structural abnormalities, adenoidal hypertrophy, tumors, and chronic rhinosinusitis.

Most guidelines for AR recommend testing for an IgE-mediated mechanism.[2,4,5] This strategy is important especially when allergen immunotherapy (AIT) is being considered. Most patients, however, are tested in the effort to suggest an IgE-mediated mechanism as the cause of their disease and to recommend avoidance measures. Avoidance of offending allergens is logical, but seems to be effective only if absolute avoidance can be achieved. For example, dust mite avoidance in high-altitude cities, such as Denver, is successful because dust mites don't exist in this environment. However, avoidance measures in locations with dust mites reduce the allergen load but do not add significantly to the positive effects of pharmacotherapy. "Sticky" allergens like cat can be transported to schools by other children who have cats in their homes, causing symptoms even in the cat-allergic child whose parents eliminate the cat from their home. Because most patients respond to pharmacotherapy, which is safe and effective, trying pharmacotherapy first is a cost-effective strategy.

PATHOPHYSIOLOGY OF ALLERGIC RHINITIS

The pathophysiologic mechanisms involved in AR begin with sensitization of the nasal mucosa to allergens that are common in the environment.[6] The sensitization process involves interactions among antigen-presenting cells, T lymphocytes, and B cells and leads to the production of antigen-specific IgE antibodies, which then localize to mast cells and basophils. IgE can also bind to low-affinity receptors on other cells, but their precise function is not elucidated. Exposure to allergens after sensitization cross-links specific IgE receptors on mast cells, resulting in their activation. Degranulation releases inflammatory mediators such as histamine that cause immediate nasal allergic symptoms, including sneezing, rhinorrhea, itching, and nasal congestion. Other proinflammatory substances are also generated after antigen exposure by mast cells, which may play a role in the inflammatory process that follows the immediate reaction to allergens. Most characteristic of the inflammatory process are eosinophils and their chemical products and cytokines. Studies show that mast cells play a role in promoting ongoing inflammation and the local production of IgE, which can further amplify inflammation through a mast cell–IgE-Fc epsilon receptor I cascade.[7–11]

Cytokines are also generated by lymphocytes, which are abundant in both resting and stimulated nasal mucosa. Cytokines upregulate adhesion molecules on the vascular endothelium, which leads to the migration of inflammatory cells into the site of tissue inflammation.[12,13] Various cytokines promote chemotaxis and survival of recruited inflammatory cells and lead to a secondary immune response by virtue of their capacity to promote IgE synthesis by B cells. Furthermore, the role of epithelial cells as immune mediators has added a newer understanding of the way these cells, through either direct cell-to-cell interaction or mediators like cytokines and chemokines, can regulate other cells like dendritic cells, mast cells, and T cells.

The nervous system amplifies the allergic reaction by central and peripheral reflexes that result in changes at sites distant from those of allergen deposition such as the eyes, sinuses, and lower airway.[14] Importantly, these inflammatory changes lower the threshold of mucosal responsiveness to various specific and nonspecific stimuli, making allergic patients more susceptible and hyperresponsive to stimuli to which they are exposed daily, as well as to subsequent exposure to allergens, referred to as priming.[15,16]

TREATMENT OF ALLERGIC RHINITIS

Pharmacotherapy is the mainstay of treatment for AR.[2] Much information is available about the effectiveness and safety of pharmacotherapy, but there is little information on the impact of these treatments on the comorbidities of AR.

Antihistamines

Histamine-1 (H_1) receptor antagonist antihistamines are classified as first generation, or sedating, and second generation, or nonsedating. The first-generation antihistamines are effective but have undesirable side effects because of their lack of selectivity, their ability to cross the blood-brain barrier, and subsequent nonspecific stimulation of other receptors. Among these are sedation, anticholinergic effects, and functional and performance impairment. Second-generation antihistamines are less lipophilic than first-generation H_1 antihistamines and do not penetrate the blood-brain barrier. Therefore, they generally produce no more somnolence than does a placebo. Their greater receptor selectivity also reduces the incidence of anticholinergic side effects.

Azelastine, a phthalazinone derivative, is an intranasal preparation, the efficacy of which is comparable to that of oral antihistamines, but with a faster onset of action. It causes some somnolence and can be associated with a bad taste. Pantanase is another topical intranasal antihistamine available in the United States.

All antihistamines are effective to treat AR and differ principally in their side effects, duration of action, and cost. H_1 receptor antagonists are most effective in treating sneezing, nasal and ocular pruritus, and rhinorrhea associated with AR, but they have little or no effect on nasal congestion. Thus, they are often prescribed in combination with a decongestant.

Decongestants

Decongestants exert their effect through stimulation of α_1- or α_2-adrenergic receptors. Oral decongestants exert their effects directly and by stimulating norepinephrine release. They can be prescribed separately or in combination with antihistamines. Current recommendations suggest that decongestants should not be used in patients with uncontrolled hypertension, in those with severe coronary artery disease, or in patients receiving monoamine oxidase inhibitors. Decongestants should be prescribed with caution to patients with diabetes, hyperthyroidism, closed-angle glaucoma, coronary artery disease, cardiac insufficiency, prostatic hypertrophy, or urinary retention. Their major side effect is insomnia, which occurs in approximately 25% of patients.

Topical decongestants are effective in reducing nasal congestion, regardless of the cause. These include catecholamines (such as phenylephrine) and imidazole derivatives (such as xylometazoline or oxymetazoline). Prolonged use, however, can lead to rhinitis medicamentosa. These agents are best reserved for cases in which nasal congestion is so severe that it precludes the use of other topical preparations such as INS, or to allow more restful sleep during acute exacerbations. Seizures have occurred in children given these medications intranasally.

A topical decongestant without the potential to cause rhinitis medicamentosa is needed. Although there are individuals who clearly develop rhinitis medicamentosa, the frequency of this phenomenon is unknown. Two studies have suggested that topical glucocorticosteroids (GCSs) prevent its development when they are used concurrently with topical nasal decongestants.[17,18]

Topical Intranasal Glucocorticosteroids

Topical intranasal GCSs are the most potent medications for the treatment of AR. These agents profoundly reduce multiple aspects of the inflammatory response to allergen. In contrast to systemic GCS, treatment with INS reduces the acute nasal response to allergen challenge, as shown by a reduction in symptoms and in the levels of recovered inflammatory mediators in nasal secretions. This observation relates to the fact that the number of mast cells near the nasal mucosal surface is reduced, decreasing the number of targets for allergen. Treatment with INS also reduces symptoms, the levels of mediators, and cellular infiltration during the late-phase response to allergen challenge, as well as the priming response to allergen. This inhibits hyperresponsiveness to nonantigenic stimuli such as histamine. INSs prevent the increase in mast cells and inflammatory cells seen during seasonal exposure to allergen. Furthermore, they suppress the seasonal increase in specific IgE antibodies during the ragweed season. A direct vasoconstrictor effect of topical glucocorticoids, found in the skin, does not occur in the nasal mucosa.[19]

Although differences in the potency of receptor binding among these molecules can be demonstrated in vitro and in certain in vivo models, none of these variations translates into major clinical differences. Their onset of action is as short as 1 day, with most preparations having a noticeable clinical effect by 3 days and a peak effect by 2 weeks. These medications work best with continued use, as opposed to intermittent, as-needed use. However, there is evidence that they are effective when used intermittently and more effective than antihistamines used as needed.[20] In the United States, there are many different INS formulations available, as either an aqueous spray or a hydrofluoroalkane (HFA)-propelled aerosol. HFA aerosols are as effective as aqueous preparations and offer a novel form of delivery, with no leakage from the nose or posterior pharyngeal drip.[21,22]

Side effects of INS are relatively rare. The most frequent is nasal irritation, which occurs in approximately 5% of patients. This manifests as a nasal burning sensation or sneezing. In general, 2% of patients have blood-tinged secretions either because of the medication or because of the delivery system. Septal perforations are reported but are extremely rare. Nasal biopsies after prolonged use of these agents do not demonstrate thinning of the nasal epithelium; in fact, the mucosa looks healthier than the mucosa of untreated patients who have perennial AR.[23] Mucosal superinfection with *Candida albicans*, which is occasionally found with the use of topical, oral inhaled GCS to treat asthma, is not a significant problem in the nose, in part because the normal pH of the nose is 5.5, thus inhibiting the growth of these organisms.

Systemic side effects of GCS are a matter of concern. Dexamethasone, the first INS available in the United States, had measurable systemic absorption, leading to adrenal suppression after prolonged use. Preparations now available have lower systemic absorption and, at the standard doses used for the treatment of AR, no detectable effects on the hypothalamic-pituitary-adrenal axis. A reduction in bone growth in children is a concern. This problem, however, has been studied in asthmatic children, and most studies suggest a small effect with high doses that exceed those recommended for intranasal use. Also, absorption of a topical GCS from the lungs is about four-fold greater than that of the same dose given intranasally.[24]

A study in asthmatic children given intranasal budesonide shows that the loss in prepubescent growth carries over into adult height.[25] Data in clinicaltrials.gov show that an INS with low bioavailability, fluticasone furoate, reduces growth by 0.27 cm, a small, clinically irrelevant but statistically significant difference, suggesting some systemic absorption.[26] Therefore, for long-term use in children, a topical GCS with low bioavailability, administered in the lowest dose necessary to provide relief of symptoms, is advisable and safe. The FDA package insert recommendations state that the growth of pediatric patients receiving INS should be monitored.

Formulations of INS in comparative trials with cromolyn, antihistamines, or montelukast are more potent in relieving nasal symptoms.[2] The addition of oral antihistamines to INS was thought to benefit ocular symptoms, although a meta-analysis shows that antihistamines and INS have equivalent effects. Studies combining a topical intranasal antihistamine with an INS show additive effectiveness.[27]

Systemic Corticosteroids

Clinical practice suggests that oral GCSs reduce symptoms during seasonal allergies, but this is not documented in placebo-controlled trials. Such medications are usually administered to patients during severe exacerbations of AR, when total nasal obstruction prevents the use of INS. Furthermore, these medications are used successfully in combination with antibiotics to treat sinus infections, which can complicate exacerbations of AR. The effectiveness of depot injections of GCS is comparable to that of short-term oral prednisone therapy, whereas GCS injections into the turbinates are clinically effective but are rarely used because of a small associated risk for blindness with injections of GGS.

Cromolyn Sodium

Cromolyn is available over the counter as a 4% solution for intranasal use and is clinically effective to treat AR. It exerts a protective effect on the allergic response when given four to six times daily before the onset of symptoms. The need for frequent dosing limits compliance. However, the safety profile makes it an attractive treatment modality, especially for children and pregnant women or when a patient knows he or she will be exposed to an animal to which he or she is allergic.

Anticholinergic Drugs

Anticholinergic medications inhibit parasympathetic stimulation of glandular secretions by competing for muscarinic receptors. They are highly effective in reducing watery rhinorrhea, but have no effect on other symptoms of AR. The clinical benefit of anticholinergic agents is limited primarily to the treatment of patients with rhinitis, allergic or nonallergic, in whom anterior watery rhinorrhea is the predominant complaint. They are also effective for treating gustatory rhinitis and for rhinitis associated with exposure to cold air (skier's rhinitis).

Leukotriene Modifiers

Two clinically available leukotriene modifiers, zafirlukast and montelukast, improve the symptoms of AR. Their effectiveness is approximately equivalent to that of an H_1 antihistamine. Many patients with asthma also have AR, and therefore leukotriene modifiers are effective for patients with both diseases. They also have a GCS-sparing effect for asthma. The 5-lipoxygenase inhibitor zileuton (Zyflo CR, Cornerstone Therapeutics, Cary, NC) is used to treat asthma and also should be effective for AR. Liver function needs to be monitored when this agent is used.

Combinations of Agents

Because patients do not always obtain complete symptomatic improvement with use of a single pharmacologic agent, clinicians often prescribe multiple medications. However, data supporting this practice are limited. The addition of an intranasal anticholinergic agent to an INS increases the effect on rhinorrhea.[28] Several studies fail to show that the combination of an oral antihistamine and an INS is better than an INS alone, although this combination is frequently prescribed.[29] In contrast, the addition of a topical intranasal antihistamine and an INS has additive efficacy, and a single-canister combination of azelastine plus fluticasone propionate is now approved for use by the FDA.[27] The combination of an antihistamine plus a leukotriene modifier was successful in small studies, but two large clinical trials failed to demonstrate efficacy greater than that of either one or the other components, montelukast and loratadine.

Studies show additive efficacy of antihistamines with oral decongestants. INS and ocular antihistamines are plausible for residual ocular symptoms after the use of an INS fails to adequately reduce symptoms. Leukotriene modifiers added to INS show no significant additive benefit.[30] The combination of an INS and a topical decongestant shows an additive benefit.[17,18] For those patients who partially respond to INS, clinicians frequently prescribe additional medications based on residual symptoms. The only caveat is that one should consider other diagnoses before adding multiple medications to treat the same disease.

Allergen Immunotherapy

The exact mode by which AIT achieves efficacy remains to be fully elucidated. Mechanistically, AIT causes immune deviation from a helper T-cell type 2 (T_H2) to a T_H1 cytokine profile and upregulation of regulatory T cells, thereby reducing the production of IgE and increasing the production of IgG. It offers relief of all nasal and ocular symptoms of AR. Patients must be advised that AIT offers control of symptoms, but efficacy is slow to begin and, unlike pharmacotherapy, is effective only for the allergens for which the patient is being treated. Discontinuation of successful AIT is followed by persistent clinical efficacy, the only such treatment for AR known to alter the natural history of the disease. This statement is true for both subcutaneous and sublingual use.[31] Moreover, AIT can reduce the development of comorbidities, such as asthma, and reduce the likelihood of new allergen sensitization.

The choice of allergens to be included in a vaccine must be considered only after a careful diagnostic workup so that the treatment extract contains all of the allergens responsible for the allergic symptoms. AIT of symptomatic asthmatic patients should be administered only with extreme caution because these patients have the greatest risk of a serious systemic allergic reaction. It should not be started during pregnancy because of the risk for inducing a systemic allergic reaction and anaphylaxis.

AIT efficacy requires optimal doses of allergen. Patients who do not achieve symptomatic improvement within 1 year should be reevaluated or therapy discontinued. No information is available on the length of time over which AIT should be continued, but most physicians treat for 3 to 5 years, after which patients can remain asymptomatic for years.

Although death from subcutaneous AIT is uncommon (the risk is estimated at 1 fatality for every 2 million or more injections), a waiting period of at least 30 minutes following administration of the injection is recommended for all patients, with longer intervals appropriate for high-risk patients.[32] Concern about mortality has led to the development of other forms of AIT, such as the sublingual form. There are data supporting its efficacy to treat AR and allergic asthma, its safety, and its lasting effects after discontinuation.

COMORBIDITIES

Besides causing symptoms and a negative impact on QOL, AR is associated with a variety of comorbid conditions (Figure 18.1). The

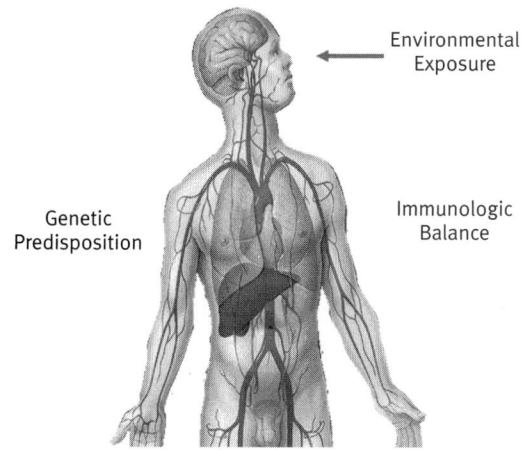

FIGURE 18.1 Comorbidities of allergic rhinitis. See Color Plate 5 in insert.

following sections comment on some of the comorbid conditions.

Conjunctivitis

Although often referred to as AR, this disease usually involves eye as well as nasal symptoms; hence, the more appropriate term may be *allergic rhinoconjunctivitis*. In fact, epidemiologic data show that ocular symptoms, defined as "episodes of watery, itchy eyes," affect 40% of the U.S. adult population, with up to 75% of those having severe disease.[33] Ocular symptoms are not only common but also distressing for allergy sufferers, with more than 50% stating that their watery and red, itchy eyes were moderately to extremely bothersome in the Allergies in America survey.[1]

The pathophysiologic mechanisms involved in the generation of ocular symptoms in patients with AR deserve special attention. These symptoms most likely result both from the direct effects of allergen deposition onto the conjunctiva and from nasal-ocular reflexes. Another possibility is that the nasal allergic reaction leads to the release of mediators from the nasal mucosa, upregulating circulatory inflammatory cells, which when attracted to the eye are primed to release more biochemical mediators and cause more severe symptoms.

The nasal-ocular reflex response is a means of explaining the beneficial effect of INS on eye symptoms in patients with AR. Nasal allergen challenge induces histamine release at the site, causing both nasonasal and nasal-ocular reflexes. This allergen-induced reflex is blocked by an H_1 receptor antagonist applied at the site of the challenge.[34] These observations support the hypothesis that eye symptoms can arise from a nasal-ocular reflex mechanism.

Pretreatment with an INS blocked the influx of eosinophils and the nasonasal and nasal-ocular reflexes in another nasal challenge study.[35] These findings not only support the nasal-ocular reflex as a mechanism of inducing eye symptoms during the allergy season but also suggest a mechanism by which INSs can affect the eye symptoms of AR without being systemically absorbed; that is, they reduce inflammation, which primes the reflex. The use of a topical antihistamine does not affect eye symptoms following nasal challenge with allergen. The importance of the nasal-ocular reflex for seasonal exposure to pollens is also supported by a park study in which subjects wore nasal filters, which reduced both nasal and ocular symptoms.[36] Additional support for the importance of the nasal-ocular reflex to eye symptoms during seasonal exposure is the observation that INS significantly reduces eye symptoms.[37]

Asthma

AR occurs in more than 75% of asthmatic patients, and 20% of these patients have asthma.[2] Additionally, the onset of AR precedes the onset of asthma in longitudinal studies. These observations suggest that the two entities are linked; the question is how. One theory is that shared environmental influences, such as smoking, allergen exposure, and viral infections, affect both the upper and lower airways.

As the entryway to the respiratory system, the nasal passages and, by proxy, the sinuses connected to them are potentially at risk for injury from toxic substances in the air (Figure 18.2). Approximately 9,000 liters of air pass through the nose daily, and a variety of pollutants may cause detrimental effects. These pollutants can affect nasal reflexes, mucociliary clearance, epithelial damage,

Allergic Rhinitis • 237

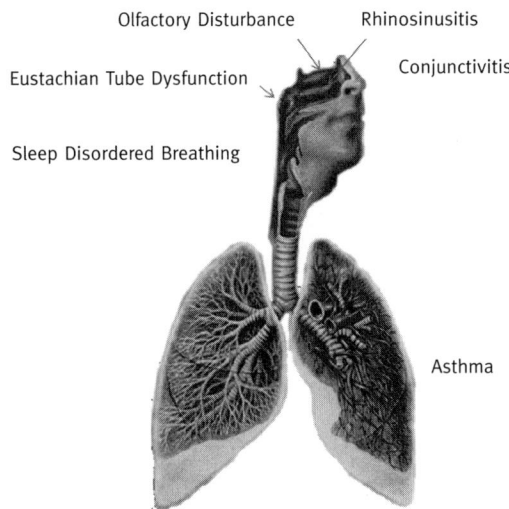

FIGURE 18.2 Comorbidities may exist if different body areas share genetic predispositions, environmental exposure, or immunologic imbalances. See Color Plate 6 in insert.

immune responses, and changes in nasal airflow.[38]

Pollutants theoretically can cause airway disease through multiple mechanisms, including induction or modulation of inflammatory responses and stimulation of nerve reflexes.[39] Air pollution, its effects on airway inflammation and allergy, and genetic susceptibility to these effects are the subjects of intense research interest. First, responses mediated by the trigeminal nerve exist for many substances that cause nasal irritation. These include paper, coffee, borax, and fiberglass dust. As a consequence, reflex neurogenic inflammation, which sets the stage for a chronic mucosal disease state, is established. Second, resistance to nasal airflow is increased with exposure to sulfur dioxide and tobacco smoke in sensitive patients. Additionally, many substances cause mucociliary clearance impairment, another factor that predisposes to stasis of secretions. Third, inflammatory responses to airborne pollutants may induce immunologic or toxic responses. Cigarette smoke, nicotine, capsaicin, ether, and formaldehyde can cause the release of neuropeptides such as substance P from the nasal mucosa, with resultant inflammation. Cigarette smoke inhibits neutral endopeptidase, an enzyme involved in the degradation of neuropeptides in lung tissue,
possibly leading to increased or chronic inflammation. Immunotoxic effects of pollutants include compromised phagocytic and killing ability, possibly leading to chronic infection or inflammation. Lastly, direct toxic effects on the sinonasal epithelium represent another mechanism that could lead to the development of disease in the sinonasal tract.

Because people in the developed world spend most of their time indoors, exposure to indoor pollutants remains an important concern. The pollutants most commonly considered inside buildings include nitrogen dioxide (NO_2), formaldehyde, sulfur dioxide (SO_2), aromatic hydrocarbons, and tobacco smoke. Organic substances such as molds and bacterial endotoxins in ventilation systems represent yet another potential environmental exposure that may be important.

NO_2, produced by the combustion of household cooking gas, is a known indoor pollutant associated with respiratory illness in epidemiologic studies.[40] High exposure to NO_2 can theoretically cause lung injury and a decrease in defense mechanisms in the lungs. Exposure to NO_2 can potentiate the effect of exposure to allergen.[41]

Formaldehyde, commonly found in construction materials, is implicated in carcinogenesis as well as the "sick-building syndrome"; it is also known to irritate the mucous membranes.[40] Ozone (O_3) is a naturally occurring, highly reactive, irritating gas recognized by the U.S. Environmental Protection Agency as an important public health hazard. It causes respiratory symptoms, alterations in pulmonary function, and lower airway inflammation. Deleterious effects of O_3 on the nose include epithelial disruption and increased permeability; inflammatory cell influx; proliferative and secretory responses; release of cytokines, cyclooxygenase, and lipoxygenase products; decreased mucociliary clearance; and a priming effect on the late-phase response to allergen challenge. Allergic asthmatic patients challenged intranasally with house dust mite allergen and exposed to ozone show an increase in eosinophils and inflammatory cytokines after 4 hours.[42]

SO_2 emission, primarily from electrical power generating plants, but also associated with indoor kerosene heaters, represents another important indoor pollutant. SO_2 produces bronchoconstriction, and short exposures lead to increased nasal airway resistance.[43]

Although 4,000 chemicals are identified in tobacco smoke, the actual number may be greater than 100,000.[44] At least 60 are carcinogens, including formaldehyde. Other chemicals, such as nicotine and carbon monoxide, interfere with normal cell development. Irritants, such as acrolein, formaldehyde, ammonia, nitrogen oxides, toluene, phenol, and pyridine, are also present in microgram amounts. The amount of smoke inhaled into the nasal cavity will be a portion of the side-stream smoke (inhaled from smoke emanating from the burning tip into the atmosphere instead of going through the cigarette into the mouth); the amount may vary because some subjects exhale smoke through the nose. Cigarette smoke is associated with a statistically significant increase in nasal airway resistance in subjects reporting sensitivity to smoke.

Ocular and nasal symptoms are related to nicotine exposure and cotinine excretion. There may be analogous effects on ears, as seen in studies linking smoking to chronic otitis media in children, given that both are mucosal inflammatory diseases. Although they are not discussed further in this review, ear diseases and symptoms are commonly associated with AR, most of them related to Eustachian tube dysfunction secondary to nasal inflammation with drainage over the torus tubarius.

Other mechanisms can explain the link between asthma and AR in addition to the direct effect of environmental factors on both the upper and lower airways (Figure 18.3).[45] There could be a shared water transport defect. The loss of nasal function could move the normal physiologic functions of warming, filtering, and humidifying of air to the lower airway, something that does not normally occur; evaporative water loss is believed to be a mechanism causing exercise-induced bronchospasm. Aspiration of upper-airway secretions into the lower airway occurs in a neurologically impaired host but should not occur in normal individuals. Whether the clearing of postnasal secretions imitates a cough or triggers a reflex is in question; neurologic reflexes from the nose to the lung are described. One study shows that changes in the nose lead to inflammatory changes in the lungs, and vice versa.[46] Another hypothesis for the upper airway affecting the lower airway is that allergic inflammation in the nose releases cytokines that affect cells in the bone marrow and systemic circulation. For example, the local release of interleukin-5 stimulates the bone marrow to produce more eosinophils. Other cytokines released from the nasal mucosa can prime circulating cells so that when they are recruited into the lungs, they release more inflammatory mediators, thus exacerbating asthma. Combinations of these mechanisms could contribute to this interrelationship.

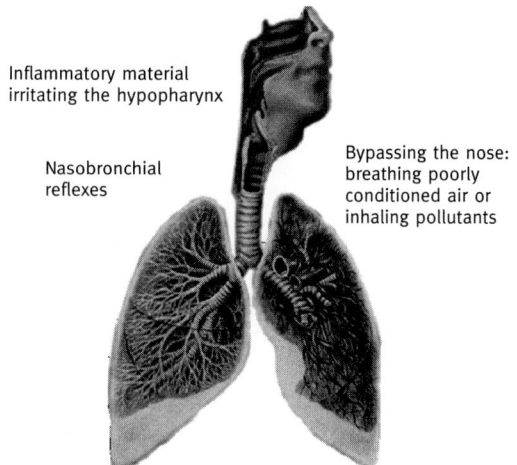

FIGURE 18.3 Postulated mechanisms by which the upper airway may affect the lower airway. See Color Plate 7 in insert.

Another way to address the interactions between AR and asthma is to assess the impact of treatment on AR. Systemic treatments affect physiologic processes in both the upper and lower airways, making interpretation of any effect on one airway versus the other somewhat difficult. INSs have had a variable impact on asthma.[47] Some studies suggest that they have an impact on seasonal exacerbations and bronchial hyperresponsiveness and that treatment with INS seems to decrease emergency department visits for asthma. An ongoing trial of asthmatic subjects randomized to either placebo or an INS may provide a more definitive answer about the utility of INS in the treatment of asthma.

Surgical intervention for chronic sinusitis and subsequent improvement in asthma suggests that improvement of upper airway disease positively affects lower airway disease.[48]

Sleep

The impact of AR on sleep, which includes trouble falling asleep, difficulty staying asleep, and not feeling that one has had a good night's sleep, is a major problem. Microarousal during sleep caused by nasal obstruction contributes to sleep-associated problems. Problems with sleep negatively affect QOL, and treatment with INS helps correct sleep disturbances in patients who have AR. Nasal obstruction and hence AR contribute minimally to sleep apnea.[49]

Acute and Chronic Sinusitis

Allergic inflammation appears to contribute to the pathogenesis of both acute and chronic rhinosinusitis.[48] Data from a number of clinical studies support this association even though no adequately controlled studies have been conducted on the incidence of chronic rhinosinusitis in patients with AR. Patients undergoing sinus surgery are found to have an incidence of atopy between 50% and 94%; however, these data are confounded by referral pattern bias. Nevertheless, they suggest a significant clinical overlap between AR and chronic rhinosinusitis.

Complementing these findings are studies showing a high prevalence of sinus disease in patients with AR. For example, 60% of subjects with rhinitis due to ragweed during the pollen season have sinus mucosal abnormalities as demonstrated on computed tomography scan.[50] Analysis by other means, such as magnetic resonance imaging, also demonstrates increased evidence of sinus mucosal abnormalities during major pollinating seasons.

Savolainen found the incidence of allergy to be 25% in a group of 224 patients who had acute maxillary rhinosinusitis, which was significantly greater than the 16% incidence in a control group.[51] Holzmann and colleagues reported an increased prevalence of AR in children who had orbital complications of acute rhinosinusitis, and these complications occurred especially during pollinating seasons.[52] Chen and colleagues found the prevalence of rhinosinusitis to be significantly higher in children with AR than in children without allergy in a study involving 8,723 children.[53]

Another example of a link between allergy and chronic rhinosinusitis is found in data correlating the severity of disease, as documented by imaging techniques, with markers of allergy, including eosinophilia and specific IgE to inhalant allergens.[54] A follow-up study shows a highly significant correlation between peripheral eosinophil counts and extent of sinus disease. These data suggest that sinus inflammation, documented by imaging, correlates with known mediators of allergic inflammation.

There are few data on the mechanisms by which AR increases susceptibility to chronic rhinosinusitis. The classic explanation is that AR alters sinus physiology, leading to ostial obstruction. Blockage then prevents normal drainage and ventilation of the sinuses, causing accumulation of mucus, serum transudation, and decreased oxygenation with resultant impairment of mucociliary transport, stasis of secretions, and susceptibility to bacterial overgrowth.

The direct effects of pollen on the sinus mucosa, because of problems of access to the paranasal sinuses, are conceptually difficult to understand. Mucociliary transport carries mucus out of the sinuses; thus, allergens deposited near the sinus ostia would be cleared away from the sinuses, into the nose. Fungal spores and hyphae, however, are found in sinuses, suggesting that mucosal sinus inflammation could be a direct response to these allergens. A study that gives support to the theory that material from the nasal passages can reach the sinuses demonstrates that contrast material instilled into the nasopharynx could be insufflated into the sinuses by blowing the nose.[55]

Studies linking viral infection to airway disease support the theory that these infections predispose to chronic mucosal inflammation. Buchman and colleagues showed that allergy is associated with viral upper respiratory tract infections and causes asthma exacerbation.[56] Like shared environmental exposures, viral responses in the upper and lower airways may explain the epidemiologic data linking these two airways.

Inflammatory cells and their mediators orchestrate the inflammatory and immunologic responses in both chronic rhinosinusitis and AR. Similar perturbations of the immune system by both diseases could explain this association. Allergic rhinitis and chronic rhinosinusitis share similar inflammatory cell infiltrates (e.g., eosinophils, mast cells, and T lymphocytes), the major effector cells in both diseases. Eosinophils, known to be involved in allergic inflammation, are the predominant inflammatory cell in patients with chronic rhinosinusitis.

Lymphocytes are important components of the inflammatory cells found in chronic rhinosinusitis. Helper T cells contribute to the pathophysiology of both AR and chronic rhinosinusitis. The involvement of T lymphocytes in sinus inflammation suggests that polarization of these cells into T_H1 and T_H2 effectors may influence disease expression. For example, T_H2 polarization may be associated with nasal polyps, whereas T_H1 is associated with chronic sinusitis without polyps. However, the similarities in the variety of different cells found in the repertoire of immune responses implicated in allergic disease and in chronic rhinosinusitis suggests that similar mechanisms may be involved in the pathology of both diseases.

UNMET, FUTURE RESEARCH NEEDS

1. Understanding the contribution of the multiple inflammatory cascades described in allergic pathophysiology will help direct avenues for new treatments. An example of how understanding pathophysiology affects disease management is the role of neural involvement in the development of the ocular symptoms of AR.

2. It is also important to determine whether AR is a heterogeneous disease with multiple endotypes. Current treatment paradigms work on the assumption that AR is a homogeneous disease with a single pathophysiology.

3. From a diagnostic perspective, it is easy to determine who has a positive in vivo or in vitro allergy test. The challenge is to determine the role of allergy in the patient's disease.

4. Many more patients have positive skin tests than have AR. An important question is the reverse of the prior statement. In how many patients with symptoms of rhinitis and a positive skin test are the results of the skin test relevant to the symptoms? Moving from the treatment of isolated disease to the treatment of comorbidities, the topic of this book, it must be understood whether AR and asthma are comorbid conditions one with the other and how these two diseases interrelate and share inflammatory responses, especially to environmental allergens and substances. When this link is better understood, more rational treatment strategies can be devised for patients with both diseases.

CONCLUSION

Allergic rhinitis is both the most common atopic disease and comorbid condition of asthma. It can be seasonal or perennial or intermittent versus persistent. It is an IgE mediated disease and presents with the following symptoms: sneezing, rhinorrhea, and nasal itching and congestion. Allergic rhinitis predisposes to the pathogenesis of both acute and chronic rhinosinusitis, also comorbid conditions of asthma. Treatment of allergic rhinitis primarily consists of avoidance, use of antihistamines, decongestants, intranasal glucocorticosteroids and antihistamines, and allergen immunotherapy.

REFERENCES

1. Meltzer EO, Blaiss MS, Naclerio RM, et al. Burden of allergic rhinitis: allergies in America, Latin America, and Asia-Pacific adult surveys. *Allergy Asthma Proc.* 2012;33:S113–S141.
2. Bousquet J, Schünemann HJ, Zuberbier T, et al., in collaboration with the WHO Collaborating Center of Asthma and Rhinitis (Montpellier). Development and implementation of guidelines in allergic rhinitis: an ARIA-GA²LEN paper. *Allergy.* 2010;65:1212–1221.
3. Arbes SJ Jr, Gergen PJ, Elliott L, Zeldin DC. Prevalences of positive skin test responses to 10 common allergens in the US population: results from the third National Health and Nutrition Examination Survey. *J Allergy Clin Immunol.* 2005;116:377–383.
4. Moscato G, Vandenplas O, Van Wijk RG, et al., for the European Academy of Allergology and Clinical Immunology. EAACI position paper on occupational rhinitis. *Respir Res.* 2009;10:16.
5. Min Y-G. The pathophysiology, diagnosis and treatment of allergic rhinitis. *Allergy Asthma Immunol Res.* 2010;2(2):65–76.

6. Baroody FM, Naclerio RM. Immunology of the upper airway pathophysiology and treatment of allergic rhinitis. In: Flint PW, Haughey BH, Lund VJ, et al., eds. *Otolaryngology—Head and Neck Surgery.* 5th ed. Philadelphia: Mosby Elsevier; 2010:597–623.
7. Pawankar R, Okuda M, Yssel H, et al. Nasal mast cells in perennial allergic rhinitis exhibit increased expression of the FcepsilonRI, CD40L, IL-4, and IL-13, and can induce IgE synthesis in B cells. *J Clin Invest.* 1997;99: 1492–1499.
8. Pawankar R, Ra C. IgE-FC epsilonRI-mast cell axis in the allergic cycle. *Clin Exp Allergy.* 1998;3:6–14.
9. Durham SR, Gould HJ, Hamid QA. Local IgE production in nasal allergy. *Int Arch Allergy Immunol.* 1997;113:128–130.
10. Pawankar R, Yamagishi S, Yagi T. Revisiting the roles of mast cells in allergic rhinitis and its relation to local IgE synthesis. *Am J Rhinol.* 2000;14:309–317.
11. Yamaguchi M, Sayama K, Yano K, et al. IgE enhances Fc epsilon receptor I expression and IgE-dependent release of histamine and lipid mediators from human umbilical cord blood-derived mast cells: synergistic effect of IL-4 and IgE on human mast cell Fc epsilon receptor I expression and mediator release. *J Immunol.* 1999;162:5455–5465.
12. Takizawa R, Pawankar R, Yamagishi S, Takenaka H, Yagi T. Increased expression of HLA-DR and CD86 in nasal epithelial cells in allergic rhinitis: antigen presentation to T cells and up-regulation by diesel exhaust particles. *Clin Exp Allergy.* 2007;37:420–423.
13. Pawankar R. Epithelial cells as immunoregulators in allergic airway diseases. *Curr Opin Allergy Clin Immunol.* 2002;2:1–5.
14. Baroody FM, Naclerio RM. Nasal-ocular reflexes and their role in the management of allergic rhinoconjunctivitis with intranasal steroids. *World Allergy Org.* 2011;4:S1–S5.
15. Wachs M, Proud D, Lichtenstein LM, Kagey-Sobotka A, Norman PS, Naclerio RM. Observations on the pathogenesis of nasal priming. *J Allergy Clin Immunol.* 1989;84:492–501.
16. Walden SM, Proud D, Lichtenstein LM, Kagey-Sobotka A, Naclerio RM. Antigen-provoked increase in histamine reactivity: observations on mechanisms. *Am Rev Respir Dis.* 1991;143:642–648.
17. Rael E, Ramey J, Lockey RF. Oxymetazoline hydrochloride combined with mometasone nasal spray for persistent nasal congestion (pilot study). *WAO J.* 2011;4(3):65–67.
18. Baroody FM, Brown D, Gavanescu L, DeTineo M, Naclerio RM. Oxymetazoline adds to the effectiveness of fluticasone furoate in the treatment of perennial allergic rhinitis. *J Allergy Clin Immunol.* 2011;127:927–934.
19. Sahin-Yilmaz A, Naclerio RM. Allergic rhinitis. In: Snow JB, Wackym PA, eds. *Ballenger's Otorhinolaryngology Head and Neck Surgery.* 17th ed. Shelton, CT: BC Decker, People's Medical Publishing House; 2009:531–550.
20. Kaszuba SM, Baroody FM, deTineo M, Haney L, Blair C, Naclerio RM. Superiority of an intranasal corticosteroid compared to an oral antihistamine in the as needed treatment of seasonal allergic rhinitis. *Arch Intern Med.* 2001;161:2581–2587.
21. Berger WE, Mohar DE, LaForce C, et al. A 26-week tolerability study of ciclesonide nasal aerosol in patients with perennial allergic rhinitis. *Am J Rhinol Allergy.* 2012;26(4):302–307.
22. Meltzer EO, Jacobs RL, LaForce CF, Kelley CL, Dunbar SA, Tantry SK. Safety and efficacy of once-daily treatment with beclomethasone dipropionate nasal aerosol in subjects with perennial allergic rhinitis. *Allergy Asthma Proc.* 2012;33(3):249–257.
23. Baroody FM, Cheng C-C, Moylan B, et al. Fluticasone propionate aqueous nasal spray does not lead to nasal mucosal atrophy. *Arch Otolaryngol Head Neck Surg.* 2001;127:193–199.
24. Grainger CI, Saunders M, Buttini F, et al. Critical characteristics for corticosteroid solution metered dose inhaler bioequivalence. *Mol Pharm.* 2012;9(3):563–569.
25. Kelly HW, Sternberg AL, Lescher R, et al., for the CAMP Research Group. Effect of inhaled glucocorticoids in childhood on adult height. *N Engl J Med.* 2012;367(10):904–912.
26. Fluticasone Furoate nasal spray (VERAMYST) long term pediatric growth study. ClinicalTrials.gov Identifier: NCT00570492.
27. Meltzer EO, LaForce C, Ratner P, Price D, Ginsberg D, Carr W. MP29-02 (a novel intranasal formulation of azelastine hydrochloride and fluticasone propionate) in the treatment of seasonal allergic rhinitis: a randomized, double-blind, placebo-controlled trial of efficacy and safety. *Allergy Asthma Proc.* 2012;33(4):324–332.
28. Naclerio R. Anticholinergic drugs in nonallergic rhinitis. *WAO J.* 2009;2:162–165.
29. Chauhan B, Patel M, Padhc H, Nivsarkar M. Combination therapeutic approach for asthma and allergic rhinitis. *Curr Clin Pharmacol.* 2008;3(3):185–197.
30. Esteitie R, deTineo M, Naclerio RM, Baroody FM. Effect of the addition of montelukast to

fluticasone propionate for the treatment of perennial allergic rhinitis. *Ann Allergy Asthma Immunol.* 2010;105:155–161.
31. Canonica GW, Bousquet J, Casale T, et al., eds. WAO Position Paper on sublingual immunotherapy. *WAO J.* 2009;22(11):223–281.
32. Cox L, Nelson H, Lockey RF, eds. Allergen immunotherapy: a practice parameter third update. *J Allergy Clin Immunol.* 2011;127(1):S1–S55.
33. Naclerio R, Baroody F. What has the relief of allergic conjunctivitis by intranasal steroids taught us about the pathophysiology of allergic rhinoconjunctivitis? *Clin Exp Allergy Rev.* 2009;9:11–17.
34. Baroody FB, Foster KA, Markaryan A, deTineo M, Naclerio RM. Nasal-ocular reflexes contribute to eye symptoms in patients with allergic rhinitis. *Ann Allergy Asthma Immunol.* 2008;100:194–199.
35. Baroody FM, Shenaq D, DeTineo M, Wang J, Naclerio RM. Fluticasone furoate nasal spray reduces the nasal ocular reflex: a mechanism for the efficacy of topical steroids in controlling allergic eye symptoms. *J Allergy Clin Immunol.* 2009;123:1342–1348.
36. O'Meara TJ, Sercombe JK, Morgan G, Reddel HK, Xuan W, Tovey ER. The reduction of rhinitis symptoms by nasal filters during natural exposure to ragweed and grass pollen. *Allergy.* 2005;60:529–532.
37. Kaiser HD, Naclerio RM, Given J, Toler TN, Ellsworth A, Philpot EE. Fluticasone furoate nasal spray: a single treatment option for the symptoms of seasonal allergic rhinitis. *J Allergy Clin Immunol.* 2007;119:1430–1437.
38. Bernstein JA, Alexis N, Barnes C, et al. Health effects of air pollution. *J Allergy Clin Immunol.* 2004;114(5):1116–1123.
39. Boushey HA. Air pollution. In: Getchell TV, Nadel JA, eds. *Textbook of Respiratory Medicine*, Vol. 1, 2nd ed. Philadelphia: WB Saunders; 1994:2032–2045.
40. Garrett MH, Hooper MA, Hooper BM. Respiratory symptoms in children and indoor exposure to nitrogen dioxide and gas stoves. *Am J Respir Crit Care Med.* 1998;158(3):891–895.
41. Saxon A, Diaz-Sanchez D. Air pollution and allergy: you are what you breathe. *Nat Immunol.* 2005;6(3):223–226.
42. Peden DB, Setzer RW Jr., Devlin RB. Ozone exposure has both a priming effect on allergen-induced responses and an intrinsic inflammatory action in the nasal airways of perennially allergic asthmatics. *Am J Respir Crit Care Med.* 1995;151(5):1336–1345.
43. Koenig JQ, Morgan MS, Horike M, et al. The effects of sulfur oxides on nasal and lung function in adolescents with extrinsic asthma. *J Allergy Clin Immunol.* 1985;76(6):813–818.
44. National Cancer Institute. *Smoking and tobacco control monograph 10: Health effects of exposure to environmental tobacco smoke.* Bethesda, MD: NCI; 1999. Retrieved August 30, 2004, from http://cancercontrol.cancer.gov/tcrb/monographs/10/index.html.
45. Naclerio RM. Immune effector cells and their mediators in the pathogenesis of rhinitis. Immunobiology of asthma and rhinitis: pathogenic factors and therapeutic options. American Thoracic Society Workshop Summary. *Am J Respir Crit Care Med.* 1999;160:1778–1787.
46. Braunstahl GJ, Fokkens WJ, Overbeek SE, Klein Jan A, Hoogsteden HC, Prins JB. Mucosal and systemic inflammatory changes in allergic rhinitis and asthma: a comparison between upper and lower airways. *Clin Exp Allergy.* 2003;33(5):579–587.
47. Schenkel EJ, Berger WE. Treatment of allergic rhinitis with intranasal steroids and their effects on the lower airway. *Pediatr Ann.* 2000;29(7):422–424.
48. Pinto JM, Naclerio RM. Environmental and allergic factors in chronic rhinosinusitis. In: Hamilos DL, Baroody FM, eds. *Chronic Rhinosinusitis.* New York: Taylor and Francis; 2007:25–49.
49. Lunn M, Craig T. Rhinitis and sleep. *Sleep Med Rev.* 2011;15(5):293–299.
50. Naclerio RM, deTineo Marcella, Baroody FM. Ragweed allergic rhinitis and the paranasal sinuses: a CT scan study. *Arch Otolaryngol Head Neck Surg.* 1997;123:193–196.
51. Savolainen S. Allergy in patients with acute maxillary sinusitis. *Allergy.* 1989;44(2):116–122.
52. Holzmann D, Willi U, Nadal D. Allergic rhinitis as a risk factor for orbital complication of acute rhinosinusitis in children. *Am J Rhinol.* 2001;15(6);387–390.
53. Chen CF, Wu KG, Hsu MC, et al. Prevalence and relationship between allergic diseases and infectious diseases. *J Microbiol Immunol Infect.* 2001;34(1):57–62.
54. Newman LJ, Platts-Mills TA, Phillips C, et al. Chronic sinusitis: relationship of computed tomography findings to allergy, asthma, and eosinophilia. *JAMA.* 1994;271(5):363–367.
55. Gwaltney JM, Hendley JO, Phillips CD, et al. Nose blowing propels nasal fluid into the paranasal sinuses. *Clin Infect Dis.* 2000;30(2):387–391.
56. Buchman CA, Doyle WJ, Pilcher O, et al. Nasal and otologic effects of experimental respiratory syncytial virus infection in adults. *Am J Otolaryngol.* 2002;23(2):70–75.

19

NONALLERGIC RHINOPATHIES AND LOWER AIRWAY SYNDROMES

COMORBID

James N. Baraniuk, Michael S. Blaiss, and Debendra Pattanaik

KEY POINTS

- Nonallergic rhinitis is a heterogeneous disease consisting of a wide variety of entities that present with persistent nasal symptoms.
- Idiopathic nonallergic rhinopathy, previously known as "vasomotor rhinitis," is the most common form of nonallergic rhinitis.
- Among rhinitis patients, the prevalence of nonallergic rhinitis is about 20% to 40%, and it is more common among adults and has a female predominance.
- Nonallergic rhinitis is a significant risk factor for the development of bronchial hyperresponsiveness and asthma. Several large epidemiologic and cohort studies confirm that the risk for asthma increases by two- to three-fold among nonallergic rhinitis patients.
- Autonomic dysfunction, entopy (local immune response not detectable by systemic testing), and changes in nasal microbiome are important pathophysiologic mechanisms involved in nonallergic rhinitis.
- Persistent and perennial nasal congestion, postnasal drip, facial pressure, and throat clearing are classic symptoms. These symptoms are often triggered by nonspecific environmental agents.
- History and physical examination in the presence of negative skin prick test or serum-specific immunoglobulin E confirms the diagnosis of nonallergic rhinitis. Detailed analysis of coexisting secondary diseases, local nasal structural abnormalities, and concomitant medications can help one arrive at the diagnosis.
- Lifestyle modifications, including avoidance of smoking and other known triggering factors, can play an essential role in symptom relief.
- Topical nasal corticosteroids are effective in a subset of nonallergic rhinitis patients

associated with nasal eosinophilia. They are not effective in relieving rhinorrhea or nasal congestion triggered by nonspecific stimuli.
- Topical antihistamines, such as azelastine, and the anticholinergic agent ipratropium bromide, can also be useful in selected patients with nasal congestion and rhinorrhea.
- Other agents, such as menthol and topical capsaicin, hold promise for the future.

INTRODUCTION

"United airways" has become a slogan verging on dogma. The concept gained momentum with the realization that the unifying atopic pathophysiology of the nose and tracheobronchial tree leads to coexistent allergic rhinitis (AR) and allergic asthma, respectively. Including non-allergic mechanisms in the differential diagnosis of comorbid rhinitides with reversible and irreversible lower airway obstructive entities is more problematic (Table 19.1).[1] Although the nose and foregut-derived tracheobronchial tree have distinct embryonic origins, they share exposure to air, pseudostratified epithelium with extensive submucosal glands, common elements of the innate and acquired mucosal immune systems, and extensive nociceptive

Table 19.1. One Airway, One Disease?

DIFFERENTIAL DIAGNOSIS OF RHINITIS	BRONCHIAL EQUIVALENT (?) / ASTHMA
Atopy	
Extrinsic rhinitis	"Extrinsic Asthma"
T_H2 lymphocytes, IgE, mast cells, eosinophils	
Allergic rhinitis	Allergic asthma
Inflammation, Mucosal Hyperresponsiveness, Reversible Airways Obstruction	
Nonallergic rhinitis with inflammation	"Intrinsic Asthmas"
Nonallergic rhinitis with eosinophilia syndrome (NARES)	Nonallergic asthma with eosinophilia syndrome; eosinophilic bronchitis
Chronic rhinosinusitis with polyposis	Triad asthma or aspirin exacerbated respiratory disease
Nonresponsive rhinosinusitis?	Steroid-dependent asthma
± Polyposis?	Churg-Strauss syndrome variant?
Viral rhinitis	Viral bronchitis
Bacterial rhinosinusitis	Acute/chronic bronchitis; bronchiectasis
Anaphylaxis	Acute sudden death
Reactive upper airway dysfunction syndrome	Reactive airway disorder syndrome
Nonallergic rhinitis without inflammation	Bronchial hyperresponsiveness?
Vasomotor rhinitis	Irritant airways
Irritant rhinitis	Chronic cough
Multiple chemical sensitivity syndrome	Chemical sensitivity
Fundamental Difference in Approach	
SPLITTERS	LUMPERS
Primary pathology of rhinitis syndromes	Final common pathway to bronchospasm
The rhinitides	The asthmas
Allergic Rhinobronchitis?	

and autonomic nervous system sensors and controls. Mechanisms affecting both anatomic sites are likely to develop comorbid disease. Anatomic differences contribute to discrete pathologic conditions as allowed by the boney box of the nasal cavity versus the cartilaginous walls and elastic alveolar interstitial tethers for bronchi and bronchioles. The diverse pathologic states of the nasal mucosa and their relationships with bronchial hyperresponsiveness are the focus of the remainder of this discussion.

CLINICAL FEATURES

The tendency to group all rhinitides having negative skin tests and the absence of nasal eosinophilia into one nonallergic rhinitis (NAR) classification for comparison with AR leads to a heterogeneous presentation and epidemiology. NAR is prevalent in younger pediatric age groups but is often described as having an adult onset with a female predominance.[2] Symptoms are generally persistent and dominated by nasal congestion, facial pressure, rhinorrhea, postnasal drip, and throat clearing with cough.[3] Specific pollen exposures do not cause symptoms.[4] However, seasonal exacerbations in NAR may result from shifts in temperature, humidity, barometric pressure, or airborne particulate loads (e.g., smoke from burning stubble or other fires, other pollution).[5] This mucosal irritant sensitivity may be confused with seasonal allergic reactivity. By comparison, AR patients experience more pruritus of the nose, conjunctivae, and palate as well as sneezing and rhinorrhea.[3,6-8] Cyclic allergen-induced mast cell degranulation can lead to large variations in these symptoms and in the magnitude of nasal airflow obstruction as measured by peak nasal inspiratory flow rates. AR is associated with elevated nasal eosinophil counts and beneficial clinical response to antihistamines. Both NAR and severe AR are associated with decreased quality of life.[9]

The two major NAR symptoms occur on a spectrum of "runners," who have wet rhinorrhea, to "blockers," who have nasal congestion and blockage to airflow with minimal rhinorrhea.[7] Rhinorrhea patients generally have enhanced cholinergic glandular secretory responses[10] and benefit from anticholinergic drugs. Blockers complain of subjective fullness that may be related to interoceptive and nociceptive mucosal neuron hypersensitivity to innocuous stimuli.[7] This dichotomy may only explain the ends of the spectrum and not the congestion plus rhinorrhea experienced by most NAR subjects. Intermittent symptoms may be triggered by cold air exposures, ingestion of certain foods or beverages, irritant chemicals, strong emotions, and changes in menstrual and other hormone levels.[4] An important caveat is that complaints of nasal fullness may not be confirmed by objective congestion with obstruction to nasal airflow, especially in children.[11,12]

Physical examination of the upper airways may show swollen erythematous turbinates in NAR, compared with pale swollen turbinates present in AR patients. Nasal secretions may vary from clear to mucoid, but colored discharge is more likely an indication of underlying infection. Abnormal nasal physical findings are more common in categories of NAR secondary to structural abnormalities, eosinophilic rhinitis, vasculitis, granulomatous infection, and autoimmune disorders. Nasal crusting, widening of the nares, and a foul odor may indicate atrophic rhinitis.

DIAGNOSIS

The patient's history must be consistent with nasal complaints, such as histamine-related pruritus and sneezing, that suggest AR or persistent congestion and rhinorrhea when exposed to environmental tobacco smoke, odorants, cleaning compounds, or changes in air temperature or barometric pressure, more typical of NAR. The critical discriminating factor is negative skin and serologic tests for relevant allergens in NAR. After atopy is excluded, it is necessary to investigate the history further for clues into the differential diagnosis of NAR. Because the mechanisms contributing to NAR may also be present in AR, it is possible to have antihistamine- and glucocorticoid-resistant AR that is termed *mixed rhinitis*.[2]

Questionnaires may assist in distinguishing between AR and NAR. Patients with symptom onset after age 35 years, a positive history of symptoms induced by perfumes and fragrances, and a negative history of seasonality, cat-induced, or familial rhinitis symptoms have a more than 95% likelihood of having NAR.[13] The Cincinnati Irritant Index Scale rates 21 different irritants from 0 (no symptoms) to 10 (severe symptoms) for upper respiratory symptoms and headaches.[14] The irritant triggers are ammonia, antiperspirants, bleach, cold air, cooking and frying odors, cosmetics, crude oils, fresh newsprints, hairsprays, smog, cleaning products, mildew odors, paints, perfumes, pine odor, soap powders, solvents, varnish, weather changes, tobacco smoke, and wood smoke. This questionnaire identifies irritant sensitivity but will not identify NAR patients when an irritant is not involved. Nasal provocation with irritants and measurements of changes in acoustic rhinometry, nasal inspiratory peak flows, or anterior rhinomanometry may be useful and analogous to bronchial provocations.

Cold dry air (CDA) causes nasal obstruction in both NAR and AR subjects but has no significant dose-dependent effects on nonrhinitic persons.[15,16] Nasal responses include rhinorrhea, decreased peak nasal inspiratory flow, and reduced minimal cross-sectional area by acoustic rhinometry.[17] CDA provocation in environmental challenge chambers permits investigation of the specific mechanisms responsible for the mucosal responses in NAR.[18] As with sensitivity to irritants, NAR subjects who are most sensitive to cold weather or air conditioning tend to respond the most during CDA provocation. Weather, temperature, and CDA-sensitive NAR may be refractory to topical nasal glucocorticoid treatment.[18] The occupational exposure of working in a cold storage facility can induce rhinitis, sore throat, cough, and bronchial hyperresponsiveness.[19] It is not known whether chemical coolants or other airborne irritants contribute to the airway changes. Cold air in the nasal cavity can activate cold-sensitive receptors that generate reflex-mediated bronchoconstriction in asthmatic patients.[20]

This raises a critical issue: does epidemiologic evidence link syndromes of NAR to asthma and bronchoconstriction? It is important to establish the prevalences of AR, NAR, and specific lung diseases in order to identify risk factors and shared pathophysiologic mechanisms. The prevalence of NAR was 8% at age 4 years and decreased to 6% by age 8 years in a birth cohort of 2,024 Swedish children.[21] Seven-year-old children from Denmark were assessed for rhinitis symptoms, positive skin tests or other evidence of atopy, and bronchial hyperresponsiveness.[22] Rhinitis was present in 105 subjects, with no symptoms in 185 others. Systemic allergy and AR were present in 36% and NAR in 64% of the subjects. Asthma was diagnosed in 21% of AR, 20% of NAR, and 5% of nonrhinitis control children. AR was distinguished by bronchial hyperresponsiveness, higher end expiratory nitric oxide levels (FeNO), eczema and other systemic manifestations of atopy, and greater itch and watery discharge with allergen exposure. Danish adults with positive rhinitis questionnaires had allergy tests that identified 77% as AR and 23% as NAR.[3] Note that the relative rate of AR to NAR changed from about 1:2 in children to 3:1 in adults. NAR was associated with female gender (odds ratio [OR] = 2.05 [1.31 to 3.20]; 95% confidence interval [CI]; P = .002), persistent symptoms within the last 4 weeks (OR = 1.88 [1.23 to 2.89]; P = .003), and recurring headaches (OR = 1.94 [1.12 to 3.37]; P = .019).[3] However, NAR subjects were less likely than AR patients to have airway hyperresponsiveness (OR = 0.40 [0.24 to 0.66]; P < .001) or food allergy (OR = 0.40 [0.19 to 0.36]; P = .009). Asthma was found in 33% of AR patients. Again, NAR and AR subjects had equivalent congestion and rhinorrhea, whereas AR subjects had more allergen-associated itch and sneezing. Other reports suggest that 70% of NAR cases occur in adults, with prevalences as high as 20% to 40% in some industrialized countries. A case series of 686 patients attending a Portuguese allergy clinic identified NAR in 28% and found that asthma was more frequent in NAR than AR.[23]

The OR for asthma in Danish adults with NAR was 2.51 (1.87 to 3.37).[24] In addition, they were also at risk for chronic bronchitis (OR = 2.27 [1.85 to 2.79]) and had decreased ratios of forced expiratory volume in 1 second

(FEV$_1$) to forced vital capacity (FVC), or FEV1/FVC, and decreased FEV$_1$ values. The association with chronic bronchitis was greater for NAR than AR, and with asthma it was greater for AR than NAR.

A case series of 108 subjects with more than 4 weeks of rhinitis complaints in Turin, Italy, found AR in 39%, NAR in 21%, and chronic rhinosinusitis (CRS) in 40%.[25] Asthma was diagnosed in 33% of AR, 9% of NAR, and 40% of CRS subjects. Both the AR and CRS groups had significantly elevated exhaled NO levels, suggesting ongoing bronchial inflammation.

The European Community Respiratory Health Survey assessed the incidence of asthma in AR and NAR adults over an 8.8-year period.[26] New cases of asthma were diagnosed by physicians. Atopy was defined by skin test positivity to mites, cat, *Alternaria*, *Cladosporium*, grass, birch, *Parietaria*, olive, or ragweed. The cumulative incidence of asthma was 2.2% overall. Incidences were 1.1% in adult controls, 1.9% with atopy only, 3.1% in NAR, and 4.0% for AR. After controlling for country, gender, baseline age, body mass index, FEV$_1$, log total immunoglobulin E (IgE), family history of asthma, and smoking, the adjusted relative risk for asthma was 2.71 (1.64 to 4.46) for NAR, 3.53 (2.11 to 5.91) for AR, and 1.63 (0.82 to 3.24) for atopy without rhinitis. Further analysis indicates an even stronger association of NAR and asthma (OR = 11.6; 95% CI = 6.2 to 21.9).[27]

The Tucson Epidemiologic Study of Obstructive Lung Disease supported this finding. AR and NAR each increased the risk for asthma three-fold after stratification of other variables.[28] Subjects with more widespread irritant rhinitis complaints are more likely to have asthma.[29]

These studies have several important implications. Rhinitis, even in the absence of atopy, was a predictor of adult-onset asthma. Asthmatic symptoms do not differentiate between AR and NAR.[6] The rate of AR to NAR based on systemic measures of atopy increased from children to adults, suggesting a potential transition of NAR to AR or high incidence of new cases of AR in adults.[30] Development of bronchial hyperresponsiveness may be more closely linked to atopic helper T-cell type 2 (T$_H$2)–IgE–mast cell and CRS eosinophilic inflammatory mechanisms compared with the broad spectrum of other mechanisms in NAR. CRS phenotypes and the severity of bronchial hyperresponsiveness may depend on the pathogenic mechanisms responsible for polyposis, glandular hypertrophy, aspirin/NSAID sensitivity, humoral immunodeficiency, eosinophilia, and atopy and their expression in both the nasal and bronchial mucosa.

DIFFERENTIAL DIAGNOSIS

There are numerous causes of nasal symptoms with negative allergy tests (NAR).[31] Although specific case designation criteria are not developed, many types can be identified by their unique features through a detailed history and physician examination. This process is often an algorithm to guide potential therapies. The most prevalent form of NAR remains idiopathic nonallergic rhinopathy (iNAR, 60%), a condition defined by what it is not: nonallergic, noneosinophilic, and noninfectious.[32] Formerly known as vasomotor rhinitis, it is associated with little evidence to support any vascular, neuromotor, secretory, or other pathophysiologic mechanism. Without the legitimacy of specific affirmative diagnostic criteria, biomarkers, or regulatory recognition (e.g., U.S. Food and Drug Administration), iNAR has remained a clinical challenge. A broader approach proposes that iNAR is part of a spectrum of "functional" interoceptive mucosal dysregulation disorders. This perspective requires assessing the entire patient instead of that portion visible through a rhinoscope. Exclusions based on the specific settings and mechanisms of infectious, occupational, hormonal, drug-induced, gustatory, and other cholinergic forms of NAR further restricts the scope of iNAR.[33]

The remainder of the differential includes NAR with eosinophilia syndrome (NARES) (≥5% nasal eosinophilia, 33% of cases), CRS (16%), "hidden allergy" with elevated IgE to unknown allergens (12%), blood eosinophilic nonallergic rhinitis syndrome (BENARS) (4%), and hypothyroidism (2%).[34] This differential diagnosis suggests that rhinitis can be classified by pathophysiologic mechanisms and

Table 19.2. Differential Diagnosis of Eosinophil—Predominant Rhinopathies

Nonallergic rhinitis with eosinophilia syndrome (NARES)
Blood eosinophil with nonallergic rhinitis syndrome (BENARS)
Chronic eosinophilic sinusitis syndromes
Chronic rhinosinusitis with nasal polyposis and eosinophilia
Aspirin/nonsteroidal antiinflammatory drug (NSAID) sensitivity
Triad asthma of reversible airflow obstruction, chronic rhinosinusitis with nasal polyps, and NSAID sensitivity
Fungal sinusitis syndromes
Occupational rhinitis with eosinophilia (non-IgE mediated)
Churg-Strauss syndrome with eosinophilic granuloma
Eosinophilic granuloma

the predominant effector leukocytes recruited to the mucosa.[35] Many of the rhinitides have analogs in the bronchial tract (see Table 19.1) and are discussed elsewhere in this text.

Nonallergic eosinophilic mechanisms are active in NARES, BENARS, aspirin and nonsteroidal antiinflammatory drug sensitivity, and chronic eosinophilic fungal rhinosinusitis (Table 19.2). Nasal lavage interleukin-4 (IL-4), IL-6, and granulocyte colony-stimulating factor were increased in NARES compared with AR and NAR. Methacholine bronchial hyperresponsiveness was present in 46% of NARES patients who had a negative history of respiratory symptoms or asthma.[36] Bronchial hyperresponsiveness was associated with increased sputum eosinophils but not with the severity of the nasal inflammatory process. Nasal eosinophilia syndromes may be associated with the spectrum of eosinophilic bronchitis that encompasses cough variant asthma, chronic cough, episodic symptoms without asthma, and some cases of chronic obstructive pulmonary disease.[37]

Neutrophilic inflammation is typical of bacterial infection and may involve innate immune, complement, lipopolysaccharide, and lipotechoic acid–induced toll-like receptor pathway activation (Table 19.3). Necrotic-type damage to the nasal and tracheobronchial

Table 19.3. Differential Diagnosis of Neutrophil-Predominant Rhinopathies

Acute and recurrent bacterial rhinosinusitis
Nasal polyps in cystic fibrosis
HIV/AIDS-related infectious rhinosinusitis
Humoral immunodeficiencies of IgA, IgE, IgG subclasses and common variable hypogammaglobulinemia
Young's syndrome of sinopulmonary disease, azoospermia, and nasal polyps
Kartagener's syndrome of bronchiectasis, chronic sinusitis, nasal polyps and immotile cilia
Foreign body
Corrosive occupational rhinitis
Superantigen rhinitis with neutrophilia
Pollution-induced neutrophilic mucositis with epithelial and ciliary dysplasia (e.g., Mexico City children)

Table 19.4. Differential Diagnosis of Rhinopathies with Complex Cellular Infiltrates or Temporal Evolution of Inflammation

Common cold syndromes
Granulomatous and vasculitis diseases
    Wegener's granulomatosis
    Midline granuloma
    Sarcoidosis
Granulomatous infections
    Tuberculosis
    Leprosy
    Syphilis
Autoimmune disorders
    Relapsing polychondritis
    Systemic lupus erythematosus
    Sjögren's syndrome
Atrophic rhinitis
Postoperative denuded rhinopathy (no normal mucosa remaining)
Senile rhinitis
Ozena
Basophilic/metachromatic rhinitis
Chronic rhinosinusitis without nasal polyps due to glandular hypertrophy
Occupational toxic exposures leading to transient neutrophilia and persistent epithelial metaplasia

---

epithelium by pollutants (e.g., Mexico City children[38]), industrial chemicals, and other inhaled toxicants may release IL-8 and other neutrophilic chemokines and cause microvillous epithelial metaplasia. IL-8 is released from mucosal epithelial cells.[39]

Other cellular patterns evolve during the course of viral and autoimmune rhinitis (Table 19.4). For viral rhinitis, the typical signs and symptoms of an infection, such as low-grade fever and purulent nasal drainage in conjunction with a duration of less than 2 weeks, usually confirm the diagnosis. IL-11 may participate in the pathogenesis of viral rhinitis.[40] Children with common colds who have elevated IL-11 concentrations in their nasal secretions are more likely to develop asthma. The asthmatic subset has significantly increased IL-11 lavage levels over those who do not develop wheezing. Increased relative adenoid size is associated in childhood NAR with asthma, but the inflammatory mechanisms are not known.[41]

Basophilic rhinitis is thought to be rare because of the low numbers of metachromatic cells that are present in lavage fluid or scrapings. More detailed studies demonstrate surface basophilic cells in 5% of normal controls, 14% of patients with CRS without nasal polyps, 65% with nasal polyps, and 91% of AR.[42] Metachromatic cells are present in 80% of tracheotomized patients, 90% of patients with atrophic rhinitis, and 100% of patients with a tumor or irradiation treatment of the nasal cavity.

Occupational rhinitis reduces worker productivity.[43] It may be mediated by several mechanisms that are shared with occupational asthma.[44] Nasal provocations with some triggers generally give eosinophilic responses within 15 minutes, suggesting an atopic mechanism. Monitoring symptoms and nasal peak inspiratory flow in and out of the workplace is valuable to document cause and effect. The greatest risk for occupational rhinitis is among furriers, followed by bakers; livestock breeders; food-processing workers; veterinarians; farmers; assemblers of electrical, electronic, and telecommunication products; and boat builders.[45] Olfaction and sensory irritation are cofactors in the perception of air quality and can make it difficult to identify occupational triggers. This may be a particular problem in certain buildings where malodorants and irritants from fungal, bacterial, or other chemical sources can trigger the nasal sentinel function of NAR subjects.[46] Nasal obstruction has been induced by inhaling acetic acid vapor, ammonia, chlorine gas, environmental tobacco smoke, volatile organic compounds (VOCs), vapors from carbonless copy paper, and SO_2. Disrupted mucociliary clearance is observed with SO_2 and environmental tobacco smoke. Ozone and VOCs can induce neutrophilic inflammation. Lymphocytic occupational rhinitis has complex mechanisms with modulation of interferon-γ, T_H1, CD8+, and regulatory T lymphocytes in the tissue and peripheral blood.[47] Avoidance of the occupational trigger by modifying the workplace to decrease exposure, increasing ventilation, use of filtering masks, or removing the subject from the adverse exposure is beneficial.

Structural anomalies of cartilage atrophy and rhinophyma contribute to dysfunction of the anterior nasal valve and nasal fullness and obstruction to airflow (Table 19.5). Laxity of the fleshy, lateral nasal wall with collapse into the anterior nasal valve may contribute to obstructed airflow, particularly in elderly people.

Turbinate hypertrophy with submucosal thickening may be due to submucosal gland hyperplasia (CRS without nasal polyps),[48,49] or potentially interstitial connective tissue deposition. Despite being the rationale for many cases of surgical extirpation, the histopathology and mechanisms underlying the irreversible increase in turbinate volume are just beginning to be explored. If associated with sinusitis, this entity may be regarded as CRS without nasal polyps. Epidermal growth factor (erbB) proteins 1, 2, 3, and 4 are elevated in nasal glands and epithelial cells.[50] Glandular erbB1 is correlated with tissue eosinophilia, so it may be more important in NARES. Epithelial cell nerve growth factor is increased and brain-derived neurotrophic factor is decreased in CRS.[51] The hypertrophy recurs after surgery, although ultrasound ablation may promote the regrowth of healthy epithelium.[52] Postoperative nasal glucocorticoid lavage is a valuable adjunct to prevent recurrence.

Hormonal changes in pregnancy cause mucosal edema, nasal congestion, rhinorrhea, and sneezing in 20% to 40% of women (Table 19.6).[53] The onset can be at any time during gestation, with the 13th to 21st weeks being most problematic. Symptoms end precipitously with delivery of the baby or placenta. Numerous hormones may play roles, including prostaglandin H, vasoactive intestinal peptide, estrogen, progesterone, and relaxin. It likely that the combination leads to synergistic glandular exocytosis and vasodilation. The best treatments are saline irrigations, exercise, and mechanical alar dilators. Sympathomimetic decongestants provide only temporary relief.

Thyroid hormone is required for adrenergic receptor function. Thyroxine induces β_1 and β_2 receptors in many tissues. Hypothyroidism may be associated with mucosal vasodilation from the loss of sympathetic vasoconstrictor activity. Autoimmune thyroid disease may be present in 14.7% of NAR, 10.4% of AR, and 9.9% of adults, with a 2:1 female predominance.[54]

A detailed history of medication use and symptoms[55] is especially pertinent in patients using excessive amounts of topical decongestant nasal sprays in the absence of purulent sinusitis. Rhinitis medicamentosa continues to be a concern with prolonged use of high doses of topical α-adrenergic agonists. Symptoms begin with mild nasal stuffiness that initially responds to the drug.[56] However, rebound mucosal swelling develops when the decongestive effect has disappeared. In the face of continued perceptions of congestion, patients gradually start using larger doses at more frequent intervals. In many cases, the patient is unaware of the condition, thus entering a vicious cycle of self-treatment. Careful questioning may be required for diagnosis. The pathophysiology is not clear but may involve

Table 19.5. Differential Diagnosis of Nasal Structural Anomalies

Deviated septum with osteomeatal occlusion

Turbinate hypertrophy with increased connective tissue

Osteomeatal complex variants

Choanal atresia

Tumors (benign and neoplastic)

Adenoidal hypertrophy with recurrent infections

Loss of nasal cartilage with sagging of the nasal tip and deformation of the anterior nasal valve

Hypertrophy of fleshy components of the anterior nasal valve (e.g., rhinophyma)

Atrophic complications of excessive surgical excision of mucosa

Cerebrospinal fluid rhinorrhea

Table 19.6. Differential Diagnosis of Hormonal and Drug-Related Rhinopathies

Pregnancy (estrogen and progesterone)

Hypothyroidism

Acromegaly

β-Adrenergic antagonists

α-Adrenergic antagonists (reserpine, α-methyldopa, guanethidine, phentolamine, prazosin)

Phosphodiesterase inhibitors for erectile dysfunction

Rhinitis medicamentosa

Chronic topical α-adrenergic agonist abuse

Cocaine abuse

Chlorpromazine

Protease inhibitors

Angiotensin-converting enzyme inhibitors (ACEIs)

Dipeptidylpeptidase IV (DDP IV) inhibitors (sitagliptin)

---

vasodilation and edema. It is possible that subjects may have as yet undefined genetic risk factors leading to adrenergic receptor dysfunction. Management requires withdrawal of topical decongestants, treatment of the underlying rhinitis, and topical corticosteroids to reduce the rebound swelling. Symptoms are exacerbated by the preservative benzalkonium chloride, so treatments should avoid this chemical. Although the entity is a well-regarded clinical finding, this rebound hypersensitivity has been difficult to identify in prospective studies. Coadministration of oxymetazoline with a nasal glucocorticoid increases treatment effectiveness and reduces the likelihood of rhinitis medicamentosa.[57,58] Other medications linked to rhinitis include β-blockers, calcium channel blockers, and other antihypertensives. Nasal congestion can be a side effect of α-adrenoceptor antagonists used for benign prostatic hyperplasia and phosphodiesterase-5 inhibitors for erectile dysfunction.

Atrophic rhinitis is characterized by nasal crusting, widening of the passages in the nose, a foul smell, and the patient's loss of sense of smell. The progressive atrophy leads to the loss of the normal secretory and humidifying functions of the nose. The primary condition is linked to *Klebsiella ozaenae* infecting females at the time of puberty in arid countries. Secondary causes include overaggressive nasosinus surgery, radiation, trauma, and granulomatous and infectious diseases. A computed tomography scan commonly shows loss of the nasal turbinates in atrophic rhinitis.

"Entopy" is perhaps one of the most important and controversial new aspects of NAR. Entopy is the hypothesis that local nasal production of IgE and reactivity to allergens occur without systemic atopy.[59] This condition may explain intermittent seasonal and persistent NAR and glucocorticoid-responsive NAR subjects.[60] It is tempting to consider that a similar situation may develop in "intrinsic asthma." Previous studies on small nasal biopsies in very strictly defined perennial nonallergic rhinitis subjects who had been treated with glucocorticoids show no significant differences for nasal mucosal lymphocytes, antigen-presenting cells, macrophages, monocytes, mast cells, or other IgE-positive cells compared with nonrhinitic controls.[61–63] Only 2 of 65 had nasal eosinophilia.

Autonomic dysfunction is associated with iNAR.[64] This and other features may allow for positive diagnostic criteria rather than the current diagnosis by exclusion (Table 19.7). Symptoms of rhinorrhea and subjective fullness were similar to allergic rhinitis, but headache was more common and severe.[65] Discharge was more commonly watery than mucoid (71% vs. 29%). Half of the subjects reported bilateral nasal obstruction. Headaches may have migraine qualities[66] or midfacial pain syndrome that is more similar to tension-type headaches.[67] Patients describe nasal pressure, heaviness, or tightness and may say that their nostrils feel blocked even though there is no obstruction to nasal airflow or reduction in nasal airspace volumes. Regions of pain and tenderness to manual palpation[68] are generally symmetrical and affect the bridge of the nose and periorbital and maxillary regions. "Sinus headache" is a misnomer because this type of headache is defined by the presence

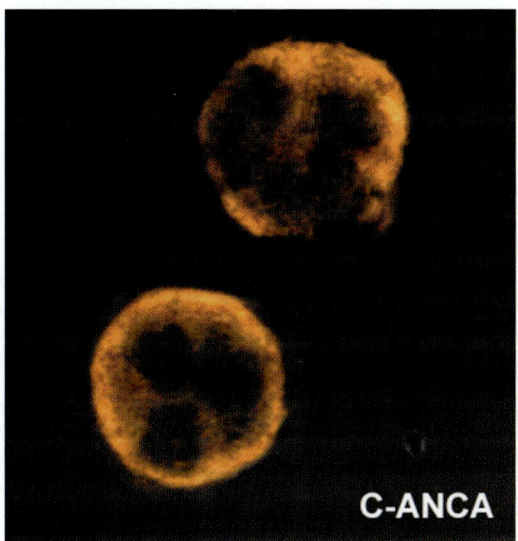

PLATE 1   This is a high-powered fluorescent microscopic view of a slide demonstrating antineutrophil cytoplasmic antibody (ANCA). Dried neutrophils are overlaid with a serum sample from a test subject, followed by antihuman antibody labeled with a fluorescent tag. The typical binding pattern shows fluorescence greater in the peripheral cytoplasm in granulomatosis with polyangiitis (Wegener's granulomatosis), as seen in this figure, and more perinuclear in eosinophilic granulomatosis with polyangiitis (Churg-Strauss syndrome) and microscopic polyangiitis. This immunofluorescent test is more sensitive than identification of specific antibodies, usually for proteinase 3 (granulomatosis with polyangiitis) or myeloperoxidase (microscopic polyangiitis or eosinophilic granulomatosis with polyangiitis), although confirmation of specific antibodies is a more specific test.

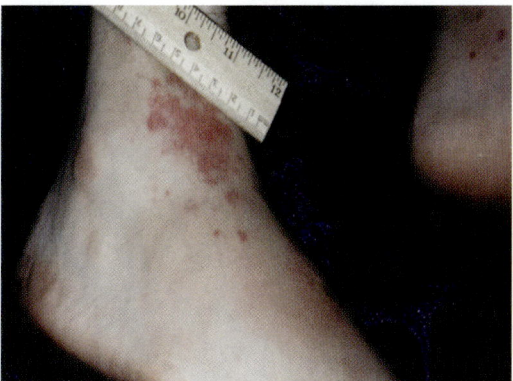

PLATE 2   A skin rash in a young male with eosinophilic granulomatosis with polyangiitis (EGPA, or Churg-Strauss syndrome). EGPA may affect variable-sized blood vessels and in dermatologic manifestations may resemble hypersensitivity vasculitis with palpable purpura.

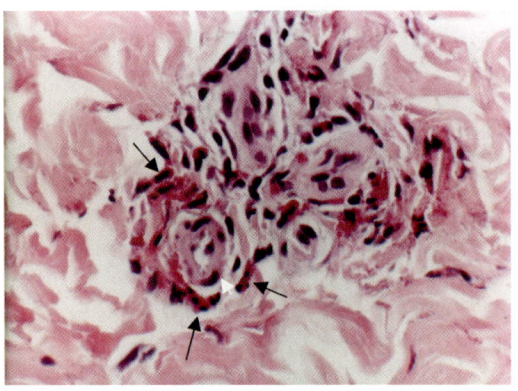

PLATE 3 A skin biopsy from a subject with eosinophilic granulomatosis with polyangiitis (EGPA, or Churg-Strauss syndrome). This is a high-power view with hematoxylin and eosin staining. Eosinophil infiltration of the tissue (black arrows) and of the small vessels (white arrowhead) in the subcutaneous tissue is seen. Granulomas are not noted, and with early diagnosis, this is often the case.

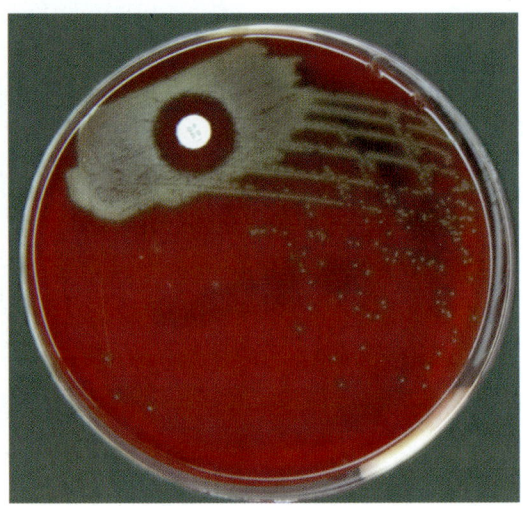

PLATE 4 Culture of Streptococcus pneumoniae on blood agar with an inhibition zone around the optochin disk.

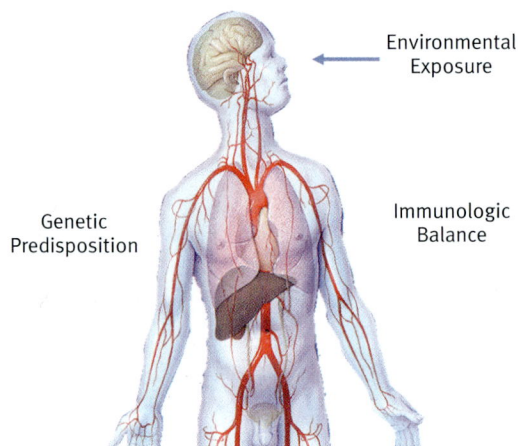

PLATE 5 Comorbidities of allergic rhinitis.

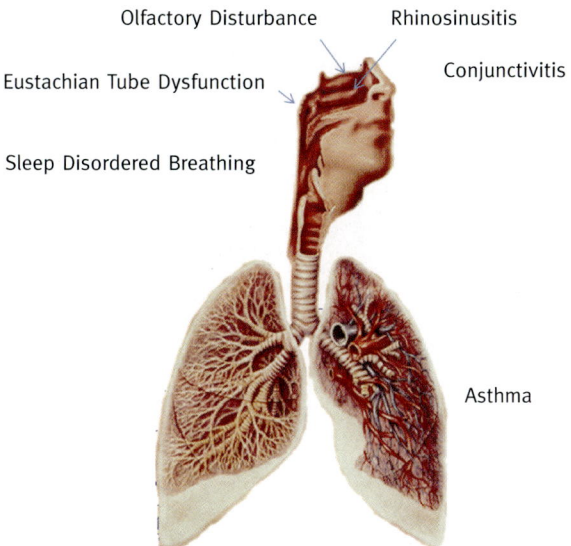

PLATE 6 Comorbidities may exist if different body areas share genetic predispositions, environmental exposure, or immunologic imbalances.

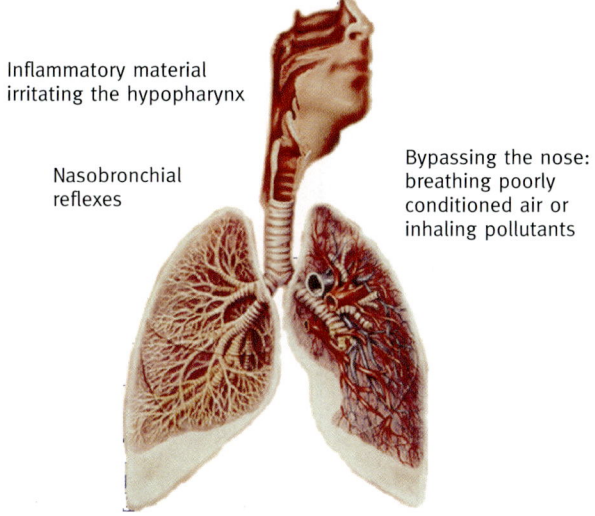

PLATE 7 Postulated mechanisms by which the upper airway may affect the lower airway.

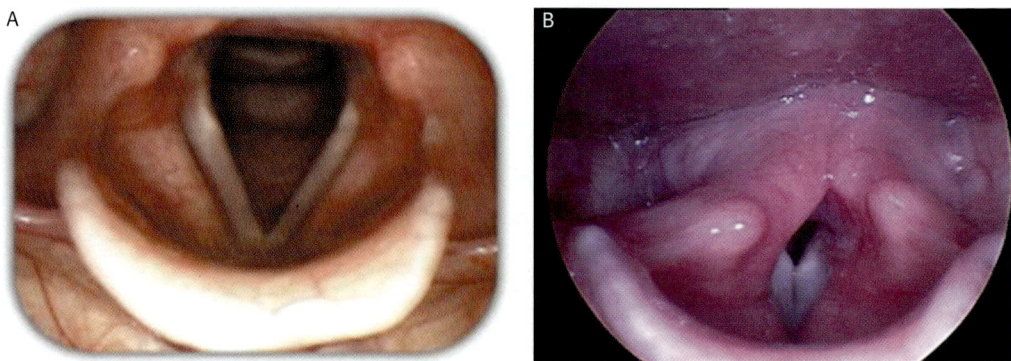

PLATE 8 Normal vocal fold abduction and paroxysmal vocal fold adduction. A, Normal abduction of vocal folds during inhalation. B, Paroxysmal adduction of vocal folds during inhalation with a characteristic posterior diamond-shaped glottis deformity.

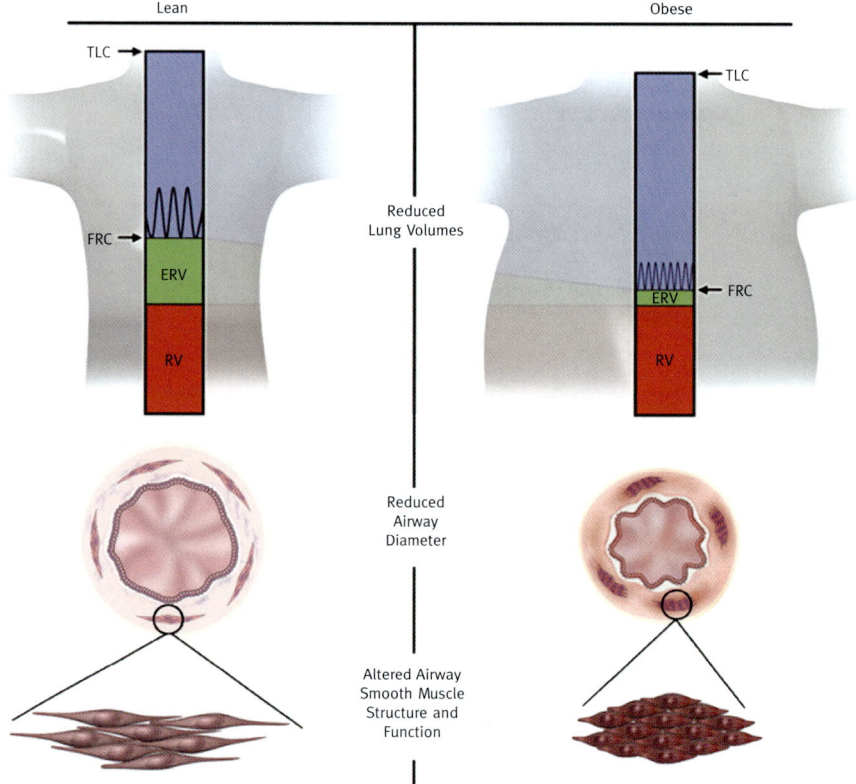

PLATE 9 Obesity leads to alterations of lung volumes, particularly expiratory reserve volume (ERV) and FRC, leading to a rapid, shallow breathing pattern that occurs close to closing volume. Obesity also causes reduced peripheral airway diameter, which can lead to increased airway hyperresponsiveness due to alterations of smooth muscle structure and function. RV, residual volume; TLC, total lung capacity. (From Beuther DA, Weiss ST, Sutherland ER. Obesity and asthma. Am J Respir Crit Care Med. 2006;174[2]:112–119.)

Table 19.7. Differential Diagnosis of Neurologic Rhinopathies

Absent sympathetic vasoconstriction (Horner's syndrome)
Vidian neurectomy
Cholinergic rhinitis
Hyperactive cholinergic parasympathetic function with excessive mucous exocytosis
Gustatory rhinitis (afferent–efferent reflex hyperactivity; "salsa sniffles")
Cold dry air–induced rhinorrhea (skier's rhinitis)
Nociceptive rhinitis/irritant rhinitis with increased nociceptive afferent nerve sensitivity to particulate, volatile organic compound, and chemical agents (weather changes, tobacco smoke, perfumes)
Hyperactivity of normal nasal reflexes (bright light–induced rhinorrhea)
Migraine-related rhinorrhea and lacrimation
Interoceptive disorders
Nonallergic rhinitis of chronic fatigue syndrome and allied interoceptive, hyperalgesia, and autonomic dysfunction syndromes

---

of acute sinusitis.[69] Symptoms typically begin as intermittent episodes with no clear provoking or exacerbating events and progress to a continuous ache. Analgesics, antibiotics, and intranasal glucocorticosteroids are ineffective unless there is a strong, prolonged placebo effect. A 6-month course of low-dose amitriptyline (20 mg) is beneficial. The mechanism and locus of action are unknown. Lightheadedness was common in iNAR (67%), but vertigo was not (17%).[65] This symptom may be related to orthostatic hypotension and other cardiovascular and sympathetic nervous system dysfunction. Palpitations are present in 72%. Concomitant irritable bowel syndrome (88%) and gastroesophageal reflux (62%) suggest that nonallergic rhinitis may be part of a larger pattern of "functional" or interoceptive, autonomic, and other mucosal organ dysfunction syndromes. One symptom of relevance is dyspnea, which is present in asthma and common in the neurologic nonallergic rhinitis of chronic fatigue syndrome.[69]

LIFESTYLE AND BEHAVIORAL MODIFICATION STRATEGIES

Although limiting the exposure to some of the triggers is often beyond one's control, there are others that can be modified on an individual basis. Avoidance of both active and passive smoking is highly recommended. Individuals with rhinorrhea secondary to alcohol ingestion should avoid alcohol. Subjects with gustatory rhinitis would benefit from avoiding triggering foods or could use prophylactic anticholinergic nasal spray (ipratropium bromide). Exposure to strong perfumes or colognes or chemicals should be avoided as much as possible. During periods of heavy pollution, it is advisable to drive cars with the windows and vents closed.

PHARMACOLOGIC TREATMENT

Topical glucocorticoids have been tested in NAR but are of little benefit unless eosinophilia is present.[32,60,62,63]

Cholinergic glandular secretion is probably the most important single tonically active influence regulating glandular exocytosis in the respiratory tract. This reflex provides the rationale for the use of anticholinergic antagonists for hypersecretory rhinitis regardless of the initial pathology. Certain skiers or subjects who jog in the winter have chronic rhinorrhea and may wear a protective mask or limit their activities in such cold weather.[70]

Irritant sensitivity due to nociceptive nerve hyperalgesia and peripheral sensitization provide an attractive potential mechanism for iNAR. Unpleasant hickory smoke and pleasant vanilla odors activate blood flow to olfactory regions of the frontal cortex.[71] This is blocked with nasal azelastine.

The challenges of diagnosing and treating iNAR have direct effects on physician perceptions of the effectiveness of rhinitis treatment.[72] Many drugs that are effective in AR have no benefit in NAR. This can be frustrating for both the physician and the patient. Intranasal glucocorticoid sprays are not efficacious for iNAR associated with weather and temperature changes or for congestion symptoms.[73] Topical antihistamines may have value, as indicated by testing in cold dry air (CDA) exposure chambers.

Of the potential drugs affecting nociceptive neural receptors, the transient receptor potential melanostatin-4 agonist menthol shows the most promise. Menthol activates a cooling sensation through Aδ nerves. In a patent nostril, the rapid flow of inhaled air causes epithelial surface water to evaporate. This leads to a net decrease in the mucosal temperature that is conveyed by Aδ nerves to the brainstem respiratory centers. This, in turn, results in a reduction in the work of breathing and perception of general airway patency. Conversely, nasal obstruction by inflammation, structural collapse, mucoid secretions, turbinate hypertrophy, or nasal packing leads to sensations of dyspnea and potentially to apnea.

Another beneficial nutraceutical is capsaicin, the picante essence of chili peppers. Several protocols have been tested in iNAR and indicate safety and efficacy for topical use.[74,75] Sinus Buster, a proprietary homeopathic preparation of *Capsicum annum* and eucalyptol, improved nasal congestion, cutaneous sinus region pain and pressure sensations, and headache after 5 minutes that persisted for 60 minutes.[76] As current prescription drugs become proprietary and are used in various combinations,[77] it is possible that new preparations may be value for treatment of the neurogenic discomfort of iNAR.

It is hoped that the next few years will bring the introduction of new pharmaceuticals that modulate these neural functions and treat iNAR. In addition, future guidelines should evolve to provide more exact explanations to physicians and other health care professionals and algorithms for patient care.[7,45]

Neurobiologic Insights

Calcitonin gene–related peptide is the likely mediator of vasodilation in human nasal mucosa and responsible for the venous sinusoid swelling that blocks nasal airflow. Nasal trigeminal nociceptive neurons enter the pons through the sensory root and turn caudally in the trigeminal spinal tract to terminate in the pars caudalis of the nucleus of the spinal tract in the lower medulla and upper three cervical segments of the spinal cord. Glossopharyngeal afferents innervate the posterior third of the tongue, upper pharynx, tonsils, eustachian tube, and middle ear, and so are relevant to rhinitis. These thermosensitive and nociceptive neurons terminate in the dorsal portion of the trigeminal spinal tract. Pars caudalis interneurons cross the midline to enter the trigeminothalamic tract and terminate in the medial part of the ventral posterior thalamic nucleus. Painful and strong thermal stimuli are appreciated at the thalamic level. Tertiary neural relays to the lower third of the parietal cortical somesthetic areas provide for localization of nasal stimuli. Activation of these central registries is responsible for the sensations of itch and congestion that are the hallmarks of AR. Afferent neurons from mucosal surfaces that do not convey pain are said to be interoceptive. Persistent activation eventually stimulates the posterior insula, which acts as the somatosensory cortex for interoceptors and nociceptors. Communications to the anterior insula may be triggered by severe and persistent interoceptive input and lead to avoidance behaviors such as the allergic salute, chronic habitual sniffing and throat clearing, disruption of train of thought and working memory leading to impaired cognition, emotional lability and fatigue through connections to the limbic system, and resetting of neuroendocrine and autonomic systems through the hypothalamus. The insula is also activated during asthma and bronchial provocations, providing a common central mechanism to link rhinitis and bronchoconstrictive disease.

UNMET, FUTURE RESEARCH NEEDS

1. Continued evaluation of entopy will determine the impact of evolving allergic inflammation in the differential diagnosis of NAR. This is relevant to the adult onset of nasal complaints. Immunotherapy based on the results of allergen nasal provocations may be useful in this subgroup. The characteristics of the nasal immune response in entopy may be different from typical eosinophilic AR. This would be consistent with the generally poor response found with nasal glucocorticoids in those with negative allergy skin tests and presumed NAR. Alternative antiinflammatory therapies are necessary.

2. The mechanisms responsible for the sensation of congestion are not understood. The interactions between airborne exposures, epithelial cell responses, and activation of chemoreceptors on peripheral nerve endings are likely to be complex, but these interactions offer new therapeutic targets for preventing the initiation of interoceptive sensations. Spinal sensitization of the central trigeminal synapses in the brainstem and upper cervical spinal cord may be amenable to modulation with drugs active at glutaminergic and other receptors that participate in this relay. Functional imaging in NAR subjects may reveal alterations in the pathways of the ascending trigeminal interneurons between the brainstem and the somatosensory regions of the insula and parietal cortex. It is conceivable that the congestion complaints of NAR are analogous to phantom limb pain, with dysfunction of central registries leading to perceptions of nasal irritation without nasal mucosal inflammation. This line of investigation may offer insights into chemical irritant hypersensitivity but may also require a broad reappraisal of the standing hypotheses to include nasal symptoms secondary to central neural dysfunction.

3. Topical nasal capsaicin treatment, in general, is successful at reducing sensations of congestion. Additional studies of the distribution of transient receptor potential vanilloid-1 and other capsaicin-binding sites on nerve endings, epithelium, and cells within venous sinusoids are warranted to better understand this phenomenon and to develop more selective and effective drug treatments.

4. CDA appears to be a suitable trigger of NAR for drug study case designation and potentially for diagnosis in research studies. The mechanism of this effect is still unclear. Activation of the "cooling" menthol receptor (TRPM4) induces a sensation of nasal patency. In contrast, TRP ankyrin 1 and other "cold pain" sensors may be responsible for NAR symptoms.

5. The biology of adrenergic receptors on nasal vessels and nerve endings will be important in understanding risk factors for rhinitis medicamentosa. Dual therapy aimed at activation of α-adrenergic and glucocorticoid receptors improves treatment efficacy in AR.[57,58] Effectiveness in NAR requires further testing.

6. Topical antihistamines are used for NAR but require more rigorous study. It remains to be determined whether the actual targets of these drugs in NAR are histamine receptors or other signaling pathways. Will these drugs be beneficial for the small proportion of NAR subjects who have a marginal increase in mucosal metachromatic cells?

7. The prevalence and pathophysiology of NAR in elderly people has been debated but requires more rigorous study to determine the impact on quality of life and mechanistic similarities with iNAR.

8. These novel mechanisms of NAR and congestion should also be assessed in the tracheobronchial tree and for dyspnea because neurologic or other processes may account for mucosal inflammatory and central perceptive changes referable to both regions of the airway.

9. The case definition for iNAR remains one of exclusion of atopy, eosinophilia, infection, and other inflammatory mechanisms. The search continues for readily available diagnostic tests and objective biomarkers.

CONCLUSION

Progress has been made in understanding the mechanisms that contribute to the differential diagnosis of rhinitis in the absence of atopy. However, translation of these new data into diagnostic and treatment modalities is challenging. New findings of progressive nasal allergy (entopy), potential microbiome alterations, and neurologic and autonomic alterations in iNAR may lead to an even broader differential, but one that sharpens our focus on specific treatable aspects of this disease.

REFERENCES

1. Staevska MT, Baraniuk JN. Differential diagnosis of persistent nonallergic rhinitis and rhinosinusitis syndromes. *Clin Allergy Immunol.* 2007;19:35–53.
2. Settipane RA, Lieberman P. Update on nonallergic rhinitis. *Ann Allergy Asthma Immunol.* 2001;86(5):494–507.
3. Molgaard E, Thomsen SF, Lund T, Pedersen L, Nolte H, Backer V. Differences between allergic and nonallergic rhinitis in a large sample of adolescents and adults. *Allergy.* 2007;62(9):1033–1037.
4. Scarupa MD, Kaliner MA. Non-allergic rhinitis, with a focus on vasomotor rhinitis: clinical importance, differential diagnosis, and effective treatment recommendations. *WAO J.* 2009;2(3):20–25.
5. Wedback A, Enbom H, Eriksson NE, Moverare R, Malcus I. Seasonal nonallergic rhinitis (SNAR): a new disease entity? A clinical and immunological comparison between SNAR, seasonal allergic rhinitis and persistent non allergic rhinitis. *Rhinology.* 2005;43:86–92.
6. Lindberg S, Malm L. Comparison of allergic rhinitis and vasomotor rhinitis patients on the basis of a computer questionnaire. *Allergy.* 1993;48:602–607.
7. Dykewicz MS, Fineman S, Skoner DP. Diagnosis and management of rhinitis: complete guidelines of the joint task force on practice parameters in allergy, asthma and immunology. American Academy of Allergy, Asthma and Immunology. *Ann Allergy Asthma Immunol.* 1998;81:478–518.
8. Di Lorenzo G, Pacor ML, Amodio E, et al. Differences and similarities between allergic and nonallergic rhinitis in a large sample of adult patients with rhinitis symptoms. *Int Arch Allergy Immunol.* 2011;155(3):263–270.
9. Hellgren J. Quality of life in nonallergic rhinitis. *Clin Allergy Immunol.* 2007;19:383–387.
10. Stjarne P, Lundblad L, Lundberg JM, Anggard A. Capsaicin and nicotine sensitive afferent neurons and nasal secretion in healthy human volunteers and in patients with vasomotor rhinitis. *Br J Pharmacol.* 1989;96:693–701.
11. Chawes BL, Kreiner-Møller E, Bisgaard H. Objective assessments of allergic and non-allergic rhinitis in young children. *Allergy.* 2009;64(10):1547–1553.
12. Erwin EA, Faust RA, Platts-Mills TA, Borish L. Epidemiological analysis of chronic rhinitis in pediatric patients. *Am J Rhinol Allergy.* 2011;25(5):327–332.
13. Brandt D, Bernstein JA. Questionnaire evaluation and risk factor identification for nonallergic vasomotor rhinitis. *Ann Allergy Asthma Immunol.* 2006;96(4):526–532.
14. Bernstein JA. Characteristics of nonallergic vasomotor rhinitis. *WAO J.* 2009;2:102–105.
15. Braat JP, Mulder PG, Fokkens WJ, van Wijk RG, Rijntjes E. Intranasal cold dry air is superior to histamine challenge in determining the presence and degree of nasal hyperreactivity in nonallergic noninfectious perennial rhinitis. *Am J Respir Crit Care Med.* 1998;157(6 Pt 1):1748–1755.
16. Van Gerven L, Boeckxstaens G, Jorissen M, Fokkens W, Hellings PW. Short-time cold dry air exposure: A useful diagnostic tool for nasal hyperresponsiveness. *Laryngoscope.* 2012;122(12);2615–2620.
17. Bernstein JA, Salapatek AM, Lee JS, et al. Provocation of nonallergic rhinitis subjects in response to simulated weather conditions using an environmental exposure chamber model. *Allergy Asthma Proc.* 2012;33(4):333–340.
18. Jacobs R, Lieberman P, Kent E, Silvey M, Locantore N, Philpot EE. Weather/temperature-sensitive vasomotor rhinitis may be refractory to intranasal corticosteroid treatment. *Allergy Asthma Proc.* 2009;30(2):120–127.
19. Jammes Y, Delvolgo-Gori MJ, Badier M, Guillot C, Gazazian G, Parlenti L. One-year occupational exposure to a cold environment alters lung function. *Arch Environ Health.* 2002;57(4):360–365.
20. Fontanari P, Zattara-Hartmann MC, Burnet H, Jammes Y. Nasal eupnoeic inhalation of cold, dry air increases airway resistance in asthmatic patients. *Eur Respir J.* 1997;10(10):2250–2254.
21. Westman M, Stjärne P, Asarnoj A, et al. Natural course and comorbidities of allergic and non-allergic rhinitis in children. *J Allergy Clin Immunol.* 2012;129(2):403–408.
22. Chawes BL, Bønnelykke K, Kreiner-Møller E, Bisgaard H. Children with allergic and nonallergic rhinitis have a similar risk of asthma. *J Allergy Clin Immunol.* 2010;126(3):567–573.e1–8.
23. Lourenco O, Fonseca AM, Taborda-Barata L. Asthma is more frequently associated with

non-allergic than allergic rhinitis in Portuguese patients. *Rhinology*. 2009;47(2):207–213.
24. Håkansson K, von Buchwald C, Thomsen SF, Thyssen JP, Backer V, Linneberg A. Nonallergic rhinitis and its association with smoking and lower airway disease: a general population study. *Am J Rhinol Allergy*. 2011;25(1):25–29.
25. Rolla G, Guida G, Heffler E, et al. Diagnostic classification of persistent rhinitis and its relationship to exhaled nitric oxide and asthma: a clinical study of a consecutive series of patients. *Chest*. 2007;131(5):1345–1352.
26. Shaaban R, Zureik M, Soussan D, et al. Rhinitis and onset of asthma: a longitudinal population-based study. *Lancet*. 2008;372:1049–1057.
27. Leynaert B, Bousquet J, Neukirch C, Liard R, Neukirch F. Perennial rhinitis: an independent risk factor for asthma in nonatopic subjects: results from the European Community Respiratory Health Survey. *J Allergy Clin Immunol*. 1999;104(2 Pt 1):301–304.
28. Guerra S, Sherrill DL, Martinez FD, Barbee RA. Rhinitis as an independent risk factor for adult-onset asthma. *J Allergy Clin Immunol*. 2002;109(3):419–425.
29. Bernstein JA, Levin LS, Al-Shuik E, Martin VT. Clinical characteristics of chronic rhinitis patients with high vs low irritant trigger burdens. *Ann Allergy Asthma Immunol*. 2012;109(3):173–178.
30. Rondon C, Dona I, Torres MJ, Campo P, Blanca M. Evolution of patients with nonallergic rhinitis supports conversion to allergic rhinitis. *J Allergy Clin Immunol*. 2009;123(5):1098–1102.
31. Kaliner MA. Classification of nonallergic rhinitis syndromes with a focus on vasomotor rhinitis, proposed to be known henceforth as nonallergic rhinopathy. *WAO J*. 2009;2:98–101.
32. Blom HM, Godthelp T, Fokkens WJ, KleinJan A, Mulder PG, Rijntjes E. The effect of nasal steroid aqueous spray on nasal complaint scores and cellular infiltrates in the nasal mucosa of patients with nonallergic, noninfectious perennial rhinitis. *J Allergy Clin Immunol*. 1997;100(6 Pt 1):739–747.
33. Tran NP, Vickery J, Blaiss MS. Management of rhinitis: allergic and non-allergic. *Allergy Asthma Immunol Res*. 2011;3(3):148–156.
34. Settipane GA, Klein DE. Non allergic rhinitis: demography of eosinophils in nasal smear, blood total eosinophil counts and IgE levels. *N Engl Reg Allergy Proc*. 1985;6(4):363–366.
35. Canakcioglu S, Tahamiler R, Saritzali G, et al. Evaluation of nasal cytology in subjects with chronic rhinitis: a 7-year study. *Am J Otolaryngol*. 2009;30(5):312–317.
36. Leone C, Teodoro C, Pelucchi A, et al. Bronchial responsiveness and airway inflammation in patients with nonallergic rhinitis with eosinophilia syndrome. *J Allergy Clin Immunol*. 1997;100(6 Pt 1):775–780.
37. Gibson PG, Fujimura M, Niimi A. Eosinophilic bronchitis: clinical manifestations and implications for treatment. *Thorax*. 2002;57(2):178–182.
38. Calderón-Garcidueñas L, Valencia-Salazar G, Rodríguez-Alcaraz A, et al. Ultrastructural nasal pathology in children chronically and sequentially exposed to air pollutants. *Am J Respir Cell Mol Biol*. 2001;24(2):132–138.
39. Yoon BN, Choi NG, Lee HS, Cho KS, Roh HJ. Induction of interleukin-8 from nasal epithelial cells during bacterial infection: the role of IL-8 for neutrophil recruitment in chronic rhinosinusitis. *Mediators Inflamm*. 2010;2010:813610.
40. Einarsson O, Geba GP, Zhou Z, et al. Interleukin-11 in respiratory inflammation. *Ann N Y Acad Sci*. 1995;762:31–40.
41. Nuhoglu C, Nuhoglu Y, Bankaoglu M, Ceran O. A retrospective analysis of adenoidal size in children with allergic rhinitis and nonallergic idiopathic rhinitis. *Asian Pac J Allergy Immunol*. 2010;28(2–3):136–140.
42. Sakaguchi K, Okuda M, Ushijima K, Sakaguchi Y, Tanigaito Y. Study of nasal surface basophilic cells in patients with nasal polyp. *Acta Otolaryngol Suppl*. 1986;430:28–33.
43. Hellgren J, Torén K. Nonallergic occupational rhinitis. *Clin Allergy Immunol*. 2007;19:241–248.
44. Castano R, Gautrin D, Thériault G, Trudeau C, Ghezzo H, Malo JL. Occupational rhinitis in workers investigated for occupational asthma. *Thorax*. 2009;64(1):50–54.
45. Moscato G, Siracusa A. Rhinitis guidelines and implications for occupational rhinitis. *Curr Opin Allergy Clin Immunol*. 2009;9(2):110.
46. Shusterman D, Murphy MA. Nasal hyperreactivity in allergic and non-allergic rhinitis: a potential risk factor for non-specific building-related illness. *Indoor Air*. 2007;17(4):328–333.
47. Mamessier E, Milhe F, Guillot C, et al. T-cell activation in occupational asthma and rhinitis. *Allergy*. 2007;62(2):162–169.
48. Malekzadeh S, Hamburger MD, Whelan PJ, Biedlingmaier JF, Baraniuk JN. Density of middle turbinate subepithelial mucous glands in patients with chronic rhinosinusitis. *Otolaryngol Head Neck Surg*. 2002;127(3):190–195.

49. Baraniuk JN, Casado B, Malekzadeh S. Differentiating osteomeatal complex disease and chronic rhinosinusitis from nonallergic rhinitis. *Clin Allergy Immunol.* 2007;19:115–146.
50. Nguyen KH, Suzuki H, Wakasugi T, et al. Expression of epidermal growth factors, erbBs, in the nasal mucosa of patients with chronic hypertrophic rhinitis. *ORL J Otorhinolaryngol Relat Spec.* 2012;74(2):57–63.
51. Coffey CS, Mulligan RM, Schlosser RJ. Mucosal expression of nerve growth factor and brain-derived neurotrophic factor in chronic rhinosinusitis. *Am J Rhinol Allergy.* 2009;23(6):571–574.
52. Gindros G, Kantas I, Balatsouras DG, et al. Mucosal changes in chronic hypertrophic rhinitis after surgical turbinate reduction. *Eur Arch Otorhinolaryngol.* 2009;266(9):1409–1416.
53. Dzieciolowska-Baran E, Teul-Swiniarska I, Gawlikowska-Sroka A, Poziomkowska-Gesicka I, Zietek Z. Rhinitis as a cause of respiratory disorders during pregnancy. *Adv Exp Med Biol.* 2013;755:213–220.
54. Reisacher WR. Prevalence of autoimmune thyroid disease in chronic rhinitis. *Ear Nose Throat J.* 2008;87(9):524–527.
55. Varghese M, Glaum MC, Lockey RF. Drug-induced rhinitis. *Clin Exp Allergy.* 2010;40(3):381–384.
56. Graf P. Rhinitis medicamentosa: a review of causes and treatment. *Treat Respir Med.* 2005;4(1):21–29.
57. Baroody FM, Brown D, Gavanescu L, DeTineo M, Naclerio RM. Oxymetazoline adds to the effectiveness of fluticasone furoate in the treatment of perennial allergic rhinitis. *J Allergy Clin Immunol.* 2011;127(4):927–934.
58. Rael EL, Ramey J, Lockey RF. Oxymetazoline hydrochloride combined with mometasone nasal spray for persistent nasal congestion (pilot study). *WAO J.* 2011;4(3):65–67.
59. Powe DG, Jagger C, Kleinjan A, Carney AS, Jenkins D, Jones NS. "Entopy": localized mucosal allergic disease in the absence of systemic responses for atopy. *Clin Exp Allergy.* 2003;33:1374–1379.
60. Small P, Black M, Frenkiel S. Effects of treatment with beclomethasone dipropionate in subpopulations of perennial rhinitis patients. *J Allergy Clin Immunol.* 1982;70:178–182.
61. van Rijswijk JB, Blom HM, KleinJan A, Mulder PGH, Rijntjes E, Fokkens WJ. Inflammatory cells seem not to be involved in idiopathic rhinitis. *Rhinology.* 2003;41(1):25–30.
62. Blom HM, Godthelp T, Fokkens WJ, KleinJan A, Mulder PG, Rijntjes E. The effect of nasal steroid aqueous spray on nasal complaint scores and cellular infiltrates in the nasal mucosa of patients with nonallergic, noninfectious perennial rhinitis. *J Allergy Clin Immunol.* 1997;100:739–747.
63. Lundblad L, Sipila P, Farstad T, Drozdziewicz D. Mometasone furoate nasal spray in the treatment of perennial non-allergic rhinitis: a Nordic, multicenter, randomized, double-blind, placebo-controlled study. *Acta Otolaryngol.* 2001;121:505–509.
64. Malcomson KG. The vasomotor activities of the nasal mucous membrane. *J Laryngol Otol.* 1959;73:73–98.
65. Elsheikh MN, Badran HM. Dysautonomia rhinitis: associated otolaryngologic manifestations and characterization based on autonomic function tests. *Acta Otolaryngol.* 2006;126:1206–1212.
66. Ravindran MK, Zheng Y, Timbol C, Merck SJ, Baraniuk JN. Migraine headaches in chronic fatigue syndrome (CFS). *BMC Neurol.* 2011;11:30.
67. Jones NS. Midfacial segment pain: implications for rhinitis and sinusitis. *Curr Allergy Asthma Rep.* 2004;4:187–192.
68. Naranch K, Park Y-J, Repka-Ramirez SM, Velarde A, Clauw D, Baraniuk JN. A tender sinus does not always mean sinusitis. *Otolaryngol Head Neck Surg.* 2002;127:387–397.
69. Baraniuk JN, Zheng Y. Relationships among rhinitis, fibromyalgia, and chronic fatigue. *Allergy Asthma Proc.* 2010;31(3):169–178.
70. Silvers WS. The skier's nose: a model of cold-induced rhinorrhea. *Ann Allergy.* 1991;67(1):32–36.
71. Bernstein JA, Hastings L, Boespflug EL, Allendorfer JB, Lamy M, Eliassen JC. Alteration of brain activation patterns in nonallergic rhinitis patients using functional magnetic resonance imaging before and after treatment with intranasal azelastine. *Ann Allergy Asthma Immunol.* 2011;106(6):527–532.
72. Meltzer EO, Nathan RA, Derebery J, et al. Physician perceptions of the treatment and management of allergic and nonallergic rhinitis. *Allergy Asthma Proc.* 2009;30(1):75–83.
73. Jacobs R, Lieberman P, Kent E, Silvey M, Locantore N, Philpot EE. Weather/temperature-sensitive vasomotor rhinitis may be refractory to intranasal corticosteroid treatment. *Allergy Asthma Proc.* 2009;30(2):120–127.
74. Blom HM, Van Rijswijk JB, Garrelds IM, Mulder PG, Timmermans T, Gerth van Wijk R. Intranasal capsaicin is efficacious in

non-allergic, non-infectious perennial rhinitis: a placebo-controlled study. *Clin Exp Allergy.* 1997;27(7):796–801.
75. Van Rijswijk JB, Boeke EL, Keizer JM, Mulder PG, Blom HM, Fokkens WJ. Intranasal capsaicin reduces nasal hyperreactivity in idiopathic rhinitis: a double-blind randomized application regimen study. *Allergy.* 2003;58(8): 754–761.
76. Bernstein JA, Davis BP, Picard JK, Cooper JP, Zheng S, Levin LS. A randomized, double-blind, parallel trial comparing capsaicin nasal spray with placebo in subjects with a significant component of nonallergic rhinitis. *Ann Allergy Asthma Immunol.* 2011;107(2):171–178.
77. Yuta A, Baraniuk JN. Therapeutic approaches to mucous hypersecretion. *Curr. Allergy Asthma Rep.* 2005;5:243–251.

20

INFECTIOUS COMORBIDITIES OF ASTHMA IN THE UPPER AIRWAY

Claus Bachert and Griet Vandeplas

KEY POINTS

- Virus-induced infectious rhinitis (also known as the common cold) and postviral rhinosinusitis are frequent diseases of the upper airways. Only in a minority of cases is there evolution to acute bacterial rhinosinusitis. Restrictive use of antibiotics is therefore important to prevent bacterial resistance.
- Chronic rhinosinusitis (CRS) is not an infectious but rather an inflammatory disorder, which can be subdivided into CRS without and with nasal polyps (CRSs/wNP). The factors leading to disease chronicity are not completely understood.
- The influence of *Staphylococcus aureus* as a disease-modifying factor in chronic rhinosinusitis with nasal polyps (CRSwNP) is established. Immunoglobulin E formation to staphylococcal superantigens is a predictor for comorbid asthma in patients with CRSwNP.
- Fungal rhinosinusitis is an endemic condition and may lead to an immune response in selected cases, called *allergic fungal rhinosinusitis*.

INTRODUCTION: CONCEPT OF THE "UNITED AIRWAY"

The upper and lower airways show similarities in mucosal structure and in the generation of innate and adaptive immune responses (Chapter 19). The airways are continuously exposed to environmental pollutants, such as cigarette smoke and microorganisms, including viruses, bacteria, and fungi. These microorganisms may succeed in breaking through the natural mucosal barriers, leading to disease. This may lead to an acute infection but may also, for reasons that are not understood, lead to chronic airway disease. The interaction between the microbiome and the mucosal immunity is a focus of interest, linking the upper and lower airways in acute as well as chronic diseases.

Studies of the microbiome and its impact on airway mucosa demonstrate the complexity and richness of microbial colonization. Viral or bacterial infections may disturb the delicate balance between germs and the airway mucosa, as can an immune deficiency. This can lead to the breakdown of the epithelial barrier, consequently adversely affecting the immune response. Often, several factors in an individual patient are responsible for the resultant acute or chronic airway disease.

MUCOSAL BARRIER

The upper airway respiratory mucosa is composed of ciliated, pseudostratified columnar epithelial cells and goblet mucus cells. This mucosa layer is covered by mucus in which microbes, dust, and irritant particles are easily confined. The mucus is propulsed from the sinuses into the nasal cavity and the posterior pharynx, thanks to the mucociliary clearance mechanisms, where it is swallowed. The nose provides a large mucosal surface with a mucus layer to trap particles and heats, cools, and humidifies passing air. There are erectile vascular plexuses in the nasal submucosa that promote swelling and increased mucus production following exposure to irritants, temperature changes, and other environmental substances. The paranasal sinuses are bony chambers lined with the same mucosa. Every sinus has an ostium through which mucus drains into the nasal cavity. The maxillary and frontal and anterior ethmoidal sinuses drain into the middle meatus, beneath the middle turbinate. The sphenoidal and posterior ethmoidal sinuses drain into the superior meatus, beneath the superior turbinate, or drain medial to the superior turbinate.

After a microorganism enters the body, it comes in contact with the innate immune system, comprising the complement system, lysozymes, and defensins, and finally with the adaptive immune system, comprising both humoral and cell-mediated immunity. Beneath the mucosal surface, inflammatory cells, such as dendritic cells, macrophages, lymphocytes, plasma cells, neutrophils, basophils, mast cells, and others, orchestrate an inflammatory response if the innate immune system fails to eliminate the organism. In response to certain triggers, chemical mediators, such as histamine, leukotrienes, platelet-activating-factor, and kinins, are released from these cells to cause sneezing, mucus secretion, mucociliary clearance, and other physiologic responses in an effort to eliminate offending agents from the upper airway.[1,2]

INFECTIOUS RHINITIS

Pathophysiology

The nasal and paranasal cavities are connected, and any infectious agent will affect both, as occurs with infectious rhinosinusitis. The most frequent airway infection is the virus-induced common cold. Symptoms are caused by the interplay between viral replication and the host's immunologic and inflammatory responses. Within the first several days, there is increased concentration of inflammatory mediators in nasal secretions. These include kinins, leukotrienes, histamine, interferons, interleukin-1 (IL-1), IL-6, IL-8, tumor necrosis factor, and RANTES (regulated on activation, normal T-cell expressed and secreted). The release of interferons and chemokines, the activation of T cells, and the migration of predominantly neutrophilic granulocytes results in the suppression of viral replication and a temporary inflammation of the mucosa, which normally resolves without further consequence. Viral infections of the nasal mucosa lead to epithelial disruption, vasodilatation, and increased vascular permeability, causing edema with obstruction of the nose and sinuses and rhinorrhea. The number of goblet cells increases, and ciliated cells decreases, with increased mucous gland secretion and sneezing. These changes increase the risk for a secondary bacterial infection.[3]

The most common viruses associated with the common cold are rhinoviruses, accounting for about 50% of such infections and usually causing mild illness. Other viruses include coronaviruses, influenza viruses, parainfluenza viruses, adenovirus, respiratory syncytial virus, and enterovirus.[2,4,5] Transmission of viruses that cause the common cold occurs primarily by hand contact with secretions that contain the virus, small-particle aerosols, or direct contamination from large-particle aerosols from an infected individual.[3] Allergic rhinitis predisposes individuals to more frequent and severe viral rhinosinusitis.

Clinical Features

The common cold typically begins with a sore throat, associated with general malaise. Low-grade fever can be present during the first several days and gradually resolves, followed by increased sneezing, rhinorrhea, and nasal congestion. The nasal secretions are usually clear but can be thick and purulent. Viral rhinitis can extend to the lower airways, leading to cough, bronchitis, and an exacerbation of asthma and chronic obstructive pulmonary disease (COPD). It can also cause eustachian tube dysfunction, considered an important factor in the pathogenesis of acute otitis media. The incubation period varies depending on the virus; symptoms typically peak within 2 to 3 days of onset, gradually decline thereafter, and usually resolve within 10 to 14 days. An increase in symptoms after 5 days or persistence of symptoms over 10 days usually indicates a secondary infection or acute rhinosinusitis (ARS; see later).[6]

Epidemiology

The common cold is the most frequent type of infection in humans. Despite being benign, it causes an enormous economic burden for the health care system and absenteeism from work, school, and daycare centers. The average adult experiences two to five colds per year, but the rates are higher in younger adults, especially in women 20 to 34 years of age. This increase in young adult women, not seen in the same age group in men, is probably related to the greater exposure of women in this age group to young children. Thereafter, there is a general decline in the number of infections as age increases. There is considerable seasonal variation in the occurrence of common colds, with a higher prevalence in the autumn and winter months because of the seasonality of certain viruses. Rhinoviruses are isolated the whole year through, whereas parainfluenza viruses peak in autumn and early winter, adenovirus in autumn and winter, and influenza and respiratory syncytial viruses in winter.[5]

Infectious Rhinitis in Children

Children experience six to eight viral infections per year, with fever as the most frequent symptom. Infections are rare in the first 6 months because of maternal antibodies and increase during the second 6 months of life. After age 1 to 2 years, the common cold is most prevalent. There is a decline throughout the rest of childhood.[5] Children in daycare are at higher risk for respiratory illnesses.

Link with Asthma and Chronic Obstructive Pulmonary Disease

Viral respiratory tract infections are the most frequent cause of an acute asthma exacerbation and are associated with 80% to 85% of pediatric[7] and 80% of adult asthma exacerbations.[8] Rhinoviruses account for two-thirds of these infections. Coronavirus is the next most common cause but seems to result in less severe asthma exacerbations. In the lower airways of asthmatic patients, ICAM-1, the main receptor molecule for rhinoviruses, is upregulated, possibly accounting for the increased susceptibility to viral infection. Atopic asthmatic patients are not at greater risk than healthy individuals for rhinoviral infections, but they do suffer from more frequent respiratory tract infections in the lower airways that are more severe and last longer.[9] In vitro studies show that epithelial cells from asthmatic patients efficiently replicate rhinoviruses, whereas those from healthy individuals do not. The virus load in asthmatic patients is strongly correlated with the severity of both lower respiratory symptoms and increases in bronchial hyperreactivity. Decreased helper T-cell type 1 (T_H1) responses (interferon-γ and IL-12), considered to be protective for rhinovirus-induced illness, and augmented T_H2 responses (IL-4, IL-5, and IL-13) are responsible for more severe virus-induced asthma symptoms.[10] Consequentially, treating asthmatic patients with anti–immunoglobulin

E (IgE) and controlling the T_H2 response lead to improved asthma control, reduced need for asthma control medications, and near elimination of seasonal peaks in exacerbations induced by viral infections.[11]

Individuals with COPD are also at risk for viral infections. Although the frequency of viral respiratory tract infections is similar in patients with or without COPD, the use of medical resources, including hospital admissions and visits to emergency clinics, during viral respiratory illnesses is substantially increased in these patients.

Diagnosis and Differential Diagnosis

The diagnosis of a common cold is simple and based on the history and clinical signs and symptoms. There is no need for imaging or other diagnostic studies in the absence of complications. Isolation and identification of the causative virus have little value in clinical practice.

Infectious rhinitis should be differentiated from other types of rhinitis, such as allergic rhinitis, which is based on a history of atopy and exacerbation on allergen exposure. Ocular symptoms and nasal itching are more likely associated with allergic rhinitis, whereas mucopurulent discharge, facial pain, and anosmia are more likely associated with infectious rhinitis. Specific serum IgE and skin prick test (SPT) results can be used to help differentiate between the two.[2] Nonallergic, noninfectious "vasomotor" rhinitis manifests as chronic nasal symptoms not caused by an allergic or infectious process (Chapter 19). Symptoms include nasal obstruction and/or increased secretions, typically in response to changes in temperature, strong odors, passive tobacco smoke, alcohol, and emotional factors. Nonallergic rhinitis with eosinophilia syndrome is characterized by perennial nasal symptoms, particularly nasal congestion, sneezing, profuse watery rhinorrhea, nasal pruritus, and occasionally anosmia. Nasal smears demonstrate eosinophils, but patients lack evidence of allergic rhinitis. The existence of this entity is under debate; local allergy or allergy without a positive specific IgE in vitro or positive skin prick test (SPT) may be excluded by doing a nasal provocation test with the suspected allergen. The use of α-adrenergic decongestants for more than 10 days may induce rebound nasal congestion or rhinitis medicamentosa. Hormonal rhinitis and rhinitis gravidarum are mostly temporary forms of rhinitis that cease with the use of estrogen or with delivery. Atrophic rhinitis is characterized by crust formation, mucosal atrophy, and bacterial colonization.

Complications

Bacterial superinfection is the most common complication of viral rhinitis, occurring in 0.5% to 2.0% of the cases and resulting in acute bacterial rhinosinusitis (ABRS). Acute otitis media is the most common bacterial complication of colds in children, occurring in up to 20% of cases. Studies indicate that respiratory viruses play a crucial role in the development of acute otitis media, and detection rates of different viruses in the middle-ear fluid suggest that at least some viruses actively contribute to this inflammatory process.[3]

Treatment

PREVENTION

Prevention of the spread of viruses by proper hand hygiene, avoiding handshakes, and sharing objects can help prevent viral infections. Vaccination is impossible because of the large number of serologically distinct viral agents that cause the common cold. However, there is a vaccine commercially available for influenza, recommended for all age groups above 6 months of age for the injection and 2 years to 49 years for the attenuated nasal vaccine. The prophylactic use of vitamin C supplements fails to reduce the incidence of colds in the normal population but may reduce the duration and severity of a cold in selected individuals under physical and environmental stress. Air pollution, cigarette smoke, and the allergic diathesis are associated with impaired ciliary function, predisposing patients to colds.[2]

PHARMACOLOGIC

Watchful waiting and symptomatic relief of pain, cough, and malaise are generally recommended to treat the common cold. Analgesics, short-term local or oral decongestants, and isotonic saline irrigations can be helpful.[2] With new-generation influenza-specific antivirals (zanamivir, oseltamivir), the duration of clinical illness can be reduced by 1 to 2 days when the appropriate medication is started within 48 hours of the onset of symptoms.[3] Intranasal and oral glucocorticoids do not help, and antibiotics are contraindicated because they are not effective against viruses.

ACUTE RHINOSINUSITIS

Sinusitis is the inflammation of one or more of the paranasal sinuses. *Rhinosinusitis* is a more appropriate term than *sinusitis* in recognition of the continuity between the nose and paranasal sinuses in infectious and inflammatory diseases.[12,13]

Pathophysiology

Acute rhinosinusitis (ARS) primarily occurs after a viral respiratory tract infection and is subdivided into postviral rhinosinusitis and ABRS. They usually appear one after the other.

POSTVIRAL RHINOSINUSITIS

The difference between viral and postviral rhinosinusitis is the fact that a viral infection leads to inflammation in the nasal and paranasal mucosa and persists for several days after the viral replication ceases. Postviral rhinosinusitis is an increase in symptoms after 5 days from the onset of an infection or persistent symptoms after 10 days and for less than 12 weeks' duration.

ACUTE BACTERIAL RHINOSINUSITIS

Bacterial superinfection should be suspected when at least three of the following occur: initial improvement followed by worsening symptoms ("double sickening"); body temperature higher than 38°C; unilateral facial and tooth pain; elevated inflammatory parameters in the blood; and discolored discharge, often with unilateral predominance.[2,6,14] Secondary bacterial infection is thought to occur only in a small percentage of cases (0.5% to 2.0%). Factors associated with ABRS include a preceding viral infection, ciliary impairment, allergy, laryngopharyngeal reflux, *Helicobacter pylori* infection, nasotracheal intubation, and the presence or history of a nasogastric tube. The most common bacteria belong to the "infernal trio" and include *Streptococcus pneumoniae*, *Haemophilus influenzae*, and *Moraxella catarrhalis*. If the ARS does not resolve and the infection persists, anaerobic oropharyngeal flora and bacteria (i.e., *S. aureus* and *Pseudomonas aeruginosa*) predominate.[2]

Clinical Features

Acute rhinosinusitis is defined as anterior and/or posterior purulent nasal discharge with nasal obstruction or facial or dental pain, pressure, or fullness of up to 12 weeks' duration. Additional signs and symptoms include fever, cough, fatigue (malaise), hyposomia, anosmia, maxillary dental pain, and ear fullness or pressure. Although the general presentation of postviral rhinosinusitis and ABRS can be similar, a particular emphasis on the duration and severity of symptoms can help differentiate bacterial from viral illness.[6]

Epidemiology

Prevalence rates of ARS are between 6% and 15%. The primary cause is a viral infection; of all patients with a viral rhinitis-rhinosinusitis, 0.5% to 2.0% eventually develop ABRS. Prevalence of ARS is higher in winter months and in environments with higher air pollution. Allergic inflammation and cigarette smoke exposure are also associated with higher prevalence rates, possibly owing to alterations in ciliary motility and function. The role of laryngopharyngeal reflux in ARS remains unclear. Chronic concomitant diseases in children, poor mental health, and anatomic variations are also associated with an increased likelihood of ARS.[2]

Diagnosis

The diagnosis of ARS is based on clinical findings alone, without the use of special imaging techniques or laboratory tests. The diagnostic criteria are purulent nasal discharge with nasal obstruction or facial pain, pressure, or fullness of up to 12 weeks' duration. In the past, the term "subacute" ARS was used to describe symptoms between 4 to 8[4,6] and 4 to 12 weeks,[2] but this term has been abandoned in the latest European Position Paper on Rhinosinusitis and Nasal Polyps (EP²OS) guidelines because of the small size of the subgroup. Anterior rhinoscopy may be performed to examine the nasal mucosa for swelling and erythema, pus, and posterior nasal discharge; however, nasal endoscopy is usually not necessary to make the diagnosis. Also, the teeth and gingiva should be checked for inflammation or abscess formation to exclude dentogenic sinusitis or oroantral fistulas. Radiography is neither useful nor cost-effective, and computed tomography (CT) is not routinely recommended but is the preferred imaging option in cases of severe disease, an immunocompromised state, suspected complications, or alternative diagnosis or before surgery.[14] Nasal culture is also not generally recommended, except in the event of complications or treatment failure.[15] Sinus puncture is recommended in acute episodes refractory to treatment or for rapid and accurate identification of the causative organism in immunocompromised patients. Tests to assess for immunodeficiency include quantitative immunoglobulins and specific antibody titers, HIV testing, and other immune parameters to rule out primary or secondary immunodeficiency in suspected cases of recurrent sinusitis.

Treatment Options

The outcome of ARS can be self-limited or result in serious morbidity and mortality, depending on the infectious organism and immune competency. The appropriate treatment is to identify those patients who need medical treatment (i.e., antibiotics, intranasal glucocorticoids, or other medications) and those who need surgery in a timely fashion.

LIFESTYLE

See earlier discussion of infectious rhinitis.

PHARMACOLOGIC

"Watchful waiting" and symptomatic relief, in particular managing the discomfort associated with the disease, are recommended for mild cases of ARS. Nasal decongestants and isotonic saline irrigations are recommended.[2,16] Intranasal corticosteroids are effective to treat the inflammatory aspects and are indicated as monotherapy or, in severe cases, in combination with antibiotics.[17] The appropriate use of antibiotics depends on the symptoms, severity, and duration of the infection (e.g., antibiotics should be considered when the patient's problem fails to improve after 10 days, worsens after 5 days, and includes severe symptoms, including temperature >38°C, facial pain, and periorbital swelling). Amoxicillin is the first-choice drug and should be given for 10 to 14 days.[18] As previously stated, most ARS is viral in etiology and resolves without antibiotic use. The unnecessary use of antibiotics should be avoided because of the risk for adverse effects and the increasing problem of antimicrobial resistance. In addition, antibiotics do not reduce the risk for complications associated with ABRS.

When no improvement occurs after 48 hours of treatment, a consultation with a specialist is indicated. Hospitalization, nasal endoscopy, and appropriate imaging and cultures should be considered. Other adjunctive therapy, such as the use of antihistamines, mucolytics, and expectorants, may provide symptomatic relief in some cases. Recurrent ARS should be treated like any other ARS, but a more extensive workup is indicated to identify an underlying predisposition for this disease.

SURGICAL

Surgical intervention is primarily indicated in patients who have complications or severe frontal headaches refractory to medical therapy.

Complications in Acute Rhinosinusitis

Periorbital edema, displaced globe, double vision, ophthalmoplegia, reduced visual acuity, severe unilateral or bilateral frontal headache, frontal swelling, cranial nerve palsies, signs of meningitis, and focal neurologic signs are alarm signals.[2,12] Severe complications of ABRS include orbital (preseptal cellulitis, orbital cellulitis, orbital abscess), intracranial (cavernous vein thrombosis, encephalitis, meningitis, epidural or subdural abscess, brain abscess), or osseous (osteomyelitis) involvement. Such patients should be immediately referred to an otolaryngologist for nasal endoscopy, to obtain appropriate imaging tests and cultures, and hospitalization. Intravenous antibiotics and possible surgery may be necessary.[2]

Acute Rhinosinusitis in Children

The diagnosis of ARS in children is similar to that in adults. However, children are more susceptible to complications. Orbital complications are especially common in adolescents and need appropriate management to avoid blindness.[2]

Link with Asthma and Chronic Obstructive Pulmonary Disease

See earlier discussion of infectious rhinitis.

CHRONIC RHINOSINUSITIS

Chronic rhinosinusitis (CRS) is a heterogeneous group of inflammatory diseases of the nose and paranasal cavities and is defined by the EP²OS diagnostic criteria as the presence of at least two of the following: nasal obstruction, nasal secretion and/or postnasal drip, headache and/or facial pain or pressure, and a reduced sense of smell. Symptoms should be present for more than 12 weeks, with at least one symptom including nasal obstruction or nasal secretion. The impact of CRS on quality of life and work productivity is often underestimated. CRS can be stratified based on disease severity by using a visual analog scale (VAS) of 0 (no complaints) to 10 (most severe complaints) or based on the intranasal appearance in CRS without (*sine*) nasal polyps (CRSsNP) and with nasal polyps (CRSwNP).[2] Evidence points to notable differences between CRSsNP and CRSwNP in mucosal remodeling and the inflammation pattern. Cluster analyses are underway to further classify disease endotypes within these clinical phenotypes, potentially resulting in different treatment regimens for each subgroup.

Pathophysiology

Little is known about the pathophysiology of CRS and the factors that can lead to its chronicity. It is best considered as a multifactorial chronic inflammatory disorder in which allergy, mucosal dysfunction, and complex bacterial communities play a role. Anatomic abnormalities of the nose and paranasal cavities may also lead to obstruction of the osteomeatal complex; however, evidence is lacking that this is a major factor in most cases of CRS.

CHRONIC RHINOSINUSITIS WITHOUT NASAL POLYPS

The subcategory of CRSsNP is characterized by fibrosis, basement membrane thickening, goblet cell hyperplasia, subepithelial edema, and a mononuclear cell infiltration. It is a predominantly neutrophilic T_H1-biased inflammatory disease in which interferon-γ and transforming growth factor-β1 (TGF-β1) play key roles, causing an upregulation of collagen synthesis. There is a high regulatory T-cell activity and a mild inflammatory signature[13] (Figure 20.1).

CHRONIC RHINOSINUSITIS WITH NASAL POLYPS

Nasal polyps, pale smooth structures usually emanating bilaterally from the ostiomeatal complex and the skull base of both sides of the nose, are characterized by an eosinophilic T_H2-biased inflammatory disease, driven by IL-5 and eotaxin, which are responsible for the chemotaxis, activation, and survival of eosinophils.[19] TGF-ß, its receptors, and the number of regulatory T cells are downregulated in this disease. There is a lack of adequate collagen synthesis, resulting in edematous stroma and deposition of albumin, pseudocyst formation, and subepithelial and perivascular inflammatory cell infiltration[13] (see Figure 20.1).

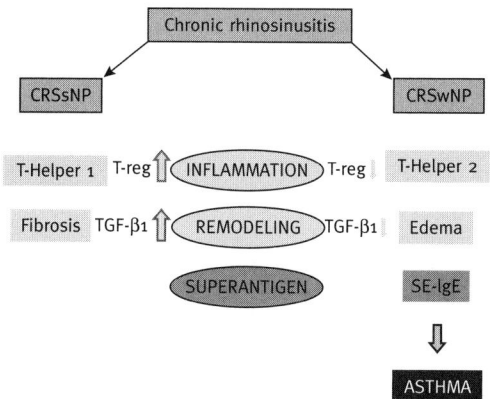

FIGURE 20.1 CRSsNP and CRSwNP are two phenotypes of chronic rhinosinusitis with different inflammatory and remodeling parameters. CRSsNP, chronic rhinosinusitis without nasal polyps; CRSwNP, chronic rhinosinusitis with nasal polyps; SE-IgE, specific IgE antibodies to *Staphylococcus aureus* enterotoxins; TGF-β1, transforming growth factor-β1; T-reg, regulatory T cell.

There is considerable heterogeneity based on predominant biomarkers within the subgroup of CRSwNP. Bachert and colleagues subdivided patients with nasal polyps into three groups depending on their total IgE concentrations and the presence of specific IgE antibodies against staphylococcal superantigens in tissue homogenates. Total IgE correlated with a higher comorbidity of asthma and aspirin sensitivity, whereas atopy to inhalant allergens was not related to total or specific IgE. No effect of atopy was found on any of the mediators or cytokines in the polyp group, questioning the role of common allergens in nasal polyp pathophysiology.[19] The same group also studied the effect of eosinophilic and neutrophilic types of inflammation and polyclonal IgE in nasal polyps from white and Asian patients to elucidate the inflammatory phenotype linking nasal polyps with asthma.[20] CRSwNP is orchestrated by T_H2 cells, with IL-5 as a major cytokine expressed in 83% of the Belgian nasal polyp patients in white subjects. IL-5 results in increased eosinophilic chemotaxis, activation, and survival and an eosinophilic type of inflammation, which is associated with IgE formation. However, only 16% of the Asian subjects with nasal polyps expressed IL-5, and less than 10% had the eosinophilic type of inflammation. The predominant effector T cell is the Th17 cell, with IL-17 as the key cytokine resulting in a predominance of neutrophils in these polyp patients. Such classification should lead to differential treatment regimens. Mucosal IgE in nasal polyp tissue activates mast cells; it is postulated that superantigen-induced polyclonal IgE in airway disease contributes to chronic inflammation by continuously activating mast cells. High mucosal IgE concentrations (>1,442 kU/L) are associated with asthma comorbidity in polyp patients.[20]

Biofilm

Microbial colonization of the sinuses in CRS is often characterized by the presence of polymicrobial bacterial biofilms, which adhere to the mucosa and serve as a reservoir for planktonic germs that may repeatedly invade the mucosa. Biofilms can protect pathogens from the host immune response and antibiotic therapies and permit bacteria to persist as a low-grade infection within the sinus mucosa; this may result in poor outcomes with conventional therapies. To assess the microbiome, DNA pyrosequencing is more sensitive and diverse than is obtaining a culture to detect microbes in the middle meatus, especially for certain genera, such as anaerobes. Studies suggest that subjects with CRS have different microbial communities with more *S. aureus*, whereas healthy individuals with normal sinuses are lightly colonized by commensal microorganisms. Antibiotic therapy may induce changes in the sinonasal microbiomes of CRS patients.[21] *Staphylococcus aureus* in biofilms is associated with an eosinophilic type of CRSwNP and may contribute to the T_H2 signature[22]; alternatively, activated macrophages in a T_H2 environment may allow it to colonize the mucosa owing to a deficit in phagocytosis.[23]

Staphylococcus aureus Superantigen

Staphylococcus aureus commonly colonizes the nose, with up to one-third of Europians identified as lifelong carriers of coagulase-positive organisms.[13] It is considered an aggravating and disease-modifying factor in CRSwNP. Patients with nasal polyps have increased colonization rates; for example, Van Zele and colleagues report such colonization in more than 60% of polyp patients and in up to 87% of the subgroup with asthma and aspirin sensitivity. This compares with control individuals and patients with CRSsNP, who had colonization rates of 33% and 27%, respectively.[24] *Staphylococcus aureus* may not only colonize the nasal mucosa, but it may also invade and reside in or form biofilms. Using peptide nucleic acid-fluorescence in situ hybridization, Corriveau and colleagues showed that *S. aureus* can create an intramucosal reservoir in polyp tissues from patients with aspirin-exacerbated respiratory disease (AERD).[25]

Staphylococcus aureus secretes enterotoxins that act like superantigens. A superantigen is able to activate T cells without undergoing processing by antigen-presenting cells by binding to the T-cell receptor through its variable β-chain, independent from the antigen-specific groove. This leads to strong immune reactions and a polyclonal activation of T and B cells, as well as the activation of structural and inflammatory cells. Superantigens amplify the T_H2 polarization and inhibit regulatory T-cell function and related cytokine production. Also, the enterotoxins are able to activate plasma cells and induce IgG4 and polyclonal IgE formation to multiple inhalant and noninhalant allergens, resulting in a high total IgE concentration in polyp tissue. Specific IgE antibodies to *S. aureus* enterotoxin (SE-IgE) are present in 28% of polyp samples, with rates as high as 80% in the subgroup with AERD. In contrast, only 15% of the control individuals and 6% of the patients with CRSsNP produce SE-IgE.[24] Other studies confirm that the presence of SE-IgE in the polyp mucosal tissue bears a significant risk for comorbid asthma.[20,26] These findings suggest a role for *S. aureus* enterotoxins as disease modifiers, especially in CRSwNP. *S. aureus* enterotoxin B contributes to the continuous mast cell degranulation, further shifting the cytokine pattern toward T_H2-type cytokines while disfavoring the regulatory T cytokines, IL-10 and TGF-β, released in nasal polyps.[27]

Clinical Features

In contrast to the pathologic diversity, the clinical presentation of CRS is quite nonspecific. It is not clear to what extent the pathological differences are reflected in the clinical presentation of CRS patients, since histologically and immunologically the differences are great but the clinical features are less distinct. The main diagnostic criteria are the presence of at least two of the following symptoms: nasal obstruction, nasal secretion and/or postnasal drip, headache and/or facial pain or pressure, and reduction in the sense of smell, with the presence of symptoms for more than 12 weeks during the past year without complete resolution of symptoms between episodes.[2,28] Pain appears to be less of a feature of CRSwNP compared with ARS or CRSsNP. There are additional minor symptoms, including ear pain or pressure, halitosis, dental pain, cough, fever, and fatigue, apart from the main signs and symptoms of this disease. Prolonged duration of rhinosinusitis symptoms (i.e., >8 to 12 weeks) is the primary reason to evaluate a patient for CRS. It is a general belief that nasal polyp patients have higher symptom scores with more olfactory dysfunction and that CRSsNP patients complain of more facial pain.[29] CRS has a significant impact on the patient's quality of life.

Diagnosis

In contrast to ARS, the clinical signs of CRS are not sufficient to make a diagnosis. In addition to the diagnostic criteria (see earlier), nasal endoscopy or a CT scan is necessary to support the diagnosis. The visualization of nasal polyps by nasal endoscopy, ideally after decongesting the nasal cavity, permits the diagnosis of CRSwNP. CRSsNP is diagnosed by visualizing mucopurulent discharge or edema found in the middle meatus or spheno ethmoid recesss.

When the findings on nasal endoscopy are equivocal, a CT scan is necessary before proceeding with surgery (Figure 20.2). Visualization of mucosal changes within the ostiomeatal complex and/or sinuses confirms the diagnosis of CRS. However, up to 42.5% of CT scans demonstrate sinus abnormalities in asymptomatic adults, with mucosal thickening

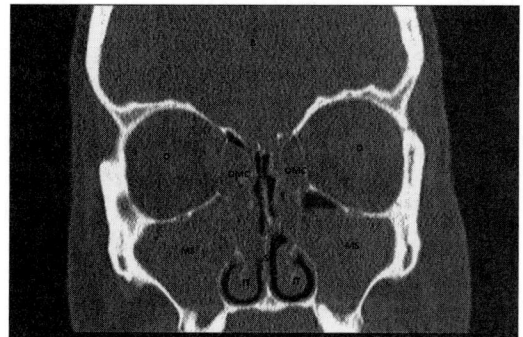

FIGURE 20.2 Coronal computed tomographic image of a patient with CRSwNP. B, brain; IT, inferior turbinate; MS, maxillary sinus; O; orbit; OMC, ostiomeatal complex; S, nasal septum.

most often identified in the ethmoid sinuses.[30] Such findings highlight the importance of correlating the clinical presentation with imaging results. Fungal disease, tumors, or extensions into the brain may require magnetic resonance imaging. Plain radiographic imaging is not beneficial to evaluate suspected CRS.[12]

Allergic rhinitis is a comorbidity of CRS because up to 60% of CRS patients are sensitized as determined by SPT or serum specific IgE measurements.[12] Allergic rhinitis as a comorbidity needs to be included in the management of such patients.

Other factors that need to be excluded include cystic fibrosis, immunodeficiencies, and ciliary dyskinesia. Other diseases should be considered when symptoms are unilateral: malignant or benign tumors, juvenile angiofibroma, antrochoanal polyps, and inverted papilloma. When headaches are the predominant complaint, the differential diagnosis should include migraine, tension headaches, cluster headaches, neuralgia, and problems with the teeth. Furthermore, underlying diseases need to be considered, such as Churg-Strauss syndrome, characterized by severe asthma, nasal polyps, eosinophilia, and eosinophilic vasculitis with granulomas (Chapter 2). About 50% of these patients are anti–neutrophil cytoplasmic antibody positive.

Epidemiology

The Global Allergy and Asthma Network of Excellence (GA$_2$LEN) performed a multicentered study to determine the prevalence of CRS, based on almost 60,000 questionnaires from 19 centers in 12 European countries. It concluded that the overall prevalence of CRS by EP^{2}OS criteria was 10.9%, ranging from 6.9% to 27.1%. Higher prevalences were recorded in the younger age group, in females, and in southern countries of Europe.[31] In the United States, CRS affects approximately 12.5% of the population.[32] CRS also affects an increasing proportion of the adult population until the sixth decade of life and then declines. Of all CRS patients, 20% to 33% have nasal polyps, 60% to 65% have CRS without nasal polyps, and 8% to 12% have allergic fungal sinusitis.

Comorbidities

Allergic rhinitis occurs in up to 60% of CRS patients, and patients are typically sensitized to perennial versus seasonal allergens. Primary ciliary dyskinesia (PCD) is a rare autosomal recessive disorder in which the mucosal cilia do not beat in a coordinated pattern. PCD is associated with chronic upper airway problems that begin from the first days of life and include chronic nasal discharge and bronchiectasis. The diagnosis can be confirmed by examining a mucosal biopsy sample under electron microscopy.[2] Up to 50% of patients with cystic fibrosis develop nasal polyps in the first decade of life. Gastroesophageal reflux disease is also suggested as a cause of sinusitis.[4]

Link with Asthma

The association between chronic rhinosinusitis and asthma has long been appreciated, although the pathophysiology of this link is not understood. Various mechanisms are proposed, including nasopharyngeal bronchial reflex, pulmonary aspiration of inflammatory cells and mediators through mucopurulent material, and the inhalation of dry (not appropriately humidified) cold air.[4] Studies in both children and adults suggest that the appropriate treatment of CRS results in objective and subjective improvement of asthma.[33] The Severe Asthma Research Program identified five different asthma phenotypes using cluster analysis. Up to 45% of the total cohort reported chronic sinus disease, with a higher prevalence in clusters in the higher age group. In one cluster, representing a nonatopic late-onset asthma group, nearly half of the patients reported prior sinus surgery.[34] The incidence of self-reported allergic rhinitis and rhinosinusitis in asthma patients was evaluated using the data of two cohorts. Of the 2,500 participants with bronchial asthma, 41% to 51% reported rhinosinusitis, and 35% reported both allergic rhinitis and rhinosinusitis on a questionnaire. Concomitant rhinosinusitis was associated with worse asthma, cough, quality of life, and sleep quality and an increased number of asthma exacerbations in one of the cohorts. The burden of symptoms was more pronounced in those with more severe asthma at baseline.[35] The link with allergic rhinitis and asthma could be explained by the common atopic pathway. However, asthma also occurs in nonatopic patients, and this group appears to develop more severe forms of asthma with concomitant CRS.

In a study performed in CRSwNP patients, the presence of SE-IgE and IL-5 and an increased total IgE concentration within the polyp tissue were identified as predictors of comorbid asthma.[20] Consequently, mean serum SE-IgE concentrations were found to be increased in patients with severe refractory asthma compared with patients with nonsevere asthma and controls. Moreover, asthmatic patients with an immune response to staphylococcal enterotoxins had a significantly higher serum total IgE, reduced lung function, and more hospitalizations within the past 12 months. This was not true for grass pollen– or house dust mite–specific IgE, which suggests that this effect is not purely due to the atopic diathesis. Staphylococcal enterotoxins could explain the elevated total IgE levels in nonatopic patients with severe asthma.[26]

Aspirin Intolerance

Aspirin and other nonsteroidal antiinflammatory drug (NSAID) intolerance should be suspected in patients with nasal polyps and asthma. The prevalence of AERD is about 8% in the CRSwNP group, significantly higher than in controls or CRSsNP. Polyps occur in more than 50% of patients with AERD. The intolerance to aspirin is thought to be secondary to alterations in the arachidonic acid metabolism. AERD usually develops first, with persistent rhinitis appearing during the third decade, followed by the onset of asthma, aspirin intolerance, and nasal polyposis. In about half of these patients, asthma is severe and glucocorticoid dependent. It is more common in females and nonatopic patients. The diagnosis of aspirin sensitivity is dependent on either a clear history of at least two aspirin/NSAID-induced reactions or by aspirin challenge, most reliably by the oral route. When present, patients should be warned to avoid drugs with cyclooxygenase-1 inhibitory activity. Aspirin desensitization can be considered. Sinus surgery is known to be associated with high relapse rates in AERD patients.[12]

Treatment Options

Because CRS is so heterogeneous, it is difficult to create general guidelines for its treatment. Goals for treatment include reduction of mucosal edema, reestablishment of sinus ventilation, and eradication of pathogens.[18]

LIFESTYLE

Studies describe an association of CRS with smoking in a dose-dependent manner, probably secondary to smoke-induced impaired mucociliary function; smoking cessation should be encouraged in patients with CRS.[31]

Avoiding upper respiratory tract infections by good hygiene practices also makes sense. Allergen avoidance is important in patients with comorbid allergic rhinitis. Air pollution is undesirable because it can impair mucociliary clearance.

PHARMACOLOGIC

CRSsNP. The management for mild symptoms (VAS score 0–3) and minimal mucosal disease follows a step-wise order starting with intranasal corticosteroids with nasal saline lavage[18] (Table 20.1). In cases with

Table 20.1. Evidence-Based Treatment Evidence and Recommendations for Adults with Chronic Rhinosinusitis without Nasal Polyps*†

THERAPY	LEVEL	GRADE OF RECOMMENDATION	RELEVANCE
Steroid—topical	Ia	A	Yes
Nasal saline irrigation	Ia	A	Yes
Bacterial lysates (OM-85 BV)	Ib	A	Unclear
Oral antibiotic therapy short term, <4 wk	II	B	During exacerbation
Oral antibiotic therapy long term, ≥12wk‡	Ib	C	Yes, especially if IgE is not elevated
Steroid—oral	IV	C	Unclear
Mucolytics	III	C	No
Proton pump inhibitors	III	D	No
Decongestant oral/topical	No data on single use	D	No
Allergen avoidance in allergic patients	IV	D	Yes
Oral antihistamine added in allergic patients	No data	D	No
Herbal and probiotics	No data	D	No
Immunotherapy	No data	D	No
Probiotics	Ib (−)§	A (−)	No
Antimycotics—topical	Ib (−)	A (−)	No
Antimycotics—systemic	No data	A (−)	No
Antibiotics—topical	Ib (−)	A (−)¶	No

* Some of these studies also included patients with CRS with nasal polyps.
† Acute exacerbations of CRS should be treated like acute rhinosinusitis.
‡ Level of evidence for macrolides in all patients with CRSsNP is Ib, and strength of recommendation is C, because the two double-blind placebo-controlled studies are contradictory; indications exist for better efficacy in CRSsNP patients with normal IgE and the recommendation A. No randomized controlled trials exist for other antibiotics.
§ Ib (−): Ib study with a negative outcome.
¶ A(−): grade A recommendation *not* to use.
From Fokkens WJ, Lund VJ, Mullol J, et al. EPOS 2012: European position paper on rhinosinusitis and nasal polyps 2012: a summary for otorhinolaryngologists. *Rhinology.* 2012;50(1):1–12.

improvement, the patients continue this treatment. If the condition does not improve within 3 months, a culture should be performed and long-term oral antibiotics prescribed, preferably macrolides. Treatment improvement with macrolides occurs gradually and may be partially due to their antiinflammatory properties. In cases with a lack of response after 3 months, a CT scan is advised, if not done before, to confirm the diagnosis, and sinus surgery should be considered. Initial management for moderate to severe symptoms (VAS score >3 to 10) with mucosal disease at endoscopy should include the following: start nasal lavage, topical corticosteroids, a culture, and long-term macrolides; if no response is seen within 3 months, a CT scan and surgery are warranted. Acute exacerbations of CRS should be treated as acute rhinosinusitis. The appropriate treatment of underlying allergic rhinitis is also recommended.[2]

CRSwNP. In patients with CRSwNP and symptoms of mild severity (VAS score 0 to 3) and minimal mucosal disease at endoscopy, treatment with a topical corticosteroid is recommended (Table 20.2). Glucocorticoid nasal drop and spray solutions are both effective, but the head-down instillation method with glucocorticoid drops appears to be a superior means to reach the ostiomeatal complex and skull base, which is the origin of nasal polyps. Treatment should be continued with follow-up every 6 months if improvement occurs within 3 months. If no improvement occurs within 3 months, a CT scan is recommended and the patient should be evaluated for surgery. With moderate severity (VAS

Table 20.2. Evidence-Based Treatment Evidence and Recommendations for Adults with Chronic Rhinosinusitis with Nasal Polyps*

THERAPY	LEVEL	GRADE OF RECOMMENDATION	RELEVANCE
Topical steroids	Ia	A	Yes
Oral steroids	Ia	A	Yes
Oral antibiotics short term, <4 wk	Ib and Ib(−)	C†	Yes, small effect
Oral antibiotics long term, ≥12 wk	III	C	Yes, especially if IgE is not elevated, small effect
Capsaicin	II	C	No
Proton pump inhibitors	II	C	No
Aspirin desensitization	II	C	Unclear
Furosemide	III	D	No
Immunosuppressants	IV	D	No
Nasal saline irrigation	Ib, no data in single use	D	Unclear
Topical antibiotics	No data	D	No
Anti–IL-5	No data	D	No
Phytotherapy	No data	D	No
Decongestant topical/oral	No data in single use	D	No
Mucolytics	No data	D	No
Oral antihistamine in allergic patients	No data	D	No
Antimycotics—topical	Ia (−)‡	A (−)	No
Antimycotics—systemic	Ib (−)§	A (−)¶	No
Antileukotrienes	Ib (−)	A (−)	No
Anti-IgE	Ib (−)	A (−)	No

*Some of these studies also included patients with CRS with nasal polyps.
†Short-term antibiotics show one positive and one negative study. Therefore, recommendation C.
‡Ia (−): Ia level of evidence that treatment is *not* effective.
§Ib (−): Ib study with a negative outcome.
¶A (−): grade A recommendation *not* to use.
From Fokkens WJ, Lund VJ, Mullol J, et al. EPOS 2012: European position paper on rhinosinusitis and nasal polyps 2012: a summary for otorhinolaryngologists. *Rhinology.* 2012;50(1):1–12.

score >3 to 7) with mucosal disease at endoscopy, topical corticosteroids, preferably drops, are recommended, and long-term treatment with doxycycline should be considered. When treatment is successful, intranasal corticosteroids should be continued and the patient followed every 6 months. If no improvement occurs, a CT scan is recommended with appropriate surgery. Severe cases of CRS with nasal polyps (VAS score >7 to 10) should initially be managed with a 3-week tapering course of oral glucocorticosteroids in combination with topical corticosteroids. Glucocorticoid therapy temporarily decreases mucosal inflammation, restores the sense of smell, and reduces the size of nasal polyps. After 1 month of improvement, the patient should be continued on topical corticosteroids and doxycycline. Once again, when improvement does not occur, an appropriate CT and surgical intervention may be necessary.[2]

Alternative treatment approaches are necessary for patients who have recurrent problems following surgery and have comorbid asthma. Anti–IL-5 (reslizumab, mepolizumab) and anti-IgE (omalizumab) have been tried in pilot studies[36,37] for such patients based on the roles of IL-5 and IgE in subjects with severe polyposis. Response rates to such treatments range from 50% to 80%; the use of biomarkers hopefully will increase the preselection of responders versus nonresponders.

SURGICAL

Functional endoscopic sinus surgery is minimally invasive surgery in which sinus air cells are opened under direct visualization. Indications for such surgery include persistence of CRS despite medical therapy to correct anatomic deformities believed to contribute to the disease and surgically removing nasal polyp tissue. The goal of such surgery is to restore patency of the ostiomeatal unit and improve sinus ventilation and drainage by enhancing the normal function of the mucociliary clearance system.[38] A conservative mucosa-sparing approach is advocated in CRSsNP, whereas the complete removal of polyp tissue is the goal with CRSwNP.

Long-term follow-up and maintenance treatment with intranasal corticosteroids and saline irrigation are recommended to reduce the recurrence rate. In nasal polyp patients, the long-term use of postoperative doxycycline is advocated in patients with nasal polyps.[39] Extensive surgery, including frontal sinus surgery, may be needed in selected patients who do not respond to appropriate medical and surgical intervention.

Chronic Rhinosinusitis in Children

Maxillary and ethmoidal sinuses are partially developed at birth; the frontal sinus begins to develop after the fourth year of life. The maxillary sinuses increase significantly in size after secondary dentition. Diagnostic criteria for CRS in children are the presence of two or more of the following symptoms, one of which should be either nasal blockage or nasal discharge: nasal blockage, nasal discharge, facial pain and pressure, and cough for 12 weeks or longer duration. As in adults, endoscopic examination is recommended. Plain radiographs are not recommended, and a CT scan is only recommended in children before surgery.[2] CT scan studies demonstrated that sinus opacification, mainly of maxillary and ethmoidal sinuses, occurs in 50% of symptomatic as well as asymptomatic children. The presence of sinus opacification decreases gradually with age, whereas the prevalence of allergy and anatomic abnormalities tend to increase.[40,41]

Recurrent acute and chronic sinusitis can be associated with other underlying diseases, which include immunodeficiency, cystic fibrosis, asthma, PCD, gastroesophageal reflux, allergic rhinitis, or other conditions associated with the obstruction of sinus ostia such as nasal polyps or a foreign body. Quantitative sweat chloride and genetic testing for cystic fibrosis should be considered when nasal polyps and/or colonization of the nose and sinuses with *Pseudomonas* species occur early in life.[4] Medical treatment using nasal saline irrigation and topical corticosteroids in mild cases (VAS score 0 to 3) and long-term antibiotics in persistent or moderate to severe cases (VAS score >3 to 10) is preferable in children.

When failure occurs after 3 months of therapy, rhinoscopy and a CT scan and the need for adenoidectomy and/or sinus irrigation should be considered. Endoscopic sinus surgery in children should be reserved for those with severe problems who fail medical therapy.[2]

FUNGAL RHINOSINUSITIS

Fungal spores are ubiquitous and are continuously inhaled and deposited in the airway mucosa. Fungi are present in the nose in the most human subjects from the beginning days of life. *Aspergillus, Penicillium, Cladosporium, Candida, Aureobasidium,* and *Alternaria* are the most frequently found species. Although they rarely are pathogenic in healthy individuals, they may cause human disease in others. The noninvasive versus the invasive forms of fungal rhinosinusitis are more common.[42]

Noninvasive

Fungal hyphae in noninvasive fungal rhinosinusitis do not penetrate the mucosal barrier but reside within the sinus lumen primarily in immunocompetent subjects. They can be further differentiated into "fungal balls," with persistent fungi within the sinuses not associated with an immune reaction, or allergic fungal sinusitis (AFS), an immune reaction associated with high levels of IgE.[43]

FUNGAL BALL

Fungal ball, previously termed *sinus mycetoma,* is present in 3.7% of all sinus surgeries. It is a noninvasive condition in which many devitalized fungal hyphae are found compressed into a thick exudate or ball within a sinus cavity. In general, only one sinus is affected. It occurs in patients with previous sinus surgery, oral-sinus fistula, history of cancer chemotherapy, and sometimes without any predisposing factor. Surgical evacuation is curative.[43]

ALLERGIC FUNGAL SINUSITIS

The incidence of AFS is 6% to 9% in patients with CRS and higher in warmer climates. Patients with this disease are immunocompetent and often atopic and sensitized to multiple aeroallergens, including the fungus cultured during surgery. There is a strong IgE-mediated hypersensitivity response in the presence of extramucosal sinus fungal hyphae. This, together with the presence of eosinophils in the mucin, has led to the name "allergic," although the etiology of the reaction may not be allergic at all. Both the histopathology and the immunopathology of AFS strongly resemble the characteristics of allergic bronchopulmonary aspergillosis, but total serum IgE levels are usually not as high.

The Bent and Kuhn diagnostic criteria include fungus-specific IgE by SPT or serology; the presence of documented nasal polyposis; characteristic CT findings; eosinophilic mucin and inflammation; and a positive fungal stain of mucin or on the surface of tissue removed during surgery with no histologic evidence of invasive fungal disease.[44] The sinus mucosa demonstrates eosinophilic-lymphocytic inflammation without evidence for mucosal fungal invasion, such as mucosal necrosis, granuloma formation, or giant cells on histopathology. Allergic mucin is an ill-defined pathologic entity with the appearance of a peanut buttery viscoelastic, eosinophil-rich material. The histopathologic features include high concretions of pyknotic eosinophils and sparse numbers of fungal hyphae. Attempts to identify specific fungal species using fungal stains of allergic mucin are often unreliable. Diagnosis requires culture of intraoperative material and typically shows fungi such as *Bipolaris spicifera, Curvularia lunata,* or *Aspergillus* species.[45] The allergic mucin and associated hypertrophic sinus mucosa may occasionally expand and extend through the sinus wall into the orbit or cranium, resulting from bone resorption secondary to the pressure from the expanding fungal mass. The sinus CT scan shows evidence of extensive rhinosinusitis often with evidence of erosions and expansion of the bony sinus walls and areas of hyperattenuation with abnormal paranasal sinuses (Figure 20.3). AFS typically affects multiple sinuses.

Treatment requires surgical clearing with removal of all obstructing fungus-containing mucin and diseased hypertrophic mucosa. The disease commonly reoccurs, so long-term

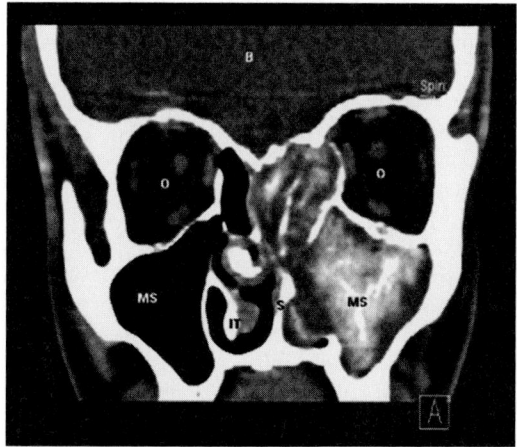

FIGURE 20.3 Coronal computed tomographic (CT) image of a patient with allergic fungal sinusitis. The sinus CT scan shows evidence of erosions and expansion of the bony sinus walls and areas of hyperattenuation within abnormal paranasal sinuses. B, brain; IT, inferior turbinate; MS, maxillary sinus; O, orbit; S, nasal septum.

follow-up is necessary. Longer term use of oral corticosteroids is often required for AFS just as it is for ABPA. Topical nasal corticosteroids are also indicated. Systemic antifungal drugs are not an effective treatment for AFS.[43]

Invasive

Invasive forms of fungal rhinosinusitis are rare and occur in immunocompromised hosts, mostly in India, Africa, and Saudi Arabia.

ACUTE NECROTIZING RHINOSINUSITIS

In this form of invasive fungal RS, formerly known as mucormycosis, the infection often begins with fever, a nasal eschar, or paranasal anesthesia. Although *Rhizopus* species are a common offender, virtually any fungi can be involved in this disease. It primarily occurs in immunocompromised patients, the main reason for a poor prognosis. Rapid spread of the fungal infection from the sinonasal mucosa to surrounding soft tissues and bone with widespread facial tissue necrosis leads to high morbidity and mortality. Wide surgical debridement of infected and devitalized tissues in combination with antifungal drug therapy is urgently required.[43,45]

CHRONIC INVASIVE FUNGAL RHINOSINUSITIS

This form of fungal rhinosinusitis is less aggressive and also occurs in patients with an increased susceptibility to infection, such as patients with diabetes mellitus. Ethmoid fungal infection commonly causes periorbital tissue invasion or the orbital apex syndrome. Treatment requires systemic antifungal drugs and surgical debridement. The infection often recurs and can be difficult to eliminate.[43]

GRANULOMATOUS INVASIVE (INDOLENT) FUNGAL RHINOSINUSITIS

Invading fungal hyphae are well contained within necrotizing granulomas at the surface of the sinus mucosa. There is no significant tissue invasion by fungi outside of these granulomas. Patients are immunocompetent, and the most common predisposing risk factor is previous sinus surgery for some form of chronic recurring rhinosinusitus.[43] Sinus mucosal resection may be curative, but systemic antifungal medications are commonly used postoperatively to ensure complete resolution of the fungal infection when the histopathologic diagnosis is available.[45]

Fungi as a Cause of All Chronic Rhinosinusitis

Fungi were postulated as a potential cause of all CRS in the late 1990s. However, the presence of fungal hyphae in nasal secretions of CRS patients does not imply a causal relationship, and several studies find topical and systemic antifungal treatments ineffective to treat the disease.[42,46]

UNMET, FUTURE RESEARCH NEEDS

1. There is need for large multicenter studies investigating the link between lower and upper airways to better understand the

pathophysiology of this link for allergic and nonallergic asthma.

2. The upper airways should always be evaluated during clinical investigation of asthma, especially with respect to exacerbations and severe disease. Assessing total serum IgE and SE-IgE should be part of the standard workup of asthmatic patients because they are important to determine the impact of upper airway disease and superantigens on severe asthma.

3. A cluster analysis of CRS, based on clinical and immune markers, is needed. This information may lead to a better idea of prognosis and permit identification of phenotypes and endotypes and of the response of these phenotypes and endotypes to innovative therapies, including biologic therapies.

4. The distribution of CRS phenotypes and endotypes may not be identical throughout the world; disease subgroups and the impact of the microbiome on these subgroups should be identified and evaluated.

5. New therapeutic options, including antibiotic or anti-IgE strategies, should be tested for patients with high total serum IgE, based on polyclonal activation by superantigens, independent of the allergic status.

CONCLUSION

The link between the upper and lower airways is no longer a matter of debate. Acute or chronic disease of the upper airways and colonization by microorganisms such as *S. aureus* leads to worsening of asthma symptoms. Asthmatic patients also are known to be more prone to developing CRS. Proper treatment of upper airway pathology, both medically and surgically, results in objective and subjective improvement of asthma. Understanding upper airway disease and its impact on asthma will provide new insights, not only in the pathogenesis of asthma, but also in its treatment.

REFERENCES

1. Glovsky MM. Upper airways involvement in bronchial asthma. *Curr Opin Pulm Med*. 1998;4(1):54–58.
2. Fokkens WJ, Lund VJ, Mullol J, et al. EPOS 2012: European position paper on rhinosinusitis and nasal polyps 2012: a summary for otorhinolaryngologists. *Rhinology*. 2012;50(1):1–12.
3. Heikkinen T, Jarvinen A. The common cold. *Lancet*. 2003;361(9351):51–59.
4. Slavin RG, Spector SL, Bernstein IL, et al. The diagnosis and management of sinusitis: a practice parameter update. *J Allergy Clin Immunol*. 2005;116(6 Suppl):S13–S47.
5. Monto AS, Sullivan KM. Acute respiratory illness in the community: frequency of illness and the agents involved. *Epidemiol Infect*. 1993;110(1):145–160.
6. Rosenfeld RM, Andes D, Bhattacharyya N, et al. Clinical practice guideline: adult sinusitis. *Otolaryngol Head Neck Surg*. 2007;137(3 Suppl):S1–S31.
7. Johnston SL, Pattemore PK, Sanderson G, et al. Community study of role of viral infections in exacerbations of asthma in 9-11 year old children. *BMJ*. 1995;310(6989):1225–1229.
8. Nicholson KG, Kent J, Ireland DC. Respiratory viruses and exacerbations of asthma in adults. *BMJ*. 1993;307(6910):982–986.
9. Corne JM, Marshall C, Smith S, et al. Frequency, severity, and duration of rhinovirus infections in asthmatic and non-asthmatic individuals: a longitudinal cohort study. *Lancet*. 2002;359(9309):831–834.
10. Message SD, Laza-Stanca V, Mallia P, et al. Rhinovirus-induced lower respiratory illness is increased in asthma and related to virus load and Th1/2 cytokine and IL-10 production. *Proc Natl Acad Sci U S A*. 2008;105(36):13562–13567.
11. Busse WW, Morgan WJ, Gergen PJ, et al. Randomized trial of omalizumab (anti-IgE) for asthma in inner-city children. *N Engl J Med*. 2011;364(11):1005–1015.
12. Scadding GK, Durham SR, Mirakian R, et al. BSACI guidelines for the management of rhinosinusitis and nasal polyposis. *Clin Exp Allergy*. 2008;38(2):260–275.
13. Van Crombruggen K, Zhang N, Gevaert P, Tomassen P, Bachert C. Pathogenesis of chronic rhinosinusitis: inflammation. *J Allergy Clin Immunol*. 2011;128(4):728–732.
14. Meltzer EO, Hamilos DL. Rhinosinusitis diagnosis and management for the clinician: a synopsis of recent consensus guidelines. *Mayo Clin Proc*. 2011;86(5):427–443.
15. Fokkens W, Lund V, Mullol J, for the European Position Paper on Rhinositus and Nasal Polyps Group. European position paper on rhinosinusitis and nasal polyps 2007. *Rhinol Suppl*. 2007;20:1–136.

16. Jund R, Mondliger M, Steindl H, et al. Clinical efficacy of a dry extract of five herbal drugs in acute viral rhinosinusitis. *Rhinology*. 2012;50(4):417–426.
17. Meltzer EO, Bachert C, Staudinger H. Treating acute rhinosinusitis: comparing efficacy and safety of mometasone furoate nasal spray, amoxicillin, and placebo. *J Allergy Clin Immunol*. 2005;116(6):1289–1295.
18. Chan Y, Kuhn FA. An update on the classifications, diagnosis, and treatment of rhinosinusitis. *Curr Opin Otolaryngol Head Neck Surg*. 2009;17(3):204–208.
19. Bachert C, Gevaert P, Holtappels G, Johansson SG, van Cauwenberge P. Total and specific IgE in nasal polyps is related to local eosinophilic inflammation. *J Allergy Clin Immunol*. 2001;107(4):607–614.
20. Bachert C, Zhang N, Holtapels G, et al. Presence of IL-5 protein and IgE antibodies to staphylococcal enterotoxins in nasal polyps is associated with comorbid asthma. *J Allergy Clin Immunol*. 2010;126(5):962–968, 8 e1–6.
21. Feazel LM, Robertson CE, Ramakrishnan VR, Frank DN. Microbiome complexity and Staphylococcus aureus in chronic rhinosinusitis. *Laryngoscope*. 2012;122(2):467–472.
22. Foreman A, Holtappels G, Psaltis AJ, et al. Adaptive immune responses in Staphylococcus aureus biofilm-associated chronic rhinosinusitis. *Allergy*. 2011;66(11):1449–1456.
23. Krysko O, Holtappels G, Zhang N, et al. Alternatively activated macrophages and impaired phagocytosis of S. aureus in chronic rhinosinusitis. *Allergy*. 2011;66(3):396–403.
24. Van Zele T, Gevaert P, Watelet JB, et al. Staphylococcus aureus colonization and IgE antibody formation to enterotoxins is increased in nasal polyposis. *J Allergy Clin Immunol*. 2004;114(4):981–983.
25. Corriveau MN, Zhang N, Holtappels G, Van Roy N, Bachert C. Detection of *Staphylococcus aureus* in nasal tissue with peptide nucleic acid-fluorescence in situ hybridization. *Am J Rhinol Allergy*. 2009;23(5):461–465.
26. Kowalski ML, Cieslak M, Perez-Novo CA, Makowska JS, Bachert C. Clinical and immunological determinants of severe/refractory asthma (SRA): association with staphylococcal superantigen-specific IgE antibodies. *Allergy*. 2011;66(1):32–38.
27. Patou J, Gevaert P, Van Zele T, Holtappels G, van Cauwenberge P, Bachert C. Staphylococcus aureus enterotoxin B, protein A, and lipoteichoic acid stimulations in nasal polyps. *J Allergy Clin Immunol*. 2008;121(1):110–115.
28. Bachert C, Van Bruaene N, Toskala E, et al. Important research questions in allergy and related diseases: 3-chronic rhinosinusitis and nasal polyposis—a GALEN study. *Allergy*. 2009;64(4):520–533.
29. Litvack JR, Fong K, Mace J, James KE, Smith TL. Predictors of olfactory dysfunction in patients with chronic rhinosinusitis. *Laryngoscope*. 2008;118(12):2225–2230.
30. Havas TE, Motbey JA, Gullane PJ. Prevalence of incidental abnormalities on computed tomographic scans of the paranasal sinuses. *Arch Otolaryngol Head Neck Surg*. 1988;114(8):856–859.
31. Hastan D, Fokkens WJ, Bachert C, et al. Chronic rhinosinusitis in Europe: an underestimated disease. A GA(2)LEN study. *Allergy*. 2011;66(9):1216–1223.
32. Hamilos DL. Chronic rhinosinusitis: epidemiology and medical management. *J Allergy Clin Immunol*. 2011;128(4):693–707.
33. Rachelefsky GS, Katz RM, Siegel SC. Chronic sinus disease with associated reactive airway disease in children. *Pediatrics*. 1984;73(4):526–529.
34. Moore WC, Meyers DA, Wenzel SE, et al. Identification of asthma phenotypes using cluster analysis in the Severe Asthma Research Program. *Am J Respir Crit Care Med*. 2010;181(4):315–323.
35. Dixon AE, Kaminsky DA, Holbrook JT, Wise RA, Shade DM, Irvin CG. Allergic rhinitis and sinusitis in asthma: differential effects on symptoms and pulmonary function. *Chest*. 2006;130(2):429–435.
36. Gevaert P, Van Bruaene N, Cattaert T, et al. Mepolizumab, a humanized anti-IL-5 mAb, as a treatment option for severe nasal polyposis. *J Allergy Clin Immunol*. 2011;128(5): 989–995 e1–8.
37. Gevaert P, Calus L, Van Zele T, et al. Omalizumab is effective in allergic and nonallergic patients with nasal polyps and asthma. *J Allergy Clin Immunol*. 2013;131(1):110–116 e1.
38. Stammberger H, Posawetz W. Functional endoscopic sinus surgery: concept, indications and results of the Messerklinger technique. *Eur Arch Otorhinolaryngol*. 1990;247(2):63–76.
39. Van Zele T, Gevaert P, Holtappels G, et al. Oral steroids and doxycycline: two different approaches to treat nasal polyps. *J Allergy Clin Immunol*. 2010;125(5):1069–1076 e4.
40. Diament MJ, Senac MO Jr, Gilsanz V, Baker S, Gillespie T, Larsson S. Prevalence of incidental

paranasal sinuses opacification in pediatric patients: a CT study. *J Comput Assist Tomogr.* 1987;11(3):426–431.

41. van der Veken PJ, Clement PA, Buisseret T, Desprechins B, Kaufman L, Derde MP. CT scan study of the incidence of sinus involvement and nasal anatomic variations in 196 children. *Rhinology.* 1990;28(3):177–184.

42. Fokkens WJ, Ebbens F, van Drunen CM. Fungus: a role in pathophysiology of chronic rhinosinusitis, disease modifier, a treatment target, or no role at all? *Immunol Allergy Clin N Am.* 2009;29(4):677–688.

43. Schubert MS. Allergic fungal sinusitis. *Clin Rev Allergy Immunol.* 2006;30(3):205–216.

44. Bent JP 3rd, Kuhn FA. Diagnosis of allergic fungal sinusitis. *Otolaryngol Head Neck Surg.* 1994;111(5):580–588.

45. Schubert MS. Allergic fungal sinusitis: pathophysiology, diagnosis and management. *Med Mycol.* 2009;47(Suppl 1):S324–S330.

46. Sacks PL, Harvey RJ, Rimmer J, Gallagher RM, Sacks R. Topical and systemic antifungal therapy for the symptomatic treatment of chronic rhinosinusitis. *Cochrane Database Syst Rev.* 2011;8:CD008263.

21

NASAL POLYPS AND CHRONIC RHINOSINUSITIS

COMORBID

Hae-Sim Park, Mario Sánchez-Borges, Seung Youp Shin, and Marek L. Kowalski

KEY POINTS

- Chronic rhinosinusitis with nasal polyps is a common comorbid condition of asthma.
- Chronic rhinosinusitis with nasal polyps is usually characterized by nasal blockage or obstruction, nasal discharge, and olfactory dysfunction.
- Some patients with chronic rhinosinusitis with nasal polyps and asthma react to aspirin and other nonsteroidal anti-inflammatory drugs, usually with acute rhinorrhea, nasal congestion and an asthma exacerbation. Such reactions can be life threatening. These drugs should be avoided in such patients.
- Medical treatment is the treatment of choice for patients with chronic rhinosinusitis with nasal polyposis.
- Most data indicate that both medical and surgical treatment of chronic rhinosinusitis with or without nasal polyps improves asthma outcomes.

INTRODUCTION

Nasal polyps (NPs) are outgrowths of the upper airway mucosa that arise from the ethmoidal sinuses, the middle turbinate, or the maxillary sinuses and are characterized by inflammatory cell infiltration, structural modifications in the epithelium (e.g., goblet cell hyperplasia), and changes in the lamina propria (accumulation of extracellular matrix proteins, edema, and glandular hyperplasia). Based on morphology and localization, at least two types of NPs can be distinguished, antrochoanal and ethmoidal, but the bilateral type of NP is associated with eosinophilic inflammation of the airway mucosa and bronchial asthma.[1] NPs are rarely a separate entity and most commonly arise from underlying inflammation of the sinus mucosa, as with chronic rhinosinusitis (CRS), and may coexist with bronchial asthma with cystic fibrosis, Kartegener's syndrome, or Wegener's granulomatosis (granulomatosis

Table 21.1. Differential Characteristics of Chronic Rhinosinusitis with Nasal Polyps and without Nasal Polyps in Association with Asthma

	CRSwNP	CRSsNP
Association with asthma	Strong	Medium/weak
Symptoms	Nasal obstruction	Headache
	Loss of smell	Postnasal drip
Histopathology	Eosinophilia	Mononuclear cells, neutrophils
T-cell polarization	T_H2 type	T_H1 type
Cytokines increased in sinus mucosa	IL-4, IL-5, IL-25, IL-33, CCL18, and eotaxin-3	IFN-γ, IL-32, and TGF-β1
Regulatory T cells/factors	FOXP3 decreased	FOXP3 normal
Remodeling with collagen formation	Absent	Present

CCL18, chemokine ligand 18; FOXP3, forkhead box P3; IFN-γ, interferon-γ; IL, interleukin; TGF-β1, transforming growth factor-β1; T_H1, helper T cell type 1; T_H2, helper T cell type 2.

polyangiitis) in a minority of cases. Thus it seems more appropriate not to discuss NPs in the context of asthma comorbidities separately, but rather to consider NPs as a hallmark of chronic inflammatory diseases of the sinus mucosa.

CRS is a heterogeneous disorder and may be associated with NPs (CRSwNP) or not (CRSsNP).[2] Both forms of CRS, with and without NPs, are considered distinct entities with a different pathophysiology, specific inflammatory cells or cytokine patterns, and variation in remodeling tendencies. CRSwNP is characterized by eosinophilic inflammation influenced by helper T-cell type 2 (T_H2) cytokines, downregulation of regulatory T cells, and decreased transforming growth factor-β (TGF-β) expression in the paranasal mucosa. Evidence of T_H2 bias toward eosinophilic inflammation is provided by increased expression of interleukin-5 (IL-5) and local immunoglobulin E (IgE) generation in NP tissue, and may be a risk factor for asthma development. In contrast, predominantly neutrophilic inflammation resulting from Th1/Th17 cells occurs in patients with CRSsNP, associated with normal regulatory T cells and increased TGF-β expression.[3] Excess tissue repair and fibrosis formation (remodeling) are probably a consequence of TGF-β activity (Table 21.1). However, this form of CRS is less likely to be associated with bronchial asthma.

NASAL POLYPOSIS AND CHRONIC RHINOSINUSITIS AS A COMORBID CONDITION WITH ASTHMA

X-rays of paranasal sinuses are abnormal in 31% to 75% of children and adults with asthma, compared with 15% to 26% of normal, asymptomatic individuals, and mucosal thickening can be visualized by computed tomography (CT) scans in 74% of asthmatic patients.[4] Thirty to fifty percent of patients with CRS may suffer from bronchial asthma. Asthma is more prevalent in white European patients (with mostly eosinophilic polyps) than in Asian patients, who mostly exhibit neutrophilic CRSwNP.[5] The Global Allergy and Asthma Network of Excellence conducted a questionnaire in a representative sample of more than 52,000 adults living in Europe to assess the presence of asthma and CRS defined by the European Position Paper on Rhinosinusitis and Nasal Polyps criteria.[6] That study demonstrated a strong association between asthma and CRS (adjusted odds ratio [OR], 3.47; 95% confidence interval [CI], 3.20 to 3.76) at all ages. Asthmatic patients with CRS are also more likely to have NPs than nonasthmatic patients (57.6% vs. 25%).[7] Although it is widely accepted that the presence of CRS and/or NP aggravates the course of asthma, few studies support such a perspective. CRS has been associated with lower airway disease, particularly asthma, which may reflect increased asthma severity.[8] In another study, CRS was related to more severe asthma as defined by higher medication use and lower forced expiratory volume in one second (FEV_1).[9] A cross-sectional analysis of prospectively collected data in 187 patients with CRS demonstrated that increased asthma severity is associated with radiologic severity of CRS and a greater prevalence of NPs. Indirect evidence for the association between CRSwNP and asthma severity arises from analysis of patients with aspirin-exacerbated respiratory disease (AERD), who usually suffer from pansinusitis with recurrent NPs. The presence of aspirin hypersensitivity is a risk factor for difficult-to-treat asthma. Patients with AERD have persistent asthma of greater than average severity and require greater use of medication than subjects without AERD, including dependence on corticosteroids.[10,11]

The pathogenesis of CRS and NP has not been fully elucidated. Although IgE sensitization is more prevalent in patients with CRSwNP (30% of patients with NP have atopy), disease severity and intensity of underlying eosinophilic inflammation in the upper airways are independent of allergic sensitization.[12] However, both upper and lower airway inflammation also occur in subjects without NPs. It has been postulated that mucosal inflammation may represent either a local or systemic immunologic response to environmental stimuli such as air pollution, active or second-hand cigarette smoke, or infections (viral, bacterial, or fungal). Development of local inflammatory responses and NP formation may reflect abnormalities in host innate and adaptive response to these heterogeneous, external stimuli.[13] Although both fungal and bacterial antigens were implicated by earlier studies, data suggest a role for *Staphylococcus aureus* enterotoxins (SEs) in the pathogenesis of CRSwNP. The incidence of staphylococcal colonization in CRSwNP is 64%, which is twice as frequent as in CRSsNP,[14] and it increases to 87% in subjects with asthma and AERD. Furthermore, specific IgE to SEs is increased in NP tissue compared with normal mucosa and further increased in NPs from subjects with AERD.[15] It has been postulated that SE superantigens by means of T-cell activation induce polyclonal IgE production by local B cells, resulting in continuous activation of eosinophils and mast cells and development of inflammation underlying CRSwNP.

The mechanisms linking the pathophysiology of upper airway diseases (CRSwNP) with the development and/or aggravation of lower airway inflammatory disease (bronchial asthma) have not been elucidated. Although several hypotheses explaining the comorbid association between CRS and asthma have been proposed (Table 21.2), limited

Table 21.2. Possible Mechanisms Linking Chronic Rhinosinusitis with Nasal Polyps and Bronchial Asthma

Neurogenic reflex
Loss of the protective function of the nose (mouth breathing)
Aspiration of nasal secretions into the lower airway
Common triggers operating in the background of an impaired innate immune response
- Infectious agents (fungal, bacterial, viral)
- Allergens
- Other environmental factors (e.g., tobacco smoke)

Activation of systemic inflammation and involvement of bone-marrow-derived inflammatory cells, particularly eosinophils experimental data are available. The role of neural reflexes, mouth breathing, or aspiration of paranasal secretions into the lower airways has not been supported with plausible experimental data from human models. A similar set of etiologic factors (infectious or environmental) has been implicated in the development of CRS and bronchial asthma, suggesting that these triggers may act in concert to initiate upper and lower airway eosinophilic inflammation in susceptible individuals. Experimental data have accumulated to support the role for SEs as superantigens to induce a local immunologic response and generate SEs specific to IgE with subsequent development of eosinophilic inflammation in the upper and lower airways. The presence of sIgE to SE in nasal tissue constitutes a significant risk factor (OR, 7.78) for the development of bronchial asthma, and the serum level of SE-specific IgE is almost three times higher in patients with severe asthma compared with those with non-severe asthma, suggesting associations among the immune response, enterotoxins, and airway inflammation.

Clinical Features, Diagnosis, and Differential Diagnosis

Typical clinical symptoms of CRSwNP are nasal blockage or obstruction, nasal discharge, and olfactory dysfunction. Reduced or lost sense of smell may be a leading symptom in patients with NP, although it occurs in CRSsNP, albeit less commonly. Conversely, facial pain is rare in patients with NP. The clinical course of CRSwNP is characterized by recurring episodes of symptom exacerbation often accompanied by bacterial infections with mucopurulent nasal discharge, malaise, and elevated temperature. NPs, particularly in patients with asthma, recur after surgery. CRS with or without NPs may affect the quality of life (QOL) of patients and impair their work or school performance.

A subpopulation of individuals with CRSwNP reacts to aspirin and other nonsteroidal antiinflammatory drugs with acute upper (rhinorrhea and congestion) and usually lower (asthma exacerbation) respiratory symptoms.[16] These subjects present with an underlying chronic inflammatory airway disorder manifesting as CRS and usually as bronchial asthma. This condition is referred to as the aspirin triad and more recently as AERD. In patients with AERD, CRS usually has a protracted course and is complicated by mucosal hypertrophy and NP formation.[17] On CT, mucosal hypertrophy is present in up to 100% of patients, and the frequency of NPs may be as high as 90%.[18] NPs usually recur after surgery; the recurrence rate in patients with AERD following endoscopic sinus surgery is almost 10 times greater than that in aspirin-tolerant patients.[19] A subgroup of patients with AERD may not have asthma but will manifest a reaction to aspirin exclusively in the upper respiratory tract. However, the clinical picture of nasal disease (hypertrophic rhinosinusitis) in these patients is similar to that observed in patients with AERD.

The diagnosis of CRSwNP is based on symptoms, endoscopic findings, and CT abnormalities. Nasal endoscopy may reveal edema and mucosal obstruction, mucopurulent discharge, and/or NPs. Characteristic CT changes include mucosal hypertrophy within the ostiomeatal complex and/or sinuses and mucosal thickening or opacification. The differential diagnosis of CRSwNP should include specific disorders that may predispose the patient to the development of NPs, such as ciliary dysfunction, cystic fibrosis, or immune deficiency, typically characterized by noneosinophilic polyps. The possibility of fungal or bacterial sinus infections resistant to treatment should also be investigated.

LIFESTYLE AND BURDEN OF RHINOSINUSITIS

Based on the SF-36, a questionnaire that determines health-related QOL, CRS has a negative impact on several aspects of QOL, with a greater impact on social functioning than chronic heart failure, angina, or back pain.[20,21] Patients with CRSwNP tend to report better QOL than those with CRSsNP, despite worse CT and endoscopy scores.[22] However, patients with CRSwNP and asthma have poorer QOL than CRSwNP patients without asthma. AERD also has a negative effect on QOL.[23] Based on patient-reported outcomes, QOL improves in patients with CRSwNP after both medical and surgical interventions.[24,25] Treatment with a short course of oral corticosteroids (7 to 10 days, 0.2 to 0.5 mg/kg/day of prednisone or equivalent) followed by intranasal corticosteroids (INS) improves QOL of patients with CRSwNP.

The economic burden of CRSwNP in the United States has been estimated to be $5.78 billion USD/year.[26] In North America, direct costs spent for CRS are $2,609/patient per year, whereas in Europe direct costs are $1,861/patient per year. Patients with CRS incur 43% more ambulatory and 25% more urgent care visits and require 43% more prescriptions than normal subjects without CRS.[27] (in the United States). The highest costs involve patients with recurrent polyps after surgery.[28] A meta-analysis of 21 studies with 2,070 patients who underwent functional endoscopic sinus surgery (FESS) showed greater improvement of nasal obstruction, facial pain, and postnasal discharge but less improvement of hyposmia and headache.[29]

TREATMENT

Pharmacologic

Medications presently recommended for treating CRSwNP include corticosteroids (topical and systemic), oral antibiotics, and nasal saline irrigation (Table 21.1).[1] Additionally, oral antihistamines (for allergic patients with CRSwNP) and leukotriene antagonists are recommended by the British Society of Allergy and Clinical Immunology.[30] Factors that negatively influence the outcome of treatment in patients with CRSwNP include the extent of the disease, presence of asthma, AERD, cystic fibrosis, and biofilm formation, which can be examined by optical microscopy.

CORTICOSTEROIDS

Corticosteroids constitute the first-line medical treatment for CRSwNP. They are administered topically (intranasally) or systemically, and topical treatment should be prolonged owing to the chronic nature of the disease.

INTRANASAL CORTICOSTEROIDS

Patients with CRSwNP experience improved symptoms and other patient-reported outcomes when treated with INS. INSs improve nasal function and are generally safe. Clinical efficacy is similar for all INSs, although agents with increased first-pass hepatic clearance have fewer systemic side effects for equivalent efficacy. A meta-analysis of 39 studies demonstrated significant benefits for symptoms, polyp size, polyp recurrence, and nasal expiratory peak flow rate with INS treatment compared to placebo. Significant improvements were observed for pooled combined symptom scores and the proportion of responders.[31] INSs administered after sinus surgery have a greater effect on reducing polyp size than in patients without surgery, although symptoms and nasal airflow do not differ. The most common adverse effects of INS are epistaxis and nasal dryness. Other side effects, such as inhibition of the hypothalamic-pituitary-adrenal axis, are rare, and no effects on child growth occur if steroids with low systemic bioavailability are used once or twice daily.

SYSTEMIC CORTICOSTEROIDS

These drugs also have significant benefits on various outcomes, including polyp size, nasal symptom scores, and nasal expiratory peak flow rate. Short courses of systemic corticosteroids (7 to 14 days of 0.2 to 0.5 mg/kg/day of prednisone or equivalent) are used in patients with severe NP not controlled by INS. Systemic corticosteroids are also used with INS as medical polypectomy in the case of a limited response to initial therapy with INS, before endoscopic surgery and in the postoperative state to reduce polyp recurrence. The European position paper on CRSwNP recommends the following scheme for medical polypectomy: 0.5 mg/kg/day prednisolone in the morning for 5 to 10 days plus two betamethasone nasal drops/nostril three times daily in the head upside-down position for 5 days, then twice daily until the bottle runs out.[1] Long-term maintenance with fluticasone (400 µg daily) or mometasone (200 µg daily) is recommended. Side effects of oral corticosteroids depend on the dose and duration of treatment, and the most relevant side effects are suppression of the hypothalamic-pituitary-adrenal axis, alterations in bone metabolism with bone loss, and growth retardation in children. Bisphosphonate therapy coincident with systemic corticosteroid treatment may help prevent bone loss but has not been evaluated in controlled trials.

SHORT- AND INTERMEDIATE-TERM ANTIBIOTICS

The theoretical framework for using antibiotics in patients with NP is the production of disease-modifying enterotoxins by microorganisms in the polyp tissue (generally *Staphylococcus*). A 20-day course of doxycycline induces a significant but small effect on polyp size and improvement in postnasal discharge compared to placebo.[31]

LONG-TERM ANTIBIOTICS

This approach is based on the antiinflammatory effect demonstrated for some antibiotics, mainly from the macrolide group, and mediated by inhibition of the nuclear factor-κB transcription factor. Studies conducted with clarithromycin and roxithromycin administered for at least 3 months showed some reduction of polyp size and symptoms. The observed effects, although moderate, were more sustained than those of systemic corticosteroids. Efficacy of macrolides appears to be less in patients with severe abnormalities on CT scans, asthma, low IgE levels, and polyps with increased eosinophil infiltration.[32,33]

OTHER MEDICAL THERAPIES

Insufficient evidence is available to recommend nasal vasoconstrictors, mucolytic agents, leukotriene modifiers, anti-IgE, anti-IL5, antihistamines, antimycotics, immunosuppressants, furosemide, aspirin desensitization, proton pump inhibitors, or capsaicin for nasal polyposis. A practical approach for treating CRSwNP was recommended in the EPOS 2007 guidelines based on symptom severity according to a visual analog scale as summarized by Meltzer and Hamilos[34] (Table 21.3).

Surgical Treatment

Sinus surgery may be indicated in patients who fail to improve after a trial of maximum medical therapy. FESS is the preferred method and involves clearance of polyps and polypoid mucosa and opening the sinus ostia. Removing inflammatory tissue results in improved symptoms, sinus ventilation, and mucociliary clearance.

The long-term efficacy of surgery is influenced by the postoperative medical regimen. A prolonged reduction in nasal symptoms and improved QOL were demonstrated in a review of 33 trials of FESS with postoperative medical management.[35] Significant improvement in QOL was also observed in a prospective cohort study including 3,128 patients who completed the sinonasal outcome test-22 questionnaire.[36] Prolonged postoperative medical treatment with INS improves outcomes after FESS.[35,37–39] Surgery is less successful in patients with AERD, asthma, cystic fibrosis, or pansinus disease than in aspirin-tolerant individuals.[40]

Effects of Chronic Rhinosinusitis and Nasal Polyp Treatment on Asthma

Most evidence suggests a beneficial effect of both medical and surgical treatment of CRS on asthma outcomes, including improving overall asthma control, reducing exhaled nitric oxide, and increasing FEV_1.[30,31,41–43] Polypectomy results in subjective improvement of asthma, improves respiratory function, decreases the use of corticosteroids, and does not aggravate or induce asthma.

UNMET, FUTURE RESEARCH NEEDS

1. Further studies are needed to clarify the definition and to develop diagnosis and management strategies for CRSwNP associated with asthma.

Table 21.3. Treatment of Chronic Rhinosinusitis with Nasal Polyps According to Evidence-Based Medicine

DRUG	LEVEL OF EVIDENCE	GRADE OF RECOMMENDATION		CLINICAL RELEVANCE	
	EPOS	BSACI	EPOS	BSACI	EPOS
Intranasal corticosteroids	Ia	A	A	Yes	Yes
Oral corticosteroids	Ia	A	A	Yes	Yes
Oral antibiotics, short term (<4 wk)	Ib	D	C	No	Yes
Oral antibiotics, long term (>12 wk)	III	D	C	Yes	Yes
Oral antihistamine*	No data	A	D	Yes	No
Nasal saline douche	Ib	A	D	Yes	Yes
Antileukotrienes	Ib (–)	C	A (–)	Yes	No

*In allergic patients.
BSACI, British Society of Allergy and Clinical Immunology; EPOS, European Position Paper on Rhinosinusitis and Nasal Polyps.
Grades of Recommendations:
  A. At least one metaanalysis, systematic review, or randomized controlled trial (RCT) rated as Ia and directly applicable to the target population, OR a systematic review of RCTs or a body of evidence consisting principally of studies rated as Ib directly applicable to the target population and demonstrating overall consistency of results
  B. A body of evidence including studies rated as IIa directly applicable to the target population and demonstrating overall consistency of results, OR extrapolated evidence from studies rated as Ia or Ib
  C. A body of evidence including studies rated as IIb directly applicable to the target population and demonstrating overall consistency of results, OR extrapolated evidence from studies rated as IIa
  D. Evidence level III or IV, OR extrapolated evidence from studies rated as IIb Modified from References 31 and 32.

2. Although the immunologic diversity in inflammatory parameters seems to stand in contrast to the universal clinical presentation of NPs, knowledge of the disease phenotype is of potential importance for development and application of highly individualized therapeutics.

3. Subphenotyping of CRSwNP by cluster analysis in which ethnic differences and comorbid asthma phenotypes are considered is needed. New therapeutic approaches should be tailored to the CRSsNP or the CRSwNP patient subgroup.

4. Comorbidities and confounding conditions in patients with asthma could affect their clinical course. Therefore, identifying specific disease subgroups using biomarkers is a challenging task for future research.

5. Possible selective targets include prostanoid receptor antagonists and biologics that target T_H2-biased and SE-IgE–positive subjects.

CONCLUSION

CRS and NP are major comorbid conditions of bronchial asthma. CRSwNP occurs in the setting of CRS characterized by T_H2 and eosinophilic inflammation. Therefore, CRSwNP is considered an entity separate from CRSsNP. Previous studies demonstrated a strong association between asthma and CRS, and patients with asthma and CRS are more likely to have NPs. The presence of CRSwNP can increase asthma severity, and effective medical management can improve asthma outcomes, including overall lung function and asthma control and drug requirements. Surgery should be reserved for select patients with inadequate response to medical management or with medication intolerance or side effects. Future research may further elucidate the pathophysiology of CRS and NP, which may in turn lead to the development of more effective treatment modalities.

REFERENCES

1. Fokkens WJ, Lund VJ, Mullol J, et al. EPOS 2012: European position paper on rhinosinusitis and nasal polyps 2012: a summary for otorhinolaryngologists. *Rhinology.* 2012;50:1–12.
2. Huvenne W, van Bruaene N, Zhang N, et al. Chronic rhinosinusitis with and without nasal polyps: what is the difference? *Curr Allergy Asthma Rep.* 2009;9:213–220.
3. Van Crombruggen K, Zhang N, Gevaert P, Tomassen P, Bachert C. Pathogenesis of chronic rhinosinusitis: inflammation. *J Allergy Clin Immunol.* 2011;128:728–732.
4. Slavin RG. The upper and lower airways: the epidemiological and pathophysiological connection. *Allergy Asthma Proc.* 2008;29:553–556.
5. Zhang N, Van Zele T, Perez-Novo C, et al. Different types of T-effector cells orchestrate mucosal inflammation in chronic sinus disease. *J Allergy Clin Immunol.* 2008;122:961–968.
6. Jarvis D, Newson R, Lotvall J, et al. Asthma in adults and its association with chronic rhinosinusitis: the GA2LEN survey in Europe. *Allergy.* 2012;67:91–98.
7. Pearlman AN, Chandra RK, Chang D, et al. Relationships between severity of chronic rhinosinusitis and nasal polyposis, asthma, and atopy. *Am J Rhinol Allergy.* 2009;23:145–148.
8. Lötvall J, Ekerljung L, Lundbäck B. Multi-symptom asthma is closely related to nasal blockage, rhinorrhea and symptoms of chronic rhinosinusitis: evidence from the West Sweden Asthma Study. *Respir Res.* 2010;26(11):163.
9. Aazami A, Sharghi A, Ghofrani M, Anari H, Habibzadeh E. Rhinosinusitis predispose asthmatic patients to severe bronchial asthma. *Iran J Allergy Asthma Immunol.* 2009;8:199–203.
10. Kowalski ML, Cieślak M, Pérez-Novo CA, Makowska JS, Bachert C. Clinical and immunological determinants of severe/refractory asthma (SRA): association with Staphylococcal superantigen-specific IgE antibodies. *Allergy.* 2011;66:32–38.
11. Palikhe NS, Kim JH, Park HS. Update on recent advances in the management of aspirin exacerbated respiratory disease. *Yonsei Med J.* 2009;50:744–750.
12. Robinson S, Douglas R, Wormald PJ. The relationship between atopy and chronic rhinosinusitis. *Am J Rhinol.* 2006;20:625–628.
13. Tan BK, Schleimer RP, Kern RC. Perspectives on the etiology of chronic rhinosinusitis. *Curr Opin Otolaryngol Head Neck Surg.* 2010;18:21–26.
14. Tomassen P, Van Zele T, Zhang N, et al. Pathophysiology of chronic rhinosinusitis. *Proc Am Thorac Soc.* 2011;8:115–120.
15. Pérez-Novo CA, Kowalski ML, Kuna P, et al. Aspirin sensitivity and IgE antibodies to Staphylococcus aureus enterotoxins in nasal polyposis: studies on the relationship. *Int Arch Allergy Immunol.* 2004;133:255–260.
16. Stevenson DD, Szczeklik A. Clinical and pathologic perspectives on aspirin sensitivity and asthma. *J Allergy Clin Immunol.* 2006;118:773–786.
17. Chang JE, White A, Simon RA, Stevenson DD. Aspirin-exacerbated respiratory disease: burden of disease. *Allergy Asthma Proc.* 2012;33:117–121.
18. Kowalski ML, Bienkiewicz B, Kordek P, et al. Nasal polyposis in aspirin-hypersensitive patients with asthma (aspirin triad) and aspirin-tolerant patients. *Allergy Clin Immunol Int.* 2003;6:246–250.
19. Kim JE, Kountakis SE. The prevalence of Samter's triad in patients undergoing functional endoscopic sinus surgery. *Ear Nose Throat J.* 2007;86:396–399.
20. Gliklich RE, Metson R. The health impact of chronic sinusitis in patients seeking otolaryngologic care. *Otolaryngol Head Neck Surg.* 1995;113:104–109.
21. Radenne F, Lamblin C, Vandezande LM, et al. Quality of life in nasal polyposis. *J Allergy Clin Immunol.* 1999;104:79–84.
22. Poetker DM, Mendolia-Loffredo S, Smith TL. Outcomes of endoscopic sinus surgery for chronic rhinosinusitis associated with sinonasal polyposis. *Am J Rhinol.* 2007;21:84–88.
23. Alobid I, Benitez P, Bernal-Sprekelsen M, Guilemany JM, Picado C, Mullol J. The impact of asthma and aspirin sensitivity on quality of life of patients with nasal polyposis. *Qual Life Res.* 2005;14:789–793.
24. Alobid I, Benitez P, Bernal-Sprekelsen M, et al. Nasal polyposis and its impact on quality of life: comparison between the effects of medical and surgical treatments. *Allergy.* 2005;60:452–458.
25. Mace JC, Michael YL, Carlson NE, Litvack JR, Smith TL. Correlations between endoscopy scores and quality-of-life changes after sinus surgery. *Arch Otolaryngol Head Neck Surg.* 2010;136:340–346.
26. Ray NF. Healthcare expenditures for sinusitis in 1996: contributions of asthma, rhinitis, and other airway disorders. *J Allergy Clin Immunol.* 1999;103:408–414.

27. Murphy MP, Fishman P, Short SO, Sullivan SD, Yueh B, Weymuller EA Jr. Health care utilization and cost among adults with chronic rhinosinusitis enrolled in a health maintenance organization. *Otolaryngol Head Neck Surg.* 2002;127:367–376.
28. Bhattacharyya N. Assessing the additional disease burden of polyps in chronic rhinosinusitis. *Ann Otol Rhinol Laryngol.* 2009;118:185–189.
29. Chester AC. Symptom outcomes following endoscopic sinus surgery. *Curr Opin Otolaryngol Head Neck Surg.* 2009;17:50–58.
30. Scadding GK, Durham SR, Mirakian R, et al. BSACI Guidelines for the Management of Rhinosinusitis and Nasal Polyposis. *Clin Exp Allergy.* 2007;38:260–275.
31. Van Zele T, Gevaert P, Holtappels G, Beule A, Wormald PJ, Mayr S. Oral steroids and doxycycline: two different approaches to treat nasal polyps. *J Allergy Clin Immunol.* 2010;125:1069–1076.
32. Wallwork B, Coman W, Mackay-Sim A, Greiff L, Cervin A. A double-blind, randomized, placebo-controlled trial of macrolide in the treatment of chronic rhinosinusitis. *Laryngoscope.* 2006;116:189–193.
33. Haruna S, Shimada C, Ozawa M, Fukami S, Moriyama H. A study of poor responders for long-term, low-dose macrolide administration for chronic sinusitis. *Rhinology.* 2009;47:66–71.
34. Meltzer EO, Hamilos DL. Rhinosinusitis diagnosis and management for the clinician: a synopsis of recent consensus guidelines. *Mayo Clin Proc.* 2011;86:427–443.
35. Dalziel K, Stein K, Round A, Garside R, Royle P. Systematic review of endoscopic sinus surgery for nasal polyps. *Health Technol Assess.* 2003;7:1–159.
36. Hopkins C, Slack R, Lund V, Brown P, Copley L, Browne J. Long-term outcomes from the English national comparative audit of surgery for nasal polyposis and chronic rhinosinusitis. *Laryngoscope.* 2009;119:2459–2465.
37. Ragab SM, Lund VJ, Scadding G, Saleh HA, Khalifa MA. Impact of chronic rhinosinusitis therapy on quality of life. A prospective randomized controlled trial. *Rhinology.* 2010;48:305–311.
38. Alobid I, Benitez P, Bernal-Sprekelsen M, Roca J, Alonso J, Picado C. Nasal polyposis and its impact on quality of life: comparison between the effects of medical and surgical treatments. *Allergy.* 2005;60:452–458.
39. Rowe-Jones JM, Medcalf M, Durham SR, Richards DH, Mackay IS. Functional endoscopic sinus surgery: 5 year follow up and results of a prospective, randomised, stratified, double-blind, placebo controlled study of postoperative fluticasone propionate aqueous nasal spray. *Rhinology.* 2005;43:2–10.
40. Gosepath J, Hoffmann F, Schafer D, Amedee RG, Mann WJ. Aspirin intolerance in patients with chronic sinusitis. *ORL Otorhinolaringol Relat Spec.* 1999;61:146–150.
41. Lund VJ. The effect of sinonasal surgery on asthma. *Allergy.* 1999;54(Suppl 57):141–145.
42. Scadding G. The effect of medical treatment of sinusitis upon concomitant asthma. *Allergy.* 1999;54(Suppl 57):136–140.
43. Dunlop G, Scadding GK, Lund VJ. The effect of endoscopic sinus surgery on asthma: management of patients with chronic rhinosinusitis, nasal polyposis, and asthma. *Am J Rhinol.* 1999;13:261–265.

22

VOCAL CORD DYSFUNCTION AND PARADOXICAL VOCAL FOLD MOTION DISORDER

COMORBID, COEXISTING, AND DIFFERENTIAL DIAGNOSIS

Roger W. Fox and Mark C. Glaum

KEY POINTS

- Vocal cord dysfunction (VCD), also termed paradoxical vocal fold motion disorder, is a syndrome with many names and presents with varied clinical manifestations.
- VCD is a common masquerader of asthma and may coexist with it and other respiratory conditions.
- VCD is often unrecognized and, as a consequence, results in misdiagnosis and unnecessary exposure to medications.
- Diagnosis of VCD relies on clinical history, inspiratory flow–volume loops, and visualization of vocal cord motion by rhinolaryngoscopy.
- The treatment of VCD requires a multidisciplinary approach relying on elimination of triggers, treatment of comorbid conditions, and consultation with a speech pathologist.

INTRODUCTION

Asthma is a common respiratory problem. An important question the physician should ask is whether symptoms suggestive of persistent asthma despite appropriate use of effective medical treatment are really asthma. Vocal cord dysfunction (VCD) or paradoxical vocal fold motion disorder is an important differential diagnosis increasingly recognized during the past several decades. The importance of VCD as an asthma comorbidity is highlighted in the most recent version of National Heart, Lung and Blood Institute guidelines for the diagnosis and management of asthma.[1] VCD can present in a variety of forms that mimic allergic disorders, including chronic cough and recurrent angioedema of the throat as well as asthma (Table 22.1). This chapter focuses on VCD as it relates to symptoms that suggest asthma and provides specific information to help with the evaluation of VCD.

Table 22.1. Differential Diagnosis of Shortness of Breath Due to Airway Dysfunction

Poorly controlled asthma
Paroxysmal laryngospasm
Vocal cord dysfunction
Laryngeal angioedema
Vocal cord paralysis
Exercise-induced bronchospasm
Structural lesion causing intermittent obstruction
Tracheal stenosis
Laryngomalacia

Table 22.2. Symptoms of Vocal Cord Dysfunction

- Dry cough
- Chest and/or throat tightness
- Shortness of breath, difficulty breathing
- Voice change, intermittent hoarseness, dysphonia
- Frequent throat clearing, globus pharyngeus, choking
- Exercise-induced wheezing, inspiratory stridor
- Wheezing, stridor
- Feeling they are "breathing through a straw"
- Difficulty with inhalation and/or exhalation
- Sensation of panic

PRESENTATION OF VOCAL CORD DYSFUNCTION IN ASTHMA

VCD is characterized by paroxysmal vocal fold adduction during respiration, particularly inspiration but also expiration. This narrowing of the larynx restricts the airway opening, leading to episodic dyspnea, wheezing, cough, and/or inspiratory stridor that can be mistaken for asthma (Table 22.2). The upper airway sound produced by the laryngeal narrowing can be transmitted to the lungs, resulting in a generalized wheeze. The physician should auscultate over the larynx and compare with auscultation over the chest to appreciate the source of the sounds. Many triggers of VCD overlap with those of asthma (Table 22.3). A consequence of misdiagnosing VCD as asthma is long-term, unnecessary treatment for asthma. The dramatic, acute presentation of VCD may lead to emergency department treatment or hospitalization with aggressive, ineffective medical treatment. Many physicians fail to distinguish VCD from asthma because of the similarity of symptoms and lack of experience with or consideration of VCD. Exercise-induced VCD is a distinct phenotype with symptoms that only occur with strenuous exercise, and unlike in exercise-induced asthma (exercise-induced bronchospasm [EIB]), the respiratory symptoms develop suddenly and resolve quickly without bronchodilator treatment.

HISTORICAL PERSPECTIVE AND NOMENCLATURE

The first description of a disorder of the laryngeal muscles resulting in "hysterical croup" appeared in a textbook published in 1842.[2] In 1902 Sir William Osler wrote about this unusual disorder as a "spasm of muscles [that] may occur with violent inspiratory efforts and great distress."[3] Over the subsequent years, the literature has given various names to this disorder, including episodic laryngeal dyskinesis, Munchausen's stridor, factitious asthma, functional laryngeal obstruction, spasmodic croup,

Table 22.3. Triggers of Vocal Cord Dysfunction

- Laryngopharyngeal or gastroesophageal reflux
- Postnasal drip, sinus drainage
- Noxious odors, fumes, smoke
- Exercise
- Anxiety, stress
- Upper respiratory tract infections
- Temperature, humidity fluctuations

emotional laryngeal wheezing, and irritable larynx syndrome.[4-7] In 1983 Christopher reported the comprehensive evaluation of five patients treated for uncontrolled asthma and referred to this condition as "vocal cord dysfunction syndrome." Diagnosis of this condition was made using rhinolaryngoscopy and flow loop pulmonary function tests (Figure 22.1).[8]

A spectrum of disorders involves abnormal vocal fold motion during breathing, and many experts believe a better and more accurate description of this condition is *paradoxical vocal fold motion disorder* (PVFMD) because both the vocal folds (true vocal cords) and the ventricular folds (false vocal cords) may participate. Although PVFMD may describe the pathophysiology more accurately, VCD is the most commonly used term in clinical practice and is recognized as a specific diagnosis. Therefore, VCD will be used in this chapter.

VOCAL CORD ANATOMY AND FUNCTION

The larynx is an organ that is important for phonation and singing, but it also has the very important function of protecting against inhaling toxic substances or aspirating foreign

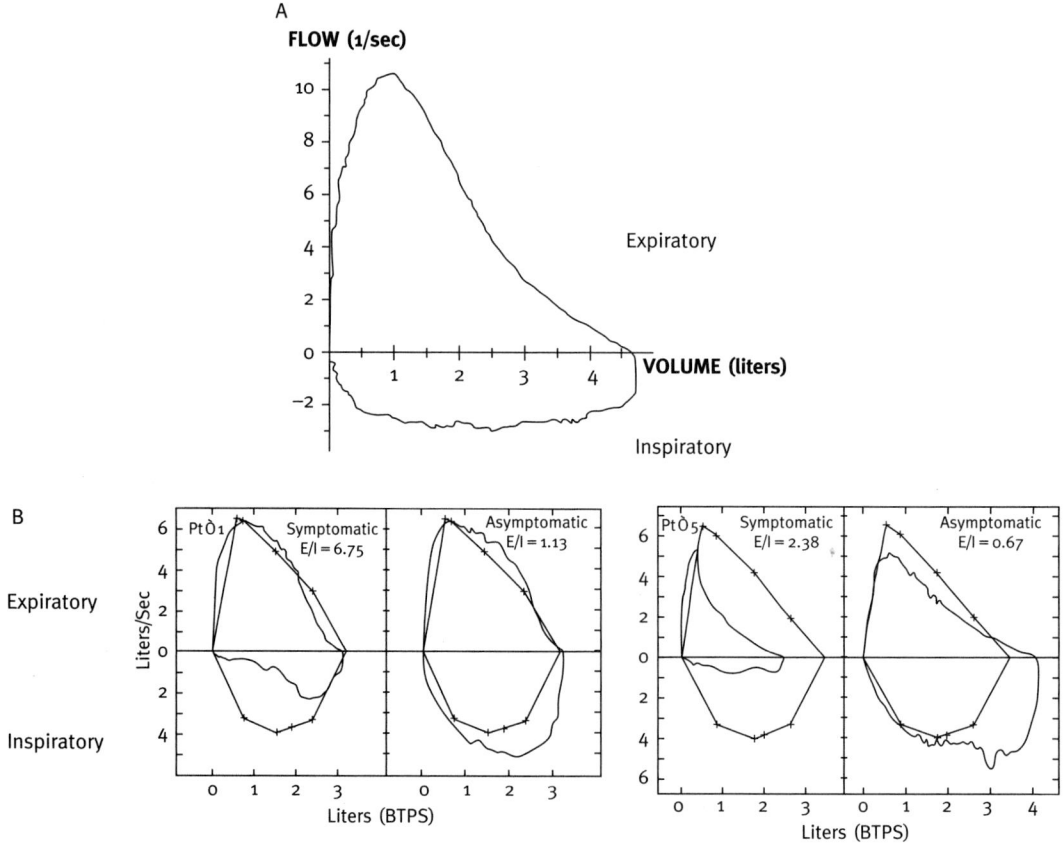

FIGURE 22.1 **A,** Representative flow–volume loop showing normal forced expiratory volume (tracing above abscissa) and flattened inspiratory portion of flow–volume loop (tracing below abscissa) demonstrating extrathoracic obstruction suggestive of vocal cord dysfunction. **B,** Representative maximum inspiratory and expiratory flow–volume relationship in two patients (*left*) and (*right*) during symptomatic and asymptomatic periods. *Thin lines* connecting crosses show predicted values; *bold lines* indicate actual measurements. BTPS, standardized to barometric pressure at sea level, body temperature, saturated with water vapor: body temperature and pressure, saturated; E/I, expiratory-to-inspiratory ratio. (Christopher KL, Wood RP 2nd, Eckert RC, et al. *N Engl J Med.* 1983;308:1566–1570.)

bodies or liquids into the lungs. The larynx is a valve separating the hypopharynx and esophagus from the trachea. The glottis consists of the true vocal cords and false vocal folds. The principal muscle for vocal cord abduction is the posterior cricoarytenoid muscle (PCA). Adduction is performed mainly by the lateral cricoarytenoid muscle (LCA). During normal ventilation, the glottic opening is controlled through the medullary respiratory center by the vagus nerve, leading to the contraction of the PCA muscle and abduction of the vocal cords. During normal expiration, there is a decrease in the tonic activity of the PCA muscle and contraction of the LCA muscle, resulting in slight narrowing of the glottis opening.

EPIDEMIOLOGY

The overall incidence of VCD in the general population is not defined. Different studies have reported variable incidences in various groups of symptomatic individuals with respiratory complaints. For example, in a military cohort study of exertional dyspnea, 12% had VCD.[9] In a retrospective study of 148 elite and recreational athletes referred to a tertiary care asthma center for exercise-related respiratory complaints, 70% were diagnosed with VCD with or without asthma.[10] In another study of 111 Olympic athletes with EIB, 5% had VCD.[11] In 1995, the National Jewish Asthma Center published an article on refractory asthmatic patients evaluated at their center, disclosing that 10% of these individuals had no asthma but had VCD alone. Thirty percent of patients with difficult-to-treat asthma had both VCD and asthma.[12]

Although VCD affects mainly children and young adults, there is a reported 2:1 female predominance.[13] VCD is likely underreported or misdiagnosed, so the true incidence and prevalence in the general population might be higher than anticipated. In certain specialties such as allergy/immunology, pulmonary medicine, and otolaryngology, the diagnosis is more frequently recognized because of familiarity with the syndrome and accessibility to rhinolaryngoscopy and pulmonary function testing.

PATHOGENESIS

The pathogenesis of VCD is uncertain, and there is likely no single cause. Both organic causes, such as gastroesophageal reflux disease (GERD), postnasal drip, and inhaled irritants, and nonorganic causes, such as psychological or emotional triggers, have been identified. VCD includes a spectrum of symptoms and triggers that result in shortness of breath and cough. Therefore, each patient needs a complete history and physical examination to ascertain the presence of this disorder. Multiple factors likely contribute to ongoing VCD symptoms. One proposed pathogenic mechanism is laryngeal hyperresponsiveness.[14] Inflammatory or irritant stimuli can cause transient or long-lasting laryngeal narrowing that contributes to stridor and transmitted wheezing heard by auscultation of the chest. Recurrent laryngeal stimulation may lead to autonomic imbalance maintained by central brain regions in the medulla that are postsynaptically connected to the larynx. Both the true and false cords derive motor innervation from the vagus nerve, whereas the sensory fibers from M3 muscarinic receptors in the laryngeal mucosa pass through the vagus to the medulla. With persistent imbalance of these autonomic responses, irritants and psychological stimuli induce local reflexes contributing to airway narrowing in the glottis.

ETIOLOGY

Numerous respiratory tract irritants, such as smoke, gases, vapors, dust, airborne pollutants, and odors, have been linked to VCD. Other conditions contributing to VCD include GERD, sinusitis, and allergic rhinitis associated with postnasal drip. Irritant-induced VCD is postulated to result from a reflex adduction of the vocal folds as a protective reflex. GERD may cause posterior glottic changes of erythema and edema of the arytenoids and interarytenoid area. This finding in a patient with VCD is suggestive, but not necessarily diagnostic, of GERD causing the VCD. An adequate trial of antireflux therapy with symptom improvement or a pH probe study would validate the role of GERD.

Clinically, patients with GERD-induced VCD generally respond to antireflux therapy over several months. However, laryngeal hyperreactivity is slow to respond to therapy. Some patients seem to develop VCD after harsh, prolonged coughing episodes from bronchitis. Another phenotype is spontaneously recurring VCD, triggered by talking or eating, both stimulating the hypersensitive larynx. The role of psychogenic factors as an etiology or a contributing trigger for VCD has been discussed in many reports and reviews on the topic.[15,16]

Certainly, individuals suffering with VCD will display anxiety and concern for their well-being. Patients with VCD who undergo psychological evaluations and receive treatment for underlying psychological issues may experience improvement in VCD symptoms. Some associated diagnoses include conversion reaction, major depression, obsessive-compulsive disorder, and anxiety.

A study describes workers who developed symptoms of dyspnea in the cleanup of the World Trade Center disaster site and who were subsequently diagnosed with VCD.[17] These workers were exposed to many respiratory irritants and considerable emotional stressors, and this combination of triggers was thought to contribute to their VCD. It is not clear why only certain individuals were affected.

Normal psychological stress can also contribute to VCD. For example, an adolescent competitive athlete under severe social stresses, such as may result from the responsibility of serving as captain of the squad or from efforts to earn a college scholarship, diagnosed with recent onset of EIB may in fact have VCD. One report failed to document a greater incidence of psychological dysfunction in adolescents with VCD compared with asthmatic controls.[18] Therefore, many VCD patients do not have psychological factors causing this disorder. Often the speech pathologist during vocal therapy can allay some of the fears and teach relaxation techniques to reduce the tension in the throat.

Other factors associated with VCD include trauma to the larynx from intubation during surgery, injury to the recurrent laryngeal nerve, or neuromuscular disorders (Parkinson's disease, amyotrophic lateral sclerosis, paroxysmal laryngospasm). Tracheomalacia, subglottic stenosis, and vocal cord polyps are also included in the differential diagnosis of VCD (see Table 22.1). These conditions do not result in VCD but could either enhance the symptoms or emulate VCD.

CLINICAL FEATURES AND DIAGNOSIS

Many of the symptoms of VCD overlap with asthma, and the clinician must consider VCD in the differential diagnosis, particularly if the asthma is difficult to control. Certain features may suggest VCD rather than asthma, such as a predominant symptom complex of chronic throat clearing, cough, and dysphonia. VCD symptoms may also be intermittent and not always associated with specific environmental exposure. Individuals with intermittent VCD symptoms may be sensitive to a variety of irritants or unrecognized provocateurs with sudden onset of respiratory complaints (see Table 22.3). Bronchodilators delivered by inhalation, particularly metered-dose inhalers, may not give the patient any relief immediately, whereas a nebulized solution of a bronchodilator may be beneficial. The therapeutic effect of nebulized medications may be related to the soothing effect of the mist rather than any pharmacologic effect because β-agonists have no effect on the larynx.

A high index of suspicion for the diagnosis of VCD is needed to avoid unnecessary medical treatment, morbidity, and hospitalizations that often occur with this condition. The clinician should consider VCD when the asthmatic patient indicates that bronchodilators do not help and there is no sputum production. In these cases, the history often is atypical for asthma or allergic respiratory disease. The patient may have inspiratory stridor, point to the throat where the constriction is located, and complain about tightness of the upper chest or throat and air hunger, with inability to get enough air into the lungs. These symptoms may occur sporadically and resolve quickly, particularly if the patient is distracted. Usually there is an absence of respiratory symptoms during sleep. The patient may be complaining of respiratory symptoms but have a physical examination that is remarkably unrevealing of wheezes or abnormal breath sounds other than those transmitted from the throat. Pulse oximetry and pulsus paradoxus are normal during an attack. At the time of symptoms, a flow loop and spirometry may suggest the diagnosis by identifying the inspiratory cutoff or flattening of the flow loop, often with a sawtooth appearance on the inspiratory phase reflecting the laryngospasm of VCD (see Figure 22.1). The sensitivity of the flow–volume loop in the absence of acute symptoms is low. Fiberoptic rhinolaryngoscopy is an important tool in establishing the diagnosis of VCD. During an episode or symptomatic phase of VCD, the observation of the adduction of the vocal folds and vocal cords confirms the clinical diagnosis (Figure 22.2). Both the pulmonary function tests and the upper airway endoscopy may be completely normal in the asymptomatic individual. There are no standardized provocation tests to induce VCD, although some patients may develop an attack by performing vigorous forced exhalation or inhalation. Care must be taken not to touch the vocal cords with the rhinolaryngoscope because this can induce a glottic reflex. Chest x-ray or imaging of the throat is not helpful except to exclude other conditions.

MANAGEMENT

At the time of the initial diagnosis of this condition, the patient needs to be reassured about VCD (Table 22.4), and the clinician must define whether the patient has concomitant asthma that requires ongoing asthma therapy (Table 22.5). Asthma medication should be discontinued if concomitant asthma is not suspected. Education and relaxation techniques may allay anxiety. Panting and a forced cough may abort an episode of VCD in some instances by forcing the glottis aperture to widen. Panting activates the PCA muscle and abducts the vocal cords. Inhaled helium-oxygen mixture or nebulized lidocaine has afforded temporary relief in some patients. Inhaled anticholinergic agents, such as ipratropium, may benefit some patients with exercise-induced VCD by blocking the vagal influence on the larynx.

The mainstay of VCD treatment is evaluation and treatment by an accomplished speech pathologist. Most patients are able to overcome or control their symptoms of VCD within a few sessions of cognitive behavioral therapy with a trained therapist. Speech techniques must be practiced during asymptomatic periods to be effective during an episode. Often, the speech pathologist can help identify psychological factors and stresses that are contributing to VCD. Hypnosis and biofeedback have been reported to help some patients.

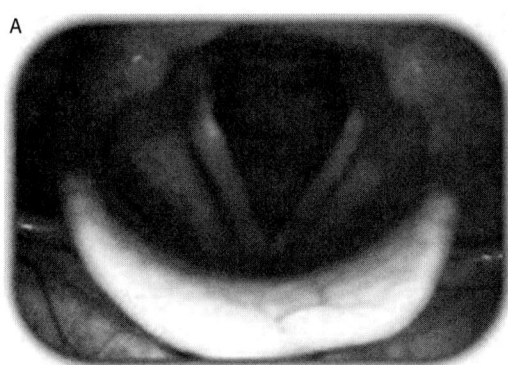
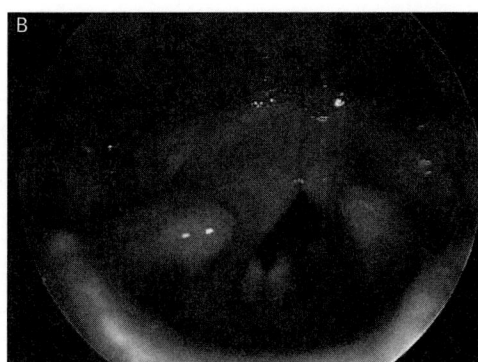

FIGURE 22.2 Normal vocal fold abduction and paroxysmal vocal fold adduction. **A,** Normal abduction of vocal folds during inhalation. **B,** Paroxysmal adduction of vocal folds during inhalation with a characteristic posterior diamond-shaped glottis deformity. See Color Plate 8 in insert.

Table 22.4. Management of Vocal Cord Dysfunction

ACUTE MANAGEMENT	LONG-TERM MANAGEMENT
Calm environment with reassurance	Speech therapy
Panting	Diaphragmatic breathing
Making an "s" sound on expiration	Wide-open mouth breathing
Heliox (70%–80% helium/20%–30% oxygen)	Psychological therapy
Sedatives	Yoga
	Hypnosis
	Biofeedback
	Pharmacotherapy
	Psychotherapy
	Discontinuation of asthma medication if no documented asthma
	Medical therapy to circumvent triggers

Psychotherapy or medications for coexisting disorders that are contributing to the VCD are necessary in some cases. Other treatments mentioned in the literature include continuous positive airway pressure to maintain an open glottis and botulinum toxin (Botox) injections into the larynx to prevent release of acetylcholine from the vagus nerve. Botox injections are only advocated for severe refractory cases not responding to conventional behavioral therapy.

PROGNOSIS

VCD is generally a self-limited disorder, although morbidity results from the use of excess medications and rarely tracheostomy for suspected laryngeal obstruction. Early diagnosis and treatment hasten the resolution of symptoms and limit the use of unnecessary medications, particularly corticosteroids. Attempts should be made to identify triggers and avoid or manage underlying causes. In patients who have been suffering with VCD for long periods, prolonged behavioral therapy is required. At least three VCD phenotypes exist: exercise induced; spontaneous and recurring; and secondary to comorbid medical problems stimulating the larynx, such as drainage from chronic upper airway disease or laryngeal irritation from GERD. In the case of the latter

Table 22.5. Differences between Vocal Cord Dysfunction and Asthma

LABORATORY TEST/STUDY	VOCAL CORD DYSFUNCTION	ASTHMA
Chest x-ray	Normal	Hyperinflation, peribronchial cuffing
Pulmonary function tests:		
1. Flow–volume loops	1. Flattened inspiratory portion of loop	1. Obstructive pattern with concavity of expiratory loop
2. Forced expiratory volume in 1 second (FEV_1)	2. Normal or decreased	2. Decreased
3. Peak expiratory flow	3. Normal or decreased	3. Decreased
4. FEV_1/forced vital capacity (FVC) ratio	4. Normal	4. Decreased

phenotype, treatment of the comorbidity, along with a discussion of measures to reduce laryngeal tension, may be sufficient to control the condition without consultation with a speech pathologist. Addressing chronic anxiety or counseling for individuals with previous trauma is helpful. The coexistence of VCD and asthma is a notable clinical challenge and requires attentive treatment of both conditions.

UNMET, FUTURE RESEARCH NEEDS

1. Greater appreciation and recognition of VCD by clinicians is needed to help minimize the impact of misdiagnosis and the use of inappropriate, unneeded pharmacotherapy and diagnostic procedures in patients with this condition. Respiratory specialists, such as allergists/immunologists, pulmonologists, and otolaryngologists, and emergency department physicians should particularly be aware of VCD because these physicians are more likely to care for individuals with symptoms unresponsive to usual therapy.

2. There is an unmet need for development of better therapeutic options to treat VCD in patients whose symptoms are resistant to available medical and behavioral therapies.

3. Future research needs to include elucidation of neural mechanisms responsible for the development of VCD and pursuit of noninvasive biological markers that would more clearly identify this condition.

CONCLUSION

Although VCD was first described in the middle of the 19th century, it remains unrecognized and misdiagnosed in clinical practice. VCD commonly masquerades as severe asthma, resulting in unnecessary morbidity, inappropriate procedures, and unwarranted use of medications with potentially harmful side effects. Diagnosis of VCD relies primarily on a thorough clinical history; however, inspiratory flow–volume loops and visualization of vocal cord movement by rhinolaryngoscopy may aid in the diagnosis. The primary modality of VCD treatment is avoidance of triggers, treatment of comorbidities, and speech therapy. Reassurance of the patient and understanding of the condition are essential to improve outcomes. A good source of patient education is www.nationaljewish.org/healthinfo/conditions/vcd.

REFERENCES

1. National Institutes of Health; National Heart, Lung, and Blood Institute; National Asthma Education and Prevention Program. Expert panel report 3: guidelines for the diagnosis and management of asthma. Bethesda: National Institutes of Health; 2007. NIH publication no. 07-4051.
2. Dunglison RD. *The Practice of Medicine: A Treatise on Special Pathology and Therapeutics.* Philadelphia: Lea and Blanchard; 1842:67.
3. Osler W. *The Principles and Practice of Medicine,* "Hysteria." New York and London: Appleton and Company; 1892:1111.
4. Patterson R, Schatz M, Horton M. Munchausen's stridor: non-organic laryngeal obstruction. *Clin Allergy.* 1974;4:307-310.
5. Downing ET, Braman SS, Fox MJ, et al. Factitious asthma: physiological approach to diagnosis. *JAMA.* 1982;248:2878-2881.
6. Morrison M, Rammage L, Emami A. The irritable larynx syndrome. *J Voice.* 1999;13:447-455.
7. Appelblatt NH, Baker SR. Functional airway obstruction: a new syndrome. *Arch Otolaryngol.* 1981;107:305-306.
8. Christopher KL, Wood RP 2nd, Eckert RC, et al. Vocal-cord dysfunction presenting as asthma. *N Engl J Med.* 1983;308:1566-1570.
9. Morris MJ, Deal LE, Bean DR, et al. Vocal cord dysfunction in patients with exertional dyspnea. *Chest.* 1999;116:1676-1682.
10. Hanks CD, Parsons J, Benninger C, et al. Etiology of dyspnea in elite and recreational athletes. *Phys Sportsmed.* 2012;40(2):28-33.
11. Rundell KW, Spiering BA. Inspiratory stridor in elite athletes. *Chest.* 2003;123:468-474.
12. Newman KB, Mason UG 3rd, Schmaling KB. Clinical features of vocal cord dysfunction. *Am J Respir Crit Care Med.* 1995;152(4):1382-1386.
13. Perkins PJ, Morris MJ. Vocal cord dysfunction induced by methacholine challenge testing. *Chest.* 2002;122:1988-1993.
14. Ayres JG, Gabbott PL. Vocal cord dysfunction and laryngeal hyperresponsiveness: a function of altered autonomic balance? *Thorax.* 2002;57:284-285.
15. Husein OF, Husein TN, Gardner R, et al. Formal psychological testing in patients

with paradoxical vocal fold dysfunction. *Laryngoscope.* 2008;118:740–747.
16. Maschka DA, Bauman NM, McCray PB, et al. A classification scheme for paradoxical vocal cord motion. *Laryngoscope.* 1997;107(11):1429–1435.
17. de la Hoz RE, Shohet MR, Bienenfeld LA, et al. Vocal cord dysfunction in former World Trade Center (WTC) rescue and recovery workers and volunteers. *Am J Indust Med.* 2008;51:161–165.
18. Gavin LA, Wamboldt M, Brugman S, et al. Psychological and family characteristics of adolescents with vocal cord dysfunction. *J Asthma.* 1998;35(5):409–417.

SECTION FIVE

GASTROINTESTINAL

23

GASTROESOPHAGEAL REFLUX

COMORBID AND COEXISTING

Promila Banerjee and Stephen J. Sontag

KEY POINTS

- Most asthmatic patients—and many patients with pulmonary symptoms—have gastroesophageal reflux (GER).
- GER plays an important role in an undefined but moderately sized subset of these patients.
- No diagnostic test can identify with certainty which patients have GER-induced or GER-exacerbated pulmonary symptoms.
- No diagnostic test can establish a definite cause-and-effect relationship between GER and pulmonary disease.
- Ambulatory esophageal pH testing can suggest, but cannot prove, the diagnosis of GER-induced pulmonary disease, and pH testing cannot be safely relied on to make clinical decisions.
- Even positive results on such direct tests as sputum inspection and scintigraphic monitoring, both of which establish reflux into the tracheobronchial tree, do not necessarily establish cause or effect and certainly cannot be used to predict outcomes.
- No diagnostic test can predict which patients will respond to antireflux therapy.
- A trial of a proton pump inhibitor (PPI) is definitely indicated to assess both subjective and objective improvement in pulmonary symptoms.
- In a trial of a PPI, the dose must be high enough to prevent silent esophageal acid exposure, and the duration of treatment must be long enough to detect subtle improvements in subjective and objective respiratory parameters.
- Antireflux surgery remains a therapeutic option and should not be withheld if GER is a reasonable suspect in asthma exacerbations.
- Although strong opinions have been voiced about whether a good response to PPI therapy predicts a good response to antireflux

surgery, the opinions, although logical, are based on personal experience and "gut feelings"; a good PPI response may not necessarily predict a good surgical response.
- Opinions that suggest that a poor response to PPIs predicts a poor response to anti-reflux surgery may also seem logical but are not based on clinical data; a poor PPI response may not necessarily predict a poor anti-reflux surgical response.

And God formed the human, of dust from the soil,
And blew into his nostrils the breath of life
And the human became a living being.
Genesis 2:7[1]

INTRODUCTION
Legend, Myth, and Possibilities

The symptoms of gastroesophageal reflux (GER) and the symptoms of pulmonary diseases have been recognized since the beginning of time. In the Garden of Eden, we are left with the untold story of whether our first man, Adam, feared his very first night because he had never before seen darkness or because he was worried about nocturnal heartburn or wheezing. Those of us who believe in a relationship between GER and pulmonary symptoms must use our imaginations when reading the Book of Genesis.

As the world evolved and humans began to develop thinking skills, a relationship between what we ate and how we felt began to take shape. Those who were endowed with the power to think began to use foods for certain medicinal purposes. In the Talmud (the 300-year collection of 3rd to 6th century commentaries on the Hebrew Bible), the treatment for annoying pulmonary symptoms usually involved some type of food. Coughing was treated with a fish oil drink,[2] and asthma was treated with three wheat cakes soaked in honey followed by a drink of undiluted wine.[3] Meanwhile, the 5th century Roman physician Aurelianus Caelius offered detailed descriptions of events that happened at night, such as nocturnal wheezing and the frequent occurrence of nocturnal asthma attacks.[4] During the 12th century, the great Jewish physician-philosopher, Moses Maimonides, firmly counseled against overeating.[5] Writing of an association between eating, lying down, and wheezing, Maimonides suggested in his *Treatise on Asthma*, that sleep was dangerous during an attack:

One should not sleep face downwards, nor on one's back, but lying on the side; at the beginning, on the left side, and the close of one's rest, on the right side. One should not go to sleep immediately after a meal, but only when three or four hours have elapsed. One should not sleep during the day.

In 1776, Nicholas Rosen von Rosenstein, the First Physician to the Swedish King, published his pediatric textbook, *The Diseases of Children and Their Remedies*, in which he discusses what he terms *the stomachic cough* of children[6]:

Such a cough is caused by the natural proclivity of children to ingest huge quantities of disgusting food that cannot be digested or changed as it ought.

Just 26 years later, William Heberden published his 1802 textbook, *The History and Cure of Diseases*[7]:

In most persons, the breath is shorter and more difficult after a meal.

Nearly a century later, Sir William Osler published his famous 1892 textbook, *The Principles and Practice of Medicine*. Osler, a genius in sociology, philosophy, and religion as well as medicine, seemed to be preparing the 20th century by warning about our eating habits[8]:

Diet, too has an important influence and in persons subject to this disease (asthma) severe paroxysms may be induced by overloading the stomach, or by taking certain articles of food.

In the same chapter, Osler again suggested that particular attention be paid to the diet of the asthmatic:

A rule of which experience generally compels them to make is to take the heavy meal in the early part of the day and not retire to bed before gastric digestion is completed.

The 20th Century

The 20th century produced scientists impervious to the realities that came before them. Ignoring the prophesy of Ecclesiastes 3,000 years earlier, "There is nothing new under the sun," the new scientists ignored the emphasis on diet and the strong references to the relationship between food, eating habits, and asthma. To them, the GER/asthma concept was difficult to swallow.

For the first half of the century, only a few scattered wheezes were heard amidst the competing voices of subspecialty medicine's bellowing burps and clamoring coughs. One of these scattered wheezes was G.W. Bray, who in 1934 regurgitated the same warnings of previous physicians regarding dietary indiscretions that led to asthmatic attacks.[9] Like those of Maimonides 800 years earlier, Bray's comments went unnoticed. It would be another quarter of a century before the medical community began to process the information that was being said. Indeed, in a 1960 review on the pulmonary complications of esophageal disease, Belsey reported on patients with GER who were prone to severe, progressive, and disabling pulmonary damage.[10] The Belsey Bandwagon had begun to roll. Within two years, Kennedy threw the gastrointestinal and pulmonary communities into spasm by suggesting that "silent" GER, although poorly recognized, was an important cause of pulmonary complications.[11] Not to be outdone, Urschel and Paulson reported in 1967 their experience in patients who were referred for hiatal hernia repair.[12]

Figure 23.1 shows the results of their 5-year experience (from 1961 to 1966) in 636 patients ranging in age from 7 months to 94 years who were referred for surgical correction of GER. Thirty-nine percent had classic reflux symptoms consisting of heartburn, indigestion, and postural aggravation without respiratory symptoms; 45% had both reflux symptoms and respiratory symptoms; and 16% had respiratory symptoms only. Thus, more than 60% of these patients, who were

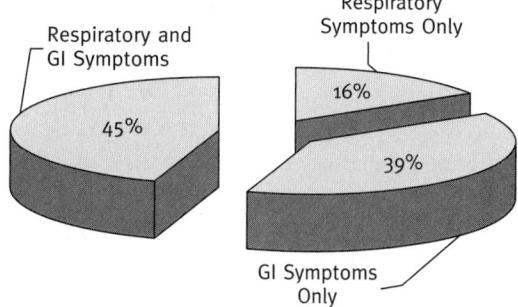

84% had classic GER symptoms	61% had respiratory symptoms
• postural aggravation (88%)	• cough (47%)
• dysphagia, choking (40%)	• bronchitis (35%)
• regurgitation (23%)	• asthma and wheezing (16%)
• nausea, vomiting (21%)	• pneumonitis (16%)
	• hemoptysis (13%)
	• hoarseness (12%)

FIGURE 23.1 Prevalence of pulmonary diseases in patients referred for hiatal hernia surgery. Although the authors were from a large surgical practice and the 636 patients had severely symptomatic GER in need of surgical repair, the results of the survey cannot be ignored: 84% had classic GER symptoms comprising heartburn, indigestion, and postural aggravation, while 61% had respiratory symptoms comprising cough (47%), bronchitis (35%), asthma and wheezing (16%), pneumonitis (16%), hemoptysis (13%), and hoarseness (12%). More than 60% had symptoms of pulmonary disease coexisting with the GER.

being referred for surgery to correct a gastroesophageal abnormality, actually had respiratory symptoms.

Nearing the end of the 1960s, the larynx—the guard to the entrance of the pulmonary cavities—received much deserved recognition when Cherry and Margulies vocalized their findings and reported that laryngeal contact ulcers, as well as other abnormalities of the voice box, might be a result of chronic GER.[13]

The Past Thirty Years

By the 1970s, the stage had been set for serious and meaningful research on the relationship between GER and asthma. In the ensuing

27 years, investigators fondled the GER/asthma concept as if they were trying to atone for the previous 2,000 years of neglect. Using a Medline search in a study on the incidence of publications that dealt with the relationship between GER and pulmonary disease, Sontag found 177 English-language publications between 1966 and 1997.[14] Half were actual studies in which some type of diagnostic procedure or intervention was undertaken, and almost 80% were published in the adult literature. The study showed that the GER/asthma relationship was not confined to the pediatric population.

DIFFICULTIES IN DETERMINING PREVALENCE OF GASTROESOPHAGEAL REFLUX IN PULMONARY PATIENTS

Study Designs and Sampling Procedures

Accurate *prevalence* studies rely on accurate recruitment of patients. For data to be meaningful and generally applicable, the population of asthmatic patients studied should represent the asthmatic population at large. Because most of the epidemiologic studies originate in large academic teaching hospitals, and because teaching hospitals and clinics are dependent on the referral of patients for treatment, the studies that report on *prevalence* rates are subject to two types of selection bias: subject selection bias and spectrum bias.[15–18] In subject selection bias, patients are unintentionally selected who have both asthma and GER or who have neither asthma nor GER. The importance of such selection bias cannot be overemphasized because the bias (although unintentional) can produce seriously misleading results. In the available studies on *prevalence* rates, the difficulty in recruiting consecutive patients was clearly an issue. Indeed, selection bias, which could not be avoided, remains a real problem in the interpretation of the results.

Spectrum bias, the second type of bias, may occur when more patients with GER than without GER volunteer for a study. Again, such a bias may be unintentional on the part of both the investigators and patients. Spectrum bias, however, rather than create an association when none exists, is more likely to lessen associations between variables. Thus, in studies reporting an association between GER and asthma, the presence of spectrum bias is more likely to lessen that association. Selection bias and spectrum bias are considered common problems in clinical samples.

A third type of bias is the hidden bias of Berkson's Fallacy—the possibility of spurious associations between diseases (GER associated with asthma) in specific studies. Because of the nature of most referral centers, it is likely that the results of prevalence studies do show Berkson's Fallacy, which states that the interplay of differential admission rates "from an underlying population to a particular study group" can result in an artificial association in the study group.[19] For instance, many patients are likely to have GER, and many patients are likely to have asthma. In tertiary hospitals and referral centers, therefore, GER and asthma are likely to occur together in the same patient—merely by chance. Such an occurrence may represent a spurious association between GER and asthma. Unfortunately, the nature of tertiary hospitals and referral centers is such that Berkson's Fallacy is difficult to avoid.

Coexistence Studies to Determine Mechanisms

Numerous authors have studied potential GER-induced asthma mechanisms and reported on the coexistence of GER and asthma in both children[20–22] and adults.[23–26] Although these studies strongly suggest a dependent relationship between GER and asthma, they were designed for the most part to clarify the mechanism by which GER might cause asthma. They were not designed to determine the prevalence of GER in the asthmatic population.

Prevalence Studies with Adequate Data

Of the 177 articles reviewed by Sontag, 18 (7 pediatric, 11 adult) contained sufficient information from which prevalence data could be extracted.[14] In general, the definitions of asthma were uniform, but the definitions of gastroesophageal reflux disease (GERD) differed considerably. For the most part, the definition of GER did reflect the presence of pathologic reflux. The terms for *prevalence* and *incidence* were often confused and used interchangeably, but for the purpose of the review, the terms were switched to reflect the proper use.

Definitions of Asthma and Gastroesophageal Reflux

ASTHMA

Most of the prevalence studies originate from pulmonary referral centers. The definition of asthma was not always given in the reports. The occurrence of wheezing and reversible airway disease, as well as the requirement for classic asthmatic therapy, indicates that almost all (if not all) of the patients enrolled in these studies truly met the accepted criteria for asthma. A few of the studies, reported by groups with a focus in gastroenterology, actually documented the asthmatic state with the methacholine bronchoprovocation test and/or the measurement of airway reversibility after bronchodilator administration.

GASTROESOPHAGEAL REFLUX DISEASE

The prevalence studies varied in their methods of determining the presence or absence of GER. The documentation of GERD was based on either direct or indirect evidence. The number of methods used to document the occurrence of GERD varied among centers and included short- and long-term pH monitoring, barium x-ray, endoscopy, and scintigraphy.

Table 23.1 shows the methods used to document the presence of GER.

PREVALENCE OF GASTROESOPHAGEAL REFLUX IN ASTHMATIC ADULTS ACCORDING TO DEFINITION OF GASTROESOPHAGEAL REFLUX

Gastroesophageal Reflux Disease Defined as Presence of Reflux Symptoms

Figure 23.2 shows the prevalence of GER symptoms in asthmatic adults in three studies with sufficient interpretable data. In the first study, Perrin-Foyalle and colleagues[27] found evidence of reflux symptoms in 65% of 150 consecutive asthmatic subjects. In the second study, Field and colleagues[28] studied 109 asthmatic subjects and 135 controls in a questionnaire-based, cross-sectional analytic study. Seventy-seven percent of the asthmatic subjects had heartburn, 55% had regurgitation, and 24% had difficulty with swallowing; 37% of the group required at least one antireflux medication, and 41% during the prior week had reflux-associated respiratory symptoms. Pulmonary symptoms occurred significantly more frequently in the asthmatic subjects than in the controls. In the third study, Sontag and colleagues[29] reported that 71% of 261 consecutive asthmatic patients had heartburn. Almost half the asthmatic patients awoke suddenly from sleep with heartburn, and 25% had nocturnal burning in the throat.

The results of these three studies, which together comprise a group of 520 asthmatic

Table 23.1. Methods Used to Document the Presence of Gastroesophageal Reflux

DIRECT EVIDENCE	INDIRECT EVIDENCE
• Short-duration esophageal pH testing	• Symptoms of gastroesophageal reflux
• Long-duration (24-hr) esophageal pH testing	• Esophageal manometry and motility
• Esophagoscopy	• Presence of hiatal hernia on standard barium x-ray
• Cine barium radiography	
• Scintigraphy	

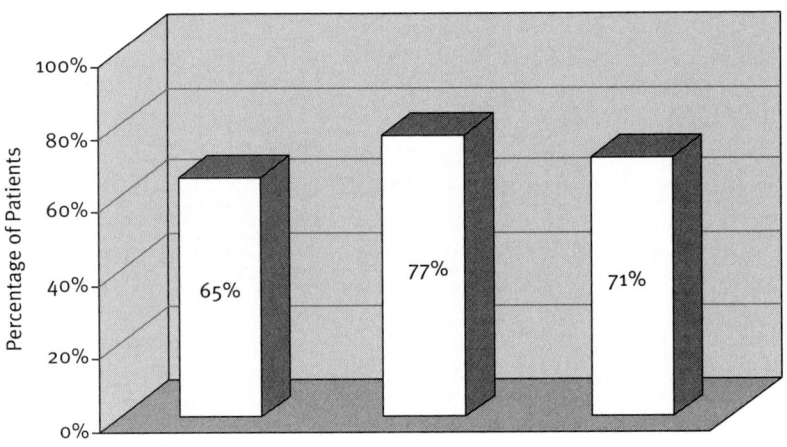

FIGURE 23.2 Prevalence of GER symptoms in asthmatics. On average, 70% of adult asthmatics admit to some type of GER symptoms.

subjects from France, Canada, and the United States, are remarkably similar. Taken as a group, 367 of the 520 patients had reflux symptoms, indicating that 71% of asthmatic patients have reflux symptoms. Despite some weaknesses in the patient-selection methods in all three studies, these reports present the most reliable data in the medical literature on GER symptoms in consecutive asthmatic patients.

Gastroesophageal Reflux Disease Defined as Presence of Abnormal Acid Reflux

Figure 23.3 shows the prevalence of abnormal acid reflux in adult asthmatic patients in seven studies comprising 628 patients from seven centers in five countries (France, Chile, Great Britain, Sweden, and the United States). The prevalence of abnormal acid reflux, as determined by pH testing, ranged from 34% to 90%.[31-36] In two of the studies,[30,31] short-term acid reflux testing was used to determine the presence of GER. These studies were conducted in the 1980s before the availability of ambulatory 24-hour pH testing. The remaining five studies[32-36] comprised 553 patients and used ambulatory 24-hour pH testing to determine abnormal GER. In all seven studies, recruitment of consecutive asthmatic subjects was suboptimal in that all depended on referral centers to enroll their patients. Nevertheless, the studies represent the most reliable data found in the literature on pH testing and the prevalence of GER in asthma. When the results of these seven studies are combined, 421 (67%) of the 628 enrolled patients had evidence of acid reflux, suggesting that two-thirds of all asthmatic patients have GER as defined by abnormal acid pH testing.

Gastroesophageal Reflux Disease Defined as the Presence of Esophageal Mucosal Disease

Figure 23.4 shows the prevalence of esophageal mucosal disease in asthmatic adults.[37] Esophageal erosions or ulcerations as seen on endoscopy were present in 39% of consecutive asthmatic patients, and 13% had

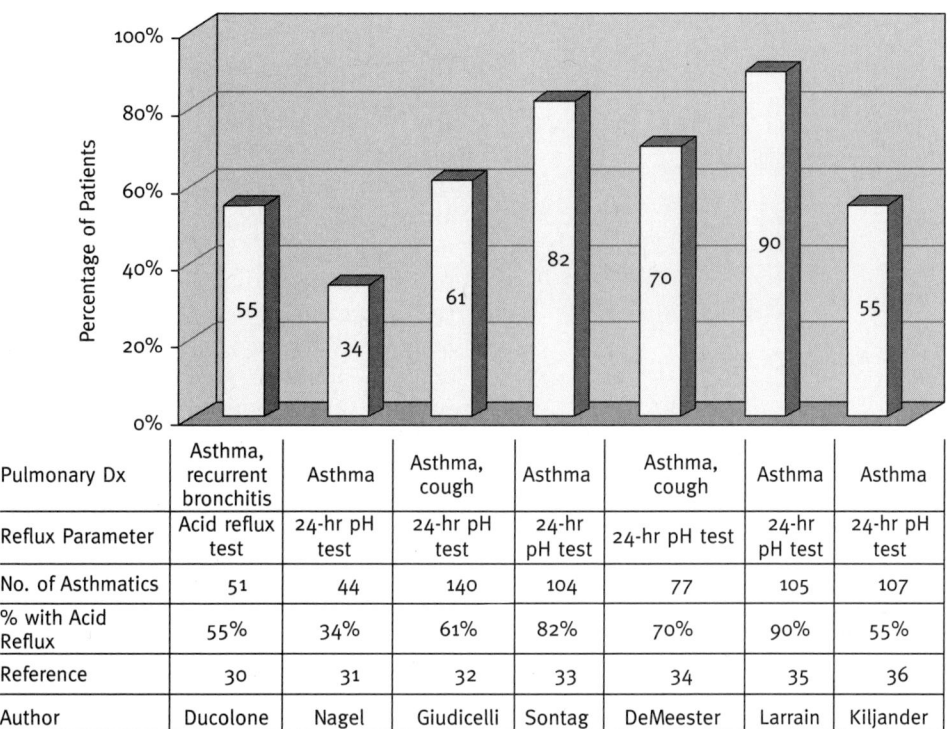

FIGURE 23.3 Prevalence of acid reflux in asthmatics. On average, 70% of adult asthmatics have GER as defined by abnormal esophageal pH testing.

Barrett's esophagus. In this study, Sontag and colleagues limited the recruitment to asthmatic subjects who were referred for endoscopy in an approved study on the prevalence of GER abnormalities in consecutive asthmatic patients. The authors eliminated from their study any patients who were referred for workup because of gastrointestinal symptoms and who were not part of the consecutive asthmatic protocol. Thus, this study appears to be one of the few that reports the prevalence of GER as it relates to esophageal mucosal disease in consecutive asthmatic patients.

Gastroesophageal Reflux Disease Defined as the Presence of Hiatal Hernia

Figure 23.5 shows three studies that used the presence of hiatal hernia as indirect evidence of the presence of GER.[37-39] In the first study, Sontag and colleagues showed that hiatal hernia was present in 58% of consecutively chosen asthmatic patients using predetermined endoscopic criteria for hiatal hernia and esophagitis.[37] In this study, all endoscopies were performed by one of two endoscopists using the same criteria for esophageal mucosal disease and the presence of hiatal hernia. In asthmatic patients with esophagitis, the hiatal hernia occurred seven times more frequently than in asthmatic patients without esophagitis, indicating that hiatal hernia in asthmatic patients is associated with more severe esophageal disease. In the second study, Mays reported on 28 patients with severe asthma, 64% of whom had hiatus hernia and 46% of whom had barium reflux.[38] In the third study, which included 15 patients with nocturnal asthma, Rodriguez-Villarruel reported a 73% prevalence rate of reflux based on a combination of barium x-ray studies, endoscopy, and technetium scintigraphy. In his report, all 11 of 15 patients had abnormal barium x-rays, indicating a 73% prevalence rate of reflux in asthmatic patients.[39] These studies were criticized by Chernow and Castell because of the lack of data demonstrating aspiration, the reliance on upper gastrointestinal series to determine GER, and the abnormally low prevalence

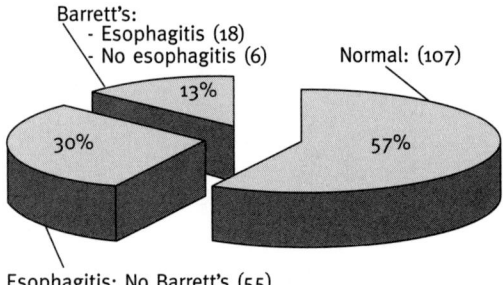

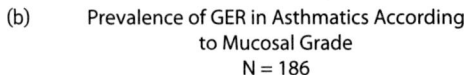

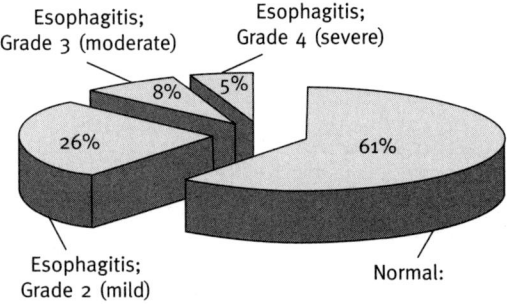

FIGURE 23.4 Prevalence of GER in asthmatics. **A,** According to esophageal mucosal disease: when Barrett's or esophagitis is considered as evidence of GER, 43% of asthmatics have GER-associated mucosal disease. **B,** According to mucosal grade: when Barrett's existing without esophagitis is considered as normal, 39% of asthmatics have GER as defined by the presence of esophagitis, and 13% have moderate to severe esophagitis.

of hiatus hernia and barium reflux in the control group.[40] Despite the criticisms, however, they concluded that the postulated relationship between GER and asthma most likely existed, but that it was premature to suggest cause and effect. When all three studies are combined, the prevalence of GER as defined by abnormal barium reflux on fluoroscopy or the presence of a hiatal hernia is 50%.

Taken together, the results of the retrospective studies, with their highly selected referral patterns, agree to a great extent with the results of the prospective epidemiologic and cross-sectional studies, which demonstrate that GER is highly prevalent in asthmatic patients.

Figure 23.6 summarizes the three prospective studies, which are part of the 12 adult prevalent studies. Approximately 75% of the asthmatic subjects have heartburn, and almost 20% awaken with nocturnal burning in the throat[29]; 80% of consecutive asthmatic patients have pathologic acid GER in either the upright or supine position, and 75% have increased frequency of reflux episodes.[33] In addition, almost 60% of consecutive asthmatic patients have hiatal hernias,[37] and almost 40% have esophageal mucosal damage from reflux.[37] Ninety percent of asthmatic patients have reflux symptoms, esophageal mucosal disease, or abnormal acid reflux. These data strongly indicate that GER is highly prevalent in consecutive asthmatic adults.

PREVALENCE OF GASTROESOPHAGEAL REFLUX IN ASTHMATIC CHILDREN

Figure 23.7 shows the prevalence of GER in asthmatic children.[41–48] The eight studies, with a total of 783 patients, report prevalence rates of GER ranging from 47% to 64%, with a mean prevalence of 56%. Although these studies suffer from the same biases in selection process as the adult studies, they provide the most reliable data available. In the first study, which is a retrospective radiographic review of 54 children with unremitting asthma, Friedman reported a 48% prevalence rate of hiatal hernia.[41] The prevalence rate was significantly higher than the 19% prevalence of hiatal hernias seen in the matched control group. Despite the known limitations of such retrospective radiographic reviews, the finding that almost 50% of the patients had a hiatal hernia is powerful evidence in support of the GER/asthma relationship. In the remaining seven studies,[42–48] pH testing was used to define the presence of GER. Four of the studies used the short-term acid reflux test, whereas three used 24-hour esophageal pH testing. Taken together, 439 of the 783 asthmatic children had evidence of GER by short-term pH testing, long-term pH testing,

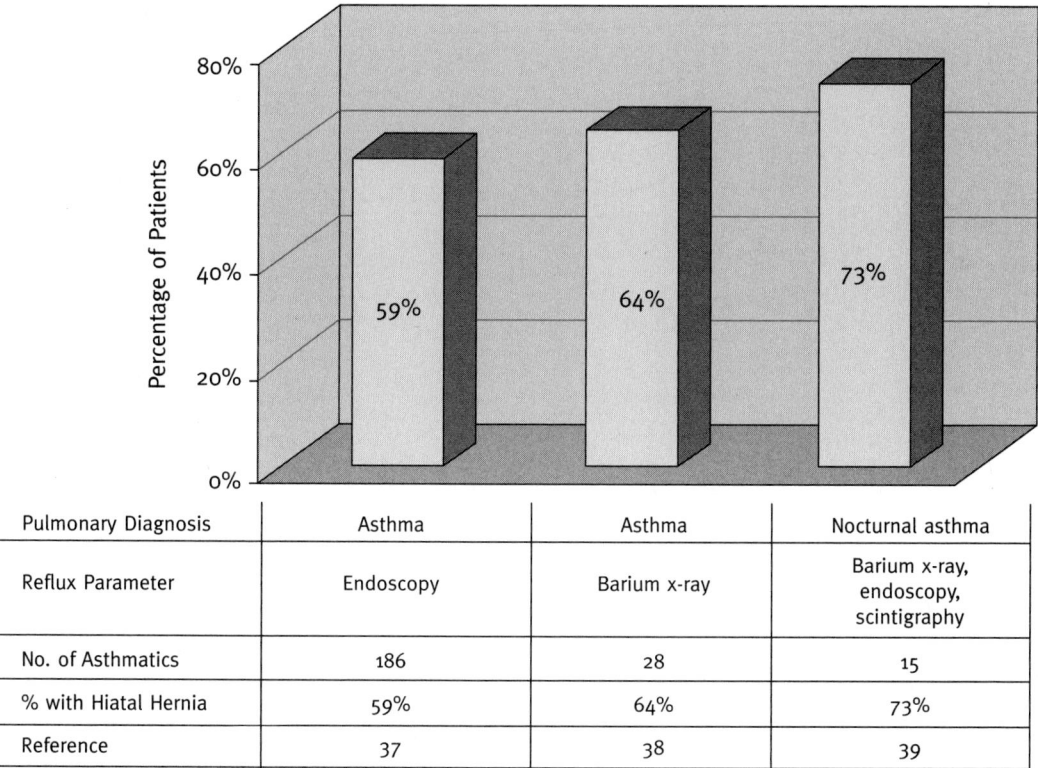

FIGURE 23.5 Prevalence of hiatal hernia in patients with asthma. On average, 66% of adult asthmatics have GER as defined by the presence of a hiatal hernia.

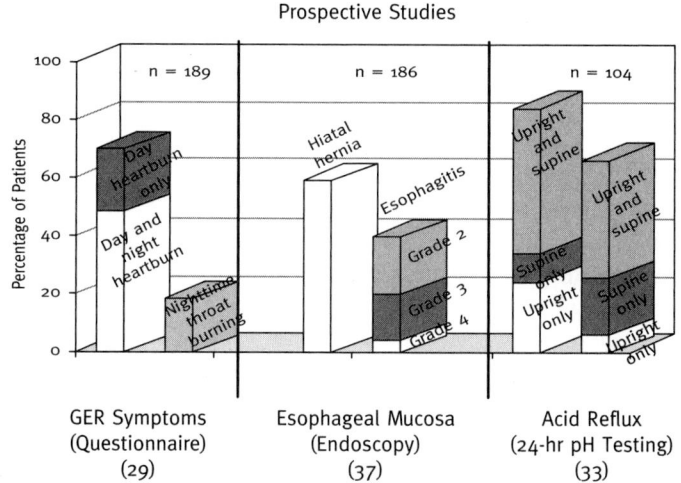

FIGURE 23.6 Prevalence of GER in consecutive asthmatics: 3 prospective studies. Three prospective studies were performed at the same institution. In all, 90% of asthmatics have at least one of the abnormal tests that are considered as indicative of GER. These data strongly indicate that GER is highly prevalent in adult asthmatics.

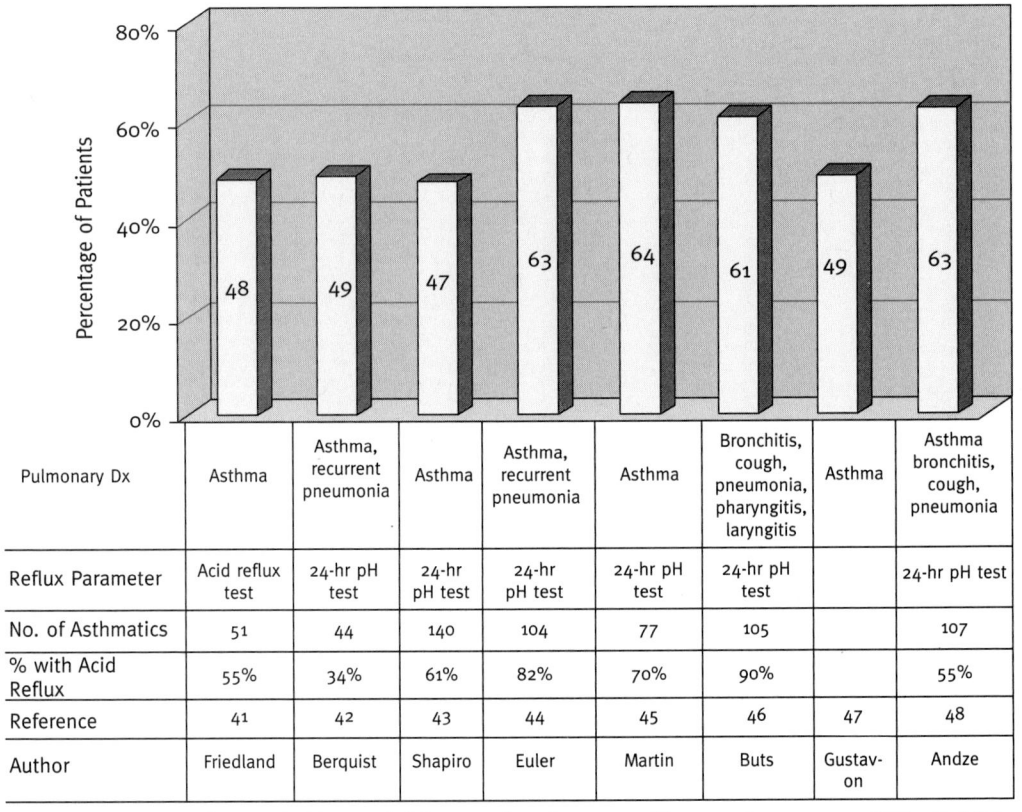

FIGURE 23.7 Prevalence of GER in children with pulmonary disease. On average, 66% of children with asthma have GER as defined by abnormal esophageal pH testing.

or radiographic evidence of hiatal hernia. Thus, the GER prevalence rate of 56% in asthmatic children is similar to that reported in asthmatic adults.

BRONCHODILATORS AND THE EFFECT ON GASTROESOPHAGEAL REFLUX

Support for the bronchodilator-induced GER concept comes from the numerous reports suggesting that asthma drug therapy relaxes the lower esophageal sphincter.[49-54] Such an effect might be expected to promote GER, and asthmatic patients who require continuous bronchodilators would likely have more GER than those who do not require bronchodilators. In addition, bronchodilators might increase the risk for nocturnal asthma because of the loss of bronchodilating effect as the drug is eliminated throughout the night.

Various studies argue against the bronchodilator-induced GER concept. Sontag and colleagues compared asthmatic subjects who received bronchodilators with those who did not receive bronchodilators.[55] The reflux patterns were similar in both groups of asthmatic patients, indicating that the reflux was indeed intrinsic to the asthma and not a result of the bronchodilator therapy.

Figure 23.8A shows the effect of asthma medications on the lower esophageal sphincter pressure, the total acid contact time, and the total reflux frequency in asthmatic subjects taking bronchodilators and asthmatic subjects taking no bronchodilators. Asthma medications had no adverse effect on any of the three reflux parameters.

Figures 23.8B and C demonstrate the effect of asthma medications, positions, and eating on the acid contact time and frequency of reflux episodes in the same two groups of asthmatic subjects—those receiving bronchodilators

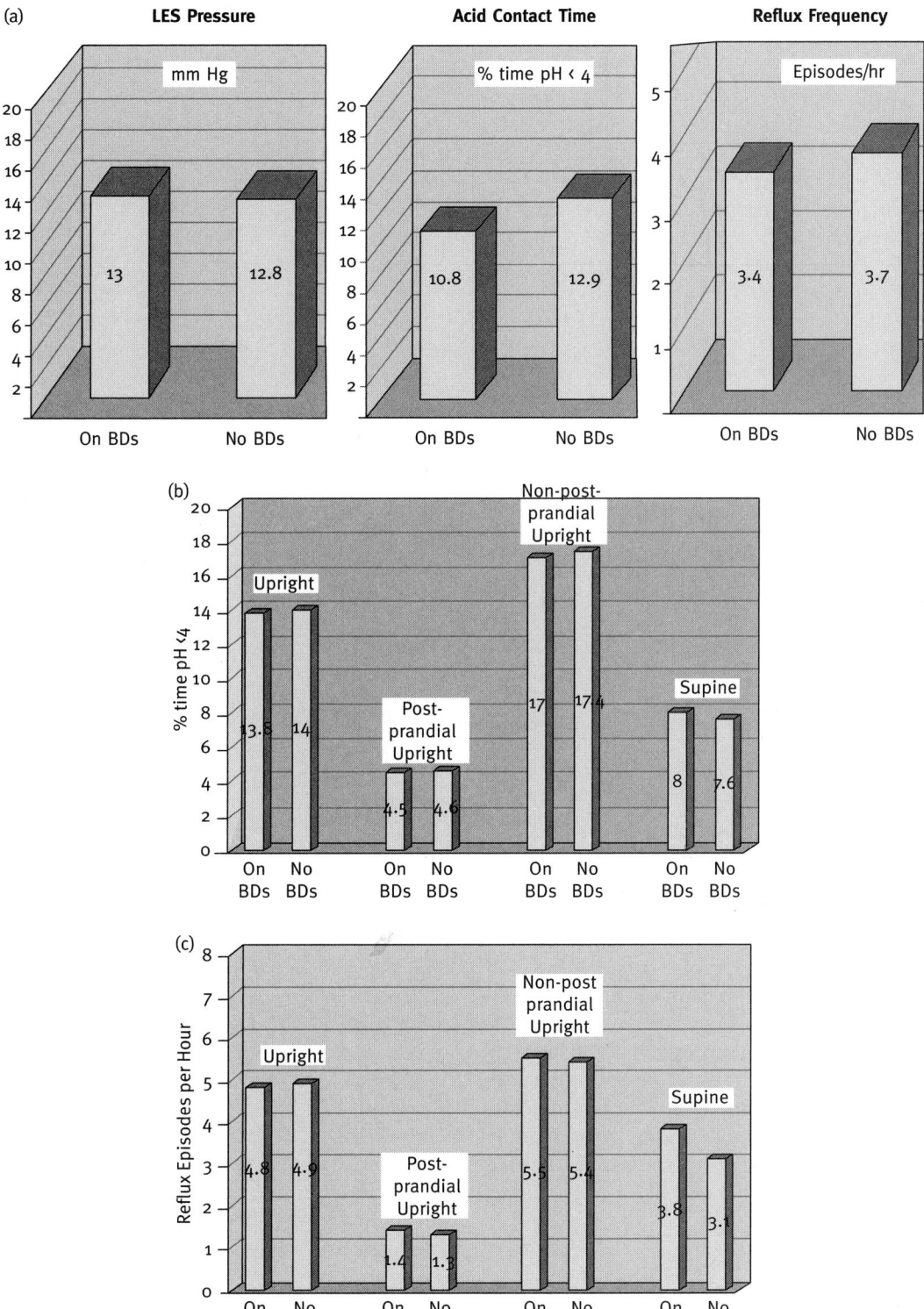

FIGURE 23.8 Effect of bronchodilator (BD) therapy **A**, on 3 GER parameters (total 24-hour period), **B**, on acid contact time before and after eating, and **C**, on reflux frequency before and after eating. The use of bronchodilator therapy in asthmatics appears to have no adverse effects on GER parameters at any time during the day or night or before or after eating. BDs, bronchodilators.

Gastroesophageal Reflux • 309

and those receiving no bronchodilators. The results show that bronchodilators do not influence any of the GER parameters during the upright, supine, postprandial, or non-postprandial periods. Asthmatic subjects receiving bronchodilators had no worse reflux than those not receiving bronchodilators, suggesting that bronchodilators do not promote postprandial or nocturnal GER.

In summary, these 24-hour esophageal pH test results obtained during the normal, everyday positions in asthmatic patients receiving bronchodilator therapy and those receiving no bronchodilator therapy suggest that GER is an intrinsic abnormality of asthma and not a result of bronchodilator-induced smooth muscle relaxation of the lower esophageal sphincter.

EFFECT OF THERAPY ON PULMONARY SYMPTOMS

Medical versus Surgical Therapy

The most compelling evidence for the existence of a close relationship between GER and pulmonary disease comes from the results of those clinical studies in which GER was adequately treated. In the several studies that report a beneficial response of asthma symptoms to acid reduction therapy with histamine-2 (H_2)-receptor antagonists,[56–58] the results are not convincing—possibly because the dosage of H_2-receptor antagonists used was inadequate to prevent reflux. The studies showing improvement or even cessation of wheezing after surgical correction of the reflux[56,59–61] provide the strongest evidence yet that GER is either a cause of or contributing factor to the asthma. It is reasonable to suggest that the dramatic improvement provided by surgery is related to the prevention not only of acid reflux but also of all gastric reflux.

Effect of Surgical Therapy on Pulmonary Disease

UNCONTROLLED SURGICAL STUDIES

Early reports of an association between GER and asthma described a reduction or even a disappearance of the asthmatic state after antireflux surgery.[12,23,26,32,34,46,60–65] In most of these studies, however, pulmonary function tests were not performed before or after surgical repair. Despite the lack of objective data, the dramatic subjective improvement reported in some of the studies (e.g., complete elimination of asthma after 20 years) cannot be ignored.

Figure 23.9 shows the results of the early studies and the more recent uncontrolled studies of antireflux surgery in asthmatic subjects. Despite the limitations of these studies, it appears that many patients have dramatic subjective improvement in asthma after surgery. In five of the studies, laparoscopic fundoplication was the procedure used in most of the patients.[66–70] Similar to the open procedures, the results were dramatic, with improvement or cure of pulmonary symptoms in 50% to 80% of patients.[71,72]

CONTROLLED SURGICAL STUDIES

Only three randomized surgical trials are reported.[56,73,74] In the first, Larrain and coworkers[56] conducted an initial 6-month study in 81 patients as well as a 5-year follow-up study. By the end of 6 months, the mean symptom and medication scores were significantly better in the surgical group and the cimetidine group than in the placebo group. The cimetidine group required less medication, and the surgical group required substantially less medication, but the placebo group required the same or more. By 5 years, only the surgical group had maintained its symptom-free status; the placebo and cimetidine groups were unchanged.

The results of the second study are shown in Figure 23.10. In this study,[73] 73 patients with both GER and asthma were randomized to receive antacids, ranitidine 150 mg three times daily, or antireflux surgery. Follow-up for up to 15 years showed that only surgical correction of reflux significantly improved pulmonary function, decreased the need for bronchodilators and prednisone, and diminished or eliminated the symptoms of asthma.

In the third study,[74] Spechler reported on 151 patients who were enrolled in a multicenter study of therapies for severe

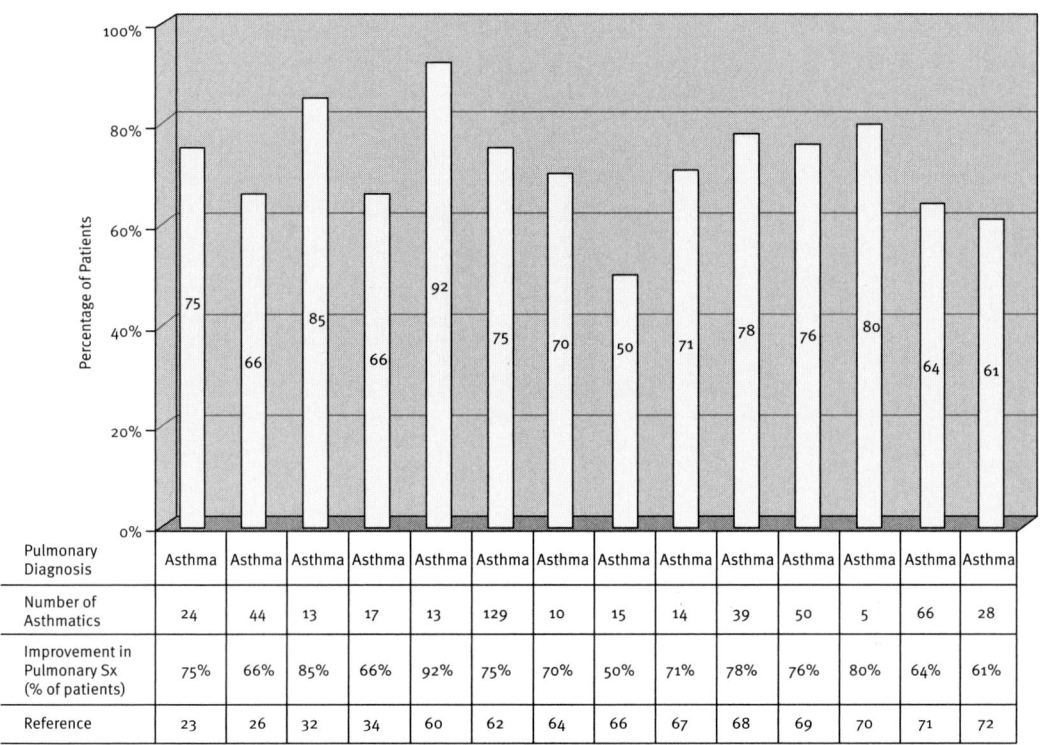

FIGURE 23.9 Effect of anti-reflux surgery on asthma symptoms in adults: 14 studies. On average, 75% of patients with pulmonary disease whose primary problem was GER and who had anti-reflux surgery because of the severe GER symptoms had improvement in their pulmonary symptoms.

GERD. The 5-year follow-up demonstrated no improvement in pulmonary function status after 1 year with either the medical or the surgical antireflux treatment. Although these results are consistent with our findings, it is important to note that the 151 patients in the severe GERD study were chosen because of GER symptoms, and if pulmonary disease was present, it was incidental and not necessarily apparent. Therefore, no real conclusions can be drawn from this large study.

DOES GASTROESOPHAGEAL REFLUX DISEASE CAUSE IDIOPATHIC PULMONARY FIBROSIS?

In the past decade, remarkably little research has added to the knowledge of the relationship between chronic pulmonary diseases and GERD. Failure to elucidate the mechanisms by which the two are related is not necessarily an indictment but rather a reflection of normal human limitations. The devastating pulmonary condition known as interstitial pulmonary fibrosis (IPF)—or interstitial lung disease (ILD)—has gotten the attention of those who believe in the GER–pulmonary disease association, if only because the treatment of IPF has been antireflux surgery followed by a lung transplantation. It has been a little more than a decade since the *New England Journal of Medicine* published a review article on pulmonary fibrosis in the Medical Progress section of the journal. In this article, the term "gastroesophageal reflux" appeared once: "Traction bronchiectasis, poor clearance of mucus, and perhaps an increased incidence of gastroesophageal reflux predispose patients with idiopathic pulmonary fibrosis to lower respiratory tract infections."[75] In the entire article, GER was never even suggested as a risk factor for IPF.

Some investigators at that time were citing older literature to support their theories. Today, without much additional knowledge

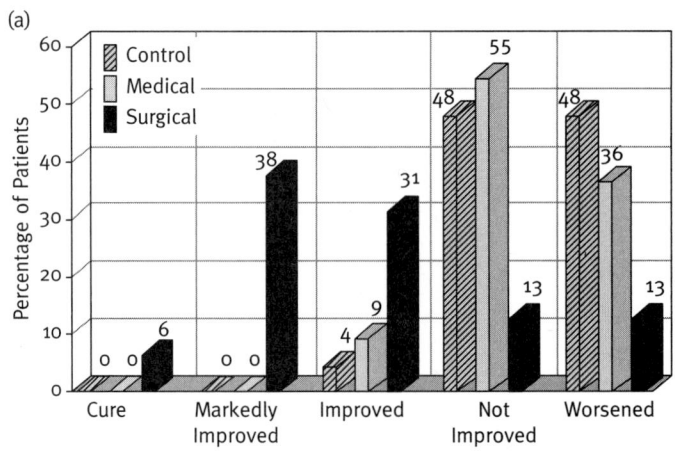

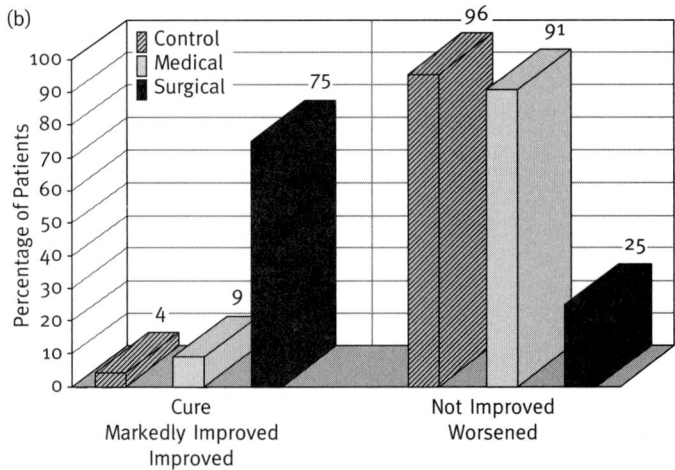

FIGURE 23.10 Overall clinical response of asthma to anti-reflux therapy. **A,** By the end of 2 years, complete cure occurred only in the surgical group and in only 6% of patients. Marked improvement or cure occurred in 44% of surgery patients and in no patients in the control or medical groups. **B,** Improvement, marked improvement, or cure in the overall asthma status occurred in 74.9% of the surgical group, 9.1% of the medical group, and 4.2% of the control group ($p < .001$, surgical vs. medical and control). The overall status worsened in 47.8% of the control group, 36.4% of the medical group, and 12.5% of the surgical group. The worsening in the surgical group was due entirely to 2 patients who died within 1 year of their surgery.

or convincing research, GER has been implicated in IPF to the point that antireflux surgery is being done before lung transplantation in order to protect the new lung from GERD-induced pulmonary disease.

In an article attempting to clarify a causal relationship between GERD and different ILDs, the investigators conducted a systematic search of the literature published between 1980 and 2010. After a review by two independent authors, each study was assigned an evidence-based rating according to a standard scoring system. Although 22 of 319 publications met the entry criteria, only 14 of 22 investigated the relationship between GERD and IPF.[76] The information resulting from this particular review study was a foregone conclusion. Anyone knowledgeable in the field knows the difficulty in demonstrating a causal relationship between any two diseases, especially two entities like GER and IPF.

Nevertheless, transplant surgeons believe in the relationship strongly enough to require antireflux surgery in patients receiving lung transplants for IPF. Furthermore, there is even the thought that if antireflux surgery performed *after* the lung transplantation improves outcomes in IPF patients by preventing aspiration of refluxed gastric acid, then antireflux surgery performed *before* the transplantation may actually obviate the need for the transplantation. Such a discovery would certainly have a powerful influence on the concept of acid GER and pulmonary disease.

THE GER/ASTHMA THEORY

If the high prevalence of GER in asthmatic patients is clinically relevant, it should be readily explainable. We suggest that the GER/asthma relationship consists of a self-propagating situation wherein reflux aggravates asthma, which in turn induces further reflux. In the early course of the disease, asthma may not be apparent because aspiration-induced pulmonary symptoms may occur infrequently—perhaps once or twice a year. With time, however, aspiration may become more frequent, and the pulmonary tree may become hypersensitive. The individual may be diagnosed as having asthma. The pulmonary tree becomes increasingly hypersensitive, and to a variety of stimuli. In such a scenario, the initial contribution of acid aspiration is no longer apparent because the primary focus is on the asthma. In any individual patient, the emphasis may be placed on the GER, if reflux symptoms predominate, or on asthma if pulmonary symptoms predominate. The result is confusion over whether a patient with severe reflux has pulmonary symptoms or whether a patient with asthma has reflux symptoms. The unending debate about whether GER is a cause of the asthma or a result of the asthma becomes the focus of attention. At such a point, the question of whether GER exists in asthmatic patients or whether pulmonary symptoms exist in refluxers is irrelevant. For the individual patient, gastric contents refluxed into the pulmonary tree is an undesirable event—whether cause or effect—and it is up to the physician to determine how such events can be stopped.

TREATMENT DECISIONS

Despite the large number of published studies on the relationship between GER and asthma, the true *prevalence* of GER in asthmatic patients must be estimated from fewer than 20 of the studies. The estimated *prevalence* is between 60% and 80% in asthmatic adults and 50% and 60% in asthmatic children. These studies comprise highly selected, referred populations that may not reflect the overall populations with asthma. Despite the limitations, however, the data likely reflect the general asthma population as much as can be expected, and clinical decisions must be based on these available data.

With the knowledge that up to 12 million asthmatic individuals live in the United States, that the vast majority of asthmatic people have GER (either symptomatic or silent), that no single diagnostic test or combination of tests will identify the asthmatic subject with GER-induced pulmonary disease, that no test results will predict which patients will respond to therapy, and that genuine improvement in overall pulmonary status and health may require a long-term steadfast commitment to medical or surgical antireflux therapy, how is a decision made on the management of GER in asthmatic people? Although certain markers are suggested as predictors of a good surgical response,[26] such as (1) onset of reflux symptoms before the onset of pulmonary symptoms, (2) the presence of nocturnal asthma, and (3) an initial pulmonary response to potent gastric acid suppression therapy,[32] it is impossible to totally rely on markers.

Perhaps the most important factor in GER and GER-induced pulmonary symptoms is the factor that is also the most ignored in discussions about mechanisms and is frequently ignored when we discuss treatment with our patients: eating before bedtime. In a recent study entitled "Asthmatics Have More Frequent Life-Threatening Reflux Symptoms Than Non-Asthmatics, and They Are Related to Bed-Time Eating,"[29] our group used an extensive questionnaire to demonstrate in a large population of asthmatic subjects and controls that the GER symptoms of burning in the throat, regurgitation, and dysphagia are significantly more prevalent in asthmatic than

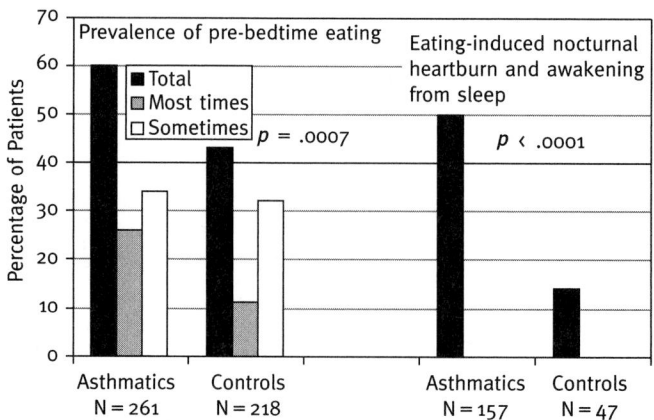

FIGURE 23.11 Heartburn characteristics. Heartburn characteristics in the subgroup of asthmatics and controls with heartburn symptoms. Up to half of the asthmatics could identify foods and activities that worsened heartburn symptoms.

nonasthmatic people, occurring in up to three times as many asthmatic people (Figures 23.11 and 23.12). More important, however, are the events that occur at nighttime during sleep that result in sudden awakening. Indeed, between midnight and 6 o'clock in the morning, one-third of the asthmatic population awakens with suffocation, cough, or wheezing that is preceded by heartburn or throat burning.

Eating before bedtime appears to be a significant negative factor in asthmatic patients with GER. Although a high percentage of both groups (60% vs. 44%) ate sometimes or most times before bedtime, the nocturnal GER symptoms associated with pulmonary disease (e.g., suffocation) were three times as frequent in asthmatic subjects as in controls. These findings suggest that eating before bedtime

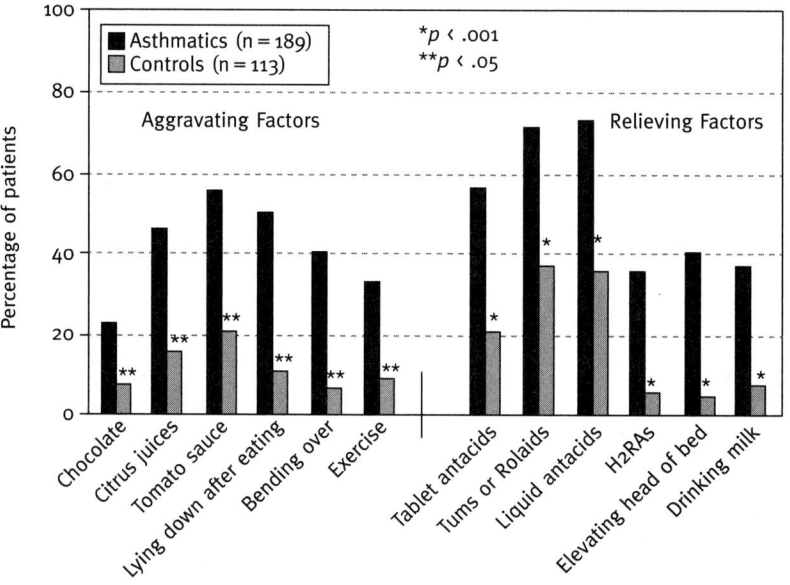

FIGURE 23.12 Prevalence of pre-bedtime eating and the effect on sleep in asthmatics and controls. Sixty percent of asthmatics and 44% of non-asthmatic controls eat before going to bed. Mean difference = 16%, 95% CI = 7.1–24.9, P = .0007. Of those who eat before bedtime, half the asthmatics, compared with only 14% of controls, had heartburn that in turn caused the sudden awakening. Mean difference = 36%, 95% CI = 23.1–48.6, P < .0001.

has more serious consequences in asthmatic than in nonasthmatic patients.

In the final analysis, it is unlikely that people will abstain from nighttime eating every night for years. Thus, the decision on treatment of GER in asthmatic patients must be based almost entirely on clinical judgment, and a trial of empirical antireflux therapy is likely the safest and most practical option.

SUMMARY

Most asthmatic people have GER, and the evidence is strong that GER plays an important role in some patients with asthma. Despite sophisticated study methods and technologically advanced diagnostic tests, the results of published studies on mechanisms fail to provide a diagnostic test with a degree of certainty great enough to identify which patients have GER-induced or GER-exacerbated asthma and which patients will respond to antireflux therapy. Indeed, even positive results on such direct tests as sputum inspection and scintigraphic monitoring, both of which establish reflux into the tracheobronchial tree, do not necessarily establish cause or effect and cannot be used to predict outcomes. Finally, the popular and frequently used ambulatory esophageal pH test (Bravo), believed by many to be the best GER test available, can only suggest, but cannot prove, the diagnosis of GER-induced asthma, and pH testing cannot be safely relied on to make our clinical decisions.

Despite extensive research on mechanisms of GER-induced pulmonary symptoms, we are still forced to fall back on "the therapeutic trial"—a trial of a proton pump inhibitor (PPI) to assess whether asthma improves subjectively and objectively. It is important to understand, however, that the therapeutic trial must use a dose high enough to prevent even silent esophageal acid exposure. The duration must be long enough to allow for detection of even subtle trends in subjective and objective respiratory improvement.

Antireflux surgery remains a therapeutic option and should not be withheld if GER is a reasonable suspect in asthma exacerbations. Although strong opinions have been voiced about whether a good response to PPI therapy predicts a good response to antireflux surgery, the opinions, although logical, are based on personal experience and "gut feelings"; a good PPI response may not necessarily predict a good surgery response, and a poor response to PPI does not necessarily predict a poor response to anti-reflux surgery.

UNMET, FUTURE RESEARCH NEEDS

1. A noninvasive method that predicts whether *any* antireflux treatment would provide long-term improvement of pulmonary symptoms
2. A method that identifies *which* antireflux therapy—medical or surgical—would provide the most improvement in pulmonary symptoms
3. Randomized long-term studies of GER treatments that compare (1) maximal PPI therapy, (2) on-demand PPI therapy, and (3) antireflux surgery in patients with pulmonary symptoms, such as cough, laryngitis, and asthma

CONCLUSION

When the method is found that predicts which patients with GER and asthma will respond to antireflux treatment, the results could be profound: fewer hospitalizations for respiratory complications, less pulmonary morbidity and mortality, less need for pulmonary medications, less time lost from work, fewer visits to a physician's office, and less illness associated with corticosteroid therapy. For the present time, however, clinical judgment and good sense are still our best friends. It is not unreasonable to urge patients to alter their lifestyle: the huge-volume, calorie-dense, high-fat meals that are eaten before bedtime are not likely to prevent GER or add to life expectancy.

REFERENCES

1. The Bible. Genesis 2:7.
2. The Talmud: Divrei Chayyim II, 52.
3. The Talmud: Gittin, 69b.
4. Aurelianus Caelius. In: *De Morbis Acutis et Chronicis*. Amsterdam: Wetstenland; 1709.

5. Maimonides M. Treatise on asthma. In: Munter S, ed. *Medical Writings of Moses Maimonides*. Philadelphia: Lippincott; 1963.
6. Rosen von Rosenstein N. On the cough of children. In: *The Diseases of Children and Their Remedies*. The Classics of Medicine Library. Birmingham, AL: LB Adams; 1776:183-190.
7. Heberden W. Asthma. In: *The History and Cure of Diseases*. The Classics of Medicine Library. Birmingham, AL: LB Adams; 1802:62-69.
8. Osler W. Bronchial asthma. In: *The Principles and Practice of Medicine*. The Classics of Medicine Library. Birmingham, AL: LB Adams; 1776:497-503.
9. Bray GW. Recent advances in the treatment of asthma and hay fever. *Practitioner*. 1934;34:368-371.
10. Belsey R. The pulmonary complications of oesophageal disease. *Br J Dis Chest*. 1960;54:342-348.
11. Kennedy JH. "Silent" gastroesophageal reflux: an important but little known cause of pulmonary complications. *Dis Chest*. 1962;42:42-45.
12. Urschel HC, Paulson DL. Gastroesophageal reflux and hiatal hernia: complications and therapy. *J Thorac Cardiovasc Surg*. 1967;53:21-32.
13. Cherry J, Margulies SI. Contact ulcer of the larynx. *Laryngoscope*. 1968;78:1937-1940.
14. Sontag SJ: The prevalence of gastroesophageal reflux disease in asthma. In: Stein M, ed. *Gastroesophageal Reflux Disease and Airway Disease*. New York: Marcel Dekker; 1999:115-138.
15. Ransohoff DF, Feinstein AR. Problems of spectrum and bias in evaluating the efficacy of diagnostic tests. *N Engl J Med*. 1978;299:926-930.
16. Philbrick JT, Horowitz RI, Feinstein AR, Langou RA, Chandler JP. The limited spectrum of patients studied in exercise test research: analyzing the tip of the iceberg. *JAMA*. 1982;248:2467-2470.
17. Feinstein AR. On blind men, elephants, spectrums, and controversies: lessons from rheumatic fever revisited. *J Chronic Dis*. 1986;39:337-342.
18. Miller TQ, Turner CW, Tinsdale RS, Posavac EJ. Disease based spectrum bias in referred samples and the relationship between type A behavior and arteriosclerosis. *J Clin Epidemiol*. 1988;41:1139-1149.
19. Berkson J. The statistical study of association between smoking and lung cancer. *Mayo Clin Proc*. 1955;30:319-324.
20. Berquist WE, Rachelefsky GS, Rowshan N, et al. Quantitative gastroesophageal reflux and pulmonary function in asthmatic children and normal adults receiving placebo, theophylline, and metaproterenol sulfate therapy. *J Allergy Clin Immunol*. 1984;73:253-258.
21. Davis RS, Larsen GL, Grunstein MM. Respiratory response to intraesophageal acid infusion in asthmatic children during sleep. *J Allergy Clin Immunol*. 1983;72:393-398.
22. Hughes DM, Spier S, Rivlin J, Levison H. Gastroesophageal reflux during sleep in asthmatic patients. *J Pediatr*. 1983;102:666-672.
23. Overholt RH, Voorhees RJ. Esophageal reflux as a trigger in asthma. *Dis Chest*. 1966;49:464-466.
24. Davis MV. Relationship between pulmonary disease, hiatal hernia, and gastroesophageal reflux. *N Y State J Med*. 1972;72:935.
25. Bretza J, Novey HS. GE reflux and asthma. *West J Med*. 1979;131:320.
26. Perrin-Fayolle M, Gormand F, Braillon G, et al. Long-term results of surgical treatment for gastroesophageal reflux in asthmatic patients. *Chest*. 1989;96:40-45.
27. Perrin-Foyalle M, Bel A, Kofman J, et al. Asthma and gastroesophageal reflux: results of a survey of over 150 cases. *Poumon Coeur*. 1980;36:225-230.
28. Field SK, Underwood M, Brant R, Cowie RL. Prevalence of gastroesophageal reflux symptoms in asthma. *Chest*. 1996;109:316-322.
29. Sontag SJ, O'Connell S, Miller TQ, Bernsen M, Seidel J. Asthmatics have more nocturnal gasping and reflux symptoms than nonasthmatics, and they are related to bedtime eating. *Am J Gastroenterol*. 2004;99:789-796.
30. Ducolone A, Vandevenne A, Jouin H, Grob JC, Coumaros D, Meyer C. Gastroesophageal reflux in patients with asthma and chronic bronchitis. *Am Rev Respir Dis*. 1987;135:327-332.
31. Nagel RA, Brown P, Perks WH, Wilson RSE, Kerr GD. Ambulatory pH monitoring of gastro-oesophageal reflux in "morning dipper" asthmatics. *BMJ*. 1988;297:1371-1373.
32. Giudicelli R, Dupin B, Surpas P, et al. Reflux gastro-oesophagien et manifestations respiratoires: attitute diagnostique, indications therapeutiques et resultats. *Ann Chir*. 1990;44:552-554.
33. Sontag S, O'Connell S, Khandelwal S, et al. Most asthmatics have gastroesophageal reflux with or without bronchodilator therapy. *Gastroenterology*. 1990;99:613-620.
34. DeMeester TR, Bonavina L, Iascone C, Courtney JV, Skinner DB. Chronic respiratory symptoms and occult gastroesophageal reflux. *Ann Surg*. 1990;211:337-345.
35. Larrain A, Carrasco E, Galleguillos F, Sepulveda R, Pope C. Medical and surgical treatment of

non-allergic asthma associated with gastroesophageal reflux. *Chest.* 1991;99:1330–1336.
36. Kiljander TO, Salomaa ER, Hietanen EK, Terho EO. Gastroesophageal reflux in asthmatics: a double-blind, placebo-controlled crossover study with omeprazole. *Chest.* 1999;116:1257–1264.
37. Sontag SJ, Schnell TG, Miller TQ, et al. Prevalence of oesophagitis in asthmatics. *Gut.* 1992;33:872–876.
38. Mays EE. Intrinsic asthma in adults, association with gastroesophageal reflux. *JAMA.* 1976;236:2626–2628.
39. Rodriguez-Villarruel H, Villarreal-Plata M, Hernandez-Contreras I, et al. Reflujo gastroesofagico associado a asthma bronquial. *Bol Md Hosp Infant Mex.* 1988;45:442.
40. Chernow B, Castell DO. Asthma and gastroesophageal reflux (letter). *JAMA.* 1977;237:2379.
41. Friedland GW, Yamate M, Marinkovich VA. Hiatal hernia and chronic unremitting asthma. *Pediatr Radiol.* 1973;1:156–160.
42. Berquist WE, Rachelefsky GS, Kadden M, et al. Gastroesophageal reflux-associated recurrent pneumonia and chronic asthma in children. *Pediatrics.* 1981;68:29–35.
43. Shapiro GG, Christie DL. Gastroesophageal reflux in steroid-dependent asthmatic youths. *Pediatrics.* 1979;63:207–212.
44. Euler AR, Byrne WJ, Ament ME, et al. Recurrent pulmonary disease in children: a complication of gastroesophageal reflux. *Pediatrics.* 1979;63:47–51.
45. Martin ME, Grunstein MM, Larsen GL. The relationship of gastroesophageal reflux to nocturnal wheezing in children with asthma. *Ann Allergy.* 1982;49:318–322.
46. Buts JP, Barudi C, Moulin D, Calus D, Cornu G, Otte JB. Prevalence and treatment of silent gastro-oesophageal reflux in children with recurrent respiratory disorders. *Eur J Pediatr.* 1986;145:396–400.
47. Gustafsson PM, Kjellman N-IM, Tibbling L. Bronchial asthma and acid reflux into the distal and proximal oesophagus. *Arch Dis Child.* 1990;65:1255–1258.
48. Andze GO, Brandt ML, St Vil D, et al. Diagnosis and treatment of gastroesophageal reflux in 500 children with respiratory symptoms: the value of pH monitoring. *J Pediatr Surg.* 1991;26:295–300.
49. Berquist WE, Rachelefsky GS, Rowshan N, Siegel SC, Katz RM, Welch M. Quantitative gastroesophageal reflux and pulmonary function in asthmatic children and normal adults receiving placebo, theophylline, and metaproterenol sulfate therapy. *J Allergy Clin Immunol.* 1984;73:253–258.
50. Mitsuhashi M, Tomomasa T, Tokuyama K, Morikawa A, Kuroume T. The evaluation of gastroesophageal reflux symptoms in patients with bronchial asthma. *Ann Allergy.* 1985;54:317–320.
51. Stein MR, Towner TG, Weber RW, et al. The effect of theophylline on the lower esophageal sphincter pressure. *Ann Allergy.* 1980;45:238–239.
52. Clemencon GH, Osterman PO. Hiatal hernia in bronchial asthma: the importance of concomitant pulmonary emphysema. *Gastroenterologia.* 1961;95:110–120.
53. DiMarino AJ, Cohen S. Effect of an oral beta 2-adrenergic agonist on lower esophageal sphincter pressure in normals and in patients with achalasia. *Dig Dis Sci.* 1982;27:1063–1066.
54. Goyal RK, Rattan S. Mechanism of the lower esophageal sphincter relaxation: action of prostaglandin E1 and theophylline. *J Clin Invest.* 1973;52:337–341.
55. Sontag S, O'Connell S, Khandelwal S, et al. Effect of positions, eating and bronchodilators on gastroesophageal reflux in asthmatics. *Dig Dis Sci.* 1990;35:849–856.
56. Larrain A, Carrasco E, Galleguillos F, Sepulveda R, Pope C. Medical and surgical treatment of non-allergic asthma associated with gastroesophageal reflux. *Chest.* 1991;99:1330–1336.
57. Ekstrom T, Tibbling L. Gastro-oesophageal reflux and triggering of bronchial asthma: a negative report. *Eur J Respir Dis.* 1987;71:177–180.
58. Harper PC, Bergner A, Kaye MD. Anti-reflux treatment for asthma: improvement in patients with associated gastroesophageal reflux. *Arch Intern Med.* 1987;147:56–60.
59. Davis RS, Larsen GL, Grunstein MM. Respiratory response to intraesophageal acid infusion in asthmatic children during sleep. *J Allergy Clin Immunol.* 1983;72:393–398.
60. Sontag SJ, O'Connell SA, Greenlee HB, et al. Is gastroesophageal reflux a factor in some asthmatics? *Am J Gastroenterol.* 1987;82:119–126.
61. Johnson DG, Syme WC, Matlak ME, Black RE, Herbst SJ. Gastro-oesophageal reflux and respiratory disease: the place of the surgeon. *Aust N Z J Surg.* 1984;54:405–415.
62. Lomasney TL. Hiatus hernia and the respiratory tract. *Ann Thorac Surg.* 1977;24:448–450.
63. Meadows CT. Clinical observations regarding sliding hiatal hernia. *Dis Chest.* 1965;47:629–631.

64. Tardiff C, Nouvet G, Denis P, Tombelaine R, Pasquis P. Surgical treatment of gastroesophageal reflux in ten patients with severe asthma. *Respiration*. 1989;56:110–115.
65. Berquist WE, Rachelefsky GS, Kadden M, et al. Gastroesophageal reflux-associated recurrent pneumonia and chronic asthma in children. *Pediatrics*. 1981;68:29–35.
66. Bittner HB, Meyers WC, Brazer SR, Pappas TN. Laparoscopic Nissen fundoplication: operative results and short-term follow-up. *Am J Surg*. 1994;167:193–200.
67. Alexander R, Kopita J, Kussin I, Pappas T, Brazer S, Kussin P. Outcome of laparoscopic Nissen fundoplication for asthma associated with refractory gastroesophageal reflux: evidence for clinical benefit at one year follow-up. *Am J Respir Crit Care Med*. 1994;149:A202.
68. Spivak H, Smith CD, Phichith A, Gallaway K, Waring PJ, Hunter JG. Asthma and gastroesophageal reflux: fundoplication decreases need for systemic corticosteroids. *Gastroenterology*. 1998;114:A1428.
69. Johnson WE, Hagen JA, DeMeester TR, et al. Outcome of respiratory symptoms after surgery on patients with gastroesophageal reflux disease. *Arch Surg*. 1996;131:489–492.
70. Hunter JG, Trus TL, Branum GD, Waring JP, Wood WC. A physiologic approach to laparoscopic fundoplication for gastroesophageal reflux disease. *Ann Surg*. 1996;223:673–687.
71. Ribet M, Pruvot FR, Mensier E, Ghoch K, Rousseau B. Gastro-oesophageal reflux and respiratory disorders treated by Hill's procedure. *Eur J Cardiothorac Surg*. 1989;3:414–418.
72. Henderson RD, Woolfe CR. Aspiration and gastroesophageal reflux. *Can J Surg*. 1978;21:352–354.
73. Sontag SJ, O'Connell S, Khandelwal S, et al. Asthmatics with gastroesophageal reflux: long-term results of a randomized trial of medical versus surgical anti-reflux therapies. *Am J Gastroenterol*. 2003;98:987–999.
74. Spechler SJ, Lee E, Ahnen D, et al. long-term outcome of medical and surgical treatments for gastroesophageal reflux disease: follow-up of a randomized controlled trial. *JAMA*. 2001;285(18):2331–2338.
75. Tobin RW, Pope CE II, Pellegrini CA, Emond MJ, Sillery J, Raghu G. Increased prevalence of gastroesophageal reflux in patients with idiopathic pulmonary fibrosis. *Am J Respir Crit Care Med*. 1998;158:1.
76. Hershcovici T, Jha LK, Johnson T, et al. The relationship between interstitial lung diseases and gastro-oesophageal reflux disease. *Aliment Pharmacol Ther*. 2011;34(11):1295–1305.

SECTION SIX

METABOLIC

24

OBESITY AND ASTHMA

COMORBID AND COEXISTING

Erick Forno, Louis-Philippe Boulet, and Juan C. Celedón

KEY POINTS

- The prevalence of asthma is increased in obese subjects.
- The mechanisms by which obesity leads to the development of asthma or affects its severity or control are incompletely understood.
- In obese individuals, asthma may represent a specific phenotype characterized by noneosinophilic airway inflammation and reduced response to asthma medications such as inhaled corticosteroids.
- Weight loss is associated with an improvement of asthma in obese patients and should be part of asthma management.
- The impact of obesity-related comorbid conditions on asthma remains to be determined.

INTRODUCTION

Obesity co-occurs with diseases affecting multiple organ systems (e.g., diabetes, atherosclerosis, and obstructive sleep apnea [OSA]). Although the co-occurrence of obesity and a particular disease (e.g., rheumatoid arthritis) may be coincidental, obesity is known to predispose to certain illnesses (e.g., diabetes type 2 [by increasing insulin resistance] and OSA [by causing narrowing of the upper airways]). Conversely, certain diseases (e.g., osteoarthritis) may lead to reduced physical activity and thus cause obesity in overweight subjects or worsen obesity in affected individuals. Quite often, the relationship between obesity and a coexisting disease is bidirectional. For example, obesity can worsen osteoarthritis of weight-bearing joints, resulting in reduced mobility and weight gain.

An association between obesity and asthma has been reported in multiple studies of children and adults. In this chapter, the existing evidence is reviewed to support a causal link between obesity and asthma, including potential mechanisms that underlie this relationship and may lead to what we and others have referred to as the "obese asthmatic" phenotype. In addition, the impact of obesity on asthma morbidity and asthma management in subjects with preexisting or coexisting asthma is discussed. Finally, future directions for research in this field are outlined.

EPIDEMIOLOGIC STUDIES

Epidemiology of Asthma

Asthma affects more than 300 million people worldwide and is a serious public health concern in the United States, where about 16 million people are currently affected.[1] The Centers for Disease Control and Prevention (CDC) estimate that the total asthma-related cost is $56 billion per year in the United States.[2] Although the overall prevalence of asthma in this country is approximately 8.2% in adults and 9.6% in children, there is profound variability by socioeconomic status and ethnicity. The economically disadvantaged and members of certain ethnic minorities (e.g., African Americans and Puerto Ricans) are disproportionally affected by asthma.[3] Moreover, the frequency of current asthma has almost tripled over the past few decades, increasing from about 3.1% in the early 1980s to 8.5% in 2010.[3,4]

Epidemiology of Obesity

Obesity is defined as a body mass index (BMI) of 30 kg/m² or greater in adults and at or above the 95th percentile in children. Overweight includes a BMI between 25 and 29.9 kg/m² for adults and between the 85th and 95th percentiles for children. In the United States, 35.7% of adults and 16.9% of children are obese; thus, more than 78 million adults and 12.5 million children are affected. A cause of major concern is that overweight, which often precedes obesity, affects an additional 34% of adults and 17% to 18% of children.[5] By comparison, in 1976 to 1980, the estimated prevalence of obesity was 5% to 6% in children and approximately 15% in adults. In 2008, the estimated direct and indirect costs of obesity were approximately $132 billion.[6]

Epidemiologic Evidence of an Association between Obesity and Asthma

Multiple studies demonstrate an association between obesity or increased BMI and asthma. Because the initial studies had a cross-sectional design,[7,8] "reverse causation" (e.g., asthma leading to reduced physical activity and weight gain) could not be excluded as a potential explanation for the observed link between obesity and asthma. However, several prospective studies and meta-analyses show that increments in adiposity[9] or BMI, as early as infancy, precede the development of asthma in children and adults[10-12] (Figure 24.1). Although it could be argued that subclinical or mild asthma could have been missed at the onset of these studies, the aggregate evidence suggests that overweight or obesity increases the risk for new-onset asthma. A different issue is whether obesity increases asthma morbidity or severity in subjects with preexisting disease; in this regard, obesity has been associated with increased symptoms, disease exacerbations, and reduced quality of life in subjects with asthma.[13]

The magnitude or significance of the association between obesity and asthma may differ according to gender, atopic status, and age. Some investigators show that in children, obesity is predominantly associated with asthma in girls,[14] but others have shown a similar link in boys.[15] A large study of Chinese adults shows that an increased BMI is significantly associated with asthma in both men and women when the disease is defined using an objective measure of airway responsiveness in addition to self-reported symptoms.[7] Similar to studies in Western countries, a female-specific association is demonstrated when asthma

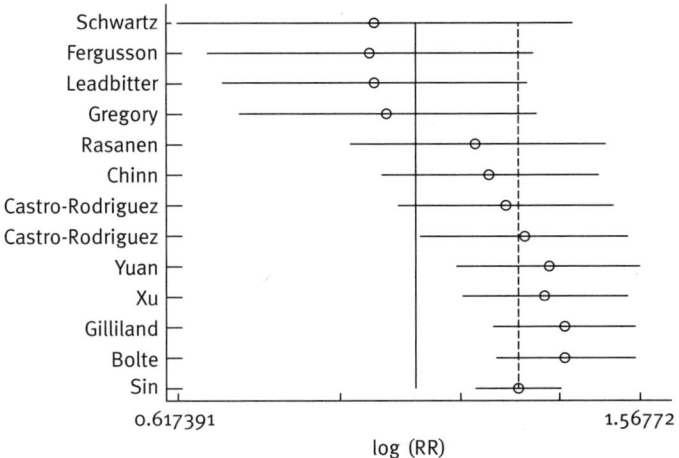

FIGURE 24.1 Cumulative meta-analysis of effect of high weight in childhood on subsequent development of asthma, in order of year of publication. (From Flaherman V, Rutherford GW. A meta-analysis of the effect of high weight on asthma. *Arch Dis Child*. 2006;91[4]:334–339.)

is defined according to self-reported physician-diagnosed asthma. This suggests that diagnostic bias may partly explain reported gender differences in the relation between obesity and asthma. Conflicting evidence also exists for obesity, atopy, and asthma. The bulk of evidence points against a role of atopy and eosinophils in the relationship between asthma and obesity, but there are some diverging reports.[12,16,17] Finally, current evidence indicates that the "obese asthmatic" phenotype may not necessarily be the same in children—in whom an obstructive airway deficit is reported[18]—as in adults, who exhibit a decrease in resting lung volumes (such as expiratory reserve volume [ERV]) or a frank restrictive pattern.[19] This phenotype of "obese asthma" also may be modified or influenced by gender and other variables.

In summary, there is ample epidemiologic evidence for an association between obesity and the subsequent development of asthma. Findings from population-based studies also support an association between obesity and increased asthma severity or reduced asthma control. The mechanisms underlying or modifying the relation between obesity and asthma or asthma severity are incompletely understood. In upcoming sections, proposed mechanisms are reviewed (Table 24.1).

PROPOSED MECHANISMS AND IMPLICATIONS FOR MANAGEMENT

Lung Mechanics and Respiratory Physiology

One of the first theories proposed to explain the distinct behavior of asthma among obese adults was that the excess adipose tissue in the chest would alter the mechanics of breathing. At rest, this extra adipose tissue would weigh down on the lungs, and during breathing, subjects would have to overcome additional resistance, leading to worsening dyspnea and other asthma symptoms. Indeed, obesity results in reductions in ERV, functional residual capacity (FRC), and other lung volumes[20] (Figure 24.2). This leads to characteristic "shallow" breathing near closing volumes, rendering obese individuals more susceptible to airway collapse and atelectasis, which would worsen their dyspnea and other respiratory symptoms.

In contrast to the restrictive ventilatory deficit reported in obese adults, several studies report an obstructive ventilatory pattern in children with increased forced expiratory volume in 1 second (FEV_1) or FVC but decreased FEV_1/FVC ratio.[18,21] Tantisira and colleagues report that the estimated effects of obesity on lung function measures are more pronounced in boys[18] and, contrary to findings in adults,

Table 24.1. Proposed Mechanisms for the Association between Asthma and Obesity

- Alteration of lung and airway mechanics
- Latching of actin–myosin bridges in airway smooth muscle cells
- Comorbidities (obstructive sleep apnea, gastroesophageal reflux disease)
- Hormonal differences
- Systemic inflammation and adipokines
- Predominantly noneosinophilic airway inflammation
- Insulin resistance and insulin-like growth factor 1
- Arginine/nitric oxide metabolism imbalance
- Vitamin D and other nutritional deficiencies
- Genetic/genomic determinants
- Decreased response to asthma medications

that the FEV_1 and FVC increase with BMI. Obese children may tend to be somewhat taller than their lean counterparts, which could explain why their lungs, and therefore their absolute flows, may be greater. However, FEV_1/FVC decreases with BMI in children, and this obstructive pattern could partly explain increased symptoms and/or greater severity of asthma in obese children.

Even if any negative impact of obesity on lung volumes were not large enough to produce symptoms, it could have other effects. Lung volume reduction decreases the tethering of the small airways in the lungs and reduces the stretching of airway smooth muscle (ASM) cells, which causes actin–myosin cross-bridges to turn from fast-cycling bridges into slow-cycling "latch" bridges.[22] Small airways may thus become "hypercontractile," increasing the risk for airflow obstruction and, perhaps, increased airway responsiveness (Figure 24.3). Whereas avoidance of deep inspiration, such as sighing, increases airway responsiveness to methacholine in nonobese individuals, such avoidance is not associated with a change in airway responsiveness in obese subjects.[23] These findings suggest that obesity negates or reduces potential protective effects of periodic deep inspiration or sighing against increased airway responsiveness, a key feature of asthma.

Comorbidities

As previously mentioned, obesity is associated with a wide range of coexisting and comorbid conditions that may affect asthma. For example, obese children and adults are at higher risk for developing gastroesophageal reflux disease (GERD).[24] Although GERD theoretically could increase airway inflammation or airway responsiveness in subjects with asthma, there is insufficient evidence to support an association between GERD and increased asthma morbidity.[25,26] Nissen fundoplication improved lung function and reduced medication use in an uncontrolled study of children with severe GERD and steroid-dependent asthma[27]; however, a multicenter clinical trial showed no beneficial effects of proton pump inhibitors on asthma in children with asymptomatic GERD.[28] Controlled studies are needed to appropriately assess whether treatment of symptomatic GERD reduces asthma morbidity in general, and in particular in obese subjects.

Overweight and obesity are associated with increased risks for OSA and symptoms

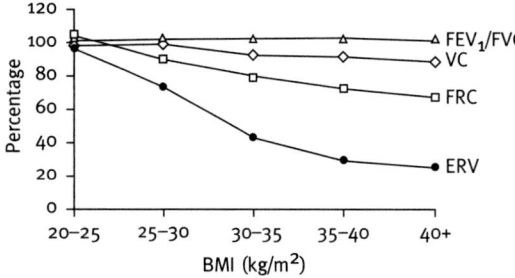

FIGURE 24.2 Effect of obesity on lung volumes. BMI, body mass index; ERV, expiratory reserve volume; FEV_1, forced expiratory volume in 1 second; FRC, functional residual capacity; FVC, forced vital capacity; VC, vital capacity. (From Sin DD, Sutherland ER. Obesity and the lung: 4. Obesity and asthma. *Thorax*. 2008;63[11]:1018–1023.)

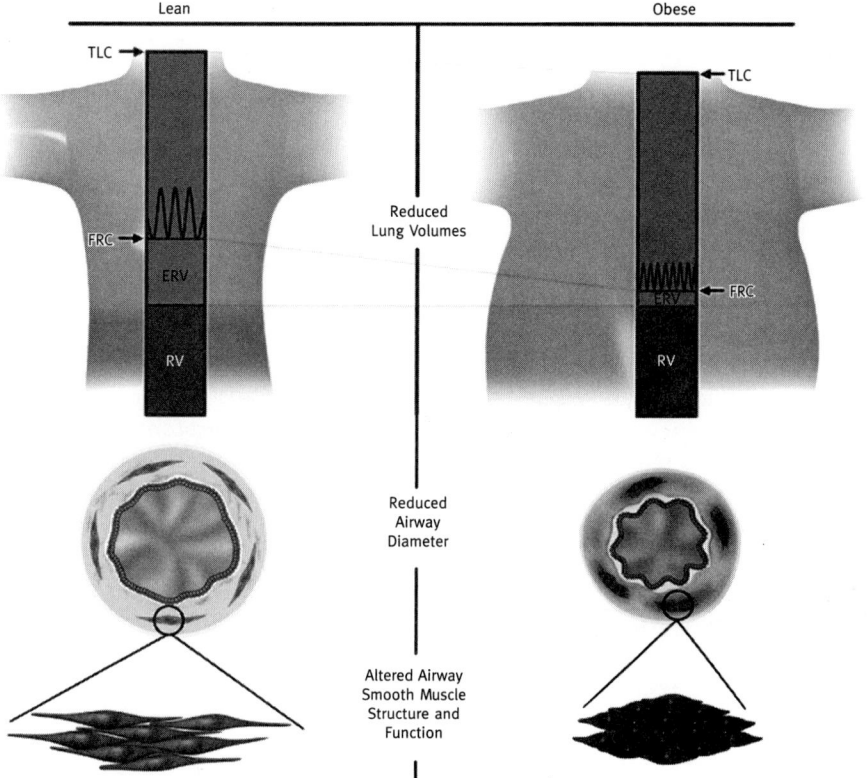

FIGURE 24.3 Obesity leads to alterations of lung volumes, particularly expiratory reserve volume (ERV) and FRC, leading to a rapid, shallow breathing pattern that occurs close to closing volume. Obesity also causes reduced peripheral airway diameter, which can lead to increased airway hyperresponsiveness due to alterations of smooth muscle structure and function. RV, residual volume; TLC, total lung capacity. See Color Plate 9 in insert. (From Beuther DA, Weiss ST, Sutherland ER. Obesity and asthma. *Am J Respir Crit Care Med.* 2006;174[2]:112–119.)

related to OSA. OSA may lead to increased airway inflammation, causing worsening and/or persistent symptoms from asthma.[29,30] An uncontrolled study of children shows that adenotonsillectomy leads not only to improvement in OSA but also to reduced asthma symptoms and decreased frequency of asthma exacerbations.[31] Although this merits further study, there are no controlled studies of the impact of treatment of OSA on asthma or "obese asthma."

Hormonal Differences

A potential modification of the effect of obesity on asthma by gender (see earlier) may be explained by hormonal differences between males and females. For example, estrogen level is associated with the development of adult-onset asthma in obese women.[32] Whereas estrogens increase eosinophil adhesion, migration, and degranulation,[33] testosterone decreases eosinophil adhesion and viability.[33] Among women, estrogens may stimulate interleukin-3 (IL-3) and IL-4 secretion in monocytes, estradiol may skew immunity toward a helper T-cell type 2 (T_H2) phenotype, and progesterone could augment airway inflammation.[34] The phenomenon of menstrual-linked asthma is recognized, whereby some women's asthma symptoms are worse or occur solely during menstruation. Aromatase, the last enzyme in the pathway that converts androgens to estrogens, is found in high concentrations in adipose tissue. This could contribute to elevated circulating levels of estrogen in obese individuals, which may in turn lead to increased eosinophilic activation and consequent worsening of airway inflammation and asthma symptoms. However, this pathway has not been adequately assessed in subjects with obesity and asthma.

Systemic Inflammation

Obesity, the metabolic syndrome, and to a certain degree overweight are associated with a state of increased systemic inflammation. This proinflammatory state could in theory translate into augmented airway inflammation, one of the main components of asthma. Several chemokines produced by adipocytes (adipokines) may have proinflammatory functions that are implicated in asthma (e.g., IL-6, eotaxin, tumor necrosis factor-α [TNF-α], leptin, and ghrelin). Other molecules implicated in asthma (transforming growth factor-β1) are not exclusive to adipose tissue but can be secreted in significant amounts by adipocytes.[35]

Adiponectin, an adipokine, has antiinflammatory properties. In murine models, higher serum adiponectin levels inhibit airway hyperresponsiveness and airway inflammation.[36] In humans, the serum adiponectin level is inversely associated with airflow obstruction, asthma symptoms, and risk for asthma exacerbations.[37] Levels of this adipokine are reduced in obese individuals. The rate of decrease of adiponectin with BMI is more pronounced among the obese than the nonobese, and it seems to vary by gender.[38]

Leptin, another adipokine, is important in the regulation of the basal metabolic rate and satiety in humans and other species.[39] Although metabolic rate and weight regulation may be its most important role, leptin increases immunoglobulin E and airway responsiveness in murine models of allergic airway inflammation.[40] Several studies show an association between leptin and measures of asthma in obese subjects, although some studies fail to report such an association.[41] At least one study reports increased leptin levels in asthma and in obesity but no obesity–asthma interaction[42]; however, this study included only women and may be underpowered to detect interactions. Finally, it is known that airway epithelial cells express leptin and adiponectin receptors; thus, it is tempting to speculate that excess adipose tissue exerts directs effects on the airways of asthmatic patients, separately and in addition to any indirect effects on asthma through systemic inflammation.

The molecular mechanisms and effects of the "low-grade proinflammatory state" of obesity and the metabolic syndrome on common illnesses such as diabetes mellitus type 2 and coronary artery disease are beginning to be understood. However, whether and how obesity influences asthma through a proinflammatory state remains largely unknown.

Atopy and Eosinophilic Inflammation

Increased BMI is associated with decreased exhaled nitric oxide (FeNO),[43] a marker of eosinophilic airway inflammation, and also with decreased sputum eosinophils[44] and increased sputum neutrophils.[17] The association between BMI and risk for asthma also seems to be stronger in nonatopic than atopic children.[12] Although obesity or increased BMI is associated with increased risk for atopy,[45,46] obesity is often associated with nonatopic asthma. These findings are consistent with theories that propose that the link between obesity and asthma is explained by either increased systemic inflammation or airway inflammation that is primarily neutrophilic and therefore nonresponsive to certain asthma medications such as inhaled corticosteroids (ICS) (see later).

Insulin Resistance and Arginine Metabolism

One of the main metabolic complications of obesity is the development of insulin resistance. Insulin resistance, and the consequent increase in free insulin-like growth factor 1 (IGF-1), profoundly affects several organ systems, including the respiratory system. Insulin and IGF-1 can directly cause ASM hypercontractility[47]; exert marked proliferative effects on lung fibroblasts, resulting in airway collagen deposition and fibrosis; and promote submucosal gland metaplasia.[48,49] Insulin resistance is associated with new-onset asthma symptoms in adults.[50]

Reduced insulin sensitivity may be coupled with increased protein turnover in obese subjects, which can raise levels of methylarginines such as asymmetrical dimethylarginine (ADMA)[49] (Figure 24.4). Increased levels of ADMA and similar molecules act as competitive inhibitors of the endothelial nitric oxide synthase (eNOS). In healthy individuals, eNOS is responsible for converting L-arginine and producing low levels of nitric oxide (NO), which regulate several homeostatic processes through cyclic guanosine monophosphate, including airway relaxation. However, increased ADMA reduces L-arginine bioavailability and inhibits eNOS, leading to decreased production of NO and impaired ASM relaxation. In addition to bronchial tone and reactivity, NO is also critical to other biologic processes, including endothelial and platelet function, as well as immune modulation. In murine models, the subcutaneous injection of ADMA leads to increased airway responsiveness and airway fibrosis.[51] Increased methylation of genes in the arginine–NO pathway is associated with increased FeNO.[52]

In summary, obesity can alter insulin and/or arginine metabolism, and this dysregulation may affect the airways. Insulin and IGF-1 may increase airway contractility and tone and spur fibroblast proliferation and collagen deposition.

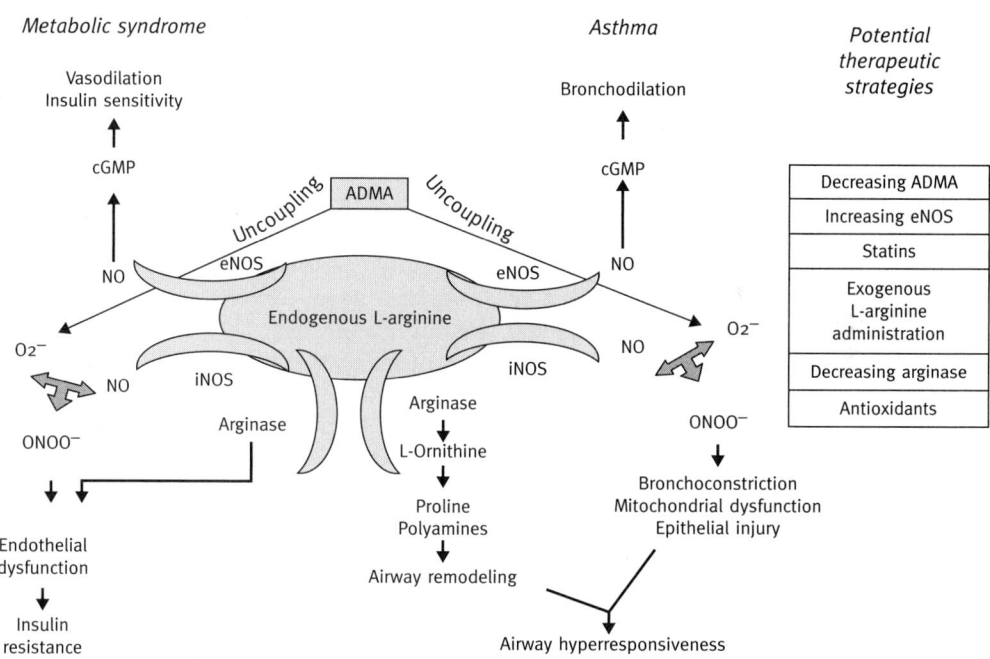

FIGURE 24.4 Schematic pathologic mirror view of L-arginine metabolism in metabolic syndrome and asthma, highlighting common features. In metabolic syndrome and asthma, the availability and utilization of endogenous L-arginine are similarly affected. Increased utilization of L-arginine by inducible nitric oxide synthase (iNOS) and arginase leads to less availability of L-arginine to endothelial nitric oxide synthase (eNOS). Diminished eNOS function is exaggerated by asymmetrical dimethylarginine (ADMA)-induced uncoupling of eNOS to form peroxynitrite. Arginase converts L-arginine into L-ornithine, which contributes to airway remodeling and endothelial dysfunction. Potential therapeutic strategies also might be similar as indicated. cGMP, cyclic guanosine monophosphate; NO, nitric oxide; O_2^- = superoxide free radicals; ONOO$^-$, peroxynitrite. (From Agrawal A, Mabalirajan U, Ahmad T, Ghosh B. Emerging interface between metabolic syndrome and asthma. Am J Respir Cell Mol Biol. 2011;44[3]:270–275.)

The insulin resistance and high protein turnover linked to obesity can lead to decreased NO, defective airway smooth muscle relaxation, airway inflammation, and perhaps immune dysregulation. Further research is needed to understand the relation among obesity, systemic or airway inflammation, and asthma.

Vitamin D

Vitamin D is implicated in the pathogenesis of asthma and asthma morbidity.[53] Low levels of vitamin D are associated with indicators of increased asthma severity or reduced asthma control, including severe asthma exacerbations, lower lung function, and increased airway responsiveness.[54,55] Because vitamin D is lipophilic, obese subjects, who have increased adipose tissue, are at higher risk for vitamin D deficiency or insufficiency.[56] Both low levels of vitamin D and overweight/obesity are associated with decreased response to inhaled corticosteroids, assessed by lung function measures such as FEV_1 in a cohort of over 1,000 asthmatic children followed for four years.[57] This suggests independent but potentially synergistic effects of obesity and vitamin D insufficiency on glucocorticosteroid responsiveness.

Experimental studies further support an effect of vitamin D on glucocorticosteroid sensitivity. When administered together with ICS, vitamin D modulates the secretion of proinflammatory cytokines by airway smooth muscle. Moreover, when CD4+ T-cell cultures from glucocorticosteroid-resistant asthmatic subjects are supplemented with vitamin D, glucocorticosteroid resistance decreases or disappears through the induction of IL-10–secreting regulatory T cells.[58] Ongoing clinical trials are examining whether vitamin D supplementation prevents the incident asthma and/or reduces asthma morbidity. Findings from these trials will be relevant to and could motivate future trials in obese subjects with asthma, who commonly have vitamin D insufficiency.

Genetic Determinants

Both asthma and obesity are common multifactorial diseases resulting from the interaction among insufficiently characterized genetic and environmental or lifestyle factors. Because obesity and asthma often co-occur, one can hypothesize that these two diseases share some genetic and/or epigenetic determinants. However, little is known about putative genetic or epigenetic determinants of asthma and obesity.

In children, single nucleotide polymorphisms (SNPs) in the leptin gene are associated with asthma using a candidate-gene approach,[59] and SNPs in the gene for protein kinase C alpha (PRKCA) have been linked to both BMI and asthma[60] using genome-wide methodology followed by a replication study. In a candidate-gene study of the TNF-α gene (TNFA), the association with asthma was stronger among nonatopic obese individuals with genotypes G/A and A/A of TNFA-308 compared with those with G/G genotype.

Other evidence of genetic mechanisms possibly shared by asthma and obesity is more indirect. For example, the genes for the $β_2$-adrenergic (ADRB2) and the glucocorticoid (NR3C1) receptors are separately implicated in pathways related to asthma and obesity, and they are both located on chromosome 5q. Similarly, polymorphisms of the fractalkine receptor gene CX3CR1 are associated with asthma, atopy, and obesity.[61,62]

Although there has been some progress in studying the possible shared genetic variants between asthma and obesity, much remains to be done. Because of the potential for false-positive results, replication of findings from previous genetic association studies of obesity and asthma is needed for proper evaluation of their significance.

Decreased Medication Response and Clinical Implications

Reducing airway inflammation is one of the main goals of asthma management, and ICS are one of the most effective antiinflammatory medications for asthma. Several studies show a decreased response among obese adults[63,64] and an impaired response to ICS in obese children with asthma (see earlier).[57] However, obese subjects with asthma do respond to systemic antiinflammatory therapies such as systemic corticosteroids and leukotriene modifiers.[63]

This phenomenon could be explained in part by reduced eosinophilic airway inflammation or increased systemic inflammation in obese subjects with asthma, as mentioned earlier. Inhaled medications, whose effects are limited to the airways, would not be effective in combatting the systemic inflammatory milieu as systemic glucocorticosteroids would. Beyond the site of action, systemic inflammation could also render obese asthmatic patients intrinsically resistant to corticosteroids. The glucocorticoid receptor has two main isoforms. The beta isoform (GRβ) strongly inhibits the active alpha isoform (GRα) by blocking the activation of glucocorticoid-responsive genes. GRβ is linked with glucocorticosteroid resistance, and cytokines associated with inflammation and obesity such as TNF-α and IL-6 regulate glucocorticoid receptor expression, with accumulation of GRβ. Genetic pathways that link asthma, obesity, and glucocorticosteroid metabolism and response, as in the case of the *CX3CR1* fractalkine receptor gene (see earlier), could also play a role. Alternatively, ICS doses commonly used in lean children may not be sufficient in obese children with asthma.

Because obese subjects may be less responsive to a safe and commonly used antiinflammatory medication (ICS) for asthma, new therapeutic approaches may be needed for "obese asthma." Such approaches may include novel and safe treatments for airway or systemic inflammation and simultaneous and aggressive management of obesity.

Weight Loss and Asthma Control

A systematic review of 15 studies concluded that medically or surgically induced weight reduction may improve asthma-related outcomes.[65] However, only five of the studies reviewed had asthma as their primary outcome. A newly published meta-analysis by the Cochrane collaboration looked at four studies of weight loss for chronic asthma and found some evidence of improvement in asthma symptom scores, lung function, quality of life, and severe exacerbations.[66] Of note, however, the studies included had several inconsistencies, and the authors presented not a pooled analysis but rather a description of significant findings in each cohort. Yet another systematic review found some evidence of benefit for weight loss in subjects with asthma but did not perform a pooled analysis because of the marked differences in the studies reviewed.[67]

Most studies included in these meta-analyses used combinations of diet and exercise, with only a handful looking at surgical interventions. Studies in adults show that bariatric surgery is associated with improved disease control, quality of life, and airway hyperresponsiveness in obese subjects with asthma,[68] and a recent study found that similar reductions in asthma symptom scores and medications and improvement in airway responsiveness and lung volumes correlated with the reduction in BMI after bariatric surgery.[69] Data on pharmaceutical weight-loss interventions for asthma are even scarcer, with only one clinical trial reported. Among 33 obese asthmatic adults, an intervention combining a low-calorie diet and weight-loss medications (orlistat and sibutramine) produced improvements in lung function, asthma symptoms, and use of asthma medication compared with controls.[70] Of note, there have been no studies of weight loss and asthma in children or adolescents.

UNMET, FUTURE RESEARCH NEEDS

1. *Phenotype definition:* Evidence suggests that "asthma" is a syndrome encompassing a variety of phenotypes that likely have different causal mechanisms (e.g., atopic vs. nonatopic asthma, eosinophilic vs. neutrophilic asthma, occupational vs. nonoccupational asthma). Similarly, obesity may be divided into subphenotypes, which may necessitate appropriate characterization using novel biomarkers or measures of adiposity different from BMI (e.g., total body fat). Defining "obese asthma" may thus be the most important next step toward improving the understanding of the link between obesity and asthma. Future studies should include objective measures of lung function and asthma severity because

obesity-related deconditioning or dyspnea may mimic asthma symptoms and thus lead to diagnostic bias.

2. *Clinical trials* are needed to further demonstrate and characterize the relation between overweight or obesity and asthma. Such trials should not only examine the effectiveness and impact of weight loss on asthma morbidity but also assess biomarkers of response to treatment because only a subset of obese subjects may experience improvement of asthma symptoms or morbidity after weight loss.

3. *Genetic studies:* Large genome-wide association studies of obesity and asthma, coupled with studies of gene expression and epigenetic regulation, should help identify any shared genetic or epigenetic control of obesity and asthma.

4. *Multidisciplinary interventions* for obesity and asthma may be most effective but need to be properly assessed in controlled studies. For example, little is known about whether and how treatment of comorbid conditions such as OSA or vitamin D insufficiency, coupled with integral and aggressive weight loss interventions, affects subjects with "obese asthma." Similarly, studies of the impact of treating insulin resistance or the metabolic syndrome in subjects with obesity and asthma are needed.

CONCLUSION

The current epidemiologic and experimental evidence for a causal association between obesity and asthma is reviewed in this chapter. Putative mechanisms underlying the association between obesity and asthma, including genetics, changes in lung mechanics and airway smooth muscle physiology, hormonal differences, and detrimental effects of comorbidities and the systemic proinflammatory state of obesity are also discussed. These proposed causal pathways are largely speculative or insufficiently studied.

Whereas obesity seems to be closely interrelated with the pathogenesis of asthma in some subjects who have the true "obese asthmatic phenotype," obesity may simply coexist with asthma in others. Proper identification of subjects with true "obese asthma" may be key to dissecting any causal mechanism. Weight loss is beneficial and should be recommended for obese adults with asthma.

REFERENCES

1. Akinbami LJ, Moorman JE, Bailey C, et al. Trends in asthma prevalence, health care use, and mortality in the United States, 2001-2010. *NCHS Data Brief*. 2012;94:1–8.
2. CDC. Asthma's impact on the nation 2012 [updated 05/03/201211/01/2012]. Available from: http://www.cdc.gov/asthma/impacts_nation/default.htm.
3. CDC. Current asthma population estimates: national health interview survey, 2010 [updated 1/30/2012Sept 20, 2012]. Current asthma population estimates—in thousands—by age, United States: National Health Interview Survey, 2010. Available from: http://www.cdc.gov/asthma/nhis/2010/table3-1.htm.
4. Moorman JE, Rudd RA, Johnson CA, et al. National surveillance for asthma—United States, 1980–2004. *Morb Mortal Wkly Rep Surveill Summ*. 2007;56(8):18–54.
5. Ogden CL, Carroll MD, Curtin LR, McDowell MA, Tabak CJ, Flegal KM. Prevalence of overweight and obesity in the United States, 1999-2004. *JAMA*. 2006;295(13):1549–1555.
6. Ramsey F, Ussery-Hall A, Garcia D, et al. Prevalence of selected risk behaviors and chronic diseases—Behavioral Risk Factor Surveillance System (BRFSS), 39 Steps Communities, United States, 2005. *MMWR Surveill Summ*. 2008;57(11):1–20.
7. Celedon JC, Palmer LJ, Litonjua AA, et al. Body mass index and asthma in adults in families of asthmatic subjects in Anqing, China. *Am J Respir Crit Care Med*. 2001;164:1835–1840.
8. Ford ES. The epidemiology of obesity and asthma. *J Allergy Clin Immunol*. 2005;115(5):897–909; quiz 10.
9. Taveras EM, Rifas-Shiman S, Camargo CA Jr, et al. Higher adiposity in infancy associated with recurrent wheeze in a prospective cohort of children. *J All Clin Immun*. 2008;121(5):1161–1166.
10. Flaherman V, Rutherford GW. A meta-analysis of the effect of high weight on asthma. *Arch Dis Child*. 2006;91(4):334–339.
11. Guh DP, Zhang W, Bansback N, Amarsi Z, Birmingham CL, Anis AH. The incidence of co-morbidities related to obesity and overweight: a systematic review and meta-analysis. *BMC Public Health*. 2009;9:88.

12. Visness CM, London SJ, Daniels JL, et al. Association of childhood obesity with atopic and nonatopic asthma: results from the National Health and Nutrition Examination Survey 1999-2006. *J Asthma*. 2010;47(7):822–829.
13. van Gent R, van der Ent CK, Rovers MM, Kimpen JL, van Essen-Zandvliet LE, de Meer G. Excessive body weight is associated with additional loss of quality of life in children with asthma. *J Allergy Clin Immunol*. 2007;119(3):591–596.
14. Guerra S, Wright AL, Morgan WJ, Sherrill DL, Holberg CJ, Martinez FD. Persistence of asthma symptoms during adolescence: role of obesity and age at the onset of puberty. *Am J Respir Crit Care Med*. 2004;170(1):78–85.
15. Mannino DM, Mott J, Ferdinands JM, et al. Boys with high body masses have an increased risk of developing asthma: findings from the National Longitudinal Survey of Youth (NLSY). *Int J Obesity*. 2006;30(1):6–13.
16. Todd DC, Armstrong S, D'Silva L, Allen CJ, Hargreave FE, Parameswaran K. Effect of obesity on airway inflammation: a cross-sectional analysis of body mass index and sputum cell counts. *Clin Exp Allergy*. 2007;37(7):1049–1054.
17. Telenga ED, Tideman SW, Kerstjens HA, et al. Obesity in asthma: more neutrophilic inflammation as a possible explanation for a reduced treatment response. *Allergy*. 2012;67(8):1060–1068.
18. Tantisira KG, Litonjua AA, Weiss ST, Fuhlbrigge AL, for the Childhood Asthma Management Program Research Group. Association of body mass with pulmonary function in the Childhood Asthma Management Program (CAMP). *Thorax*. 2003;58(12):1036–1041.
19. Sin DD, Sutherland ER. Obesity and the lung: 4. Obesity and asthma. *Thorax*. 2008;63(11):1018–1023.
20. Collins LC, Hoberty PD, Walker JF, Fletcher EC, Peiris AN. The effect of body fat distribution on pulmonary function tests. *Chest*. 1995;107(5):1298–1302.
21. Al Dabal L, Bahammam AS. Obesity hypoventilation syndrome. *Ann Thorac Med*. 2009;4(2):41–49.
22. Beuther DA, Weiss ST, Sutherland ER. Obesity and asthma. *Am J Respir Crit Care Med*. 2006;174(2):112–119.
23. Boulet LP, Turcotte H, Boulet G, Simard B, Robichaud P. Deep inspiration avoidance and airway response to methacholine: influence of body mass index. *Can Respir J*. 2005;12(7):371–376.
24. Jacobson BC, Somers SC, Fuchs CS, Kelly CP, Camargo CA Jr. Body-mass index and symptoms of gastroesophageal reflux in women. *N Engl J Med*. 2006;354(22):2340–2348.
25. Hancox RJ, Poulton R, Taylor DR, et al. Associations between respiratory symptoms, lung function and gastro-oesophageal reflux symptoms in a population-based birth cohort. *Respir Res*. 2006;7:142.
26. Shirai T, Mikamo M, Shishido Y, et al. Impaired cough-related quality of life in patients with controlled asthma with gastroesophageal reflux disease. *Ann Allergy Asthma Immunol*. 2012;108(5):379–380.
27. Rothenberg S, Cowles R. The effects of laparoscopic Nissen fundoplication on patients with severe gastroesophageal reflux disease and steroid-dependent asthma. *J Pediatr Surg*. 2012;47(6):1101–1104.
28. Holbrook JT, Wise RA, Gold BD, et al. Lansoprazole for children with poorly controlled asthma: a randomized controlled trial. *JAMA*. 2012;307(4):373–381.
29. Teodorescu M, Polomis DA, Hall SV, et al. Association of obstructive sleep apnea risk with asthma control in adults. *Chest*. 2010;138(3):543–550.
30. Verhulst SL, Aerts L, Jacobs S, et al. Sleep-disordered breathing, obesity, and airway inflammation in children and adolescents. *Chest*. 2008;134(6):1169–1175.
31. Kheirandish-Gozal L, Dayyat EA, Eid NS, Morton RL, Gozal D. Obstructive sleep apnea in poorly controlled asthmatic children: effect of adenotonsillectomy. *Pediatr Pulmonol*. 2011;46(9):913–918.
32. Troisi RJ, Speizer FE, Willett WC, Trichopoulos D, Rosner B. Menopause, postmenopausal estrogen preparations, and the risk of adult-onset asthma: a prospective cohort study. *Am J Respir Crit Care Med*. 1995;152(4 Pt 1):1183–1188.
33. Hamano N, Terada N, Maesako K, Numata T, Konno A. Effect of sex hormones on eosinophilic inflammation in nasal mucosa. *Allergy Asthma Proc*. 1998;19(5):263–269.
34. Tam A, Morrish D, Wadsworth S, Dorscheid D, Man SF, Sin DD. The role of female hormones on lung function in chronic lung diseases. *BMC Womens Health*. 2011;11:24.
35. Alessi MC, Bastelica D, Morange P, et al. Plasminogen activator inhibitor 1, transforming growth factor-beta1, and BMI are closely associated in human adipose tissue during morbid obesity. *Diabetes*. 2000;49(8):1374–1380.
36. Shore SA, Terry RD, Flynt L, Xu A, Hug C. Adiponectin attenuates allergen-induced airway

37. Kattan M, Kumar R, Bloomberg GR, et al. Asthma control, adiposity, and adipokines among inner-city adolescents. *J Allergy Clin Immunol*. 2010;125(3):584–592.
38. Ochiai H, Shirasawa T, Nishimura R, et al. High-molecular-weight adiponectin and anthropometric variables among elementary schoolchildren: a population-based cross-sectional study in Japan. *BMC Pediatr*. 2012;12(1):139.
39. Belgardt BF, Bruning JC. CNS leptin and insulin action in the control of energy homeostasis. *Ann N Y Acad Sci*. 2010;1212:97–113.
40. Johnston RA, Zhu M, Rivera-Sanchez YM, et al. Allergic airway responses in obese mice. *Am J Respir Crit Care Med*. 2007;176(7):650–658.
41. Sutherland TJ, Sears MR, McLachlan CR, Poulton R, Hancox RJ. Leptin, adiponectin, and asthma: findings from a population-based cohort study. *Ann Allergy Asthma Immunol*. 2009;103(2):101–107.
42. Sutherland TJ, Cowan JO, Young S, et al. The association between obesity and asthma: interactions between systemic and airway inflammation. *Am J Respir Crit Care Med*. 2008;178(5):469–475.
43. Komakula S, Khatri S, Mermis J, et al. Body mass index is associated with reduced exhaled nitric oxide and higher exhaled 8-isoprostanes in asthmatics. *Respir Res*. 2007;8:32.
44. van Veen IH, Ten Brinke A, Sterk PJ, Rabe KF, Bel EH. Airway inflammation in obese and non-obese patients with difficult-to-treat asthma. *Allergy*. 2008;63(5):570–574.
45. Hancox RJ, Milne BJ, Poulton R, et al. Sex differences in the relation between body mass index and asthma and atopy in a birth cohort. *Am J Respir Crit Care Med*. 2005;171(5):440–445.
46. Ouyang F, Kumar R, Pongracic J, et al. Adiposity, serum lipid levels, and allergic sensitization in Chinese men and women. *J Allergy Clin Immunol*. 2009;123(4):940–948 e10.
47. Dekkers BG, Schaafsma D, Tran T, Zaagsma J, Meurs H. Insulin-induced laminin expression promotes a hypercontractile airway smooth muscle phenotype. *Am J Respir Cell Mol Biol*. 2009;41(4):494–504.
48. Warnken M, Reitzenstein U, Sommer A, et al. Characterization of proliferative effects of insulin, insulin analogues and insulin-like growth factor-1 (IGF-1) in human lung fibroblasts. *Naunyn-Schmiedeberg Arch Pharmacol*. 2010 Dec;382(5-6):511–524.
49. Agrawal A, Mabalirajan U, Ahmad T, Ghosh B. Emerging interface between metabolic syndrome and asthma. *Am J Respir Cell Mol Biol*. 2011;44(3):270–275.
50. Thuesen BH, Husemoen LL, Hersoug LG, Pisinger C, Linneberg A. Insulin resistance as a predictor of incident asthma-like symptoms in adults. *Clin Exp Allergy*. 2009;39(5):700–707.
51. Wells SM, Buford MC, Migliaccio CT, Holian A. Elevated asymmetric dimethylarginine alters lung function and induces collagen deposition in mice. *Am J Respir Cell Mol Biol*. 2009;40(2):179–188.
52. Breton CV, Byun HM, Wang X, Salam MT, Siegmund K, Gilliland FD. DNA methylation in the ARG-NOS pathway is associated with exhaled nitric oxide in asthmatic children. *Am J Respir Crit Care Med*. 2011;184(2):191–197.
53. Paul G, Brehm JM, Alcorn JF, Holguin F, Aujla SJ, Celedon JC. Vitamin D and asthma. *Am J Respir Crit Care Med*. 2012;185(2):124–132.
54. Brehm JM, Celedon JC, Soto-Quiros ME, et al. Serum vitamin D levels and markers of severity of childhood asthma in Costa Rica. *Am J Respir Crit Care Med*. 2009;179(9):765–771.
55. Brehm JM, Acosta-Perez E, Klei L, et al. Vitamin D insufficiency and severe asthma exacerbations in Puerto Rican children. *Am J Respir Crit Care Med*. 2012;186(2):140–146.
56. Alemzadeh R, Kichler J, Babar G, Calhoun M. Hypovitaminosis D in obese children and adolescents: relationship with adiposity, insulin sensitivity, ethnicity, and season. *Metabolism*. 2008;57(2):183–191.
57. Forno E, Lescher R, Strunk R, Weiss S, Fuhlbrigge A, Celedon JC. Decreased response to inhaled steroids in overweight and obese asthmatic children. *J Allergy Clin Immunol*. 2011;127(3):741–749.
58. Xystrakis E, Kusumakar S, Boswell S, et al. Reversing the defective induction of IL-10-secreting regulatory T cells in glucocorticoid-resistant asthma patients. *J Clin Invest*. 2006;116(1):146–155.
59. Szczepankiewicz A, Breborowicz A, Sobkowiak P, Popiel A. Are genes associated with energy metabolism important in asthma and BMI? *J Asthma*. 2009;46(1):53.
60. Murphy A, Tantisira KG, Soto-Quiros ME, et al. PRKCA: a positional candidate gene for body mass index and asthma. *Am J Human Genet*. 2009;85(1):87–96.
61. Tremblay K, Lemire M, Provost V, et al. Association study between the CX3CR1 gene and asthma. *Genes Immun*. 2006;7(8):632–639.
62. Sirois-Gagnon D, Chamberland A, Perron S, Brisson D, Gaudet D, Laprise C. Association of common polymorphisms in the fractalkine

receptor (CX3CR1) with obesity. *Obesity.* 2011;19(1):222–227.
63. Peters-Golden M, Swern A, Bird SS, Hustad CM, Grant E, Edelman JM. Influence of body mass index on the response to asthma controller agents. *Eur Respir J.* 2006;27(3):495–503.
64. Sutherland ER, Camargo CA Jr, Busse WW, et al. Comparative effect of body mass index on response to asthma controller therapy. *Allergy Asthma Proc.* 2010;31(1):20–25.
65. Eneli IU, Skybo T, Camargo CA Jr. Weight loss and asthma: a systematic review. *Thorax.* 2008;63(8):671–676.
66. Adeniyi FB, Young T. Weight loss interventions for chronic asthma. *Cochrane Database Syst Rev.* 2012;7:CD009339.
67. Juel CT, Ali Z, Nilas L, Ulrik CS. Asthma and obesity: does weight loss improve asthma control? A systematic review. *J Asthma Allergy.* 2012;5:21–26.
68. Dixon AE, Pratley RE, Forgione PM, et al. Effects of obesity and bariatric surgery on airway hyperresponsiveness, asthma control, and inflammation. *J Allergy Clin Immunol.* 2011;128(3):508–515 e1–2.
69. Boulet LP, Turcotte H, Martin J, Poirier P. Effect of bariatric surgery on airway response and lung function in obese subjects with asthma. *Respir Med.* 2012;106(5):651–660.
70. Dias-Junior SA, Stelmach R, Pinto RC, Reis M, Halpern A, Cukier A. Effects of weight reduction in obese people with severe asthma: a randomised controlled study [Abstract]. *Am J Respir Crit Care Med.* 2011;183:A4314.

25

ENDOCRINE DISORDERS

COMORBID AND COEXISTING

Kyriaki Sideri and Adnan Custovic

KEY POINTS

- Asthma follows characteristic age and gender patterns, with male predominance during childhood; after puberty, the association is reversed, and females have a higher risk for asthma.
- Women are more likely to suffer from asthma symptoms in adulthood and may experience more severe asthma with higher rates of acute exacerbations, hospitalizations, and death.
- The menstrual cycle is recognized as a factor influencing the course and severity of asthma.
- Exogenous hormones in women may affect asthma, and hormonal changes may play a role in the pathogenesis of adult-onset asthma; however, the exact effect of the oral contraceptive pill and/or hormone replacement therapy in asthmatic women needs to be confirmed.
- Hyperthyroidism may increase the risk for asthma exacerbations.
- There is a potential role of testosterone replacement treatment or selective androgen receptor modulator therapy in men with asthma.
- Vitamin D may influence the course and severity of asthma owing to its role in immune system development and regulation; however, the exact strategy on how to use vitamin D in asthma management is unclear.

INTRODUCTION

Asthma affects 300 million people worldwide, and the World Health Organization estimates that this figure will reach 600 million by 2025.[1] Between 2006 and 2008, 7.8% of the U.S. population suffered from asthma; the prevalence was higher among children (9.3%)

than adults (7.3%) and among females (8.6%) than males (6.9%).[2]

The prevalence of asthma follows a characteristic age and gender pattern and reaches its highest rate during childhood with male predominance. After puberty, the gender association is reversed, and females have a higher risk for asthma.[3] In addition to gender, the menstrual cycle is recognized as a factor influencing the course and severity of asthma. However, there is a relative paucity of epidemiologic data for several other comorbidities that may have an adverse effect on asthma severity and an impact on its natural history, such as endocrine conditions related to thyroid function, Addison's disease, testosterone, and vitamin D deficiency. This relative lack of evidence is not unexpected, given the relatively small number of studies about these conditions and their possible association with asthma.

Nonetheless, several epidemiologic studies suggest an association of asthma with hormonal and metabolic disorders such as hypothyroidism and hyperthyroidism, Addison's disease, and testosterone and vitamin D deficiency. Several hypotheses have been proposed to explain these observed associations; however, the precise pathophysiologic mechanisms underpinning these findings are not yet clarified.

GENDER

Female and male asthmatic patients share the common clinical features of the disease, but the natural course of asthma differs between genders with respect to the age of onset, prevalence, morbidity, and severity. A number of studies provide conclusive evidence that the trajectory of asthma differs markedly between males and females. There is a clear male predominance in prevalence in childhood,[4] with approximately two-thirds of the asthmatic children being boys.[5] The gender ratio reverses in adolescence, and in adulthood asthma is more common among women than men.[6] It is hypothesized that this shift during adolescence may be attributed to hormonal changes that induce a diminished clinical and immunologic responsiveness.[5] This age-related shift in male and female predominance may result from possible hormonal influences on different airway characteristics, including their size, difference in degree of inflammation, and smooth muscle and vascular functions.[5] The change from male to female predominance is thought to occur very late in or beyond the pubertal phase.[7] A possible explanation is that females may experience a recurrence of childhood disease in school age but this is not recognized until years later. Alternatively, the prevalence and incidence may increase in adult women. Asthma in girls also may be underreported and underdiagnosed. The Tucson Children's Respiratory Study[8] observed that boys were significantly more likely than girls to experience both wheeze and frequent wheeze most years during the first decade of life, but girls with symptoms were less likely to see a physician and be characterized with this diagnosis. In addition, the impact of some other risk factors (e.g., obesity) may differ between genders. For example, in an unselected birth cohort study in the United Kingdom (Manchester Asthma and Allergy Study), asthma and atopy were more common in boys than girls, but the effect of body mass index (BMI) was confined to the female gender, suggesting that an increased BMI enhanced the risk for asthma in girls but not boys.[4]

Another important difference between male and female asthmatic patients is the role of allergic sensitization. This is a strong risk factor for both childhood and adult asthma,[9] and allergen exposure in allergic asthmatic patients in synergy with viral respiratory tract infections increases the risk for exacerbations and hospital admissions.[10] Leynaert and colleagues[11] reported that female sex was an independent risk factor for nonallergic asthma in an adult population-based cohort of the European Community Respiratory Health Survey (ECRHS). The results suggest that asthma is 20% more frequent in women older than 35 years and that new-onset asthma in more than 60% of women, but only 30% of men, is nonallergic. The incidence of nonallergic asthma remains higher in women throughout their reproductive life.[11] In contrast, the same study did not observe gender differences in the incidence of allergic asthma.

Data from the European Network for Understanding Mechanisms of Severe Asthma (ENFUMOSA)[12] demonstrate that the proportion of females in the severe asthma group in all participating regions of Europe is 2.8 times higher than that of males. Furthermore, atopy is inversely related to asthma severity, suggesting that atopy is less important as a predictor of adult severe asthma. The severe asthma phenotype is characterized by the presence of increased neutrophils in the circulation and in the sputum and by a diminished or suboptimal sensitivity to glucocorticosteroids. It is also of note that an unsupervised cluster analysis of asthmatic patients from Leicester, United Kingdom, suggests that there is a distinct class of late-onset, obese, noneosinophilic asthma associated predominantly with the female gender.[13]

Furthermore, there are gender disparities in relation to asthma hospitalizations and death rates. According to the U.S. Centers for Disease Control and Prevention,[14] between 1980 and 2009, females versus males consistently had a higher rate of hospitalizations because of asthma exacerbation. Hospital admissions for asthma among females increased by 4.9% per year between 1980 and 1983. In contrast, there was an average increase from 1980 to 1986 of 1% per year among males. Over the following years, the admission rates decreased by 0.9% for women and 1.6% for men, and in 2009, the hospitalization rate for females was 40% higher than for males. Moreover, in 2009, the ratio of female to male asthma deaths was 1.4, even though during the decade between 1999 and 2009, the death rate declined by approximately 5% for both genders.

Self-reported triggers for asthma exacerbations also appear to be gender specific.[12] The ENFUMOSA data reported independent associations for asthma severity among females with sinusitis, premenstrual period, aspirin intake, exercise, and the work environment. The triggers identified for men include exercise, stress, and aspirin intake.[12] Differences between genders are reported for treatment adherence. Women appear to have higher adherence than men, both for regular treatment and for rescue treatment during asthma exacerbations.[15] Females versus males have a more positive attitude toward treatment and use of inhaled corticosteroids. However, asthmatic women report more anxiety and insomnia than men.[15] A summary of the findings related to the influence of gender on asthma is presented in Table 25.1.

MENSTRUAL CYCLE

A number of studies investigated the potential role of female hormonal factors in asthma. The results are often contradictory, and the exact mechanism of interaction between the menstrual cycle and asthma is unclear. Gibbs and colleagues[16] reported that 40% of asthmatic women experience deterioration of asthma symptoms up to 5 days premenstrually, with a modest decrease in peak flow. Different

Table 25.1. Summary of Gender Influence on Asthma[3-15]

Age of onset	Male predominance in childhood; female predominance in adulthood
Risk factors	Atopic sensitization more prevalent in boys
	Obesity more often observed in girls
Specific phenotypes	Female gender association with severe asthma; late-onset, noneosinophilic asthma; nonallergic asthma
Hospitalization rate	Increased in female gender
Mortality	Increased in women
Treatment adherence	Higher adherence during exacerbations among females
Quality of life	Anxiety and insomnia more frequent in women

results were obtained by Zimmerman and colleagues,[17] who found that women during the preovulatory phase of the menstrual cycle have more frequent emergency department visits for acute exacerbations. A similar study by Brenner and colleagues[18] suggests that both the preovulatory and perimenstrual phases may induce asthma exacerbations. Although these studies provide evidence for possible asthma variation during the menstrual cycle, there is a lack of consistency about the specific time period involved.

Hormonal changes may contribute to airway pathology in women, but the exact mechanism is unclear. Estrogens are the main hormones during the follicular phase of the menstrual cycle and reach their peak with ovulation. Progesterone is secreted during the second half of the menstrual cycle by the *corpus luteum*. Both estrogens and progesterone levels are low during the perimenstrual phase of the menstrual cycle. Any hormonal imbalance may lead to irregular menstruation. The study by Swanes and colleagues[19] examined the association of asthma and allergy with irregular menstruation in more than 6,000 women of reproductive age from seven northern European centers. The prevalence of asthma and allergy was higher in women between 25 and 42 years of age with an irregular compared with regular menstrual period. One potential explanation for this finding is reverse causation; that is, asthma medication may be responsible for the hormonal imbalance, rather than irregular menstruations "causing" asthma. However, after excluding asthmatic women on regular treatment, the observed association between asthma and allergy and irregular menstruations remained significant.[19] In addition, the authors formulated an interesting hypothesis to explain these findings and suggest that a common metabolic disease, the polycystic ovary syndrome (PCOS), may be a possible reason for irregular menstruation. PCOS is associated with insulin resistance, and the latter is not only a part of the metabolic syndrome but also linked to diminished lung function.[20] The authors propose that insulin resistance might be the link between asthma and irregular menstruation[19] and also explain the previously reported association of asthma and obesity, that is, with a high BMI.[21] Another study proposes that insulin resistance is significantly associated with an increased incidence of wheezing and asthma-like symptoms in adults and is a stronger predictor than is obesity for this association.[22]

Real and colleagues[23] investigated the association of oligomenorrhea with lung function and asthma, and the influence of BMI and physical activity on this association. Oligomenorrhea is a common symptom of PCOS and is accompanied by hormonal changes and lower fertility. Irregular menstruation is associated with more asthma symptoms and with lower forced vital capacity (FVC). Furthermore, asthma symptoms increase significantly with increasing BMI, independently of menstrual irregularity, and are common in women with irregular menstruation who exercise regularly. The study concluded that oligomenorrhea, BMI, and physical activity are all independently related to asthma.

There is some evidence that exogenous hormones in women may affect asthma and that specific hormonal changes may play a role in the pathogenesis of adult-onset asthma. Jenkins and colleagues[24] reported that the risk for adult-onset asthma in women increased with parity and decreased with the use of oral contraceptive pill (OCP) (the risk decreased by an average of 7% per year of OCP use). In contrast, the U.S. Nurse Health Study showed an elevated risk for asthma in women with past use of OCP.[25] Salam and colleagues[26] observed that among women without asthma, OCP use is associated with higher risk for wheezing, but in women with a history of asthma, OCP use is associated with a markedly reduced risk for wheezing. A cross-sectional analysis in a Nordic-Baltic population investigated the association between the use of OCP and asthma and whether BMI modulates the relationship between OCP and asthma.[27] The study demonstrated that OCP use was associated with an increased risk for asthma, asthma with hay fever, and hay fever/asthma symptoms, but only among women with normal or increased BMI, and not in those with a BMI of less than 20 kg/m^2.

Table 25.2. Female Gender and Asthma Symptoms: Major Findings Related to Hormonal Changes and Exogenous Hormonal Treatment[3-6,16-32]

Infancy, childhood	Lower prevalence of asthma in females
Puberty	No significant effect of gender
Adolescence	Higher prevalence of asthma in females
Menstrual cycle–related exacerbations	No definitive correlation with a specific phase
	All phases (premenstrual, menstrual, preovulatory) related to increased asthma symptoms
Menopause	Associated with lower lung function
Oral contraceptive pill	Contradictory results
Use of hormone replacement therapy	Contradictory results

Similar inconsistencies were reported in studies of the association of hormone replacement therapy (HRT) and asthma. The Nurse Health Study showed an increase in risk for subsequent asthma among women using long-term and/or high doses of HRT.[25] Barr and colleagues[28] found HRT use to be associated with an increased rate of new physician diagnosis of asthma, but not chronic obstructive pulmonary disease. In contrast, when HRT use was studied in association with lung function, the results suggest an improvement of forced expiratory volume in 1 second (FEV_1) and lower prevalence of airway obstruction with HRT use.[29]

The summary of findings related to the hormonal changes and exogenous hormonal treatment among females with asthma are illustrated in Table 25.2.

There is some evidence to suggest that female respiratory health is related to the time frames of the beginning and the end of reproductive life. An analysis of the ECRHS II[30] reports that women reporting early menarche, at age 10 years or earlier, compared with women with menarche at age 13 years, had lower FEV_1 and FVC in adult life. Asthma was also more common among women with early menarche. This may be explained by common metabolic and hormonal factors influencing both early menarche and lung health, or alternatively by the early menarche triggering changes in airway function.[31] Insulin resistance may be a common metabolic factor related to both early menarche and asthma. Real and colleagues[32] reported in a cross-sectional analysis of the ECRHS II that menopause may be associated with lower lung function and more respiratory symptoms, especially among lean women. The authors suggest that lower lung function in menopausal women can be explained by increased insulin resistance in menopause.

HYPOTHYROIDISM, HYPERTHYROIDISM, AND ASTHMA

Asthma and thyroid disorders occasionally coexist. Both hypothyroidism and hyperthyroidism have been associated with asthma. The clinical features of hyperthyroidism range from mild symptoms to a potentially life-threatening thyrotoxicosis. The most common manifestations of the disease are associated with symptoms of sympathetic hyperactivity. Hyperthyroidism presents with palpitations, tremor, heat intolerance, anxiety, weakness, diaphoresis, and weight loss, with a normal or increased appetite. Hypercalcemia and osteoporosis, premature atrial contractions, atrial fibrillation, and shortness of breath can also occur. The physical examination may reveal important diagnostic findings such as tachycardia, exophthalmos, pretibial myxedema, thyroid enlargement, or single nodular lesions, which can be associated with more specific thyroid disorders such as Graves' disease, thyroiditis, toxic adenoma, and toxic multinodular goiter. The initial laboratory test to help diagnose thyroid disease is serum thyroid-stimulating hormone (TSH). Low levels confirm the diagnosis of primary hyperthyroidism. Further available tests include measuring thyroid hormones, such as serum free thyroxine (T_4) and free triiodothyronine (T_3).

Hypothyroidism presents with highly variable clinical symptoms and depends on the age of onset, duration, and severity. These symptoms may include fatigue, bradycardia, cold intolerance, weight gain, constipation, dry skin, myalgias, and menstrual irregularities. The diagnosis of primary hypothyroidism is based on serum TSH, which is typically high. Low levels of serum free T_4 confirm the diagnosis and help determine the therapeutic approach.

The first report of the association between asthma and thyroid disorders dates to 1929.[33] Since then, several other studies have alluded to this possible association. Thyroid goiter can be responsible for asthma-like symptoms by causing functional tracheal compression. A prospective study enrolled 153 euthyroid patients with nodular or diffuse thyroid enlargement to determine the relationship between upper airway obstruction and thyroid enlargement.[34] The authors suggest that the prevalence of upper airways obstruction is not significantly related to the type of goiter and that surgical intervention to correct tracheal compression, and consequent upper respiratory obstruction, results in the improvement of the flow–volume loop and clinical symptoms. Of note, even a unilateral, moderately enlarged thyroid gland, entrapped in the thoracic inlet, may produce severe tracheal compression and occasionally asthma-like symptoms.[35]

Hyperthyroidism is associated with asthma exacerbations.[36] Treatment of hyperthyroidism with propylthiouracil (PTU) dramatically improved asthma symptoms in a small study of five patients with severe asthma. When PTU was discontinued, patients experienced asthma exacerbations.[36] Fedrick and Baldwin,[37] over a 4-month period, found that among 890 patients with hyperthyroidism, 1 was admitted with an asthma exacerbation, whereas in 316 hypothyroid patients, two were hospitalized for asthma. The authors suggest that treatment of hypothyroidism may increase the likelihood of developing asthma symptoms. Another study of 10 thyrotoxic nonasthmatic patients did not reveal a significant change in bronchial hyperreactivity before and after treatment of their thyrotoxicosis. This suggests that changes in thyroid hormones do not induce bronchial hyperreactivity in patients without asthma.[38] In contrast, a study of 11 nonasthmatic patients with a total thyroidectomy, evaluated when mildly hyperthyroid and when hypothyroid, proposed that acute hypothyroidism increases nonspecific bronchial reactivity.[39] Asthma, as the underlying cause of death in a retrospective cohort mortality study of more than 3,500 women treated for thyrotoxicosis at the Mayo Clinic over a 20-year period, was reported for 7 women, and in 5 of these, the onset of thyrotoxicosis exacerbated symptoms of preexisting asthma.[40]

ADDISON'S DISEASE AND ASTHMA

Primary adrenal insufficiency or Addison's disease is a rare disorder with a population prevalence from 39 to 144 cases per million.[41] It is most commonly an autoimmune disease (70% to 90%), whereas other causes include infectious diseases such as tuberculosis (7% to 20%), metastatic cancer or lymphoma infiltrative disease, adrenal hemorrhage or infarction, and medications. Autoimmune-induced Addison's disease involves both humoral and cell-mediated immune mechanisms that destroy the adrenal cortex. Antibodies against several enzymes, in particular 21-hydroxylase, are found in all the three zones of the adrenal cortex, and occasionally against other endocrine organs, forming a polyglandular autoimmune syndrome. The most common clinical features of Addison's disease are constitutional symptoms such as chronic fatigue, weakness, and anorexia leading to considerable weight loss. Characteristic objective findings of the disease are hypotension and generalized hyperpigmentation prominent in areas exposed to light or to chronic friction and pressure. Furthermore, gastrointestinal symptoms are common and correlate with the severity of adrenal insufficiency. Other common symptoms include salt cravings, diffuse myalgias and arthralgias, and psychiatric symptoms, which range from mild organic brain syndrome to psychosis. The initial evaluation includes the measurement of serum cortisol, adrenocorticotropin hormone (ACTH), and electrolytes. In the presence of low levels of cortisol, common electrolytic disturbances such as hyponatremia and hyperkalemia occur. The diagnosis is made by demonstrating low cortisol levels using the ACTH stimulation test. Abdominal computed tomography is useful to investigate the cause. Efforts to identify whether adrenal insufficiency may influence the natural course of asthma began as early as 1922 and reached a peak in the early 1970s with the publication of several case reports.[42-44] Green and Lim reported two cases of asthma with substantial eosinophilia and adrenal insufficiency, one of which had a fatal outcome, and highlighted the importance of investigating the possibility of Addison's disease in patients with asthma and evidence of significant weight loss. Although not drawing conclusions about a causal relationship between adrenal insufficiency and asthma, the authors suggest that adrenal cortex function may have a protective role against asthma. Another case report describes a patient who died in status asthmaticus; necropsy revealed profuse eosinophilic infiltration of lung parenchyma, chronic adrenalitis consistent with autoimmune Addison's disease, and Hashimoto's thyroiditis.[43] In addition, it was suggested that patients with adrenal insufficiency are more susceptible to shock during severe asthma exacerbations.[44] Harris and Collins[45] reported two asthmatic patients with adrenal insufficiency who recovered completely from respiratory symptoms following administration of cortisone in adequate doses. Hence, because glucocorticoids are the treatment of choice for both asthma and Addison's disease, it was implied that adrenal insufficiency could be the underlying disease in some asthmatic patients. However, because the number of patients with asthma and coexisting Addison's disease is limited, this hypothesis remains unproved. In clinical practice, it is important to include Addison's disease in the differential diagnosis in asthmatic patients with significant weight loss, hypotension, and hyperpigmentation.

LOW TESTOSTERONE AND ASTHMA

Testosterone is produced by the adult testis and is a key hormone responsible for androgen function. Apart from the development and maintenance of secondary sexual characteristics, testosterone contributes to men's health in terms of mental function and cognition, muscle mass, bone density, and metabolism. Low levels of testosterone are commonly associated with hypogonadism and aging. A number of studies have investigated immunoregulatory functions of testosterone,[46] leading to the hypothesis that low testosterone may contribute to the pathogenesis of asthma.[47] One study suggests that testosterone causes a reduction in the proinflammatory cytokines tumor necrosis factor and interleukin-1 (IL-1) and increases in the antiinflammatory cytokine IL-10.[46] The same cytokines regulate the immune responses that have a key role in the pathogenesis of asthma. A cross-sectional study of 2,197 men investigated the relationship between sex hormones and pulmonary function and found that diminished pulmonary function is associated with lower levels of total and free testosterone.[48] Hence, it was hypothesized that testosterone replacement treatment or even selective androgen receptor modulators could be used to manage asthma.[47]

VITAMIN D DEFICIENCY AND ASTHMA

Vitamin D has an important role in the regulation of calcium homeostasis and bone metabolism. There are two main sources of vitamin D: skin synthesis as a result of sunlight (mainly ultraviolet B) and intestinal absorption. Vitamin D is metabolized to 25-hydroxyvitamin D (25OHD) in the liver, with further hydroxylation to 1,25-dihydroxyvitamin D (1,25OHD) through the enzymatic action of 1α-hydroxylase in the kidneys. 1,25HOD is the active form of vitamin D. Vitamin D deficiency can be assessed by measuring serum levels of 25OHD. During the past several years, an increasing number of studies have focused on the association of vitamin D deficiency and asthma. Hansdottir and colleagues[49] identified the enzyme 1α-hydroxylase in primary lung epithelial cells, denoting that lung parenchyma is able to synthetize the active form 1,25OHD. This study also investigated the role of the active form of 1,25OHD and vitamin D in lung and suggests that vitamin D upregulates genes in the innate immune system in response to viral infections.[49] Brehm and colleagues[50] studied the association of 25OHD and asthma exacerbations. Serum levels of 25OHD were measured in 1,024 children with mild to moderate persistent asthma who were followed over a 4-year period. Low vitamin D levels were associated with increased risk for asthma exacerbation and emergency department visits. Furthermore, children with low vitamin D levels had a lower FEV_1.

This emerging information has been used to identify potential novel therapeutic approaches to asthma. For example, the level of group-specific component (Gc) protein, involved in the metabolism of vitamin D, was found to be increased by more than five-fold compared with healthy controls in bronchoalveolar lavage, and treatment with an anti-Gc antibody reduced airway inflammation.[51] However, it remains unclear whether vitamin D replacement treatment decreases the risk for asthma exacerbations and, if so, what is the optimal vitamin D level to achieve beneficial effects.

TREATMENT

The current therapeutic approach to the treatment of asthma in association with comorbid endocrine conditions is based on the principle that each disorder is a separate entity and should be treated as such. For practicing physicians, it would be of interest to identify whether appropriate treatment of the coexisting endocrine disorder may have an effect on asthma control and whether asthma treatment affects the course of the endocrine disorder.

As the phases of the menstrual cycle affect asthma, although little is known about the exact time of asthma deterioration, it is important that physicians inquire about perimenstrual asthma and advise women to monitor their symptoms,[52] reporting possible exacerbations. Given the fact that early menarche is associated with the onset of asthma, it may be of interest to include more information about the commencement of menses in the clinical history. Menstrual irregularity and menopause may be associated with respiratory symptoms and asthma, suggesting that asthma symptoms might need closer monitoring in women with such problems.

In addition, just as hormonal and metabolic parameters may affect asthma, the literature provides some evidence about the role of PCOS and insulin resistance,[19-22] lifestyle modifications, and maintenance of BMI within normal limits. Because obese individuals (in particular females) appear more likely to experience wheezing and late-onset asthma symptoms, diet modifications aimed at maintaining normal BMI should always be considered.

Women are more likely to suffer from asthma symptoms in adulthood and may experience more severe asthma with higher rates of acute exacerbations, hospitalizations, and death. However, it is important to emphasize that the evidence specific to gender is applicable to the whole population and cannot be directly translated to individual patients with asthma.

Patients who become thyrotoxic should be closely monitored for asthma exacerbations. Physicians should consider the diagnosis of hyperthyroidism whenever asthmatic patients complain of palpitation, tachycardia, heat intolerance, diaphoresis, and other symptoms related to excessive amounts of thyroid hormones because this could potentially affect asthma control.[36] The deterioration of asthma symptoms during thyrotoxicosis might require treatment with β-agonists. Of note, PTU, widely used to treat thyrotoxicosis, could also potentially induce asthma. Although the combination of asthma and thyrotoxicosis, as described in the literature, is potentially lethal, during the past decade or so, little progress has been made in investigating this association.

There is little published evidence to inform the therapeutic approach to patients with

Addison's disease and asthma. Both asthma and Addison's disease are treated with corticosteroids, and it is reasonable to assume that glucocorticoid treatment for one disorder will improve the other. Although the comorbidity of asthma and Addison's disease is uncommon, physicians should address concerns for asthmatic patients with hyponatremia, hypotension, and weight loss, in whom Addison's disease should be suspected and appropriately investigated. It is important to remember that long-term use of high doses of glucocorticoids may induce adrenal insufficiency as a result of decreased or inadequate cortisol production from exposure of the hypothalamic-pituitary-adrenal axis to exogenous glucocorticoids.

UNMET, FUTURE RESEARCH NEEDS

1. Evaluate the role of exogenous hormones in the course of asthma.
2. Investigate the potential benefit of the OCP and/or HRT in asthmatic women.
3. Identify the most appropriate combination of estrogens and progesterone with potential beneficial effect in the management of perimenstrual asthma.
4. Examine whether treatment of PCOS could be a possible therapeutic target for both endocrine and respiratory disorders.
5. Elucidate the mechanism of asthma deterioration due to excess thyroid hormone.
6. Discover the potential threshold of thyroid hormones associated with asthma exacerbations.
7. Clarify the association of low levels of testosterone with asthma.
8. Explore the possible role of testosterone replacement treatment or selective androgen receptor modulator therapy in asthma.
9. Identify the potential benefits of vitamin D supplementation and appropriate level of vitamin D for asthma treatment.

CONCLUSION

Although the relationship of asthma and endocrine comorbid disorders is insufficiently understood, the body of evidence available provides useful information for the clinician considering these problems in evaluating a patient with asthma (Table 25.3).

Table 25.3. Potentially Useful Guidance for Clinical Practice

- Maintain normal body mass index in asthmatic children (especially in girls)
- Carefully assess girls with symptoms suggestive of asthma to minimize the risk for underdiagnosed asthma
- Obtain thorough clinical history of respiratory symptoms in women related to menstrual cycle phases, irregular menstruations, menopause, oral contraceptives, and hormone replacement therapy use
- Control asthma symptoms in hyperthyroid patients and make treatment adjustments
- Be aware of higher risk for status asthmaticus reported in patients with asthma and Addison's disease
- Investigate possible vitamin D deficiency in children with frequent asthma exacerbations

REFERENCES

1. Pawankar R, Canonica GW, Holgate ST, Lockey RF, eds. *WAO White Book on Allergy.* Milwaukee, WI: World Allergy Organization; 2011:34.
2. Frieden TR. Forward: CDC Health Disparities and Inequalities Report—United States, 2011. *MMWR CDC Surveill Summ.* 2011;60(Suppl):1–2.
3. de Marco R, Locatelli F, Sunyer J, Burney P. Differences in incidence of reported asthma related to age in men and women: a retrospective analysis of the data of the European Respiratory Health Survey. *Am J Respir Crit Care Med.* 2000;162(1):68–74.
4. Murray CS, Canoy D, Buchan I, Woodcock A, Simpson A, Custovic A. Body mass index in young children and allergic disease: gender differences in a longitudinal study. *Clin Exp Allergy.* 2011;41(1):78–85.
5. Almqvist C, Worm M, Leynaert B. Impact of gender on asthma in childhood and adolescence: a GA2LEN review. *Allergy.* 2008;63(1):47–57.

6. de Marco R, Locatelli F, Cazzoletti L, Bugianio M, Carosso A, Marinoni A. Incidence of asthma and mortality in a cohort of young adults: a 7-year prospective study. *Respir Res.* 2005;6:95.
7. Nicolai T, Illi S, Tenborg J, Kiess W, v Mutius E. Puberty and prognosis of asthma and bronchial hyper-reactivity. *Pediatr Allergy Immunol.* 2001;12(3):142–148.
8. Wright AL, Stern DA, Kauffmann F, Martinez FD. Factors influencing gender differences in the diagnosis and treatment of asthma in childhood: the Tucson Children's Respiratory Study. *Pediatr Pulmonol.* 2006;41(4):318–325.
9. Simpson BM, Custovic A, Simpson A, et al. NAC Manchester Asthma and Allergy Study (NACMAAS): risk factors for asthma and allergic disorders in adults. *Clin Exp Allergy.* 2001;31(3):391–399.
10. Murray CS, Poletti G, Kebadze T, et al. Study of modifiable risk factors for asthma exacerbations: virus infection and allergen exposure increase the risk of asthma hospital admissions in children. *Thorax.* 2006;61(5):376–382.
11. Leynaert B, Sunyer J, Garcia-Esteban R, et al. Gender differences in prevalence, diagnosis and incidence of allergic and non-allergic asthma: a population-based cohort. *Thorax.* 2012;67(7):625–631.
12. The ENFUMOSA cross-sectional European multicentre study of the clinical phenotype of chronic severe asthma. European Network for Understanding Mechanisms of Severe Asthma. *Eur Respir J.* 2003;22(3):470–477.
13. Haldar P, Pavord ID, Shaw DE, et al. Cluster analysis and clinical asthma phenotypes. *Am J Respir Crit Care Med.* 2008;178(3):218–224.
14. Moorman JE, Akinbami LJ, Bailey CM, et al. National Surveillance of Asthma: United States, 2001–2010. National Center for Health Statistics. *Vital Health Stat.* 2012;3(35).
15. Sundberg R, Toren K, Franklin KA, et al. Asthma in men and women: treatment adherence, anxiety, and quality of sleep. *Respir Med.* 2010;104(3):337–344.
16. Gibbs CJ, Coutts II, Lock R, Finnegan OC, White RJ. Premenstrual exacerbation of asthma. *Thorax.* 1984;39(11):833–836.
17. Zimmerman JL, Woodruff PG, Clark S, Camargo CA. Relation between phase of menstrual cycle and emergency department visits for acute asthma. *Am J Respir Crit Care Med.* 2000;162(2 Pt 1):512–515.
18. Brenner BE, Holmes TM, Mazal B, Camargo CA Jr. Relation between phase of the menstrual cycle and asthma presentations in the emergency department. *Thorax.* 2005;60(10):806–809.
19. Svanes C, Real FG, Gislason T, et al. Association of asthma and hay fever with irregular menstruation. *Thorax.* 2005;60(6):445–450.
20. Engström G, Hedblad B, Nilsson P, Wollmer P, Berglund G, Janzon L. Lung function, insulin resistance and incidence of cardiovascular disease: a longitudinal cohort study. *J Intern Med.* 2003;253:574–581.
21. Shore SA, Johnston RA. Obesity and asthma. *Pharmacol Ther.* 2006;110(1):83–102.
22. Thuesen BH, Husemoen LL, Hersoug LG, Pisinger C, Linneberg A. Insulin resistance as a predictor of incident asthma-like symptoms in adults. *Clin Exp Allergy.* 2009;39(5):700–707.
23. Real FG, Svanes C, Omenaas ER, et al. Menstrual irregularity and asthma and lung function. *J Allergy Clin Immunol.* 2007;120(3):557–564.
24. Jenkins MA, Dharmage SC, Flander LB, et al. Parity and decreased use of oral contraceptives as predictors of asthma in young women. *Clin Exp Allergy.* 2006;36(5):609–613.
25. Troisi RJ, Speizer FE, Willett WC, Trichopoulos D, Rosner B. Menopause, postmenopausal estrogen preparations, and the risk of adult-onset asthma: a prospective cohort study. *Am J Respir Crit Care Med.* 1995;152(4 Pt 1):1183–1188.
26. Salam MT, Wenten M, Gilliland FD. Endogenous and exogenous sex steroid hormones and asthma and wheeze in young women. *J Allergy Clin Immunol.* 2006;117(5):1001–1007.
27. Macsali F, Real FG, Omenaas ER, et al. Oral contraception, body mass index, and asthma: a cross-sectional Nordic-Baltic population survey. *J Allergy Clin Immunol.* 2009;123(2):391–397.
28. Barr RG, Wentowski CC, Grodstein F, et al. Prospective study of postmenopausal hormone use and newly diagnosed asthma and chronic obstructive pulmonary disease. *Arch Intern Med.* 2004;164(4):379–386.
29. Carlson CL, Cushman M, Enright PL, Cauley JA, Newman AB. Hormone replacement therapy is associated with higher FEV1 in elderly women. *Am J Respir Crit Care Med.* 2001;163(2):423–428.
30. Macsali F, Real FG, Plana E, et al. Early age at menarche, lung function, and adult asthma. *Am J Respir Crit Care Med.* 2011;183(1):8–14.
31. Macsali F, Svanes C, Bjorge L, Omenaas ER, Gomez Real F. Respiratory health in women: from menarche to menopause. *Expert Rev Respir Med.* 2012;6(2):187–200; quiz 201–182.
32. Real FG, Svanes C, Omenaas ER, et al. Lung function, respiratory symptoms, and the

menopausal transition. *J Allergy Clin Immunol.* 2008;121(1):72–80 e73.
33. Elliott CA. Occurrence of asthma in patients manifesting evidences of thyroid dysfunction. *Am J Surg.* 1929;7(3):333–337.
34. Gittoes NJ, Miller MR, Daykin J, Sheppard MC, Franklyn JA. Upper airways obstruction in 153 consecutive patients presenting with thyroid enlargement. *BMJ.* 1996;312(7029):484.
35. Vadasz P, Kotsis L. Surgical aspects of 175 mediastinal goiters. *Eur J Cardiothorac Surg.* 1998;14(4):393–397.
36. Settipane GA, Schoenfeld E, Hamolsky MW. Asthma and hyperthyroidism. *J Allergy Clin Immunol.* 1972;49(6):348–355.
37. Fedrick J, Baldwin JA. Thyroid disease and asthma. *BMJ.* 1977;2(6101):1539.
38. Roberts JA, McLellan AR, Alexander WD, Thomson NC. Effect of hyperthyroidism on bronchial reactivity in non-asthmatic patients. *Thorax.* 1989;44(7):603–604.
39. Wieshammer S, Keck FS, Schauffelen AC, von Beauvais H, Seibold H, Hombach V. Effects of hypothyroidism on bronchial reactivity in non-asthmatic subjects. *Thorax.* 1990;45(12): 947–950.
40. Hoffman DA, McConahey WM. Thyrotoxicosis and asthma. *Lancet.* 1982;1(8275):808.
41. Willis AC, Vince FP. The prevalence of Addison's disease in Coventry, UK. *Postgrad Med J.* 1997;73(859):286–288.
42. Green M, Lim KH. Bronchial asthma with Addison's disease. *Lancet.* 1971;1(7710): 1159–1162.
43. Sanerkin NG, El-Shaboury AH. Chronic adrenalitis with bronchial asthma. *Lancet.* 1965;2(7410):468–470.
44. Del Rio A, Noya M, Alvarez-Prechous A, De Oya JC. Addison's disease, status asthmaticus, and shock. *Lancet.* 1971;2(7715):104.
45. Harris PW, Collins JV. Bronchial asthma with Addison's disease. *Lancet.* 1971;1(7713): 1349–1350.
46. Malkin CJ, Pugh PJ, Jones RD, Kapoor D, Channer KS, Jones TH. The effect of testosterone replacement on endogenous inflammatory cytokines and lipid profiles in hypogonadal men. *J Clin Endocrinol Metab.* 2004;89(7):3313–3318.
47. Canguven O, Albayrak S. Do low testosterone levels contribute to the pathogenesis of asthma? *Med Hypotheses.* 2011;76(4):585–588.
48. Svartberg J, Schirmer H, Medbo A, Melbye H, Aasebo U. Reduced pulmonary function is associated with lower levels of endogenous total and free testosterone. The Tromso study. *Eur J Epidemiol.* 2007;22(2):107–112.
49. Hansdottir S, Monick MM, Hinde SL, Lovan N, Look DC, Hunninghake GW. Respiratory epithelial cells convert inactive vitamin D to its active form: potential effects on host defense. *J Immunol.* 2008;181(10):7090–7099.
50. Brehm JM, Schuemann B, Fuhlbrigge AL, et al. Serum vitamin D levels and severe asthma exacerbations in the Childhood Asthma Management Program study. *J Allergy Clin Immunol.* 2010;126(1):52–58.
51. Lee SH, Kim KH, Kim JM, et al. Relationship between group-specific component protein and the development of asthma. *Am J Respir Crit Care Med.* 2011;184(5):528–536.
52. Macsali F, Svanes C, Bjorge L, Omenaas ER, Gomez Real F. Respiratory health in women: from menarche to menopause. *Expert Rev Respir Med.* 2012;6(2):187–200.

26

OSTEOPENIA AND OSTEOPOROSIS

COMORBID AND COEXISTING

Joshua A. Steinberg and Andrea J. Apter

KEY POINTS

- Osteoporosis results in an increased occurrence of low-trauma fragility fractures that result in significant morbidity and mortality.
- Osteoporosis is more common in subjects with obstructive lung disease, including asthma.
- Osteoporosis is caused or aggravated by glucocorticoid therapy, particularly systemic therapy.
- Nutritional strategies and pharmacologic therapies may prevent or treat osteoporosis in asthma and are particularly important in individuals with decreased bone density, history of fractures, or treatment with systemic or high-dose inhaled glucocorticoid.
- Factors in addition to bone density should be considered when assessing risk for fracture. FRAX® or similar tools are clinically useful in this assessment.
- Risk factors for osteoporosis should be considered in all individuals with asthma.

INTRODUCTION

Osteoporosis and osteopenia are highly prevalent, metabolic disorders of bone characterized by loss of bone strength predisposing to fracture. These are silent disorders, typically symptomatic only when there is a painful or disabling fracture. Established criteria define these diseases by the severity of deficiency of bone mineral density (Table 26.1), a proxy for the quality of bone integrity.

Over the past two decades, landmark studies, suggesting that up to one in three women and one in five men older than 50 years will experience a bone fracture, have raised significant public health concerns about osteoporosis risk.[1] The U.S. incidence of fractures from weakened bone exceeds that of stroke, heart attack, and breast cancer combined.[2] This high

Table 26.1. Classification of Bone Density from Densitometry

PATIENT	CLASSIFICATION	BONE MINERAL DENSITY*
Adult	Normal	T-score ≥ −1
	Osteopenia (low bone density)	T-score < −1 and > −2.5
	Osteoporosis	T-score ≤ −2.5
	Severe (established) osteoporosis	T-score ≤ −2.5 in the presence of one or more fragility fractures
Child	Low bone mineral density for chronologic age	Z-score ≤ −2.0
	Pediatric osteoporosis	Z-score ≤ −2.0 in the presence of one or more clinically significant fractures

* The International Society for Clinical Densitometry (ISCD) recommends use of Z-scores for children, premenopausal women, and men <50 years old. T-score is a statistical comparison to an ideal young adult with peak bone mass. Z-score is a statistical comparison to an age- and gender-matched population.
Adapted from World Health Organizaiton and ISCD data.[125-128]

incidence is estimated to be rising and is projected to increase by 100 million worldwide by 2025.[1]

Similarly, asthma is a chronic disorder with extremely high prevalence. It is estimated that asthma affects at least 315 million adults worldwide.[3] Incorporation of oral and inhaled corticosteroids as the primary pharmacologic modality for symptomatic asthma control has resulted in dramatically improved outcomes for persistent asthma.[4] However, glucocorticoids have pleotropic negative effects on bone health and are the most common iatrogenic cause of secondary osteoporosis.[5,6] As a result of glucocorticoid therapy and potentially induced bone loss, risks for osteoporosis and fracture have become inextricably associated with asthma management.

Studies have identified increased comorbidity of osteoporosis among asthmatic patients. A study of Canadian provincial health utilization claims identified increased osteoporosis prevalence among asthmatic patients throughout adulthood, with a maximum absolute rate difference of 10 persons per 1,000 for patients older than 65 years.[7] A review of the U.K. General Practice Research Database identified physician-diagnosed asthmatic adults to have a relative risk for fractures of 1.5 (95% confidence interval, 1.2 to 1.9) compared with matched cohorts.[8] A study of an Italian population identified an odds ratio of osteoporosis in asthmatic patients between 1.4 and 2.0.[9]

Aims of This Chapter

This chapter describes key factors specific to asthmatic patients that directly or indirectly affect bone health. The well-established association of corticosteroid therapy with osteoporosis will be discussed, as will less commonly known and emerging osteoporosis risk factors pertinent to asthmatic patients. Additionally, osteoporosis management and therapy will be reviewed with a discussion of the role of the asthma specialist in preventing, screening for, and treating osteoporosis and osteopenia.

Definition of Fracture and Bone Loss

Fractures occur when forces applied to the bone exceed its strength. The focus of this chapter is on low-trauma fragility fractures, developing from forces that normal bone should ordinarily support. Low-trauma fractures are defined as resulting from a force less than that of a fall at standing height.[6] Osteoporotic fractures typically involve the proximal humerus, distal radius, proximal femur, and vertebral bodies.

Severity of fragility fractures ranges from asymptomatic to exceptionally disabling and life threatening. Approximately half of patients experiencing a hip fracture lose capability for independent living, and one in five die within a year of their fracture.[10] Vertebral fractures have a much higher likelihood of being asymptomatic; nearly 40% of postmenopausal women with asthma or chronic obstructive pulmonary disease (COPD) have asymptomatic vertebral fractures.[11] After an initial vertebral osteoporotic fracture, up to 20% experience another fracture in the following year. With additional fractures, the risk exponentially increases, causing what has been termed a "vertebral fracture cascade."[12]

The World Health Organization (WHO) has established the most widely accepted diagnostic criteria based on bone mineral density or history of a minimal trauma fracture (see Table 26.1). Although this classification represents the predominant means for assessing risk of future fracture, the criteria do not address multiple other factors, such as type, rate, or distribution of bone loss or other predisposing risk factors for fracture such as fall risk, age, comorbid disease, or prior use of bone-weakening medications.

Bone mineral density (BMD) is a robust marker for assessing femoral fracture risk in postmenopausal women and adult men, associated with about a two- to three-fold relative risk increase of fracture with each reduction of the standard deviation compared with the ideal bone density of a matched young adult.[13] However, these criteria have a more limited utility for predicting risk for future fracture in other populations and body regions, specifically pediatric groups and, as will be reviewed, glucocorticoid-treated patients. The WHO definition is dependent on attainment of peak bone mass between ages 18 and 30 years; thus, pediatric and young adult bone health assessment should utilize different clinicopathologic criteria.[14]

PATHOPHYSIOLOGY

Bone is a uniquely functional tissue capable of supporting structural weights, shielding organs from trauma, providing mineral storage and acid buffering, and transmitting lever forces from muscular attachments. This strength is derived from the extracellular matrix of hard, inorganic mineralized deposits, primarily calcium phosphate and organic collagen and other materials responsible for elasticity. There are two types of bone: cortical bone is compact and highly calcified, whereas centrally located cancellous (trabecular) bone is highly porous and lattice-like. Despite a static macroscopic appearance, bone tissue is metabolically dynamic and is in a state of persistent turnover. Cancellous bone, the predominant component of vertebral bodies, is more susceptible to osteoporotic weakening because of a faster rate of remodeling.

Three major bone cell types are involved in modeling the durable extracellular matrix: osteoblasts, osteocytes, and osteoclasts. Osteoblasts and osteocytes are responsible for deposition and maintenance of the extracellular matrix, whereas osteoclasts degrade the extracellular matrix. Osteoclasts are multinucleated cells that degrade the extracellular matrix through proteases and other mechanisms. Long-lived osteocytes, which originate as osteoblasts trapped within the extracellular matrix, play a critical role as mechanosensors of bone microdamage.

RISK FACTORS FOR OSTEOPOROSIS

Factors that compromise matrix development and alter the balance of remodeling constitute many of the clinical risk factors for osteoporosis and fracture. Known risk factors for osteoporosis can be broadly categorized into modifiable and nonmodifiable groups, as well as diseases associated with secondary osteoporosis (Table 26.2). Factors of particular relevance to asthmatic patients are highlighted in the following discussion.

Modifiable Risk Factors

DRUG-INDUCED OSTEOPOROSIS: GLUCOCORTICOIDS

Although the use of glucocorticoids has revolutionized asthma management, these drugs

Table 26.2. Osteoporosis Risk Factors

POTENTIALLY MODIFIABLE	NONMODIFIABLE
Body weight related: - Athletic amenorrhea - Anorexia nervosa - Obesity	**Demographics** - Female sex - Advanced age - White race
Dietary/Lifestyle - Low calcium/vitamin D intake - Lactose intolerance/milk allergy - Excess salt intake - Excess caffeine intake - Excess aluminum intake - Excess vitamin A intake - Heavy alcohol use - Smoking - Sedentary lifestyle - Total parenteral nutrition (TPN)	**Personal/Family history** - History of a non-traumatic fracture in first-degree relative - History of previous fracture as an adult
Medications - Anticonvulsants - Aromatase inhibitors - Gonadotropin-releasing hormone agonists - Chemotherapeutics - Heparins - Glucocorticoids - Phenytoin - Warfarin - Cyclosporine/tacrolimus - Antiretrovirals - Proton pump inhibitors - Depo-medroxyprogesterone - Barbituates - Methotrexate - Thyroxine (excess)	**Genetic disorders** - Osteogenesis imperfecta - Turner's and Klinefelter's syndromes - Hemochromatosis - Marfan syndrome - Cystic fibrosis - Homocystinuria - Gaucher's disease - Porphyria - Ehlers-Danlos syndrome - Hypophosphatasia - Idiopathic hypocalciuria - Glycogen storage diseases
Fall risk factors - Deconditioning - Low vision - Delirium or dementia - Environmental trip hazards	

Table 26.2. (Continued)

POTENTIALLY MODIFIABLE	NONMODIFIABLE
ASSOCIATED MEDICAL CONDITIONS	
Endocrine disorders	**Gastrointestinal disorders**
- Diabetes mellitus	- Celiac disease
- Hypogonadism	- Inflammatory bowel disease
• Pituitary disorders	- Primary biliary cirrhosis
• Orchiectomy or testosterone deficiency	- Pancreatic disease
	- Malabsorption syndromes
• Estrogen deficiency or oophorectomy before age 45 yr	**Rheumatologic disease**
	- Rheumatoid arthritis
- Hyperparathyroidism	• Inflammatory arthropathies
- Hyperthyroidism	
- Addison's disease	
- Cushing syndrome	
Other chronic disorders	**Hematologic disease**
- Renal failure (end-stage renal disease)	- Mastocytosis
- Congestive heart failure	- Multiple myeloma
- Chronic obstructive pulmonary disease	- Pernicious anemia
- Chronic immobility	- Leukemia/lymphoma
	- Thalassemia
	- Sickle cell disease

Adapted and modified from References 121–124, 129, 130.

represent a major risk factor for osteoporosis through pleiotropic effects on osteoblasts, osteocytes, and osteoclasts. Glucocorticoid-induced increased fracture risk and loss of trabecular bone were identified in asthmatic adults in 1983.[15] Since this initial observation, there have been many assessments of risks associated with the use of oral and inhaled glucocorticoids in the management of asthma.

Pathophysiology

Glucocorticoid effects on osteoblasts are critical components of bone loss.[16] Glucocorticoids inhibit replication, differentiation, and maturation of osteoblast precursors.[17] Apoptosis of osteoblasts and osteocytes is promoted through caspase 3 signaling. Production of the primary bone organic extracellular matrix constituent, type I collagen, is also reduced.[17]

There are other noteworthy actions of glucocorticoids upon osteocytes and osteoclasts. Osteoclast apoptosis is inhibited and development is promoted through glucocorticoid-mediated enhanced expression of maturation factors, including interleukin-6, macrophage colony-stimulating factor, RANK-L (receptor activator of nuclear transcription factor kappa B ligand), and downregulation of interferon-β. RANK-L is produced by osteoblasts, stromal cells, and T cells and is pertinent as a therapeutic target of pharmacotherapy. Osteocyte loss is associated with impairment of interstitial fluid flow through bone, an independent risk factor for impaired bone mineral deposition. Production of osteoprotegerin, a decoy receptor of RANK-L, is also suppressed by glucocorticoids.[17]

There are other, indirect pathophysiologic mechanisms of glucocorticoid-induced fracture risk. Glucocorticoids impair calcium absorption from the gut and resorption from the renal tubules. Gonadotropin suppression, with resultant estrogen and testosterone reduction, may also promote bone loss.[17] Steroid-induced myopathy that weakens the pelvic musculature may indirectly increase the risk for fall-induced fracture.[16]

Kinetics. Rates of bone loss due to glucocorticoids appear to occur in two phases: an early, rapid loss due to excess resorption; and a slower, more progressive phase due to impaired production.[18] Fracture risk appears to develop rapidly upon initiation of glucocorticoid therapy, with increased fracture relative risks noted even at prednisone doses of less than 10 mg/day and increased vertebral fractures with sporadic use.[19] The risk for fracture increases up to 75% within the first 3 months of therapy, usually *before* BMD decreases are evident.[20]

Dose-Response Effect. The contribution of cumulative versus daily glucocorticoid dose to risk for fracture has been studied. The relative risk (RR) for nonvertebral fracture increased from 1.45 to 1.70 from the lowest (<0.5 g glucocorticoid) to highest (>10 g glucocorticoid) tercile of cumulative dose, whereas the risk for vertebral and nonvertebral fracture doubled when the daily dose increased from less than 2.5 mg to greater than or equal to 7.5 mg/day of prednisolone.[21] A large retrospective U.K. study found that intermittent use of glucocorticoids of at least 15 mg/day with cumulative exposure of no more than 1 g had slight increases in nonfemoral fracture risk; however, the risk increased substantially (RR of 14.42 for vertebral and 3.13 for femoral fracture) with a daily dose of at least 30 mg/day and cumulative exposure of more than 5 g of oral glucocorticoids.[22] Dose response likely is important in children, but less is known. These data suggest that daily glucocorticoid dose contributes more to fracture risk than cumulative dose. Alternate-day dosing with oral glucocorticoids has been considered yet does not appear to substantially attenuate the severity of bone loss.[23-25]

Most asthmatic patients use oral glucocorticoids intermittently for asthma flares; the risks of intermittent use are less well understood than with chronic utilization. A large prospective pediatric study identified a negative dose-dependent trend of oral glucocorticoid bursts, but not inhaled glucocorticoids, on the risk for osteopenia.[26] Patients who received more than four previous glucocorticoid prescriptions were found to have a significantly increased risk (RR, 1.51) of osteoporotic fracture.[22] A study comprising primarily asthmatic children receiving four or more short courses of oral glucocorticoids had increased risk for fractures (odds ratio [OR], 1.32), particularly humeral fractures (OR, 2.17).[27] Several studies have identified reduced risks on discontinuation of active treatment.[21,22]

Asthmatic patients typically use inhaled glucocorticoids for longer durations than oral glucocorticoids. This raises concern for total cumulative glucocorticoid exposure as well as chronic adrenal axis suppression. Absorption of currently commonly used inhaled glucocorticoids into the systemic circulation occurs primarily through the pulmonary circulation or from the throat rather than the gastrointestinal tract, owing to extensive first-pass metabolism effects with most commonly used agents.[28] Specific factors that influence systemic effects include drug-specific lipophilicity and fraction of serum protein binding, as well as the proportional metered dose delivered to the lungs.

Data have been inconsistent regarding effects of lowered BMD with inhaled glucocorticoids. However, some data suggest that high doses of inhaled glucocorticoids may promote osteoporosis in adults.[29,30] A prospective cohort study in premenopausal asthmatic women identified a significant inverse association of hip and trochanteric bone density and the dose of inhaled glucocorticoids, after exclusion of patients exposed to parenteral and oral glucocorticoids.[31] Although the per-inhalation effect was negligible, the computed compounded bone loss would more than double the risk for hip fracture by age 65 years. A Cochrane meta-analysis in 2008 found no evidence for bone loss with 2 to 3 years of inhaled glucocorticoid use in asthmatic and COPD patients; however, data for longer periods of therapy were insufficient.[32]

Among pediatric populations, most studies have not identified risks of inhaled glucocorticoids on bone health, yet studies well controlled for oral glucocorticoid use and long-term use are rare.[26] Most studies show a neutral effect; however, in one study BMD of the femoral neck and lumbar spine increased in a fluticasone-treated group of children aged 6 to 14 years, perhaps confounded by increased oral glucocorticoid use in the control population.[33]

DRUG-INDUCED OSTEOPOROSIS: OTHER DRUGS

Drugs other than glucocorticoids can also promote osteoporosis (see Table 26.2).[34] Two drug classes are especially relevant for asthma patients: proton pump inhibitors (PPIs) and antiretrovirals. Despite articles disputing a therapeutic benefit for asthmatic symptoms with PPI use in pediatric and adult patients without reflux symptoms,[35,36] asthmatic patients continue to be prescribed PPIs at high rates.[37] PPIs are also preferentially prescribed to glucocorticoid users.[38] PPIs are implicated in bone loss in initial prospective studies and in multiple retrospective studies.[38-40] Proposed mechanisms include inhibition of osteoclasts vacuolar adenosine phosphatase and impaired intestinal calcium absorption. HIV patients may have a higher prevalence of asthma than the general population, as well as a roughly three-fold higher risk for osteopenia or osteoporosis.[41,42] Multiple highly active antiretroviral therapy regimens accelerate bone mineral loss independently of HIV, and protease inhibitors can increase the systemic effects of glucocorticoids due to suppression of metabolism.[43]

DIETARY-INDUCED OSTEOPOROSIS

Milk-Avoidant Populations. Milk is rich in calcium and in some regions is fortified with vitamin D, which promotes absorption of calcium from the gastrointestinal tract. However, there are multiple asthmatic populations that may intentionally avoid ingestion of milk, for reasons that can include genuine or perceived lactose intolerance.[44] Additionally, milk allergy is the most common food allergy in young children.[45] Milk-avoidant children exhibit lower BMD, reduced peak bone mass, increased risk for prepubertal fracture, and possibly increased postmenopausal BMD reduction.[46-49]

Hypovitaminosis D–Induced Osteoporosis. Insufficiency of vitamin D is highly prevalent worldwide. Insufficiency may be associated with asthmatic morbidity, due to pleotropic effects on inflammation within the respiratory tract.[50-54] Although ideal serum vitamin D levels for asthmatic patients are controversial, a vitamin D 25-OH level less than 20 ng/mL (50 nmol/mL) is associated with adverse skeletal effects.[54] One study identified 61% of patients presenting with fragility fracture to have previously undiagnosed vitamin D deficiency.[55] Low levels of the active 1,25-dihydroxyvitamin D leads to increased bone catabolism through decreased dietary calcium and phosphorous absorption and inhibition of osteoblast maturation.

Deficiency risk factors include lack of enriched foods, low solar exposure or elevated latitude, and age. Despite the association with higher latitude, hypovitaminosis D has been identified in one-third to one-half of persons in equatorial regions.[56] Hypovitaminosis D was observed to halve bone mineral accretion in asthmatic boys treated with oral glucocorticoids.[57]

CHRONIC INFLAMMATION–INDUCED OSTEOPOROSIS

Other chronic inflammatory diseases are risk factors for osteoporosis,[58] yet there are no data linking the immunopathology of asthma directly to bone loss. Data regarding systemic inflammatory changes in asthmatic patients, unlike in COPD patients, are sparse.[59] Pulmonary disease was found to be a risk factor for lower BMD independent of glucocorticoid use in a mixed male asthma and COPD population.[60] A "spillover" of local pulmonary inflammatory processes resulting in osteoporosis has been postulated in COPD.[61,62]

OBESITY AND SEDENTARY LIFESTYLE

Despite the strong association between low body weight and osteoporosis, obesity is not an apparent protective factor against osteoporotic fracture.[63] An increased frequency of ankle and upper leg fractures, as well as issues with increased risk for falls and impaired ambulation, are also probable fracture risk factors in obese patients. Research regarding the relationship between obesity and asthma suggest obesity is a risk factor for severe asthma.[64]

A sedentary lifestyle is a risk factor for osteoporosis as well; weight-bearing and impact forces induce bone strengthening mechanosensory signals. Observational studies suggest physical activity strongly reduces risk for hip fracture, by 45% in men and 38% in women; however, the relationship between type of activity and risk reduction is unclear.[65,66] Asthmatic patients may have less aerobic fitness than nonasthmatic peers, apparently related more to lifestyle than obstructive impairment.[67]

SMOKING-INDUCED OSTEOPOROSIS

Tobacco use is associated with accelerated bone loss and may be a risk factor for fracture independent of bone mineral density.[68,69] There is an association between smoking and lower BMD in both men and women, and it is a risk factor for subsequent fracture.[70] A large meta-analysis shows that active smoking increases the risk ratio for an osteoporotic fracture by 1.29 (95% confidence interval [CI] 1.13 to 1.28) and hip fracture by 1.60 (95% CI 1.27 to 2.02). One in four asthmatic people smoke,[71] and smoking has an established association with adverse asthma outcomes as well as postulated interference with response to glucocorticoid therapy.[72]

Nonmodifiable Risk Factors

Although much attention is paid to altering osteoporosis risks, the *majority* of risk is derived from nonmodifiable risk factors (see Table 26.2), particularly genetics, sex, ethnicity, and age.

SEX AND AGE

The loss of sex hormones with menopause is a substantial contributor to the increased incidence of osteoporosis in women; however, there are other variances in skeletal morphology, such as bone diameter and muscle mass, that lower the risk for fracture in males. Osteoporosis incidence is also closely associated with age. Half of women between 60 and 69 years and 87% of women older than 80 years have osteoporosis.[73] Pan-menopausal BMD assessments demonstrate that maximal bone loss rate occurs in late perimenopause through early menopause, with peak loss rates of 1.8% to 2.3% per year of the lumbar spine and 1.0% to 1.4% per year at the hip.[74]

GENETICS

Family history is a major risk factor for osteoporosis. Genetic factors account for a large variance in peak bone mass and possibly age-related bone loss. Through multiple twin studies, it has been estimated that one-fourth to more than one-half of the risk for reduced BMD may be inherited, with 50% to 85% of the variance of peak BMD associated with genetic factors.[75] Although linkage and candidate gene studies have failed to identify target factors, large genome-wide association studies have succeeded in identifying replicated loci associated with risk for fracture.[76]

RACE AND ETHNICITY

Racial and ethnic variances in BMD occur; however, differences in fracture risk have not paralleled these differences. Additionally, body weight or size accounts for some of the observed differences between racial or ethnic groups.[77] White women have higher hip fracture rates and lower BMD compared with other populations; however, in a large study of postmenopausal women, roughly 1 in 5 women of each ethnic group studied had osteoporotic-range BMD.[77]

DIAGNOSIS AND MANAGEMENT

More than 50 organizations have published formal recommendations for osteoporosis screening and management.[78] The variance in worldwide guidelines, and frequently between different organizations within each nation, reflect regionally specific prevalence of disease and availability of resources; yet this variance confounds the ideal diagnosis and management strategy. This review will focus on common features of these guidelines.

Absolute Fracture Risk Calculator

An adult's (aged 40 to 90 years) absolute 10-year probability of hip fracture or any major (spine, hip, forearm, or humerus) osteoporotic fracture can be computed using an algorithm abbreviated FRAX®. This WHO-sponsored risk calculator, which is rapidly being incorporated into national guidelines, is downloadable, available online, or accessible through country-specific, paper-based forms (http://www.shef.ac.uk/FRAX/).

Although FRAX does not supplant bone densitometry testing, there is an association of a high FRAX score with densitometric osteoporosis.[79] The majority (80%) of patients with a 10-year major osteoporotic fracture risk greater than 20% or a hip fracture risk greater than 3% had one or more T-scores in the osteoporotic range, and nearly none with fracture had normal T-scores at all measured sites. BMD measurement is important for risk assessment, but the FRAX calculator incorporates other risk factors. These other risk factors are potentially important for individuals with asthma and include the presence or absence of smoking and more than 3 months of glucocorticoid use but notably exclude some factors, such as risk of falls. Adjustment of the calculator to account for dose of glucocorticoid has been proposed.[80]

CLINICAL EXAMINATION FEATURES

There is no specific, single physical examination finding sufficient to diagnose osteoporosis without further testing.[81] However, specific physical exam findings are associated with increased risk for occult vertebral fractures (Figure 26.1). Examination tests for thoracic and lumbar fracture include the wall–occiput test (positive likelihood ratio [PLR], 4.6) and the rib–pelvis distance test (PLR, 3.8). Additionally, tooth count less than 20 (PLR, 3.4) and weight less than 51 kg (PLR, 7.3) have high predictive value. Other features on exam suggestive for osteoporotic fractures of the spine include a frail habitus, gradual height loss, goiter, and dorsal kyphosis.[81]

Densitometry Screening

Given its low cost, radiation dose, and rapid speed of assessment, dual-energy x-ray absorptiometry (DXA) is the most widely used method for determination of densitometry in adults as well as children. It is a two-dimensional assessment of bone density and has been associated with the risk for fracture in adults. Algorithms calculate the deviation of the density from that of a normal young adult to generate a T-score, used in the WHO criteria. Z-scores, in contrast, are defined as the standard deviation of BMD compared with others of the same sex and similar age. These are used in pediatric and other populations that do not have appropriate reference standards for peak bone density.[82] Other technologies, including quantitative computed tomography and quantitative ultrasound, provide distinct advantages for volumetric assessment and portability, respectively; however, they are not in routine clinical use. There is considerable debate about the ideal bone screening method and body site selection to best predict risk.

Nonpharmacologic Prevention and Treatment

A variety of lifestyle changes may improve bone density or reduce fracture risk, or both.

EXERCISE

Efficacy of exercise interventions, such as aerobic, weight-bearing, and resistance

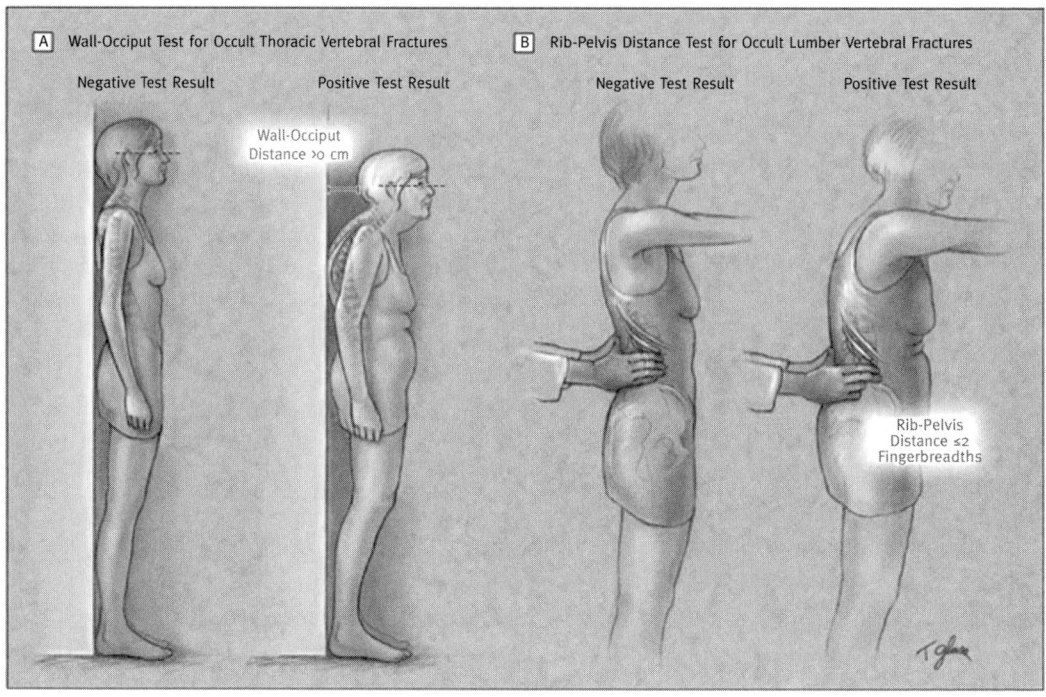

FIGURE 26.1 Clinical examination features suggestive of occult vertebral fracture. **A,** The *wall–occiput test* is used to detect occult thoracic vertebral fractures. A positive test result is defined as being unable to touch the wall with the occiput when standing with the back and heels against the wall and the head positioned such that an imaginary line from the lateral corner of the eye to the superior junction of the auricle is parallel to the floor. **B,** The *rib–pelvis distance test* is used to detect occult lumbar vertebral fractures. A positive test is defined as a distance of less than or equal to 2 fingerbreadths between the inferior margin of the ribs and the superior surface of the pelvis in the midaxillary line. © (2004) American Medical Association. All rights reserved.[125]

exercises, to increase BMD are supported in a Cochrane meta-analysis study of postmenopausal women. Walking was effective for increasing hip BMD.[83] Another meta-analysis, assessing the benefit of targeted supervised exercise, identified a benefit in children (1% to 8%) but not adults at stress-loaded sites.[84] Although exercise has been recommended for all asthmatic patients, details about the ideal activity, duration, and intensity are lacking.[67]

SMOKING CESSATION

There has been little study of the reversibility of smoking's effects on bone health. Cross-sectional studies have identified approximation of risk of quitters to never-smokers 30 years after cessation; however, BMD improvements have been identified in postmenopausal women 1 year after cessation. The effect of nicotine replacement on bone health is unknown.[69]

Nutritional and Pharmacologic Prevention and Treatment

Existing pharmacologic therapies for osteoporosis either prevent resorption or facilitate bone production. Although there is evidence of efficacy, with most studies identifying positive outcomes within 6 to 12 months after initiation, identification of those at risk for fracture and in need of preventive therapy is insufficient.[85] In 2010, only one-fifth of U.S. women 67 years and older had either BMD assessment or bone strengthening prescription in the 6 months following a fracture.[86] A review of 16 trials assessing management of osteoporosis identified investigation of fracture in less than 32% of patients. Calcium and vitamin D were only prescribed to 8% to 62% and bisphosphonates to 0.5% to 38% of patients with an osteoporotic fracture.[87] In a study of one U.S. health system network, only 41.6% of osteoporotic patients and 9.4% of females after fracture were prescribed bisphosphonates within 3 months of diagnosis.[88]

There are no guidelines for prevention of osteoporosis and fracture specific for asthmatic patients. However, recommendations for patients at risk for osteoporosis specifically from oral glucocorticoids are emerging. Seminal recommendations from the American College of Rheumatology (ACR) were revised in 2010, and similar guidelines have been developed in Holland, Japan, and Brazil.[89-92] The ACR guidelines are subsequently reviewed in detail (Table 26.3).

Calcium intake of 1,200 to 1,500 mg/day and vitamin D supplementation are advised for all patients on oral glucocorticoid therapy. The guidelines divide chronically glucocorticoid-exposed patients into two groups to determine ideal prophylactic therapy.

The first group includes men age older than 50 years and postmenopausal women, who are subdivided into low, medium, or high risk for fracture using FRAX or alternative criteria. Bisphosphonate treatment is recommended for low- and medium-risk patients if the daily dose of glucocorticoids is greater than or equal to 7.5 mg/day (prednisone equivalent). High-risk patients with any glucocorticoid exposure should receive bisphosphonates and be considered for teriparetide if the dose of glucocorticoids is more than 5 mg/day or the duration of any dose is longer than 1 month.

The second group includes premenopausal women and men younger than 50 years with known osteoporotic fracture exposed to chronic glucocorticoids. A bisphosphonate is recommended if taking at least 5 mg glucocorticoids (prednisone equivalent) a day for 1 to 3 months, and a bisphosphonate or teriparatide is a consideration for any dose of glucocorticoids anticipated for more than 3 months. Women of childbearing potential taking glucocorticoids for more than 3 months are advised to start a bisphosphonate or teriparatide if the glucocorticoid dose is at least 7.5 mg/day. Within this group, ACR guidelines did not have sufficient data to provide consensus recommendations for a glucocorticoid duration of 1 to 3 months or of more than 3 months with a dose of less than 7.5 mg/day.

There were insufficient data to make recommendations for premenopausal women and men younger than 50 years without known fracture. Modifiable nutritional factors and bone density measurements are a consideration in asthma, particularly with high-dose inhaled or intermittent oral glucocorticoid therapy.

CALCIUM AND VITAMIN D

With regard to glucocorticoid-induced osteoporosis, there is evidence from a Cochrane meta-analysis that calcium and vitamin D are more effective in slowing lumbar and forearm bone loss than calcium alone or placebo treatment[93]; however, the evidence supporting fracture prevention was not statistically significant. Specifically, in a moderate-severe asthmatic population taking at least 800 µg/day of inhaled budesonide, calcitriol (1,25-dihydroxyvitamin D) supplementation did not improve BMD.[94] Thus, calcium and vitamin D, although critical nutrients for bone health, are likely insufficient to control glucocorticoid-induced bone loss.

Worldwide dietary vitamin D intake varies considerably as a result of differences in mandated fortification of foods and the basal intake of naturally enriched foods such as fish.[95] Without mandatory food fortification, nutritional intake is typically below recommended allowances.[95] Supplementation contributes 6% to 47% of intake in some countries; however, excess supplementation can be associated with risk for harm if vitamin D intake is greater than 4,000 IU/day.[54] The 2010 joint U.S. and Canadian Institute of Medicine guidelines recommend a goal for calcium and vitamin D intake for North Americans, with variance of recommendations

Table 26.3. Summary of Major Recommendations for Glucocorticoid-Induced Osteoporosis by the American College of Rheumatology

Baseline counseling and assessment starting any dose of oral glucocorticoids, duration ≥3 months:

Weight-bearing activities

Smoking cessation

Avoidance of excessive alcohol intake (>2 drinks per day)

Nutritional counseling on calcium and vitamin D intake

Fall risk assessment

Baseline dual x-ray absorptiometry

Serum 25-hydroxyvitamin D level

Baseline height

Assessment of prevalent fragility fractures

Consider radiographic imaging of the spine or vertebral fracture assessment for those initiating or currently receiving prednisone ≥5 mg/day or its equivalent

Monitoring while on glucocorticoids ≥3 months:

Consider serial bone mineral density testing

Consider annual serum 25-hydroxyvitamin D measurement

Annual height measurement

Assessment of incident fragility fracture

Assessment of osteoporosis medication compliance

PROPHYLACTIC SUPPLEMENTATION/MEDICATION

POPULATION	RISK CATEGORIZATION	RECOMMENDED THERAPY (BASED ON GCS DOSE)
All patients on OGC		Calcium intake (supplement plus oral intake) 1,200–1,500 mg/day
Postmenopausal women or men ≥50 yr, on OGC therapy ≥3 mo	Low risk	≥7.5mg/day: alendronate or risedronate or zoledronic acid
	Medium risk	Any dose: alendronate or risedronate ≥7.5mg/day: zoledronic acid
	High risk	Any dose: alendronate or risedronate or teriparatide or zoledronic acid
Premenopausal women or men <50 yr *with* history of fracture	Duration 1–3 mo Non–childbearing potential	≥5 mg/day: alendronate or risedronate ≥7.5 mg/day: zoledronic acid

(continued)

Table 26.3. (Continued)

PROPHYLACTIC SUPPLEMENTATION/MEDICATION

POPULATION	RISK CATEGORIZATION	RECOMMENDED THERAPY (BASED ON GCS DOSE)
	Childbearing potential Duration 1–3 mo or any duration with <7.5 mg/day	No recommendations
	Non–childbearing potential Duration ≥ 3 mo	Any dose: alendronate or risedronate or zoledronic acid or teriparatide
	Childbearing potential Duration ≥ 3 mo	≥7.5 mg/day: alendronate or risedronate or teriparatide

GCS, glucocorticosteroid; OGC, oral glucocorticoid therapy.
Adapted from ACR 2010 GIOP Recommendation Clinicians Guide. http://www.rheumatology.org/practice/clinical/guidelines/ACR_2010_GIOP_Recomm_Clinicians_Guide.pdf

and upper level intakes based on age, sex, and pregnancy or lactation (Table 26.4).[54]

BISPHOSPHONATES

Bisphosphonates are the most commonly used agents for osteoporosis prevention and treatment and are the present standard of care.[96] These pyrophosphate analogs bind to bone hydroxyapatite at sites of bone remodeling and interfere with prenylation by farnesyl pyrophosphate synthase, leading to osteoclast apoptosis and inhibition of resorption.[97] There are several commercially available oral and intravenous bisphosphonates with differing side chains, which impart varied half-lives and antiresorptive potencies. Antifracture efficacy has been established with bisphosphonates for vertebral, femoral, and other nonvertebral fractures.[98] The ideal duration of therapy is debated. There is concern about residual retention of the drug in bone and the possibility of serious complications, such as esophageal cancer or ulceration, osteonecrosis of the jaw, and atypical subtrochanteric and pelvic fractures.[97]

Only a few studies of bisphosphonates have been done in asthmatic adults. No differences in BMD or fracture were observed in a large U.K. study of asthmatic men and women aged 50 to 70 years randomized to calcium, etidronate, both, or placebo treatments.[99] There are insufficient data to determine an effect on BMD or fracture risk in children.[99] Interestingly, bisphosphonate efficacy may be antagonized by glucocorticoids.[100]

PARATHYROID HORMONE

In contrast to the effect of chronic exposure, intermittently administered parathyroid hormone (PTH_{1-84}) inhibits osteoblast apoptosis and increases osteoblastogenesis. This mechanism may be pertinent for counteracting the pathophysiology of glucocorticoid-induced osteoporosis.[101,102] Teriparatide, a recombinant parathyroid hormone peptide (PTH_{1-34}), stimulates bone formation and an increase in bone mass, resulting in reduced risk for fracture at vertebral and nonvertebral sites. The drug was significantly superior in BMD augmentation and prevention of fractures compared with alendronate in an 18-month population study of primarily rheumatologic patients with glucocorticoid-induced osteoporosis.[102] Teriparatide has been incorporated into ACR management guidelines; however, it is reserved for severe cases.[96]

CALCITONIN

Intranasal calcitonin increases spinal bone mass in glucocorticoid-dependent asthmatic

Table 26.4. Dietary Reference Intakes for Calcium and Vitamin D

LIFE STAGE GROUP	CALCIUM ESTIMATED AVERAGE REQUIREMENT (MG/DAY)	RECOMMENDED DIETARY ALLOWANCE (MG/DAY)	UPPER LEVEL INTAKE (MG/DAY)	VITAMIN D ESTIMATED AVERAGE REQUIREMENT (IU/DAY)	RECOMMENDED DIETARY ALLOWANCE (IU/DAY)	UPPER LEVEL INTAKE (IU/DAY)
Infants 0–6 mo	•	•	1,000	••	••	1,000
Infants 6–12 mo	•	•	1,500	••	••	1,500
1–3 yr	500	700	2,500	400	600	2,500
4–8 yr	800	1,000	2,500	400	600	3,000
9–13 yr	1,100	1,300	3,000	400	600	4,000
14–18 yr	1,100	1,300	3,000	400	600	4,000
19–30 yr	800	1,000	2,500	400	600	4,000
31–50 yr	800	1,000	2,500	400	600	4,000
51–70-yr-old-females	1,000	1,200	2,000	400	600	4,000
>70 yr	1,000	1,200	2,000	400	800	4,000
14–18 yr, pregnant/lactating	1,100	1,300	3,000	400	600	4,000
19–50 yr, pregnant/lactating	800	1,000	2,500	400	600	4,000

• For infants, adequate intake is 200 mg/day for 0 to 6 months of age and 260 mg/day for 6 to 12 months of age.
•• For infants, adequate intake is 400 IU/day for 0 to 6 months of age and 400 IU/day for 6 to 12 months of age.
Recommended calcium and vitamin D intake. Reprinted with permission from Dietary Reference Intakes for Calcium and Vitamin D, 2011 by the National Academy of Sciences, courtesy of the National Academies Press, Washington, D.C.

patients.[103] A Cochrane meta-analysis found that calcitonin preserves bone mass in the first year of glucocorticoid therapy at the lumbar spine but not at the femoral neck.[104] Resistance may develop with daily use because of antibody binding to this hormone derived from salmon. Calcitonin nasal spray did not acutely or chronically aggravate respiratory function among asthmatic patients.[105] Calcitonin is not presently a component of most major osteoporosis management guidelines.

RANK-L ANTAGONIST

Denosumab is an injectable, fully human neutralizing antibody against RANK-L, a ligand on the surface of osteoblasts, stromal cells, and T cells, which stimulates maturation of osteoclasts by binding to RANK expressed on preosteoclasts. As an antiresorptive agent, it improves BMD and reduces the risk for vertebral fractures in postmenopausal women by 68% and femoral fractures by 40%.[106] This rate reduction is similar to that achieved with intravenous zoledronic acid and superior to that of oral bisphosphonates for vertebral fractures, and it approximates that of bisphosphonates for nonvertebral fractures. Denosumab improved BMD in a study of rheumatoid arthritis patients despite chronic prednisone of 15 mg/day or less.[107] A greater incidence of rare osteonecrosis of the jaw was observed with denosumab therapy compared with zoledronic acid.[108] Although approved in the United States and the European Union for postmenopausal and male osteoporosis, the drug is not presently recommended or approved for glucocorticoid-induced osteoporosis.

HORMONE REPLACEMENT THERAPY AND SELECTIVE ESTROGEN RECEPTOR MODULATORS

Despite its initial promotion for primary prevention of osteoporosis, large studies have failed to support routine prophylactic use of estrogen-based hormone replacement therapy (HRT) for postmenopausal osteoporosis risk reduction. Consistent observations of improved BMD with multiple types of estrogens, with a dose-response effect, are documented, yet fracture reduction was less clearly established, with a pooled risk reduction of 27% of nonvertebral fractures.[109,110] Risk for venous thromboembolism and worsened cardiovascular outcomes on HRT, identified by the Women's Health Study, have discouraged recommendation of HRT for postmenopausal osteoporosis.[43,111]

Selective estrogen receptor modulators (SERMs), which possess tissue-specific agonistic and simultaneous antagonistic estrogen activity, have been used in the prevention of osteoporosis in women. Some promote bone strength through tumor necrosis factor-α and interleukin-6 reduction and promote osteoclast apoptosis, perhaps through Fas ligand.[112] The Multiple Outcomes of Raloxifene Evaluation trial of raloxifene demonstrated durable prevention of fracture and reduction of risk for fracture, in addition to about a 2% increase in femoral and vertebral BMD.[113,114] With regard to efficacy for glucocorticoid-induced osteoporosis in women actively treated with chronic, low-dose glucocorticoids (mean, approximately 7 mg/day prednisolone), a randomized controlled trial demonstrated that raloxifene increased lumbar spine and hip, but not femoral neck, BMD by about 1% from baseline after 1 year.[115] However, there was not a statistical decrease in fracture rate. At the present time, there are no studies addressing efficacy of osteoporosis risk prevention with SERMs specifically in an asthmatic population.

Glucocorticoid Management

Because fracture risk appears to be heavily dependent on dosage and ongoing glucocorticoid therapy, clinicians should titrate therapy to the minimal glucocorticoid dose required for asthmatic symptom control and step down whenever possible. Expert Panel Report 3 asthma guidelines recommend stepping down the level of therapy after 3 months of good control; however, guidance regarding strategies for stepping down inhaled glucocorticoid therapy is minimal.[116] There is also a lack of consensus regarding duration and minimal effective oral glucocorticoid dose for asthma exacerbations, although a study found nearly all physicians treated within guidelines with less than 600 mg per 10-day course for adults and less than 2 mg/kg/day for 3 to 10 days for children younger than 11 years.[117]

Asthma-Specific Osteoporosis Risks

Most of the present osteoporosis screening and management guidelines are supported by data from adult, postmenopausal women. There is evidence that glucocorticoid-induced osteoporosis differs from postmenopausal osteoporosis, particularly regarding the predictive value of BMD for assessing fracture risk.[118] Additionally, most studies addressing glucocorticoid-induced osteoporosis include patients with severe rheumatologic disease or COPD who have different systemic inflammatory risks to bone health. Additional data regarding risks in asthmatic children and men are minimal.

Risk Reduction and Assessment in Underdeveloped Regions

Osteoporosis management in underdeveloped areas of the world is an unmet need. Osteoporosis prevalence is no less common in developing nations, and asthma is increasingly prevalent within developing nations and among poverty-stricken populations.[119,120] This is complicated by preferential oral glucocorticoid use given increased costs and restricted availability of inhaled glucocorticoids in resource-poor regions.[120] Additionally, DXA screening is presently unaffordable or inaccessible in many world regions.[119] Calcium and vitamin D supplementation and dietary enrichment are also rare in developing nations. Given these issues, additional research regarding low resource utilization tools for osteoporosis prevention, screening, and management is indicated.

UNMET, FUTURE RESEARCH NEEDS

1. Risk assessment with bone densitometry and tools such as FRAX is validated primarily with postmenopausal osteoporosis. There is a need for validated methods to better assess osteoporosis risk in asthma in asthamatic patients.

2. Glucocorticoids result in both rapid and delayed mechanisms of bone loss. The chronic use of inhaled corticosteroid with intermittent systemic glucocorticosteroids adds to the risk for osteopenia and osteoporosis. The optimal therapeutic regimen to prevent and treat glucocorticoid-induced osteoporosis is needed.

3. The role of inhaled corticosteroids in affecting bone health needs to be better quantified.

4. Limitations of bone densitometry to assess fracture risk in glucocorticoid-induced osteoporosis are suspected. Improved tests and criteria to assess risk, particularly in children and adolescents, are needed.

5. Additional research is required to determine whether asthma, independent of medications used, affects bone metabolism and risk for osteoporosis.

6. Proven measures to prevent bone loss in adults or maximize bone gain in children and adolescents are needed. Asthma spans all age groups, and correcting established bone loss is likely more difficult than preventing the development of osteoporosis.

7. Optimal nutritional factors for bone health in all age groups need to be defined in asthma. This is particularly a challenge in atopic children and adults who avoid dairy products because of perceived or documented cow's milk allergy.

CONCLUSION

Glucocorticoids are likely to remain the predominant treatment for persistent asthma among patients of all ages. Unfortunately, glucocorticoids demonstrate negative effects on bone health even at low systemic doses and even for the short durations commonly used for asthma management. Additionally, there is evidence that glucocorticoid exposure during childhood increases osteoporotic bone fracture risk in older adult populations.

As a result, clinicians should assess asthmatic patients of all ages for fracture risk, recognizing limitations of present assessment tools and guidelines. Primary prevention should include behavioral changes, nutrient enrichment, minimization of glucocorticoid total dose and cumulative exposure, and incorporation of efficacious nutritional therapy or pharmacotherapy for patients at high risk. Secondary prevention should be instituted in all asthmatic patients with a prior fracture likely related to osteoporosis. Patients at high risk for asymptomatic fracture should be screened for fracture, given the morbidity risk following an initial fracture.

Future asthma guidelines should incorporate consensus recommendations regarding osteoporosis screening and management. Additional research is warranted to better identify and minimize osteoporosis risks in asthmatic patients.

REFERENCES

1. Johnell O, Kanis JA. An estimate of the worldwide prevalence and disability associated with osteoporotic fractures. *Osteoporos Int.* 2006;17(12):1726–1733.
2. Bunta AD. It is time for everyone to own the bone. *Osteoporos Int.* 2011;22(Suppl 3):477–482.
3. To T, Stanojevic S, Moores G, et al. Global asthma prevalence in adults: findings from the cross-sectional world health survey. *BMC Public Health.* 2012;12:204.
4. National Asthma Education and Prevention Program. Expert Panel Report 3 (EPR-3): guidelines for the diagnosis and management of asthma: summary report 2007. *J Allergy Clin Immunol.* 2007;120(5 Suppl):S94–S138.
5. Weinstein RS. Clinical practice: glucocorticoid-induced bone disease. *N Engl J Med.* 2011;365(1):62–70.
6. Walker-Bone K. Recognizing and treating secondary osteoporosis. *Nat Rev Rheumatol.* 2012;8(8):480–492.
7. Gershon AS, Guan J, Wang C, Victor JC, To T. Describing and quantifying asthma comorbidity: a population study. *PLoS ONE.* 2012;7(5):e34967.
8. Soriano JB. Patterns of comorbidities in newly diagnosed COPD and asthma in primary care. *Chest.* 2005;128(4):2099–2107.
9. Cazzola M, Calzetta L, Bettoncelli G, Novelli L, Cricelli C, Rogliani P. Asthma and comorbid medical illness. *Eur Respir J.* 2011;38(1):42–49.
10. NOGG. Available at: http://www.shef.ac.uk/NOGG/NOGG_Executive_Summary.pdf. Accessed September 21, 2012.
11. Angeli A, Guglielmi G, Dovio A, et al. High prevalence of asymptomatic vertebral fractures in post-menopausal women receiving chronic glucocorticoid therapy: a cross-sectional outpatient study. *Bone.* 2006;39(2):253–259.
12. Briggs AM, Greig AM, Wark JD. The vertebral fracture cascade in osteoporosis: a review of aetiopathogenesis. *Osteoporos Int.* 2007;18(5):575–584.
13. Johnell O, Kanis JA, Oden A, et al. Predictive value of BMD for hip and other fractures. *J Bone Miner Res.* 2005;20(7):1185–1194.
14. van Kuijk C. Pediatric bone densitometry. *Radiol Clin North Am.* 2010;48(3):623–627.
15. Adinoff AD, Hollister JR. Steroid-induced fractures and bone loss in patients with asthma. *N Engl J Med.* 1983;309(5):265–268.
16. van Staa TP. The pathogenesis, epidemiology and management of glucocorticoid-induced osteoporosis. *Calcif Tissue Int.* 2006;79(3):129–137.
17. Canalis E, Mazziotti G, Giustina A, Bilezikian JP. Glucocorticoid-induced osteoporosis: pathophysiology and therapy. *Osteoporos Int.* 2007;18(10):1319–1328.
18. Mazziotti G, Angeli A, Bilezikian JP, Canalis E, Giustina A. Glucocorticoid-induced osteoporosis: an update. *Trends Endocrinol Metab.* 2006;17(4):144–149.
19. Steinbuch M, Youket TE, Cohen S. Oral glucocorticoid use is associated with an increased risk of fracture. *Osteoporos Int.* 2004;15(4):323–328.
20. van Staa TP, Laan RF, Barton IP, Cohen S, Reid DM, Cooper C. Bone density threshold and other predictors of vertebral fracture in patients receiving oral glucocorticoid therapy. *Arthritis Rheum.* 2003;48(11):3224–3229.
21. van Staa TP, Leufkens HG, Abenhaim L, Zhang B, Cooper C. Oral corticosteroids and fracture risk: relationship to daily and cumulative doses. *Rheumatology.* 2000;39(12):1383–1389.
22. De Vries F, Bracke M, Leufkens HGM, Lammers J-WJ, Cooper C, Van Staa TP. Fracture risk with intermittent high-dose oral glucocorticoid therapy. *Arthritis Rheum.* 2007;56(1):208–214.
23. Gluck OS, Murphy WA, Hahn TJ, Hahn B. Bone loss in adults receiving alternate day glucocorticoid therapy: a comparison with daily therapy. *Arthritis Rheum.* 1981;24(7):892–898.
24. Rüegsegger P, Medici TC, Anliker M. Corticosteroid-induced bone loss: a longitudinal study of alternate day therapy in patients with bronchial asthma using quantitative computed tomography. *Eur J Clin Pharmacol.* 1983;25(5):615–620.

25. Covar RA, Leung DY, McCormick D, Steelman J, Zeitler P, Spahn JD. Risk factors associated with glucocorticoid-induced adverse effects in children with severe asthma. *J Allergy Clin Immunol*. 2000;106(4):651–659.
26. Kelly HW, Van Natta ML, Covar RA, et al. Effect of long-term corticosteroid use on bone mineral density in children: a prospective longitudinal assessment in the childhood Asthma Management Program (CAMP) study. *Pediatrics*. 2008;122(1):e53–e61.
27. van Staa TP, Cooper C, Leufkens HGM, Bishop N. Children and the risk of fractures caused by oral corticosteroids. *J Bone Miner Res*. 2003;18(5):913–918.
28. Irwin RS, Richardson ND. Side effects with inhaled corticosteroids: the physician's perception. *Chest*. 2006;130(1 Suppl):41S–53S.
29. Gatti D, Senna G, Viapiana O, Rossini M, Passalacqua G, Adami S. Allergy and the bone: unexpected relationships. *Ann Allergy Asthma Immunol*. 2011;107(3):202–206.
30. Dahl R. Systemic side effects of inhaled corticosteroids in patients with asthma. *Respir Med*. 2006;100(8):1307–1317.
31. Israel E, Banerjee TR, Fitzmaurice GM, Kotlov TV, LaHive K, LeBoff MS. Effects of inhaled glucocorticoids on bone density in premenopausal women. *N Engl J Med*. 2001;345(13):941–947.
32. Jones A, Fay JK, Burr M, Stone M, Hood K, Roberts G. Inhaled corticosteroid effects on bone metabolism in asthma and mild chronic obstructive pulmonary disease. *Cochrane Database Syst Rev*. 2002;(1):CD003537.
33. Roux C, Kolta S, Desfougères J-L, Minini P, Bidat E. Long-term safety of fluticasone propionate and nedocromil sodium on bone in children with asthma. *Pediatrics*. 2003;111(6 Pt 1):e706–e713.
34. Mazziotti G, Canalis E, Giustina A. Drug-induced osteoporosis: mechanisms and clinical implications. *AJM*. 2010;123(10):877–884.
35. Writing Committee for the American Lung Association Asthma Clinical Research Centers, Holbrook JT, Wise RA, et al. Lansoprazole for children with poorly controlled asthma: a randomized controlled trial. *JAMA*. 2012;307(4):373–381.
36. Chan WW, Chiou E, Obstein KL, Tignor AS, Whitlock TL. The efficacy of proton pump inhibitors for the treatment of asthma in adults: a meta-analysis. *Arch Intern Med*. 2011;171(7):620–629.
37. Martinez FD. Children, asthma, and proton pump inhibitors: costs and perils of therapeutic creep. *JAMA*. 2012;307(4):406–407.
38. Munson JC, Wahl PM, Daniel G, Kimmel SE, Hennessy S. Factors associated with the initiation of proton pump inhibitors in corticosteroid users. *Pharmacoepidemiol Drug Saf*. 2012;21(4):366–374.
39. Fraser L-A, Leslie WD, Targownik LE, Papaioannou A, Adachi JD, for the CaMos Research Group. The effect of proton pump inhibitors on fracture risk: report from the Canadian Multicenter Osteoporosis Study. *Osteoporos Int*. 2013;24(4):1161–1168.
40. Ngamruengphong S, Leontiadis GI, Radhi S, Dentino A, Nugent K. Proton pump inhibitors and risk of fracture: a systematic review and meta-analysis of observational studies. *Am J Gastroenterol*. 2011;106(7):1209–1218, quiz 1219.
41. Gingo MR, Wenzel SE, Steele C, et al. Asthma diagnosis and airway bronchodilator response in HIV-infected patients. *J Allergy Clin Immunol*. 2012;129(3):708–714.e8.
42. Powderly WG. Osteoporosis and bone health in HIV. *Curr HIV/AIDS Rep*. 2012;9(3):218–222.
43. Brown TT, McComsey GA, King MS, Qaqish RB, Bernstein BM, da Silva BA. Loss of bone mineral density after antiretroviral therapy initiation, independent of antiretroviral regimen. *J Acquir Immune Defic Syndr*. 2009;51(5):554–561.
44. Jackson KA, Savaiano DA. Lactose maldigestion, calcium intake and osteoporosis in African-, Asian-, and Hispanic-Americans. *J Am Coll Nutr*. 2001;20(2):198S–207S.
45. Skripak JM, Matsui EC, Mudd K, Wood RA. The natural history of IgE-mediated cow's milk allergy. *J Allergy Clin Immunol*. 2007;120(5):1172–1177.
46. Black RE, Williams SM, Jones IE, Goulding A. Children who avoid drinking cow milk have low dietary calcium intakes and poor bone health. *Am J Clin Nutr*. 2002;76(3):675–680.
47. Goulding A, Rockell JEP, Black RE, Grant AM, Jones IE, Williams SM. Children who avoid drinking cow's milk are at increased risk for prepubertal bone fractures. *J Am Diet Assoc*. 2004;104(2):250–253.
48. Teegarden D, Lyle RM, Proulx WR, Johnston CC, Weaver CM. Previous milk consumption is associated with greater bone density in young women. *Am J Clin Nutr*. 1999;69(5):1014–1017.
49. Sandler RB, Slemenda CW, LaPorte RE, et al. Postmenopausal bone density and milk consumption in childhood and adolescence. *Am J Clin Nutr*. 1985;42(2):270–274.
50. Searing DA, Leung DYM. Vitamin D in atopic dermatitis, asthma and allergic diseases. *Immunol Allergy Clin North Am*. 2010;30(3):397–409.

51. Paul G, Brehm JM, Alcorn JF, Holguin F, Aujla SJ, Celedón JC. Vitamin D and asthma. *Am J Respir Crit Care Med*. 2012;185(2):124–132.
52. Brehm JM, Acosta-Pérez E, Klei L, et al. Vitamin D insufficiency and severe asthma exacerbations in Puerto Rican children. *Am J Respir Crit Care Med*. 2012;186(2):140–146.
53. Bozzetto S, Carraro S, Giordano G, Boner A, Baraldi E. Asthma, allergy and respiratory infections: the vitamin D hypothesis. *Allergy*. 2012;67(1):10–17.
54. Institute of Medicine Committee to Review Dietary Reference Intakes for Vitamin D and Calcium; Ross AC, Taylor CL, Yaktine AL, Del Valle HB, eds. *Dietary Reference Intakes for Calcium and Vitamin D*. Washington, D.C.: National Academies Press; 2011.
55. Edwards BJ, Langman CB, Bunta AD, Vicuna M, Favus M. Secondary contributors to bone loss in osteoporosis related hip fractures. *Osteoporos Int*. 2008;19(7):991–999.
56. Arabi A, El Rassi R, El-Hajj Fuleihan G. Hypovitaminosis D in developing countries: prevalence, risk factors and outcomes. *Nat Rev Endocrinol*. 2010;6(10):550–561.
57. Tse SM, Kelly HW, Litonjua AA, et al. Corticosteroid use and bone mineral accretion in children with asthma: effect modification by vitamin D. *J Allergy Clin Immunol*. 2012;130(1):53–60.e4.
58. Braun T, Schett G. Pathways for bone loss in inflammatory disease. *Curr Osteoporos Rep*. 2012;10(2):101–108.
59. Olafsdottir IS, Gislason T, Thjodleifsson B, et al. C reactive protein levels are increased in non-allergic but not allergic asthma: a multicentre epidemiological study. *Thorax*. 2005;60(6):451–454.
60. Dam T-T, Harrison S, Fink HA, Ramsdell J, Barrett-Connor E, Osteoporotic Fractures in Men (MrOS) Research Group. Bone mineral density and fractures in older men with chronic obstructive pulmonary disease or asthma. *Osteoporos Int*. 2010;21(8):1341–1349.
61. Barnes PJ, Celli BR. Systemic manifestations and comorbidities of COPD. *Eur Respir J*. 2009;33(5):1165–1185.
62. Sinden NJ, Stockley RA. Systemic inflammation and comorbidity in COPD: a result of "overspill" of inflammatory mediators from the lungs? Review of the evidence. *Thorax*. 2010;65(10):930–936.
63. Compston JE, Watts NB, Chapurlat R, et al. Obesity is not protective against fracture in postmenopausal women: GLOW. *Am J Med*. 2011;124(11):1043–1050.
64. Juel CT-B, Ali Z, Nilas L, Ulrik CS. Asthma and obesity: does weight loss improve asthma control? A systematic review. *J Asthma Allergy*. 2012;5:21–26.
65. Moayyeri A. The association between physical activity and osteoporotic fractures: a review of the evidence and implications for future research. *Ann Epidemiol*. 2008;18(11):827–835.
66. Moayyeri A, Besson H, Luben RN, Wareham NJ, Khaw K-T. The association between physical activity in different domains of life and risk of osteoporotic fractures. *Bone*. 2010;47(3):693–700.
67. Lucas S, Plattsmills T. Physical activity and exercise in asthma: relevance to etiology and treatment. *J Allergy Clin Immunol*. 2005;115(5):928–934.
68. Kanis JA, Johnell O, Oden A, et al. Smoking and fracture risk: a meta-analysis. *Osteoporos Int*. 2005;16(2):155–162.
69. Yoon V, Maalouf NM, Sakhaee K. The effects of smoking on bone metabolism. *Osteoporos Int*. 2012;23(8):2081–2092.
70. Kanis JA, Johnell O, Oden A, et al. Smoking and fracture risk: a meta-analysis. *Osteoporos Int*. 2004;16(2):155–162.
71. Cerveri I, Cazzoletti L, Corsico AG, et al. The impact of cigarette smoking on asthma: a population-based international cohort study. *Int Arch Allergy Immunol*. 2012;158(2):175–183.
72. Chaudhuri R, Livingston E, McMahon AD, Thomson L, Borland W, Thomson NC. Cigarette smoking impairs the therapeutic response to oral corticosteroids in chronic asthma. *Am J Respir Crit Care Med*. 2003;168(11):1308–1311.
73. jointcommission.org. Available at: http://www.jointcommission.org. Accessed October 28, 2012.
74. Lo JC, Burnett-Bowie S-AM, Finkelstein JS. Bone and the perimenopause. *Obstet Gynecol Clin North Am*. 2011;38(3):503–517.
75. Ralston SH, Uitterlinden AG. Genetics of osteoporosis. *Endocr Rev*. 2010;31(5):629–662.
76. Estrada K, Styrkarsdottir U, Evangelou E, et al. Genome-wide meta-analysis identifies 56 bone mineral density loci and reveals 14 loci associated with risk of fracture. *Nat Genet*. 2012;44(5):491–501.
77. Barrett-Connor E, Siris ES, Wehren LE, et al. Osteoporosis and fracture risk in women of different ethnic groups. *J Bone Miner Res*. 2005;20(2):185–194.

78. International Osteoporosis Foundation. Available at: http://www.iofbonehealth.org/national-regional-osteoporosis-guidelines. Accessed August 27, 2012.
79. Leslie WD, Majumdar SR, Lix LM, et al. High fracture probability with FRAX usually indicates densitometric osteoporosis: implications for clinical practice. Osteoporos Int. 2012;23(1):391–397.
80. Kanis JA, Johansson H, Oden A, McCloskey EV. Guidance for the adjustment of FRAX according to the dose of glucocorticoids. Osteoporos Int. 2011;22(3):809–816.
81. Green AD, Colón-Emeric CS, Bastian L, Drake MT, Lyles KW. Does this woman have osteoporosis? JAMA. 2004;292(23):2890–2900.
82. Specker BL, Schoenau E. Quantitative bone analysis in children: current methods and recommendations. J Pediatr. 2005;146(6):726–731.
83. Bonaiuti D, Shea B, Iovine R, et al. Exercise for preventing and treating osteoporosis in postmenopausal women. Cochrane Database Syst Rev. 2002;(3):CD000333.
84. Nikander R, Sievänen H, Heinonen A, Daly RM, Uusi-Rasi K, Kannus P. Targeted exercise against osteoporosis: a systematic review and meta-analysis for optimising bone strength throughout life. BMC Med. 2010;8:47.
85. Inderjeeth CA, Chan K, Kwan K, Lai M. Time to onset of efficacy in fracture reduction with current anti-osteoporosis treatments. J Bone Miner Metab. 2012;30(5):493–503.
86. SOHC-web1.pdf. ncqa.org. Available at: http://www.ncqa.org/Portals/0/SOHC-web1.pdf. Accessed October 30, 2012.
87. Elliot-Gibson V, Bogoch ER, Jamal SA, Beaton DE. Practice patterns in the diagnosis and treatment of osteoporosis after a fragility fracture: a systematic review. Osteoporos Int. 2004;15(10):767–778.
88. Asche C, Nelson R, McAdam-Marx C, Jhaveri M, Ye X. Predictors of oral bisphosphonate prescriptions in post-menopausal women with osteoporosis in a real-world setting in the USA. Osteoporos Int. 2010;21(8):1427–1436.
89. Grossman JM, Gordon R, Ranganath VK, et al. American College of Rheumatology 2010 recommendations for the prevention and treatment of glucocorticoid-induced osteoporosis. Arthritis Care Res (Hoboken). 2010;62(11):1515–1526.
90. Nawata H, Soen S, Takayanagi R, et al. Guidelines on the management and treatment of glucocorticoid-induced osteoporosis of the Japanese Society for Bone and Mineral Research (2004). J Bone Miner Metab. 2005;23(2):105–109.
91. Pereira RMR, de Carvalho JF, Paula AP, et al. Guidelines for the prevention and treatment of glucocorticoid-induced osteoporosis. Rev Bras Reumatol. 2012;52(4):580–593.
92. Abadie EC, Devogealer J-P, Ringe JD, et al. Recommendations for the registration of agents to be used in the prevention and treatment of glucocorticoid-induced osteoporosis: updated recommendations from the Group for the Respect of Ethics and Excellence in Science. Semin Arthritis Rheum. 2005;35:1–4.
93. Homik J, Suarez-Almazor ME, Shea B, Cranney A, Wells G, Tugwell P. Calcium and vitamin D for corticosteroid-induced osteoporosis. Cochrane Database Syst Rev. 2000;(2):CD000952.
94. McDonald CF, Zebaze RMD, Seeman E. Calcitriol does not prevent bone loss in patients with asthma receiving corticosteroid therapy: a double-blind placebo-controlled trial. Osteoporos Int. 2006;17(10):1546–1551.
95. Calvo MS, Whiting SJ, Barton CN. Vitamin D intake: a global perspective of current status. J Nutr. 2005;135(2):310–316.
96. Rizzoli R, Adachi JD, Cooper C, et al. Management of glucocorticoid-induced osteoporosis. Calcif Tissue Int. 2012;91(4):225–243.
97. Diab DL, Watts NB. Bisphosphonates in the treatment of osteoporosis. Endocrinol Metab Clin North Am. 2012;41(3):487–506.
98. Watts NB, Diab DL. Long-term use of bisphosphonates in osteoporosis. J Clin Endocrinol Metab. 2010;95(4):1555–1565.
99. Ward L, Tricco AC, Phuong P, et al. Bisphosphonate therapy for children and adolescents with secondary osteoporosis. Cochrane Database Syst Rev. 2007;(4):CD005324.
100. Weinstein RS, Chen J-R, Powers CC, et al. Promotion of osteoclast survival and antagonism of bisphosphonate-induced osteoclast apoptosis by glucocorticoids. J Clin Invest. 2002;109(8):1041–1048.
101. Bone H. Future directions in osteoporosis therapeutics. Endocrinol Metab Clin North Am. 2012;41(3):655–661.
102. Saag KG, Shane E, Boonen S, et al. Teriparatide or alendronate in glucocorticoid-induced osteoporosis. N Engl J Med. 2007;357(20):2028–2039.
103. Luengo M, Pons F, Martinez de Osaba MJ, Picado C. Prevention of further bone mass loss by nasal calcitonin in patients on long

term glucocorticoid therapy for asthma: a two year follow up study. *Thorax.* 1994;49(11):1099–1102.
104. Cranney A, Welch V, Adachi JD, et al. Calcitonin for the treatment and prevention of corticosteroid-induced osteoporosis. *Cochrane Database Syst Rev.* 2000;(2):CD001983.
105. Dal Negro R, Turco P, Pomari C, Trevisan F. Calcitonin nasal spray in patients with chronic asthma: a double-blind crossover study vs placebo. *Int J Clin Pharmacol Ther Toxicol.* 1991;29(4):144–146.
106. Cummings SR, Martin JS, McClung MR, et al. Denosumab for prevention of fractures in postmenopausal women with osteoporosis. *N Engl J Med.* 2009;361(8):756–765.
107. Dore RK, Cohen SB, Lane NE, et al. Effects of denosumab on bone mineral density and bone turnover in patients with rheumatoid arthritis receiving concurrent glucocorticoids or bisphosphonates. *Ann Rheum Dis.* 2010;69(5):872–875.
108. Saad F, Brown JE, Van Poznak C, et al. Incidence, risk factors, and outcomes of osteonecrosis of the jaw: integrated analysis from three blinded active-controlled phase III trials in cancer patients with bone metastases. *Ann Oncol.* 2012;23(5):1341–1347.
109. Torgerson DJ, Bell-Syer SE. Hormone replacement therapy and prevention of nonvertebral fractures: a meta-analysis of randomized trials. *JAMA.* 2001;285(22):2891–2897.
110. ahrq.gov. Available at: http://www.ahrq.gov. Accessed September 23, 2012.
111. Fraser L-A, Adachi JD. Glucocorticoid-induced osteoporosis: treatment update and review. *Ther Adv Musculoskelet Dis.* 2009;1(2):71–85.
112. Nakamura T, Imai Y, Matsumoto T, et al. Estrogen prevents bone loss via estrogen receptor alpha and induction of Fas ligand in osteoclasts. *Cell.* 2007;130(5):811–823.
113. Ettinger B, Black DM, Mitlak BH, et al. Reduction of vertebral fracture risk in postmenopausal women with osteoporosis treated with raloxifene: results from a 3-year randomized clinical trial. Multiple Outcomes of Raloxifene Evaluation (MORE) Investigators. *JAMA.* 1999;282(7):637–645.
114. Delmas PD, Ensrud KE, Adachi JD, et al. Efficacy of raloxifene on vertebral fracture risk reduction in postmenopausal women with osteoporosis: four-year results from a randomized clinical trial. *J Clin Endocrinol Metab.* 2002;87(8):3609–3617.
115. Mok CC, Ying KY, To CH, et al. Raloxifene for prevention of glucocorticoid-induced bone loss: a 12-month randomised double-blinded placebo-controlled trial. *Ann Rheum Dis.* 2011;70(5):778–784.
116. Thomas A, Lemanske RF, Jackson DJ. Approaches to stepping up and stepping down care in asthmatic patients. *J Allergy Clin Immunol.* 2011;128(5):915–924, quiz 925–926.
117. Fuhlbrigge AL, Lemanske RF, Rasouliyan L, Sorkness CA, Fish JE. Practice patterns for oral corticosteroid burst therapy in the outpatient management of acute asthma exacerbations. *Allergy Asthma Proc.* 2012;33(1):82–89.
118. Compston J, Reid DM, Boisdron J, et al. Recommendations for the registration of agents for prevention and treatment of glucocorticoid-induced osteoporosis: an update from the Group for the Respect of Ethics and Excellence in Science. *Osteoporos Int.* 2008;19:1247–1250.
119. Handa R, Ali Kalla A, Maalouf G. Osteoporosis in developing countries. *Best Pract Res Clin Rheumatol.* 2008;22(4):693–708.
120. Ait-Khaled N, Enarson DA, Bissell K, Billo NE. Access to inhaled corticosteroids is key to improving quality of care for asthma in developing countries. *Allergy.* 2007;62(3):230–236.
121. Brown JP, Josse RG. 2002 clinical practice guidelines for the diagnosis and management of osteoporosis in Canada. *CMAJ.* 2002;167(10 Suppl):S1–S34.
122. Toogood JH. Asthma and therapeutics: inhaled corticosteroids, corticosteroid osteoporosis, and the risk of fracture in chronic asthma. *Allergy Asthma Clin Immunol.* 2005;1(1):28–33.
123. Kearney DM, Lockey RF. Osteoporosis and asthma. *Ann Allergy Asthma Immunol.* 2006;96(6):769–774, quiz 775–778, 857.
124. National Clinical Guideline Centre (UK). *Osteoporosis: Fragility Fracture Risk: Osteoporosis: Assessing the Risk of Fragility Fracture.* London: Royal College of Physicians; 2012.
125. Green AD, Colón-Emeric CS, Bastian L, Drake MT, Lyles KW. Does this woman have osteoporosis? *JAMA.* 2004;292(23):2890–2900.
126. Kanis JA, Melton LJ, Christiansen C, Johnston CC, Khaltaev N. The diagnosis of osteoporosis. *J Bone Miner Res.* 1994;9(8):1137–1141.

127. Bachrach LK. Consensus and controversy regarding osteoporosis in the pediatric population. *Endocr Pract.* 2007;13(5):513–520.
128. Baim S, Leslie WD. Assessment of fracture risk. *Curr Osteoporos Rep.* 2012;10(1):28–41.
129. Ferrari S, Bianchi ML, Eisman JA, et al. Osteoporosis in young adults: pathophysiology, diagnosis, and management. *Osteoporos Int.* 2012;23(12):2735–2748.
130. Walker-Bone K. Recognizing and treating secondary osteoporosis. *Nat Rev Rheumatol.* 2012;8(8):480–492.

27

PREGNANCY

COMORBID AND COEXISTING

Jennifer A. Namazy, Michael Schatz, and Sandra Gonzalez-Diaz

KEY POINTS

- Realize that pregnant asthmatic women have a higher risk for adverse perinatal outcomes.
- Adherence to treatment, specifically inhaled corticosteroids, has been a problem for many pregnant asthmatic patients, usually due to concerns regarding the safety of these medications during pregnancy.
- Symptoms and pulmonary function need to be monitored on a monthly basis in pregnant asthmatic women so that any change in course can be matched with an appropriate change in therapy
- Patient education is an important part of managing the pregnant asthmatic woman. This includes explaining the relationship between asthma and pregnancy, identifying asthma triggers, providing training on correct use of inhalers, and establishing an asthma action plan.
- One of the most important needs for the future is the availability of further safety information for asthma medications used during pregnancy that can also account for asthma control.

INTRODUCTION

Asthma is the most common chronic medical condition to affect pregnancy, with a prevalence of self-reported asthma in the United States between 8.4% and 8.8%.[1] Asthma may adversely affect both maternal quality of life and perinatal outcomes, and pregnancy may affect the course of asthma. Management of asthma during pregnancy should optimize the health of both the mother and her baby.

EFFECT OF ASTHMA ON PREGNANCY

A meta-analysis, derived from a substantial body of literature spanning several decades and including large numbers of pregnant women (>1,000,000 for low birth weight and >250,000 for preterm labor), indicates that pregnant women with asthma are at a significantly increased risk for a range of adverse perinatal outcomes including low birth weight, small for gestational age, preterm labor and delivery, and preeclampsia.

Mechanisms postulated to explain the possible increased perinatal risks in pregnant asthmatic women demonstrated in previous studies have included (1) hypoxia and other physiologic consequences of poorly controlled asthma, (2) medications used to treat asthma, and (3) pathogenic or demographic factors associated with asthma but not actually caused by the disease or its treatment, such as abnormal placental function.

Several prospective studies[2-10] show that pregnant asthmatic patients with mild to moderate severity can have excellent maternal and fetal outcomes. In contrast, suboptimal control of asthma or more severe asthma during pregnancy may be associated with increased maternal or fetal risk.[8,11,12]

EFFECT OF PREGNANCY ON THE COURSE OF ASTHMA

Asthma may worsen, improve, or remain unchanged during pregnancy, and the overall data suggest that these various courses occur with approximately equal frequency. In a large prospective study of 1,739 pregnant asthmatic women, severity classification (based on symptoms, pulmonary function, and medication use) worsened in 30% and improved in 23% of patients during pregnancy.[13] Asthma also appears more likely to be more severe or to worsen during pregnancy in women who had more severe asthma before becoming pregnant.[14]

The course of asthma may vary by stage of pregnancy. The first trimester is generally well tolerated in asthmatic patients with infrequent acute episodes. Increased symptoms and more frequent exacerbations have been reported to occur between weeks 17 and 36 of gestation. In contrast, asthmatic women in general tend to experience fewer symptoms and less frequent asthma exacerbations during weeks 37 to 40 of pregnancy than during any earlier gestational period.[15]

The mechanisms responsible for the altered asthma course during pregnancy are unknown. The myriad pregnancy-associated changes in levels of sex hormones, cortisol, and prostaglandins may contribute to changes in asthma course during pregnancy. In addition, exposure to fetal antigens leading to alterations in immune function may predispose some pregnant asthmatic patients to worsening asthma.[16] Even fetal sex may play a role, with some data showing increased severity of symptoms in pregnancies with a female fetus.[17]

Additional factors may contribute to the clinical course of asthma during pregnancy. Pregnancy may be a source of stress for many women, and this stress can aggravate asthma. Adherence to therapy can change during pregnancy, with a corresponding change in asthma control. Most commonly observed is decreased adherence as a result of a mother's concerns about the safety of medications for the fetus (see later). For example, one study found that that less than 40% of women who classified themselves as "poorly controlled" reported use of a controller medication during pregnancy.[18]

Physician reluctance to treat may also affect the course of asthma during pregnancy. One study identified 51 pregnant women and 500 nonpregnant women presenting to the emergency department with acute asthma. Although asthma severity appeared to be similar in the two groups based on peak flow rates, pregnant women were significantly less likely to be discharged on oral corticosteroids (38% vs. 64%). Presumably related to this undertreatment, pregnant women were three times more likely than nonpregnant women to report an ongoing exacerbation 2 weeks later.[19,20]

Infections during pregnancy can certainly affect the course of gestational asthma. Some degree of decrease in cell-mediated immunity may make the pregnant patient more susceptible to viral infection, and upper respiratory tract infections are reported to be the most common precipitants of asthma exacerbations during pregnancy.[21] Sinusitis, a known asthma trigger, is up to six times more common in pregnant compared with nonpregnant women.[22] In addition, pneumonia is reported to be greater than five times more common in asthmatic than nonasthmatic women during pregnancy.[23]

DIAGNOSIS

Asthma is suspected based on the presence of typical symptoms such as wheezing, chest tightness, cough, and associated shortness of breath. The diagnosis is ideally confirmed by the demonstration of reversible airways obstruction, which most commonly is an increase in forced expiratory volume in 1 second (FEV_1) by 12% or more and at least 200 mL after an inhaled short-acting bronchodilator. In nonpregnant patients with normal pulmonary function, asthma can be confirmed by means of methacholine challenge testing. However, this type of testing is not recommended in pregnant patients. Studies suggest that an elevated fraction of exhaled nitric oxide (FeNO) can be used in pregnant women to follow asthma similar to its use in nonpregnant patients.[24] Thus, an elevated FeNO would likely support the diagnosis of asthma in pregnant patients. If the FeNO is normal or unavailable, therapeutic trials of asthma therapy, such as 2 to 4 weeks of regular inhaled corticosteroid (ICS), may be used during pregnancy in patients with possible but unconfirmed asthma.

ASSESSMENT

After the diagnosis of asthma is confirmed, the next step is the assessment of asthma severity (in patients not already on controller therapy) or assessment of control (in patients already on controller therapy) (Tables 27.1 and 27.2). Both severity and control are assessed based on frequency of symptoms, rescue therapy use, nighttime awakenings, and degree of interference with normal activity, exacerbations, and pulmonary function. Patients with intermittent asthma have short episodes of asthma, use rescue therapy less than three times per week, have nocturnal symptoms less than three times a month, and have normal pulmonary function between episodes. Patients with more frequent symptoms or who require daily asthma medications should be considered to

Table 27.1. Classification of Asthma Severity in Pregnant Patients

ASTHMA SEVERITY	SYMPTOM FREQUENCY	NIGHTTIME AWAKENING	INTERFERENCE WITH NORMAL ACTIVITY	FEV_1 OR PEAK FLOW (PREDICTED PERCENTAGE OF PERSONAL BEST)
Intermittent	2 days per week or less	Twice per month or less	None	More than 80%
Mild persistent	More than 2 days per week, but not daily	More than twice per month	Minor limitation	More than 80%
Moderate persistent	Daily symptoms	More than once per week	Some limitation	60%–80%
Severe persistent	Throughout the day	Four times per week or more	Extremely limited	Less than 60%

FEV_1, forced expiratory volume in the first second of expiration.
Data from Schatz M, Dombrowski M. ACOG practice bulletin. Clinical management guidelines for obstetrician-gynecologists number 90, February 2008: asthma in pregnancy. *Obstet Gynecol.* 2008;111:457-464.

Table 27.2. Assessment of Asthma Control in Pregnant Women

VARIABLE	WELL-CONTROLLED ASTHMA	ASTHMA NOT WELL CONTROLLED	VERY POORLY CONTROLLED ASTHMA
Frequency of symptoms	≤2 days/wk	>2 days/wk	Throughout the day
Frequency of nighttime awakening	≤2 times/mo	1–3 times/wk	≥4 times/wk
Interference with normal activity	None	Some	Extreme
Use of short-acting ß-agonist for symptom control	≤2 days/wk	>2 days/wk	Several times/day
FEV_1 or peak flow (% of the predicted or personal best value)	>80	60–80	<60
Exacerbation requiring use of systemic corticosteroid (no.)	0–1 in the past 12 mo	≥2 in the past 12 mo	≥2 in the past 12 mo

Data from Schatz M, Dombrowski M. Clinical practice: asthma in medicine. *N Engl J Med.* 2009;360:1862–1869.

have persistent asthma. Several observations support the hypothesis that uncontrolled asthma increases perinatal risks, whereas controlled asthma reduces these risks.[25,26]

A 2011 double-blind, parallel-group, controlled study by Powell and colleagues tested the measurement of FeNO to guide management of pregnant asthmatic women. The primary outcome was total asthma exacerbations. The authors found that the exacerbation rate was lower in the group using FeNO to adjust asthma therapies during pregnancy.[27]

DIFFERENTIAL DIAGNOSIS

In a patient without a previous diagnosis of asthma, asthma must be differentiated from a number of other potential causes of respiratory symptoms during pregnancy (Table 27.3). The most common differential diagnosis is dyspnea of pregnancy, which may occur in early pregnancy in approximately 70% of women. This dyspnea is usually differentiated from asthma by its lack of association with cough, wheezing, or airway obstruction. Other important masqueraders of asthma include vocal cord dysfunction; panic attacks; hyperventilation; and cough due to postnasal drip, laryngopharyngeal reflux, or angiotensin-converting enzyme inhibitor therapy. All of these can coexist with asthma. Even when these conditions coexist with asthma, their diagnosis and appropriate therapy usually reduce the patient's respiratory symptoms.

Table 27.3. Differential Diagnosis of Dyspnea during Pregnancy

Asthma
Dyspnea of pregnancy
Reflux esophagitis
Postnasal drainage
Bronchitis
Laryngeal dysfunction
Hyperventilation
Pulmonary edema
Pulmonary embolism

ASTHMA EDUCATION AND ADHERENCE

Control of maternal asthma is essential to prevent perinatal complications. It comes as no surprise that pregnant women are hesitant about continuing asthma medications during pregnancy for fear of causing untoward effects on their unborn baby. One study found that women with asthma significantly decreased their asthma medication use from 5 to 13 weeks of pregnancy. During the first trimester, there was a 23% decline in ICS prescriptions, a 13% decline in short-acting β-agonist prescriptions, and a 54% decline in rescue corticosteroid prescriptions.[28] A study found that about one-third of pregnant asthmatic women discontinued asthma medications during pregnancy, often without consulting their physicians.[29] Lim and colleagues[30] tried to elucidate the reasons for nonadherence in this particular population of patients. Data were obtained from interviews with pregnant asthmatic subjects. Concerns about medication use, specifically glucocorticosteroid use, overshadowed the potential risk for uncontrolled asthma. Many women appeared happy to rely on their reliever therapy, and many decreased their preventive therapy without consulting their doctors. Most participants complained about the lack of information available on asthma during pregnancy. Lack of support was also a common complaint. Many women felt that information they were receiving from their pharmacists, nurses, and doctors was contradictory, leading them to make their own choices about medication management. As a result, many of the participants decreased or discontinued their asthma medications or withheld doses during pregnancy. According to the studies' authors, it was clear from the interviews that women felt it would have been helpful if asthma had been discussed more by their physician or other health care professional, providing opportunities for them to pursue more reliable information.

A disappointing fact is that medical professionals can provide incorrect information. One study found that more than one-fourth of family physicians would instruct their patients to decrease or discontinue asthma medication during pregnancy when asthma was well controlled by current therapy.[31] In another study, Cimbollek and colleagues surveyed 1,000 physicians, almost half of whom were respiratory medicine and/or allergy specialists, and the other half were primary care physicians. Almost 30% of physicians would not perform spirometry in pregnant asthmatic patients, and only 64% reported that they followed the asthma guidelines in the management of pregnant asthmatic patients.[32]

Uninformed decisions by pregnant asthmatic patients or those managing their asthma may lead to exacerbations of asthma during pregnancy and potentially adverse perinatal outcomes. Therefore, asthma education is a critical component in the management of the pregnant asthmatic patient, especially regarding the potential effects of uncontrolled asthma on the baby and the self-management strategies, such as proper inhaler technique, adherence, and appropriate responses to increasing symptoms, necessary to achieve optimal control and prevent exacerbations.

PHARMACOLOGIC THERAPY

The medical management of asthma during pregnancy is not unlike that of the nonpregnant asthmatic patient. Therapy is divided into long-term control medications and rescue therapy. Long-term control medications are used for maintenance therapy to prevent asthma manifestations and include inhaled ICS agents, cromolyn, long-acting β-agonists, and leukotriene receptor antagonists and theophylline. Controller therapy should be increased in steps (Table 27.4) until adequate control is achieved. Rescue therapy, most commonly inhaled short-acting β-agonists, provides immediate relief of symptoms. Oral corticosteroids can be used either as a form of rescue therapy or as chronic therapy for severe persistent asthma.

Inhaled Corticosteroids

Inhaled corticosteroids are the mainstay of controller therapy during pregnancy. Many studies show no increased perinatal risks (including preeclampsia, preterm birth, low birth weight, and congenital malformations) associated with these medications.[9,33–38] A study of more than 4,000 women who used ICS during pregnancy found no increased risk of perinatal mortality associated with their use during pregnancy.[39] Several large

Table 27.4. Steps of Asthma Therapy during Pregnancy

STEP	PREFERRED CONTROLLER MEDICATION	ALTERNATIVE CONTROLLER MEDICATION
1	None	—
2	Low-dose ICS	LTRA, theophylline
3	Medium-dose ICS	Low-dose ICS + LABA, LTRA, or theophylline
4	Medium-dose ICS + LABA	Medium-dose ICS + LTRA or theophylline
5	High-dose ICS + LABA	—
6	High-dose ICS + LABA + oral prednisone	—

ICS, inhaled corticosteroids; LABA, long-acting β-agonists; LTRA, leukotriene-receptor antagonists.
Data from Schatz M, Dombrowski M. Clinical practice: asthma in medicine. N Engl J Med. 2009;360:1862–1869.

studies support the lack of association of ICS use with total or specific malformations.[39–42] One study[44] suggests a relationship between high-dose ICS and total malformations, but confounding by severity is a possible explanation, based on the relationships between exacerbations and congenital malformations demonstrated by the same group.[12] Lin and colleagues, in a population-based, multicenter, case-control study, found a positive association between maternal asthma use of ICS (fluticasone was the most commonly reported specific drug) and anorectal atresia (adjusted odds ratio [OR], 2.12; 95% confidence interval [CI], 1.09 to 4.12).[45]

Because it has the most published human gestational safety data, budesonide is considered the preferred ICS for the treatment of asthma during pregnancy. That is not to say that the other ICS preparations are unsafe. Therefore, ICS agents other than budesonide may be continued in patients whose asthma was well controlled by these agents before pregnancy, especially if it is thought that changing formulations may jeopardize asthma control. Doses of ICS preparations are categorized as low, medium, and high.

Inhaled β-Agonists

Inhaled short-acting β-agonists are the rescue therapy of choice for asthma during pregnancy. Inhaled albuterol is the first-choice short-acting β-agonist for pregnant women because it has been studied the most extensively,[33] although other agents may be used if uniquely helpful or well tolerated. In one case-control study, the use of bronchodilators during pregnancy was associated with an increased risk for gastroschisis among infants (OR, 2.1; 95% CI, 1.2 to 3.6).[46] In another cohort study involving 4,558 women, there was an increased risk for cardiac defects in the infants of mothers exposed to bronchodilators during pregnancy (OR, 1.4; 95% CI, 1.1 to 1.7).[40] Another case-control study also supported this association (OR, 2.20; 95% CI, 1.05 to 4.61).[47] Data from a more recent population-based, multicenter, case-control study found a positive association between maternal asthma and use of inhaled bronchodilators (albuterol was the most commonly reported specific drug) and isolated esophageal atresia (adjusted OR, 2.39; 95% CI, 1.23 to 4.66) and omphalocele (adjusted OR, 4.13; 95% CI, 1.43 to 11.95) for users of both inhaled bronchodilators and ICS preparations. However, all of these observations may be a result of confounding. Asthma exacerbations may be associated with both increased use of bronchodilators and congenital malformations. In addition, factors such as obesity or lower socioeconomic status may be associated with both more severe asthma requiring more bronchodilators and congenital malformations. In general, patients should use up to two treatments of inhaled albuterol (two to six puffs) or nebulized albuterol at 20-minute intervals for most mild to moderate symptoms; higher doses can be used for severe symptom exacerbations.

The use of long-acting β-agonists is the preferred add-on controller therapy for asthma during pregnancy. This therapy should be added in patients whose symptoms are not controlled with the use of a medium-dose ICS. Because long-acting and short-acting inhaled β-agonists have similar pharmacology and toxicology, long-acting β-agonists are expected to have a safety profile similar to that of albuterol. Two long-acting β-agonist drugs are available: salmeterol and formoterol. Limited observational data exist on their use during pregnancy. A possible association between long-acting β-agonists and an increased risk for severe and even fatal asthma exacerbations has been observed in nonpregnant patients. As a result, long-acting β-agonists are no longer recommended as monotherapy for the treatment of asthma and are available in fixed combination preparations with an ICS. Expert panels suggest that the benefits of the use of long-acting β-agonists appear to outweigh the risks as long as they are used concurrently with an ICS.[48]

Leukotriene Modifiers

Both zafirlukast and montelukast are selective leukotriene receptor antagonists indicated for the maintenance treatment of asthma. Both are pregnancy category B; however, data on the use of leukotriene receptor antagonists during pregnancy are more limited. There is one published study involving 96 patients that supports their safety during pregnancy.[49] Another study of 180 montelukast-exposed pregnancies found no increase in baseline rate of major congenital malformations.[50] From 1997 to 2006, worldwide postmarketing surveillance of montelukast identified six reports of limb reduction defects in live-born offspring of women taking montelukast during pregnancy. This was the catalyst for a retrospective insurance claims cohort study comprising approximately 12 million covered lives and more than 277,000 pregnancies linked to a live birth outcome. Reassuringly, there were no events similar to the six postmarketing surveillance events of limb reduction defects among the 1,535 infants born to mothers in the montelukast cohort.[51] Montelukast is available as a once-daily medication, with doses variable based on age. For adults, the typical dose is 10 mg daily.

Cromolyn and Theophylline

Based on the superiority of ICS agents over cromolyn and theophylline in the prevention of asthma symptoms, they are considered alternative treatments for mild persistent asthma. Theophylline is also an alternative, but not preferred, add-on treatment for moderate to severe persistent asthma. Reassuring data on the use of cromolyn and theophylline in pregnant women have been published.[48] Theophylline use is also limited by its many adverse side effects and potential drug interactions resulting in possible toxicity. Serum levels should be monitored during pregnancy and maintained between 5 and 12 μL. Cromolyn is now only available as a nebulizer solution.

Oral Corticosteroids

Some patients with severe asthma may require regular oral corticosteroid use to achieve adequate asthma control. Oral corticosteroids are also typically part of the discharge regimen after an acute asthma episode. Doses are typically 40 to 60 mg in a single dose or two divided doses for 3 to 10 days. Oral corticosteroid use has been associated with an increased risk for preterm birth[9,33] and low birth weight infants[33] in 52 of 185 exposed women. An increased risk for orofacial clefts was reported in a meta-analysis of case-control studies,[52] but this increased risk was not confirmed in a recent large cohort study.[41] Because these risks would be less than the potential risks of a severe asthma exacerbation, which include maternal or fetal mortality, oral corticosteroids are recommended when indicated for the management of severe asthma during pregnancy.[48]

UNMET, FUTURE RESEARCH NEEDS

1. The availability of further safety information for asthma medications used during pregnancy
2. Strategies to assess and improve adherence to asthma medication use during pregnancy
3. Studies addressing the safety of asthma medications that can account for asthma control
4. Studies addressing the effect of asthma control on perinatal outcomes
5. Studies addressing the use of FeNO and markers of inflammation in the management of pregnant asthmatic patients
6. Determining whether the increased risk for respiratory infections in pregnant women compared with nonpregnant women plays a role in the loss of asthma control during pregnancy, and whether it is possible to reduce the frequency of these infections
7. Understanding the mechanisms behind the change in asthma course during pregnancy and being able to predict the course in an individual patient

CONCLUSION

Asthma is a common medical problem that may worsen during pregnancy. In addition to affecting maternal quality of life, uncontrolled asthma may lead to adverse perinatal outcomes. Awareness of proper treatment options for asthma during pregnancy is important for clinicians who care for pregnant patients in order to optimize maternal and infant health.

REFERENCES

1. Kwon HL, Belanger K, Bracken MB. Asthma prevalence among pregnant and childbearing-aged women in the United States: estimates from national health surveys. *Ann Epidemiol*. 2003;13(5):317–324.
2. Triche EW, Saftlas AF, Belanger K, Leaderer BP, Bracken MB. Association of asthma diagnosis, severity, symptoms, and treatment with risk of preeclampsia. *Obstet Gynecol*. 2004;104(3):585–593.
3. Jana N, Vasishta K, Saha SC, Khunnu B. Effect of bronchial asthma on the course of pregnancy, labour and perinatal outcome. *J Obstet Gynaecol*. 1995;21(3):227–232.
4. Stenius-Aarniala BS, Hedman J, Teramo KA. Acute asthma during pregnancy. *Thorax*. 1996;51(4):411–414.
5. Minerbi-Codish I, Fraser D, Avnun L, Glezerman M, Heimer D. Influence of asthma in pregnancy on labor and the newborn. *Respiration*. 1998;65(2):130–135.
6. Mihrshahi S, Belousova E, Marks GB, Peat JK, for the Childhood Asthma Prevention Team. Pregnancy and birth outcomes in families with asthma. *J Asthma*. 2003;40(2):181–187.
7. Stenius-Aarniala B, Piirila P, Teramo K. Asthma and pregnancy: a prospective study of 198 pregnancies. *Thorax*. 1988;43(1):12–18.
8. Dombrowski MP, Schatz M, Wise R, et al. Asthma during pregnancy. *Obstet Gynecol*. 2004;103(1):5–12.
9. Bracken MB, Triche EW, Belanger K, Saftlas A, Beckett WS, Leaderer BP. Asthma symptoms, severity, and drug therapy: a prospective study of effects on 2205 pregnancies. *Obstet Gynecol*. 2003;102(4):739–752.
10. Schatz M, Zeiger RS, Hoffman CP, et al. Perinatal outcomes in the pregnancies of asthmatic women: a prospective controlled analysis. *Am J Respir Crit Care Med*. 1995;151(4):1170–1174.
11. Firoozi F, Lemiere C, Ducharme FM, et al. Effect of maternal moderate to severe asthma on perinatal outcomes. *Respir Med*. 2010;104(9):1278–1287.
12. Blais L, Forget A. Asthma exacerbations during the first trimester of pregnancy and the risk of congenital malformations among asthmatic women. *J Allergy Clin Immunol*. 2008;121(6):1379–1384, 84 e1.
13. Schatz M, Dombrowski M, Wise R. Asthma morbidity during pregnancy can be preded by severity classification. *J Allergy Clin Immunol*. 2003;112:283–288.
14. Belanger K, Hellenbrand M, Holford T, Bracken M. Effect of pregnancy on maternal asthma symptoms and medication use. *Obstet Gynecol*. 2010;115:559–567.
15. Schatz M, Harden K, Forsythe A, et al. The course of asthma during pregnancy, post-partum, and with successive pregnancies: a prospective analysis. *J Allergy Clin Immunol*. 1988;81:509–517.
16. Gluck J, Gluck P. The effect of pregnancy on the course of asthma. *Immunol Allergy Clin N Am*. 2000;20:729–743.
17. Murphy VE, Gibson PG, Smith R, Clifton VL. Asthma during pregnancy: mechanisms

and treatment implications. *Eur Respir J.* 2005;25(4):731–750.
18. Louik C, Schatz M, Hernandez-Diaz S, Werler MM, Mitchell AA. Asthma in pregnancy and its pharmacologic treatment. *Ann Allergy Asthma Immunol.* 2010;105(2):110–117.
19. Cydulka R, Emerman C, Schreiber D, Molander K, Woodruff P, Camargo C. Acute asthma among pregnant women presenting to the emergency department. *Am J Respir Crit Care Med.* 1999;160:887–892.
20. McCallister J, Benninger C, Frey H, Phillips G, Mastronarde J. Pregnancy related treatment disparities of acute asthma exacerbations in the emergency department. *Respir Med.* 2011;105(10):1434–1440.
21. Murphy VE, Gibson P, Talbot PI, Clifton VL. Severe asthma exacerbations during pregnancy. *Obstet Gynecol.* 2005;106(5 Pt 1):1046–1054.
22. Sorri M, Hartikainen A, Karja I. Rhinitis during pregnancy. *Rhinology.* 1980;18(2):83–86.
23. Munn M, Groome L, Atterbury J. Pneumonia as a complication of pregnancy. *J Matern Fetal Med.* 1999;8:151–154.
24. Tamasi L, Somoskovi A, Muller V, et al. A population-based case-control study on the effect of bronchial asthma during pregnancy for congenital abnormalities of the offspring. *J Asthma.* 2006;43(1):81–86.
25. Bakhireva LN, Schatz M, Jones KL, Chambers CD. Asthma control during pregnancy and the risk of preterm delivery or impaired fetal growth. *Ann Allergy Asthma Immunol.* 2008;101(2):137–143.
26. Schatz M, Dombrowski MP, Wise R, et al. Spirometry is related to perinatal outcomes in pregnant women with asthma. *Am J Obstet Gynecol.* 2006;194(1):120–126.
27. Powell H, Murphy VE, Taylor DR, et al. Management of asthma in pregnancy guided by measurement of fraction of exhaled nitric oxide: a double-blind, randomised controlled trial. *Lancet.* 2011;378(9795):983–990.
28. Enriquez R, Wu P, Griffin MR, et al. Cessation of asthma medication in early pregnancy. *Am J Obstet Gynecol.* 2006;195(1):149–153.
29. Sawicki E, Stewart K, Wong S, Paul E, Leung L, George J. Management of asthma by pregnant women attending an Australian maternity hospital. *Aust N Z J Obstet Gynaecol.* 2012;52(2):183–188.
30. Lim AS, Stewart K, Abramson MJ, Ryan K, George J. Asthma during pregnancy: the experiences, concerns and views of pregnant women with asthma. *J Asthma.* 2012;49(5):474–479.
31. Lim A, Stewart K, Abramson M, George J. Management of pregnant women with asthma by Australian general practitioners. *BMC Fam Pract.* 2011;12:121.
32. Cimbollek S, Plaza V, Quirce S, et al. Knowledge, attitude and adherence of Spanish healthcare professionals to asthma management recommendations during pregnancy. *Allergol Immunopathol.* 2013;41(2):114–120.
33. Schatz M, Dombrowski MP, Wise R, et al. The relationship of asthma medication use to perinatal outcomes. *J Allergy Clin Immunol.* 2004;113(6):1040–1045.
34. Schatz M, Zeiger RS, Harden K, Hoffman CC, Chilingar L, Petitti D. The safety of asthma and allergy medications during pregnancy. *J Allergy Clin Immunol.* 1997;100(3):301–306.
35. Norjavaara E, de Verdier MG. Normal pregnancy outcomes in a population-based study including 2,968 pregnant women exposed to budesonide. *J Allergy Clin Immunol.* 2003;111(4):736–742.
36. Martel MJ, Rey E, Beauchesne MF, et al. Use of inhaled corticosteroids during pregnancy and risk of pregnancy induced hypertension: nested case-control study. *BMJ.* 2005;330(7485):230.
37. Kallen B, Rydhstroem H, Aberg A. Congenital malformations after the use of inhaled budesonide in early pregnancy. *Obstet Gynecol.* 1999;93(3):392–395.
38. Bakhireva LN, Jones KL, Schatz M, Johnson D, Chambers CD, for the Organization of Teratology Information Services Research Group. Asthma medication use in pregnancy and fetal growth. *J Allergy Clin Immunol.* 2005;116(3):503–509.
39. Breton MC, Beauchesne MF, Lemiere C, Rey E, Forget A, Blais L. Risk of perinatal mortality associated with inhaled corticosteroid use for the treatment of asthma during pregnancy. *J Allergy Clin Immunol.* 2010;126(4):772–777 e2.
40. Kallen B, Otterblad Olausson P. Use of anti-asthmatic drugs during pregnancy. 3. Congenital malformations in the infants. *Eur J Clin Pharmacol.* 2007;63(4):383–388.
41. Hyiid A, Molgaard-Nielesen D. Corticosteroid use during pregnancy and the risk of orofacial clefts. *CMAJ.* 2011;183:796–804.
42. Blais L, Beauchesne MF, Rey E, Malo JL, Forget A. Use of inhaled corticosteroids during the first trimester of pregnancy and the risk of congenital malformations among women with asthma. *Thorax.* 2007;62(4):320–328.
43. Hviid A, Mølgaard-Nielsen D. Corticosteroid use during pregnancy and the risk of orofacial clefts. *CMAJ.* 2011;183:796–804.

44. Blais L, Beauchesne MF, Lemiere C, Elftouh N. High doses of inhaled corticosteroids during the first trimester of pregnancy and congenital malformations. *J Allergy Clin Immunol.* 2009;124(6):1229–1234 e4.
45. Lin S, Munsie JPW, Herdt-Losavio ML, et al. Maternal asthma medication use and the risk of selected birth defects. *Pediatrics.* 2012;129: e317–e324.
46. Lin S, Munsie J, Herdt-Losavio M, et al. Maternal asthma medication use and the risk of gastroschisis. *Am J Epidemiol.* 2008;168:73–79.
47. Lin S, Herdt-Losavio M, Gensburg L, et al. Maternal asthma medication use and the risk of congenital heart defects. *Birth Defects Res A Clin Mol Teratol.* 2009;85:161–168.
48. Busse WW. NAEPP expert panel report. Managing asthma during pregnancy: recommendations for pharmacologic treatment—2004 update. *J Allergy Clin Immunol.* 2005;115(1):34–46.
49. Bakhireva LN, Jones KL, Schatz M, et al. Safety of leukotriene receptor antagonists in pregnancy. *J Allergy Clin Immunol.* 2007;119(3): 618–625.
50. Sarkar M, Koren G, Kalra S, et al. Montelukast use during pregnancy: a multicentre, prospective, comparative study of infant outcomes. *Eur J Clin Pharmacol.* 2009;65(12):1259–1264.
51. Nelsen LM, Shields KE, Cunningham ML, et al. Congenital malformations among infants born to women receiving montelukast, inhaled corticosteroids, and other asthma medications. *J Allergy Clin Immunol.* 2012;129(1): 251–254.e6.
52. Park-Wyllie L, Mazzotta P, Pastuszak A, et al. Birth defects after maternal exposure to corticosteroids: prospective cohort study and meta-analysis of epidemiologic studies. *Teratology.* 2000;62: 385–392.

SECTION SEVEN

PSYCHOLOGICAL ISSUES

28

PSYCHOLOGICAL FACTORS

COMORBID AND COEXISTING

Fulvio Braido, Tatiana Slavyanskaya, Revaz Sepiashvili, Ilaria Baiardini, and Giorgio Walter Canonica

KEY POINTS

- Different patient-related factors may influence the unsuccessful fulfillment of optimal levels of asthma control.
- An inadequate symptom perception is a common feature in asthma patients and depends on a wide variety of cognitive and affective variables.
- Some psychological factors such as alexithymia (difficulty in identifying and describing feelings and distinguishing between feelings and bodily sensations) and coping skills may play a crucial role in influencing the course of asthma and its daily management.
- Nonadherence to prescribed treatment is a relevant issue in asthma management; its reasons vary and depend on the patient, on the disease itself, on the treatment, and on the doctor–patient relationship.
- Frustration is a relevant mechanism of psychosomatic disorders in asthma that reduces psychological adaptation to the disease and has a negative impact on rehabilitation.
- Premorbid personality and social problems are risk factors for asthma development and management.
- Modifying ineffective coping strategies is more effective in improving outcomes than increasing disease state knowledge.
- The role of hyperventilation syndrome and psychoneurovegetoimmune abnormalities may influence clinical course and psychological disorder pathogenesis.
- Because psychological factors are crucial in asthma management, the opportunity of psychological interventions (including counseling, psychoeducational programs, psychological support, or psychotherapy) should be considered.

INTRODUCTION

The aim of asthma therapy is to reach and maintain disease control, minimizing symptoms, daily activity limitation, and the risks for life-threatening exacerbations and long-term morbidity.[1] Large, population-based studies demonstrate that the achievable level of control is not always reached. For instance, the Asthma Insights and Reality in Europe (AIRE) study, which involved more than 2,800 asthma patients living in different European countries, found that more than 50% of the interviewees reported the presence of daytime symptoms and that one out of three respondents experienced asthma-related sleep problems.[2] In the International Asthma Patient Insight Research (INSPIRE) study, in which 3,415 treated asthma adults were interviewed by telephone,[3] nearly 74% of subjects used a short-acting bronchodilator every day, and 51% had at least one exacerbation that required medical treatment in the past year.

The reasons that the aims of asthma treatment are not completely achieved may depend on different factors[4] (Table 28.1). Nevertheless, the patient plays a primary role in daily asthma management. The ideas that the patient has regarding asthma, the impact of the disease on daily life, the subjective interpretation of symptoms, and therapeutic adherence depend on psychological characteristics. Moreover, the disease itself may create psychological dysfunction. The aim of this review is to explore different patient-related factors that may influence the unsuccessful fulfillment of optimal levels of asthma control.

SPECIFIC PSYCHOLOGICAL FACTORS THAT LIKELY AFFECT ASTHMA

Patients' report of symptoms constitutes an important factor in determining the diagnosis of asthma and influences the treatment plan.[1] However, self-reported symptoms poorly correlate with pulmonary function measures. Patients may exhibit limited disease severity but describe high levels of dyspnea, or vice versa. This suggests that perception is not necessarily linearly related to the sensory input but rather is modulated by subjective factors.

The proportion of patients who report difficulty in recognizing their own degree of airway obstruction ranges from 15% to 60%, depending on the measurements used.[5] Poor symptom perception may result in an inadequate management of controller therapy and a consequent overuse of reliever medication. Abnormal perception of dyspnea is related to poor health outcomes and increased costs. In a 2-year follow-up, patients with both increased and decreased symptom perception exhibited a four-fold increased rate of visits to the emergency department, a five-fold increased hospitalization rate, and a six-fold increased rate of nearly fatal or fatal asthma attacks.[6] These findings demonstrate that perception is a key factor in asthma management.

The accuracy of symptom perception is not a stable characteristic and instead depends on a wide variety of cognitive and affective variables. The medical literature suggests that factors such as emotional state, previous life experiences, attributions, contextual information, attentional and learning processes, expectation and prior asthma experiences, personality traits, and psychopathologic disturbances can profoundly affect the perception of dyspnea, often independent of airflow obstruction.

Many subjects with asthma learn to associate negative situations and emotional distress with difficult breathing and are thus likely to overperceive dyspnea. Studies in healthy volunteers and asthma patients show that subjects with high negative emotionality report more dyspnea than those with low negative emotionality. Similarly, the experimental induction of negative affective states in healthy individuals and patients increases reports of respiratory sensations such as dyspnea. The feeling of unpleasantness related to dyspnea, rather than its sensory intensity, is related to affective influences.[7] Individuals with asthma may underperceive dyspnea when experiencing a positive emotional state, potentially reducing the use of prescribed medication.[8] The discrepancy between subjective dyspnea and functional capacity, the effects of inaccurate perception on disease outcomes, and the discordance between a measure of lung function and dyspnea perception should be considered because they may suggest the need for more careful monitoring.

Table 28.1. Factors That Influence the Achievement of Asthma Control

REASONS FOR POOR CONTROL	VARIABLES	EXAMPLES
Disease related	Presence of comorbidities	Rhinitis, rhinosinusitis, gastroesophageal reflux, obstructive sleep apnea
	Exacerbating factors	Ongoing occupational or allergen exposures
Patient related	Sociodemographic factors	Female sex, education, age
	Adherence	Undertreatment, overtreatment, irregular visits to health care providers, difficulties in monitoring of symptoms, no lifestyle modifications
	Psychiatric comorbidity	Anxiety, depressive disorders
	Psychological characteristics	Alexithymia, coping style
	Perceptions	Tendency to tolerate symptoms, exacerbations, and lifestyle limits as an inevitable consequence of asthma
	Expectations	Low expectations about the possibility of controlling the disease
	Behaviors	Smoking habits
		Poor inhaler technique
	Knowledge	Inadequate or incorrect information about the disease and its treatment
Doctor related	Underdiagnosis	Limited awareness of asthma prevalence
	Knowledge of current guidelines	Lack of consciousness and familiarity about guidelines
	Attitude toward guidelines	Difficulty in accepting a particular document, or the concept of the guidelines
		Lack of confidence in personal abilities to put the recommendations into practice
		Expectations of failure in following guidelines
	Guideline implementation	Difficulty in changing deep-seated routines

CLINICAL FEATURES OF ASTHMA AND PATIENT PERCEPTION

Alexithymia

Alexithymia may play a crucial role in influencing the course of asthma and its daily management. Interesting suggestions come from the research about alexithymia,[9] a term derived from the Greek *alexis* ("no words") and *thymos* ("emotion"), which is a personality trait characterized by difficulty in identifying and describing feelings and distinguishing between feelings and bodily sensations. Individuals with alexithymia have an impaired ability to build mental representations of emotions, and therefore they misinterpret physical symptoms related to emotions (e.g., tachycardia or tremors) as symptoms of somatic disease. Alexithymia may be considered as a possible risk factor for a variety of medical conditions because it may increase susceptibility to disease development. Various instruments to detect the presence of alexithymia are available, and the most widely used is the TAS-20.[10]

Available literature concerning alexithymia and asthma helps to identify the reasons for nonoptimal disease management. Most data are focused on patients with extremely severe or nearly fatal attacks, suggesting that this personality trait is associated with disease exacerbations. A significantly higher prevalence of alexithymia occurs among patients who have experienced a nearly fatal asthma attack (36%) than among patients with matched asthma severity who have not experienced a nearly fatal attack (13%)[10] or the general population (5% to 13%). Furthermore, a study evaluating 270 asthmatic subjects during a severe attack showed that alexithymic patients reported significantly lower scores for nine symptom and sign categories on the Asthma Symptom Checklist scale.[10] These results provide evidence that alexithymic patients underestimate both physical and emotional components of asthma exacerbations, independent of the severity of the disease. A greater frequency of asthma-induced, recurrent hospitalization occurs in alexithymic patients (37.4% versus 28.4% over 6 months), suggesting that patients' difficulty in expressing symptom intensity and frequency may lead to the underestimation of asthma severity.[10] In addition, a paper by Feldman and colleagues[11] showed that higher alexithymia scores are associated with an increased report of asthma symptoms and with decreased pulmonary function, as indicated by the ratio of forced expiratory volume in 1 second (FEV_1) to forced vital capacity (FVC). Finally, the presence of alexithymia has been associated with lower levels of asthma control, poor treatment adherence, and reduced health-related quality of life (HRQoL).[12] In particular, there is a correlation between alexithymia and intentional nonadherence (i.e., the result of an active choice).[13]

In a real-life study of a large sample of asthma patients, the prevalence of alexithymia was 20%, compared with 5% to 13% in the general population, indicating that it is a common feature that characterizes almost one out of five patients with asthma.[14] Alexithymia did not correlate with disease severity but did associate with more severe disease experiences and outcomes. In alexithymic patients, asthma is less controlled, independent of the Global Initiative for Asthma (GINA) classification, and the lack of control leads to a reduced HRQoL. Also, the illness perception was different. Alexithymia altered not only the recognition of sensations and symptoms but also judgments, thoughts, and emotions related to respiratory allergy. Alexithymic asthmatic patients reported more serious negative consequences and emotions, affecting physical, psychological, and social aspects of life. Patients with alexithymia tended to perceive and to live their disease as a cyclical disorder, not a chronic condition. Alexithymia seemed also to be associated with higher levels of distress.

Coping Strategies

With the emphasis on self-management of asthma, the role of coping strategies is receiving increasing attention. The study of coping comes from psychological theories of stress management that describe how people deal with stressful events and ongoing situations.[15] Suffering from a chronic disease such as asthma predisposes individuals to a degree of stress that requires continuous personal adaptation at different levels: cognitive, emotional, behavioral, and social. Coping efforts may help one modify the situation (e.g., to improve asthma control), change the meaning of the experience (e.g., to accept the disease), or mitigate the stress related to asthma management (e.g., to be optimistic about the disease course). These relationships are not unique to asthma because other chronic disease outcomes (disease control, morbidity, mortality, quality of life) are associated with coping styles.[16]

Some researchers have distinguished coping strategies as problem focused or emotion focused. Problem-focused coping is directed toward managing or modifying a stressful situation, or it involves addressing the problem that causes distress. Emotion-focused coping directs efforts to reducing emotional distress caused by the stressful event and to managing or regulating emotions that accompany or result from the stressor.

Active coping strategies addressed directly to the problem are generally considered to be adaptive, whereas passive, emotion-focused coping is related to poor adjustment to illness.

Research suggests avoidant coping (ignoring, denying, or avoiding a problem) is associated with poor HRQoL among adult asthma patients,[17,18] whereas active coping (taking an active approach to the problem, whether cognitive or behavioral) is associated with better HRQoL scores.

Asthmatic patients with effective coping skills will experience less psychological morbidity, a feeling of greater personal control over asthma, and better long-term management of the disease.[19] These effective coping skills are characterized by maintaining a positive vision of the disease without minimizing its potential danger and by using active, cognitive strategies and flexible and diversified behaviors.

In contrast, the use of avoidance strategies is associated with a lower level of asthma control, with a worsening of clinical outcomes, and with a greater number of hospitalizations, unscheduled health care visits, and episodes of nearly fatal asthma.[20] Patients with ineffective coping strategies tend to have difficult-to-treat asthma.[21] For example, patients identified as having brittle asthma tend to delay seeking care for more than 7 days after a change in symptoms. Asthmatic subjects with avoidant strategy preferences are less adherent to medical therapy and prone to reliever drug abuse and to inadequate controller drug use.

Modifying coping strategies is more effective than enhanced disease state knowledge in improving asthma treatment outcomes. Coping skills training, based on social cognitive theory, stresses the use of adaptive coping methods and problem-solving skills. These skills can increase a subjective sense of competence and self-efficacy in dealing with a wide range of daily demands and health issues. Educational interventions aimed at improving coping strategies are effective in increasing the flexibility and functionality of the strategies, with benefits not only to asthma symptoms but also to psychological functioning, sense of well-being, and anxiety.[22]

A large, cross-sectional survey explored coping in asthma management. The aim of the study was to provide a detailed global picture of the issue, investigating the use of coping strategies of patient and physician perspectives. A total of 6,474 patients and 3,089 general practitioners were involved.[16] Active coping strategies were described by approximately one-half of the patients, whereas the physicians reported a significantly lower frequency of effective coping strategies in their patients. A similar percentage of patients and a greater percentage of physicians reported the use of negative strategies, with "rely on fate or faith" chosen more frequently by patients than physicians. Age and level of education did not seem to influence the coping style, but females were more prone to passive and avoidant behaviors. General practitioners had a greater ability than specialists to identify the use of active approaches rather than passive and avoidant ones, using the clinical opportunity to discuss the behaviors associated with effective asthma management. The degree of concordance between the choices of patients and general practitioners was only fair, indicating inadequate patient–physician communication.

Other Issues

The problems of inadequate understanding and memory, frequent in elderly people and in patients with chronic diseases, deserve special attention. Even for young patients without major comorbidities, it is sometimes difficult to remember complex treatment plans. After 5 minutes, the patient has forgotten about one-half of the verbal instructions that the physician provided; after 24 hours, the patient recalls on average only one-third of the information received from the pharmacist. The presence of psychological and psychiatric problems is a risk factor that interferes with adherence maintenance.[23] Recognizing and addressing personality issues and psychiatric disease will improve treatment outcomes.

The role of family and friends' support is crucial because they can enhance adherence to therapy through encouraging the initiation and maintenance of behaviors useful for disease management (e.g., proper use of medication, changes in habits and lifestyle). This aspect has been studied most of all in reference to children and adolescents, in whom higher levels of family support were associated with greater asthma control and quality of life and the use of most appropriate coping strategies.[24]

PHARMACOLOGIC TREATMENT: MEDICATION ADHERENCE

The problem of nonadherence to prescribed treatment is a relevant issue in asthma management: a substantial number of patients do not get the maximum benefit of medical treatment, resulting in poor health outcomes, lower sense of well-being, and increased health care costs.[25] The term "compliance" refers to how much a patient's behavior in terms of drug consumption corresponds to the doctor's prescriptions. This term involves a passive role of the patient, as "executor" of the physician's instructions.

The introduction of the term "adherence" has widened the area of observation: it refers to a collaboration between doctor and patient characterized by a positive sharing of the therapeutic choices and an internalization of the medical prescriptions by the patient.[25] Adherence is enhanced by regular visits to health care providers, along with monitoring of symptoms and reemphasis of the avoidance of aggravating factors, changes in lifestyle, and correct management of the therapeutic regimen.

Nonadherence to the therapeutic plan is a serious problem to be addressed in the management of chronic disease. The results of a survey carried out by the World Health Organization (WHO) and published in 2003[26] show that approximately 30% of patients follow medical prescriptions "correctly," 50% or less of patients partially observe them, and 20% (up to 50% in some cases) of patients demonstrate low levels of adherence. Taking into consideration bronchial asthma, adherence to treatment likely is quite low and, according to the WHO, it varies from 28% to 43%. These data indicate that more than 50% of patients do not take the prescribed medications correctly.

The chronic course of many diseases is often characterized by asymptomatic phases or periods without immediate or short-term risks. These factors contribute to nonadherence to treatment. Also, therapies whose objective is prevention are likely to lead to nonadherence because of the inability of the patient to judge value.

In one of his famous works, Roth[27] states, "If a patient declares he takes the drugs regularly, often it isn't so; if a patient declares that he sometimes forgets some dose, he is usually underestimating the deviation degree from the prescriptions; if a patient says he did not take the drugs, this is usually true." Roth provides a picture that probably is too negative: according to his idea, the patient is considered a deceiver who tries to hide his nonfulfillment, which separates him from social desirability. According to self-report of treated patients, Roth's vision is justified. The self-report usually provides unreliable data with respect to adherence or nonadherence to treatment. For instance, during a study carried out by Spector on patients suffering from asthma treated with drugs by aerosol,[28] adherence was recorded both with an electronic system that registered every inhalation and entries into a personal diary. The results show that 50% of the time, patients recorded false consumptions.

There are many causes of nonadherence. Some depend on factors external to the patient (Table 28.2), whereas others depend on patient characteristics. For example, children, adolescents, and elderly people have characteristics linked to their age that can affect adherence (i.e., children may lack motivation for understanding of the treatment, adolescents may harbor unrealistic optimism, and elderly people may have cognitive impairment).

The patient's perspective of the disease is also crucial. An inadequate understanding of asthma and naïve beliefs regarding treatment (e.g., fear of corticosteroids) are factors

Table 28.2. Causes of Nonadherence Not Dependent on the Patient

Factors linked to the patient	• Presence of physical disorders
	• Cognitive difficulties
	• Psychiatric comorbidities
	• Age (children, adolescents, and elderly patients present high risk for nonadherence)
	• Knowledge
	• Expectations
	• Social and family support
	• Coping style
Factors linked to the disease	• Chronicity
	• Symptom stability
	• Absence of symptoms
Factors linked to the treatment	• High number of daily doses
	• Presence of side effects
	• Complexity of the therapeutic regimes
	• Ease of use
	• Costs
Factors related to the doctor–patient relationship	• Bad relationship
	• Inappropriate doctor or patient behavior

that interfere with proper management. The importance of the understanding of the disease is noted in both mild and severe disease. Although symptoms are important in asthma management, the patient's perception of dyspnea will influence overuse and underuse of therapy.[29] The patient must understand that asthma is more than symptoms if adherence to preventive therapy is to be achieved.

EMOTIONAL STATE AND PSYCHOSOMATIC DISORDERS IN ASTHMA

The asthma clinical course is characterized by the combination of somatic and neurogenic symptoms and self-awareness coupled with an inflammatory airway disease. Frustration and emotional stress are of great importance because these influence symptom perception and possibly somatic pathology. Emotional responses in chronic asthma are characterized by anxiety and emotional stress, negative self-perception, hypochondriasis, and anxiety or depression. Asthma exacerbation duration and frequency increase as emotional stresses increase. Poorly controlled asthma in children is associated with intolerance of negative circumstances and limited independent productive conflict (especially domestic) resolution. All these factors contribute to personality degradation, negative experience, and destructive behavior fixation in children. As asthma severity and duration increase, anxiety and depression are supplemented with alexithymia, hypochondriasis, and asthenia. The longer the maladaptive characteristics persist, the more difficult it is to restore psychological and somatic function and coping skills.

Domestic relation disturbances are among relevant life events that are regarded as unpleasant and frustrating or emotionally stressful in patients with asthma. Pathologic abnormalities of personality traits that occur in childhood are often fixed and persist into adult life. This substantially reduces social psychological adaptation and creates a negative impact on medical rehabilitation.

PREMORBID PERSONALITY AND SOCIAL MALADAPTATION IN ASTHMATIC PATIENTS

Premorbid personality types demonstrate basic features, traits, and individual characteristics before mental disorders occur. Asthma, having both physical and emotional components, significantly affects a patient's psyche and aggravates the patient's premorbid personality. Premorbid personality aggravation by chronic psychological stress can result in abnormal individual development. Asthma duration determines psychosocial and emotional development, although some degree of emotional distress is inevitable in somatic disorders.[30]

Considering the fact that asthma occurs during the course of personality establishment (generally in the first 10 years of life), it is difficult, if not impossible, to define an "asthmatic personality type" or a child's "asthmatic character." Likewise, there are no typical premorbid traits common to asthma, although chronic anxiety is emphasized by many investigators. However, children predisposed to asthma have different combinations of certain personal characteristics and behavior abnormalities that are typical of psychosomatic patients. Unusual sensibility, anxiety, reticence, predisposition to increased frustration, distrustfulness, excitability, emotional variability, touchiness, impressionability, and negative emotional dominance, in combination with high standards and attitudes, are among personality traits observed before asthma manifestation. Psychological maladaptation in asthmatic patients is often one of four stable symptom complex variants: asthenia with physical weakness, asthenia with psychological weakness, dysthymic disorder, or psychovegetative state. In asthmatic patients, a high frequency of borderline neurotic psychological conditions is observed (62.1% in exogenous asthma, 86.7% in endogenous asthma, 75.5% in general asthma).[31] Neurotic personality types include dysthymia, anxiety with phobias, and hysterical conditions. Additional maladaptive personality characteristics in adolescent asthma include emotional instability, poor self-acceptance, stress instability, and social adaptation difficulties.[32]

Characteristic mechanisms of compensation and decompensation have an important role in somatic psychological disorders in asthma patients.[33] An introverted type of psychosomatic constitution significantly affects asthma prognosis.[34]

Family and other social factors have a negative impact on asthma in childhood. The etiology of neurosis in children is frequently linked with unfavorable family conditions due to inappropriate parental behavior. Mother's Neurotic features in the mother as well as a deficiency of emotional and physical contact between mother and child are considered ineffective pathodynamic factors.[35]

Therefore premorbid characteristics of emotional personality, constitution of a child, and low level of familiar social behavior in the premorbid period are relevant for subsequent psychopathologic development. Premorbid personality type may be important for diagnosis, prognosis, psychotherapy method selection, and rehabilitation of psychological disorders in asthma.

HYPERVENTILATING SYNDROME IN ASTHMA

Asthma is characterized by an abnormal increase in respiratory rate of predominantly thoracic breathing and bouts of significant shortness of breath. Hyperventilating with asthma can provoke an attack of breathlessness in adults and in children.[36,37]

The leading causes of hyperventilation syndrome (HVS) with asthma are neurogenic and psychogenic effects.[38] HVS is sometimes called psychogenic dyspnea or neurogenic hyperventilation.

HVS may include breathing disturbances, fainting, cephalgia, cardialgia, mental disorders, paresthesias, nausea, and, in very severe cases, tetany. Patients with HVS experience a feeling of air deficiency, breathing difficulties, chest pressure, lump in throat, chest tightness associated with an acute need for air (usually characterized by a sensation of inability to get sufficient air inhaled), and an obsessive desire to breathe deeply. Usually, breathing is rapid or deep with disorder of rhythm and regularity of respiratory cycles. Abdominal breathing is almost completely replaced by upper chest and neck breathing. HVS may be associated with emotional reactions (fear, depression, melancholy, explosions of laughter) and behavioral disorders.[39-42] The affected patient experiences panic from sensing the inability to breathe. A bout of breathlessness is accompanied by strong fear. Although air contains enough oxygen, a patient feels unsatisfied. Fear of choking generates anxiety and a sense of abandonment, which is backed by the experiences of one's peers. In children, HVS is associated with episodic severe shortness of breath, subjective feeling of lack of air, sighs, anxiety, emotional lability, headaches, heart palpitations, and pain in the abdomen during the attack. Often, attacks are associated with emotional stress or physical strain.[43] In addition to the psychological effects of HVS, asthma occurring in children after physical activity, at least partly, is a result of the effects of hyperventilation on the respiratory tract.

Objective measures of HVS have been suggested in children. These include breathing frequency and the CO_2 concentration in the final portions of the expired air (FetCCb).[44] Measuring oxygen and CO_2 concentration with an arterial blood gas may be helpful, typically with normal oxygen concentration and a respiratory alkalosis with decreased CO_2 concentration. Blood CO_2 may be decreased even between HVS episodes, suggesting that an abnormality of CO_2 detection by the carotid body may contribute to HVS. Because HVS affects many human systems and functions, the effectiveness of the treatment depends on the methods that will allow interruption of the "vicious circle" of events that trigger this syndrome. Effective treatment of HVS is multidimensional and addresses all major parts of the pathogenesis. There are three types of effects in HVS with the treatment process[45]:

1. Psychological impact on patients with HVS is achieved with the correction of two interrelated areas: cognitive and affective. Reducing the emotional tension, anxiety, worry, and fear to a large extent contributes to the patient's understanding of the physiologic mechanisms of HVS.

2. Impact on neurophysiologic and neurochemical mechanisms of HVS is provided by the prescription of psychotropic, vegetative-trophic drugs as well as medicines that reduce the increased neuromuscular excitability.

3. Effects on pulmonary function are achieved using arbitrary mechanisms of regulation of breathing. With this treatment, there are two methods that are generally used: respiratory gymnastics and the method of regulation of breathing through the use of biofeedback. Thus, the condition of asthma patients with HVS is improved by comprehensive therapy, which, in addition to bronchodilator therapy, includes breathing exercises designed to maintain the normal pattern of respiration when there is no attack. Depending on the seriousness of the problem, the treatment may be complemented by psychological consultation and psychotherapy.

PSYCHONEUROVEGETOIMMUNE ABNORMALITIES IN ASTHMA

Asthma is characterized by disturbances of central nervous system (CNS) functional status and cerebral circulatory dynamics depending on respiratory tract pathology. The association of psychoemotional abnormalities with vegetative dystonia syndrome and cerebral hemodynamic disturbances, as well as with lung ventilation-perfusion disturbances, argues that psychovegetative syndrome may be important for asthma pathogenesis.[46,47] CNS function abnormalities are observed in the course of asthma exacerbation as well as during remissions. Total left-hemispheric dominance is typical of most (75%) asthmatic patients, thus demonstrating possible psychophysiologic maladaptation in stress conditions.[34]

In moderate and severe asthma, changes in brain electrical activity, cerebral hemodynamics, and cognitive functions are observed in 75% of patients; however, these phenomena are absent in mild asthma.[48] In asthmatic children, there are significant abnormalities in cognitive functions in terms of short-term imaginative and verbal memory volume decrease (by 35% and 62%, respectively) compared with healthy children. These studies demonstrate greater neurologic system vulnerability in asthma. Neurovegetative regulation systems status is another relevant aspect of neuroimmune dysfunction in asthma. The balance of sympathetic and parasympathetic vegetative autonomic neurologic activity is abnormal in asthma. At the vegetative regulation level, parasympathetic activity (but not sympathetic, as in healthy individuals) increases in response to an emotional stress test, whereas vegetative neurologic activity that is typical of healthy persons is inactive. Asthmatic patients with baseline dominance of sympathetic activity in their vegetative tonus are characterized by high personal anxiety. Reactive anxiety increase is accompanied by sympathetic nervous system stimulation. In initial vagotonia (parasympathotonia), disease progression is more rapid and severe, whereas personal anxiety appears to be lower and depends on parasympathetic activity level at rest.[34,46]

In asthma, the basic psychoneurovegetoimmune pattern represents interaction of the immune system with individual emotional reactivity and cerebral and vegetative activity. Pathogenically relevant psychological factors such as anxiety, alexithymia, hostility, and aggression are associated with immune status.[32,49-57]

Studies provide some evidence of different system interactions and physiologic psychoimmune, neuroimmune, and vegetoimmune coupling in normal and pathologic conditions.[49] Right hemisphere frontal cortex stimuli in asthmatic patients have no effect on natural killer (CD16+) cell percentage, in contrast to healthy individuals. A decrease in the concentration of CD16+ cells is predicted as psychological defense intensity increases. Phagocyte activity is reduced; parasympathetic stimuli have no effects on phagocytosis, and its suppression is predicted by high-order neurosis. Subacute and chronic stresses affect humoral immunity and provoke regulatory dysfunction of general homeostasis. Humoral immune activation is typical of asthma. B cell (CD20+) percentage increase is expected with depression, select cortical stimulation, parasympathetic vegetative stimulation, and immunoglobulin E concentration.

The reduction of psychoneurovegetoimmune coupling in asthmatic patients represents a common biologic pattern that reflects a breaking of normal interactions between functional systems in a pathologic condition based on emotional stress. Pathologic intersystem relations prevent normal functioning of different immune system components and potentiate abnormalities. Combined disturbances of humoral immunity, psychoemotional reactivity, central and vegetative nervous system activity, pathologic intersystem relations, and significant disorganization of psychoneurovegetoimmune integration are typical.

Therefore asthma is characterized by increasing dissociation of psychoneurovegetoimmune coupling as a result of physiologic interactions between neural networks and immune system activity "autonomy." This condition is also characterized by the development of alternative psychoneurovegetoimmune coupling that reflects pathologic intersystem relations affecting the immune system.

FEATURES OF THE DIAGNOSIS, THERAPY, AND PREVENTION OF ASTHMA, TAKING INTO ACCOUNT THEIR PSYCHOSOMATIC DISORDERS

Psychological characteristics of children and adolescents suffering from asthma affect such aspects as emotional responses (anxiety, aggression, depression, hypochondriasis, hysteria, psychoasthenia, emotional instability, fragility to stress, social maladaptation), protective mechanisms, coping strategies, interpersonal relations, quality of life, and the properties of the vegetative nervous system.[58-60] Continuous age-specific dynamics, starting from the antenatal period, problems of perinatal and postnatal development of the child, and the influence of the education of mothers and families require integrated age-sensitive diagnosis and detection of psychosomatic conditions in children and adolescents. According to several authors,[34,43,47,53,61] comprehensive evaluation of the neurovegetative status of patients with asthma is

Table 28.3. Recommended Diagnostic Methods for Assessment of Neurovegetative Status of Patients with Asthma

	NAME OF METHOD	ASSIGN METHOD
1.	A method of spectral analysis of heart rate variability or cardiography	Evaluation of vegetative homeostasis
2.	Electroencephalography	Definition of bioelectric brain activity
3.	Computer rheoencephalography or duplex ultrasound scan of brain vessels	The study of cerebral blood flow
4.	Method of cognitive evoked potential	Applied to study the functions of sensor systems (somatosensory, visual, auditory) and systems of the brain responsible for cognitive processes (rational knowledge)
5.	Eysenck test	Intelligence quotient (IQ)
6.	Luscher test	Projective personality research methodology based on subjective preference of color incentives
7.	Neuropsychological testing	For early detection of encephalopathy in allergic asthma
8.	Questionnaire for the identification of alexithymia	Predisposition to alexithymia
9.	Methods for determination of the individual profile of functional brain asymmetry	To determine dominance of left or right cerebral hemispheres

appropriate and should include vegetative status and neurophysiologic and psychological examination (Table 28.3).

The increase in the incidence of asthma, increased severity of the disease, awareness of an increase in the neuropsychological pathogenesis of the disease, presence of concomitant allergic and psychological disorders, and therapeutic resistance of some patients to basic antiinflammatory drug therapy suggest that the treatment of asthma requires consideration of psychosocial factors.[61] Therefore, in some patients with asthma, psychotherapy may be necessary. The greatest effect of psychotherapeutic interventions occurs if treatment is started before the onset of irreversible pathophysiologic changes. Many psychotherapeutic options and other nondrug methods can be used for correction of psychological disorders, but these unfortunately are not sufficiently utilized. In Table 28.4, indications for various nonmedication methods of treatment and rehabilitation of patients with asthma are provided.[53]

Modern psychotherapeutic methods are individualized and are based on a biopsychosocial approach. Psychotherapy coupled with management of airway inflammation is more effective than medical management alone.[31,34,47,61] Recognition of and intervention in psychological dysfunction early in the asthma disease process may enhance the effectiveness of intervention.[46] Corrective strategies for primary psychoprophylaxis of psychosomatic diseases may include identification of the risk for the development of psychosomatic diseases, improved awareness and encouragement of expression of negative emotions, and development of skills of self-regulation.[44] Recognizing and addressing

Table 28.4. Psychopharmacologic, Psychotherapeutic, and Other Nondrug Methods of Treatment and Rehabilitation of Patients with Asthma

METHODS OF PSYCHOLOGICAL CORRECTION OF ASTHMA PATIENTS
(BASED ON THE AVAILABLE LITERATURE)

Psychopharmacotherapy	**Psychotropic drugs** (e.g., nootropic drugs, antidepressants, antipsychotics, tranquilizers)	
Psychotherapy	**Nonmedicated methods**	
Individual group/family therapy	Indications for use	Inadequate response to disease, which complicates the full rehabilitation
		Inadequate response of family members to the disease
		State of psychological crisis
		Related mental disorders
		History of personal and microsocial risk factors
		Presence in relatives of the psychosomatic models of adaptation to stress
		Existence of mental factors in etiopathogenesis of disease
		Possible secondary neurotization as a consequence of somatic disease process
		Dynamic transformation of personality features of the disease
	Varieties of therapy	Hypnosuggestive therapy
		Autogenic training
		Neurolinguistic programming
		Gestalt therapy
		Music therapy
		Game therapy
		Art therapy
		Positive psychotherapy
		Cognitive-behavioral psychotherapy
		Body-oriented psychotherapy
	Principles of group psychotherapy	Clarification of the nature of disease and its treatment
		Training in appropriate types of behavior
		Mastering the techniques of relaxation and breathing
		Having open discussion within the group
		Promoting interaction within the group

Table 28.4. (Continued)

METHODS OF PSYCHOLOGICAL CORRECTION OF ASTHMA PATIENTS
(BASED ON THE AVAILABLE LITERATURE)

Other nonmedicated methods	
Respiratory gymnastics	Autogenic training or functional training options. The process of free respiratory exercises with the gradual involvement of all muscles involved in the physical act of breathing facilitates the discharge of phlegm. This is the positive impact of respiratory gymnastics, which increases the drainage function of the bronchial tree.
Therapeutic massage	Massage helps to relieve fatigue of muscles, increase efficiency, and achieve easier phlegm discharge. Self-massage is recommended for muscles that prevent the passage of air, chest, collarbone, neck, and throat. In this way the attack can be stopped.
Climatotherapy	The question of the impact of climate change always arises when treating patients with asthma, and it is one of the most difficult to solve.
Acupuncture (the impact of using needles on biologically active points)	Acupuncture can be used in different forms and stages of bronchial asthma; it can also be recommended for antirecurrent treatment.

psychological dysfunction in asthma optimally require interaction of a psychologist or psychiatrist with the respiratory specialist.[29,46]

UNMET, FUTURE RESEARCH NEEDS

1. Asthma trials do not effectively address psychological comorbidity in trial design.
2. Improved clinical outcomes require improved recognition and strategies, particularly for anxiety and alexithymia, coping strategies, and symptom misperception.
3. Ideally, clinical trials that incorporate these challenges would provide better solutions.

CONCLUSION

Asthma is a common condition that occurs in all age groups. The chronicity and variability of the disease, coupled with the potential anxiety-provoking symptoms, result in the patient's perception of the disease being influenced by psychological comorbidities, life stressors, and patient perceptions and beliefs as well as asthma severity. The complex interaction between psychological factors and airway disease factors needs to be addressed to optimize therapy and asthma control.

ACKNOWLEDGMENTS

The authors acknowledge Dr. Marianna Bruzzone for linguistic assistance with the manuscript.

REFERENCES

1. Global Initiative for Asthma (GINA). Global strategy for asthma management and prevention, 2006. Available at: http://www.ginasthma.org. Accessed January 2010.
2. Rabe KF, Vermeire PA, Soriano JB, Maier WC. Clinical management of asthma in 1999: the Asthma Insights and Reality in Europe (AIRE) study. *Eur Respir J.* 2000;16:802–807.
3. Partridge MR, van der Molen T, Myrseth SE, Busse WW. Attitudes and actions of asthma patients on regular maintenance therapy: the INSPIRE study. *BMC Pulm Med.* 2006;6:13.

4. Haughney J, Price D, Kaplan A, et al. Achieving asthma control in practice: understanding the reasons of poor control. *Respir Med.* 2008;102:1681–1693.
5. Janssens T, Verleden G, De Peuter S, Van Diest I, Van den Bergh O. Inaccurate perception of asthma symptoms: a cognitive-affective framework and implications for asthma treatment. *Clin Psychol Rev.*
6. r-Yanay N, Weiner P. The risk of hospitalization and near-fatal and fatal asthma in relation to the perception of dyspnea. *Chest.* 2002;121:329–333.
7. von Leupoldt A, Taube K, Henkhus M, Dahme B, Magnussen H. The impact of affective states on the perception of dyspnea in patients with chronic obstructive pulmonary disease. *Biol Psychol.* 2010;84:129–134.
8. Rietveld S, van Beest I. Rollercoaster asthma: when positive emotional stress interferes with dyspnea perception. *Behav Res Ther.* 2007;45:977–987.
9. Taylor GJ, Bagby RM, Parker JDA. *Disorders of Affect Regulation: Alexithymia in Medical and Psychiatric Illness.* Cambridge, UK: Cambridge University Press; 1997:26–45.
10. Baiardini I, Abbà S, Ballauri M, Vuillermoz G, Braido F. Alexithymia and chronic diseases: the state of the art. *G Ital Med Lav Ergon.* 2011;33:A47–A52.
11. Feldman JM, Lehrer PM, Hochron SM. The predictive value of the Toronto Alexithymia Scale among patients with asthma. *J Psychosom Res.* 2002;53:1049–1052
12. Chugg K, Barton C, Antic R, Crockett A. The impact of alexithymia on asthma patient management and communication with health care providers: a pilot study. *J Asthma.* 2009;46:126–129.
13. Axelsson M, Emilsson M, Brink E, Lundgren J, Torén K, Lötvall J. Personality, adherence, asthma control and health-related quality of life in young adult asthmatics. *Respir Med.* 2009;103:1033–1040.
14. Baiardini I, Braido F, Ferraioli G, et al. Pitfalls in respiratory allergy management: alexithymia and its impact on patient-reported outcomes. *J Asthma.* 2011;48:25–32.
15. Lazarus RS, Folkman S. *Stress Appraisal and Coping.* New York: Springer; 1984.
16. Braido F, Baiardini I, Bordo A, et al. Coping with asthma: is the physician able to identify patient's behaviour? *Respir Med.* 2012;106:1625–1630.
17. Adams RJ, Wilson D, Smith BJ, Ruffin RE. Impact of coping and socioeconomic factors on quality of life in adults with asthma. *Respirology.* 2004;9:87–95.
18. Hesselink AE, Penninx BW, Schlösser MA, et al. The role of coping resources and coping style in quality of life of patients with asthma or COPD. *Qual Life Res.* 2004;13:509–518.
19. Barton C, Clarke D, Sulaiman N, Abramson M. Coping as a mediator of psychosocial impediments to optimal management and control of asthma. *Respir Med.* 2003;97:747–761.
20. Adams RJ, Smith BJ, Ruffin RE. Factors associated with hospital admissions and repeat emergency department visits for adults with asthma. *Thorax.* 2000;55:566–573.
21. Miles JF, Garden GM, Tunnicliffe WS, Cayton RM, Ayres JG. Psychological morbidity and coping skills in patients with brittle and non-brittle asthma: a case-control study. *Clin Exp Allergy.* 1997;27:1151–1159.
22. Dolinar RM, Kumar V, Coutu-Wakulczyk G, Rowe BH. Pilot study of a home-based asthma health education program. *Patient Educ Couns.* 2000;40:93–102.
23. Smith A, Krishnan JA, Bilderback A, Riekert KA, Rand CS, Bartlett SJ. Depressive symptoms and adherence to asthma therapy after hospital discharge. *Chest.* 2006;130:1034–1038.
24. Rhee H, Belyea MJ, Brasch J. Family support and asthma outcomes in adolescents: barriers to adherence as a mediator. *J Adolesc Health.* 2010;47:472–478.
25. van Dulmen S, Sluijs E, van Dijk L, de Ridder D, Heerdink R, Bensing J. Patient adherence to medical treatment: a review of reviews. *BMC Health Serv Res.* 2007;7:55.
26. Sabate E. *Adherence to Long-Term Therapies: Evidence for Action.* Geneva: World Health Organization; 2003.
27. Roth HP, Caron HS. Accuracy of doctors' estimates and patients' statements on adherence to a drug regimen. *Clin Pharmacol Ther.* 1978;23:361–370.
28. Spector SL, Kinsman R, Mawhinney H, et al. Compliance of patients with asthma with an experimental aerosolized medication: implications for controlled clinical trials. *J Allergy Clin Immunol.* 1986;77:65–70.
29. Restrepo RD, Alvarez MT, Wittnebel LD, et al. Medication adherence issues in patients treated for COPD. *Int J Chron Obstruct Pulm Dis.* 2008;3:371–384.
30. Weine AM, Vorobiev OV, Dyukov GM. Stress, depression and psychosomatic diseases. *Moscow,* 2004;12–25.
31. Baikova ES. Edge of neuro-psychiatric disorders in patients with bronchial asthma (clinic,

dynamics, prevention) [dissertation]. Tomsk, Russia: 2005:1–229.
32. Slavyanskaya TA, Sepiashvili RI. Premorbid pathological personal characteristics and social exclusion of patients with bronchial asthma. *Allergy and Immunology*. 2012;13(4):284–292.
33. Temmoeva IA. Characteristics and dynamics of clinical and pathopsychological indicators in children suffering from bronchial asthma, in the process of therapy [dissertation]. Stavropol, Russia: 2002:1–190.
34. Klyucheva MG. Bronchial asthma in adolescents: neurovegetative and psychosomatic peculiarities, rehabilitation programmes, forecast [dissertation]. Ivanovo, Russia: 2004:1–278.
35. Faure MC. *The Natural Prenatal Education: An Offer to the World Society of the 3rd Millennium*. Moscow, 2007:14.
36. Baranes T, Rossignol B, Stheneur C, Bidat E. Hyperventilation syndrome in children. *Arch Pediatr*. 2005;12:1742–1747.
37. Martínez-Moragón E, Perpiñá M, Belloch A, de Diego A. Prevalence of hyperventilation syndrome in patients treated for asthma in a pulmonology clinic. *Arch Bronchopneumol*. 2005;41:267–271.
38. De Peuter S, Van Diest I, Lemaigre V, Verleden G, Demedts M, Van den Bergh O. Dyspnea: the role of psychological processes. *Clin Psychol Rev*. 2004;24:557–581.
39. Hasler G, Gergen PJ, Kleinbaum DG, et al. Asthma and panic in young adults: a 20-year prospective community study. *Am J Respir Crit Care Med*. 2005;171:1224–1230.
40. Lee K, Noda Y, Nakano Y, et al. Interoceptive hypersensitivity and interoceptive exposure in patients with panic disorder: specificity and effectiveness. *BMC Psychiatry*. 2006;16:6–32.
41. Nardi AE, Valenca AM, Mezzasalma MA, et al. Comparison between hyperventilation and breath-holding in panic disorder: patients responsive and non-responsive to both tests. *Psychiatry Res*. 2006;15:201–208.
42. Van Diest I, Thayer JF, Vandeputte B, Van de Woestijne KP, Van den Bergh O. Anxiety and respiratory variability. *Physiol Behav*. 2006;30:189–195.
43. Ermakova EV. Changes of central regulation of airway reactivity in patients with bronchial asthma [dissertation]. Blagoveschensk, Russia: 2007:1–146.
44. Zinchenko MI. Pathogenetic aspects of therapy of hyperventilation syndrome using the respiratory biofeedback in bronchial asthma in children [dissertation]. Novosibirsk, Russia: 2007:1–105.
45. Wein AM, Moldavantz IV. *Neurogenic Hyperventilation*. Kishinev, Russia: Shtiintsa; 1988:1–182.
46. Chupak EL. Vegeto-psychological features of adolescents with bronchial asthma [dissertation]. Vladivostok, Russia: 2004:1–156.
47. Tsyuryupa VN. Pathogenetic aspects encephalopathy in patients with allergic bronchial asthma [dissertation]. Kemerovo, Russia: 2007: 1–142.
48. Webster KE, Colrain IM. P3-specific amplitude reductions to respiratory and auditory stimuli in subjects with asthma. *Am J Respir Crit Care Med*. 2002;l66:47–52.
49. Black PH. Stress and the inflammatory response: a review of neurogenic inflammation. *Brain Behav Immun*. 2002;16:622–653.
50. Maier SF. Bi-directional immune-brain communication: implications for understanding stress, pain, and cognition. *Brain Behav Immun*. 2003;17:6985.
51. Marshal GD Jr, Agarwal SK. Stress, immune regulation, and immunity: applications for asthma. *Allergy Asthma Proc*. 2000; 21(4):241–246.
52. Raison CL, Miller AH. The neuroimmunology of stress and depression. *Semin Clin Neurosychiatry*. 2001;6:277–294.
53. Slavyanskaya TA, Sepiashvili RI. Asthmatic patients with psychosomatic disorders: the features of the diagnosis and treatment. *Int J Immunorehabilitation*. 2013;15(1):5–7.
54. Trufakin SV. Pathophysiological peculiarities of psychoneurovegetoimmune relationship with immune disorders of different genesis [dissertation]. Tomsk, Russia: 2007:1–226.
55. Valeev RG. Analysis of psychoneurovegetoimmune interactions in health and in patients with bronchial asthma [dissertation]. Novosibirsk, Russia: 2007:1–155.
56. Wichers M, Maes MJ. The psychoneuroimmunopathophysiology of cytokine-induced depression in humans. *Neuropsychopharmacology*. 2002;5:375–388.
57. Wright RJ. Stress and atopic disorders. *J Allergy Clin Immunol*. 2005;116:1301–1306.
58. Baturin KA. Neurotic disorders in patients with bronchial asthma [dissertation]. Moscow, Russia: 2003:1–159.
59. Gorskaya EA. Psychological features of children and adolescents with asthma: in connection with the prevention of psychosomatic disorders [dissertation]. St. Petersburg, Russia: 2005:1–165.
60. Pekonidi AV. Autogenic training in the treatment of psychosomatic disorders in adolescents

with asthma [dissertation]. Moscow, Russia: 2005:1–97.
61. Kravtsova NA. Psychological content of the organizational forms and methods of assistance to children and adolescents with psychosomatic disorders [dissertation]. Vladivostok, Russia: 2009;1–436.
62. Krasnorutskaya ON. Psychosomatic state of child and adolescent patients with bronchial asthma [dissertation]. Voronezh, Russia: 2009:1–129.

29

ASTHMA, SUBSTANCE ABUSE, AND TOBACCO USE

COMORBID AND COEXISTING

Riccardo Polosa and Pasquale Caponnetto

KEY POINTS

- Asthma and other medical conditions are found at higher rates among patients with substance-related disorders.
- There is a growing body of evidence that patients with substance-related disorders may receive lower quality care for some medical conditions.
- Studies showed an association between marijuana smoking, worsening asthma symptoms, and acute exacerbations of bronchial asthma.
- There is an association between cocaine use and new-onset bronchospasm or recrudescence of asthma.
- Numerous reports have associated injection of heroin and inhalation of heroin with asthma exacerbations.
- Smoking accelerates decline in lung function and increases severity of airflow obstruction in asthma. It is worth noting that lung function changes can be reversed with smoking cessation.
- Many nonalcohol components of alcoholic beverages likely act as triggers for asthma in sensitized individuals.

INTRODUCTION

The *Diagnostic and Statistical Manual of Mental Disorders* (DSM) uses the term "substance use disorders" to characterize illnesses associated with drug use.[1] Commonly abused drugs are marijuana, cocaine, heroin, tobacco, and alcohol (Figure 29.1). Substance use disorders are common, with a prevalence of about 9% of the U.S. population. However, only 10% of affected individuals understand the importance of addiction treatment.[2]

Asthma remains a significant source of morbidity and mortality in the United States. Reports from the Centers for Disease

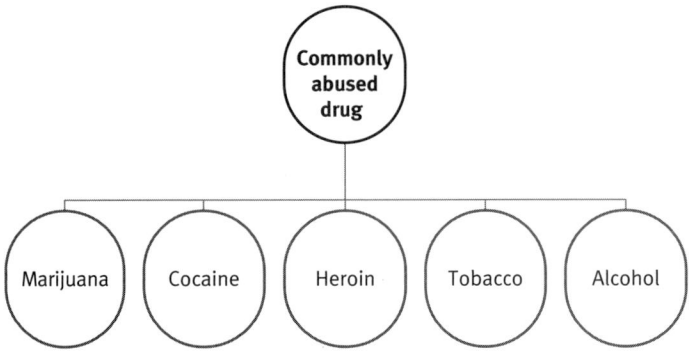

FIGURE 29.1 Drugs which cause "substance use disorders"

Control and Prevention estimate that 7.7% of Americans currently have asthma, and 11.2% will experience asthma at some point during their lifetime. In 2004, a total of 1.8 million emergency department visits, 14.7 million outpatient visits, and 497,000 hospitalizations were attributed to asthma. More than 4,000 people in the United States die from asthma each year.[3]

Asthma and other medical conditions (hypertension, diabetes, chronic liver disease, chronic obstructive pulmonary disease, pain, and stroke) are found at higher rates among patients with substance-related disorders.[3-5]

This chapter presents a review of current knowledge of relationships between asthma and substance abuse, including of marijuana, cocaine, heroin, tobacco, and alcohol (Table 29.1).

SMOKING MARIJUANA AND ASTHMA

Marijuana is derived from the cannabis plant and is intended for use as a psychoactive drug. It is smoked in the form of cigarettes or from a pipe to filter out particulate matter. Marijuana is the most commonly abused illicit substance. This drug impairs short-term memory and learning, the ability to focus, and coordination. It also increases heart rate, can harm the lungs, and may increase the risk for psychosis in vulnerable individuals.

Marijuana smoke contains similar levels of tar as tobacco smoke and up to 50% more carcinogens. Marijuana users smoke unfiltered material, inhale the smoke more deeply, and hold the smoke longer than tobacco smokers, resulting in substantially greater tar deposits in the lungs than tobacco smokers.[6]

Reports from clinical samples suggest that marijuana smokers exhibit a range of chronic respiratory symptoms.[7] In addition, marijuana users have greater utilization of outpatient medical services for respiratory and other illnesses.[8]

In view of such a high prevalence of marijuana use and the association of greater medical service utilization by its users, it is imperative for medical professionals to know about marijuana's short- and long-term consequences.

Several studies showed associations among marijuana smoking, worsening asthma symptoms, and acute exacerbations of bronchial asthma.[9] Smoking marijuana may also give rise to symptoms highly suggestive of bronchial asthma, including cough and sputum production.[10]

Physicians should question their patients carefully about marijuana use given its widespread abuse and the burden on health care it may produce by increasing the incidence of emphysema, barotrauma, inflammation, and infection. Efforts to prevent and reduce the use of marijuana, such as advising patients to quit and providing referrals for support and assistance, may have substantial public health benefits.

Table 29.1. Effects of Commonly Abused Drugs on Asthma

SUBSTANCE	EFFECT
Marijuana	Several studies showed associations among marijuana smoking, worsening asthma symptoms, and acute exacerbations of bronchial asthma.[9] Smoking marijuana may also give rise to symptoms highly suggestive of bronchial asthma, including cough and sputum production.[10]
Cocaine	Asthmatic patients who smoke cocaine may be at high risk for developing severe exacerbations of their asthma, depending on the degree of airways hyperresponsiveness, the dose of inhaled cocaine, and the nature of the contaminants inhaled during crack smoking.[15]
Heroin	Pathophysiologically, there are several reasons that heroin might induce an acute asthma exacerbation. Direct thermal injury can occur after the inhalation of heroin. The bronchoconstrictive effects of morphine, which is a metabolite of heroin, have been known since the early 1900s.[26] Bronchoconstriction after heroin use is likely because of the ability of heroin to directly cause the degranulation of mast cells, with the subsequent release of preformed inflammatory mediators, such as histamine.[27] Furthermore, under normal circumstances, asthmatic patients will increase their respiratory rate in an effort to compensate for the relative hypoxemia caused by bronchoconstriction. Because opioids cause respiratory depression, it is possible that the heroin-induced respiratory depression at least partly thwarts the ability of the body to adequately compensate, thus exacerbating the severity of an asthma attack.
Tobacco	Compared with nonsmoking asthmatic patients, smoking asthmatic patients are at risk for developing more severe symptoms and worse asthma-specific quality of life, with a huge impact on health care resources due to unscheduled doctor visits and frequent hospital admissions.[29] Moreover, cigarette smoking in asthma is associated with a higher frequency of exacerbations, increased number of life-threatening asthma attacks, and greater asthma mortality. Asthma severity is higher and asthma control is worse in asthmatic patients who smoke, the strongest association with more severe disease being observed in those with more than 20 pack-years.[30]
Alcohol	Many nonalcohol components of alcoholic beverages likely act as triggers for asthma in sensitized individuals and as such are not different from other asthma triggers. Acetaldehyde, the primary metabolite of ethanol, can trigger bronchoconstriction in asthmatic patients with genetically reduced ALDH2 activity and represents a significant trigger for asthma in certain Asian populations.

COCAINE, HEROIN, AND ASTHMA

Cocaine is a short-acting stimulant, which can lead abusers to "binge" or to take the drug many times in a single "session." Cocaine abuse can lead to severe medical consequences related to the heart (e.g., heart attack, heart failure, dilated cardiomyopathy), the respiratory system (e.g., pulmonary barotrauma, hypersensitivity pneumonitis, asthma), the nervous system (e.g., stroke), and the digestive system (e.g., gastropyloric ulcerations, gangrene, and perforation of small and large intestine).

Cocaine was used as an ingredient in tonics used to treat asthma in the last century.[11] The first report of an acute asthma exacerbation after cocaine use was made in 1932 in a young girl treated with nasal cocaine for topical anesthesia.[12] Cases of cocaine-precipitated bronchospasm, including severe or life-threatening exacerbations of bronchospasm, are described in the literature.[13] These effects are more commonly seen in cocaine use in the form of free-basing or crack smoking. Crack cocaine results in quicker absorption and euphoria than nasal insufflation or snorting and avoids the use of needles required for the intravenous (IV) route, which also provides instantaneous euphoria. Free-base is a cocaine alkaloid that melts at 98°C, vaporizes at higher temperatures, and is heat stable, thus allowing the drug to be smoked.[14] Free-base is usually prepared by mixing cocaine hydrochloride and baking soda, which is then boiled in water and cooled. The precipitate is either filtered or extracted by adding a solvent such as ether or alcohol. The cocaine remains dissolved in the solvent, which can be evaporated, leaving the relatively pure base as a residue. The simpler crack method allows the alkaloidal cocaine to precipitate without a solvent extraction method. Cocaine may then be smoked using various devices, such as a glass or regular pipe, or by mixing cocaine with tobacco or marijuana in cigarette form.[14] This method of use is most irritating to the bronchial epithelium; bronchospasm may be a result of inflammation of the respiratory epithelium by either cocaine or adulterants. Smoked cocaine base caused bronchoconstriction, whereas a similar intoxicating dose of IV cocaine did not, in a study comparing the acute effects of inhaled and IV cocaine on airway dynamics.[15] Asthmatic patients who smoke cocaine may be at high risk for developing severe exacerbations of their asthma, depending on the degree of airways hyperresponsiveness, the dose of inhaled cocaine, and the nature of the contaminants inhaled during crack smoking.[15]

The U.S. Office of National Drug Control Policy estimates that the number of chronic cocaine users is 3.6 million and that about 40% of cocaine users use cocaine in the form of crack. It is the leading cause of illicit drug-related visits to emergency departments in the United States.[16] In a prospective study by McNagny and colleagues,[16] the prevalence of cocaine use in young men presenting to an inner-city walk-in clinic was determined to be 39% by urine testing; 72% of those testing positive denied illicit drug use in the prior 3 days. Only 3 of 13 patients in a study by Rome and colleagues[17] who tested positive for cocaine actually admitted to its use. Consent was not obtained for drug screening in this study by McNagny and colleagues.[16] The results of the aforementioned study emphasize the magnitude of the cocaine epidemic and indicate the unreliability of self-reporting of illicit drug use. In another study, emergency department patients with new-onset bronchospasm were tested for cocaine metabolites, with 21 of 59 having positive results (36%).[18] This was compared with a control group of randomly selected, age- and sex-matched individuals without a history of respiratory disease, in which 15% tested positive for cocaine. This finding signifies an association between cocaine use and new-onset bronchospasm or recrudescence of asthma. In a similar study by Gaeta and Hammock,[9] 44% of asthmatic patients admitted to or tested positive for illicit drugs, compared with 20% of control patients.

Cocaine-induced asthma will primarily be observed in patients who smoke the substance because this route is associated with the most direct damage and inflammation of the bronchial epithelium.[19] Support for this theory comes from a study by Tashkin and colleagues,[15] who examined airway dynamics in patients who consumed cocaine by various routes. They observed that smoking cocaine, but not injecting it, produced acute bronchoconstriction.

The increase in prevalence of cocaine use in the United States may be an important factor responsible for increasing asthma severity and mortality, particularly in the young age group, despite major advances in available treatments. Several studies[9,18,20] point to a relatively high prevalence of cocaine use among patients with asthma exacerbation, possibly contributing to the increase in asthma morbidity.

Levine and colleagues[20] found a 42.8% prevalence of cocaine or heroin use among adult patients who had been admitted for acute asthma exacerbations to an inner-city Chicago hospital. They also found that cocaine use was associated with higher intubation rates, longer lengths of stay, and a higher likelihood of being admitted to the intensive care unit (ICU).

Levenson and colleagues[21] examined asthma deaths in Cook County, Chicago. They reported that 31.5% of asthma deaths were confounded by substance abuse or alcohol ingestion. Cocaine was the most frequently identified drug found by toxicologic analysis.

An important implication of this chapter is the importance of physicians' being alert to the possibility of cocaine as a precipitating factor for acute asthma. Patients who have been admitted to the hospital with acute asthma exacerbations in areas where illicit drug use is prevalent should be screened for the use of cocaine.

Heroin is a powerful opiate drug that produces euphoria and feelings of relaxation. It slows respiration and can increase the risk for serious infectious diseases, especially when taken intravenously. Other opioid drugs include morphine, oxycodone, and hydrocodone, which have legitimate medical uses; however, their nonmedical use or abuse can result in the same harmful consequences.

During much of the 1990s, heroin use in the United States rose steadily.[22] The current epidemic is characterized by new, young users, who increasingly report insufflation ("snorting"), rather than injection, as their sole method of use. In Chicago, New York City, Newark, and Detroit, insufflation is the most commonly reported means of heroin administration for those entering drug treatment programs.

Numerous reports have associated injection of heroin and inhalation of morphine or heroin with asthma exacerbations.[23] Hughes and Caverly[24] described three patients requiring mechanical ventilation after inhaling heroin, one of whom commonly developed acute wheezing after its use.

In the context of the current heroin epidemic, five patients with status asthmaticus associated with heroin inhalation (four from insufflation, one from smoking) were reported in Chicago.[23] These cases were characterized by preexisting asthma, the sudden onset of symptoms, relatively prolonged intubation, and eosinophilia.

Krantz and colleagues[25] examined the prevalence of drug use in asthmatic patients admitted to the ICU and compared the pattern of drug use to that of patients in the ICU who had been admitted for diabetic ketoacidosis. The authors observed that asthmatic patients in the ICU were more likely to have used heroin (60% vs. 7%; $P = .001$) than were the diabetic ketoacidosis patients.

Levine and colleagues[20] reported a surprisingly high prevalence of heroin use among adults who were admitted to an inner-city hospital for asthma exacerbation. Heroin appeared to be a risk factor for intubation.

It is probable that the high prevalence of drug use in inner-city populations contributes to the high rates of asthma exacerbations in this setting. Patients who have been admitted to the hospital with acute asthma exacerbations in areas where illicit drug use is prevalent should be screened for the use of heroin.

Pathophysiologically, there are several reasons that heroin might induce an acute asthma exacerbation. Direct thermal injury can occur after the inhalation of heroin. The bronchoconstrictive effects of morphine, which is a metabolite of heroin, have been known since the early 1900s.[26] Bronchoconstriction after heroin use is likely because of the ability of heroin to directly cause the degranulation of the mast cells, with the subsequent release of preformed inflammatory mediators, such as histamine.[27] Furthermore, under normal circumstances, asthmatic patients will increase their respiratory rate in an effort to compensate for the relative hypoxemia caused by bronchoconstriction. Because opioids cause respiratory depression, it is possible that the heroin-induced respiratory depression at least partly thwarts the ability of the body to adequately compensate, thus exacerbating the severity of an asthma attack.

TOBACCO SMOKING, ALCOHOL, AND ASTHMA

Smoking is associated with a higher incidence of asthma and is strongly predictive of the development of new-onset asthma.[28]

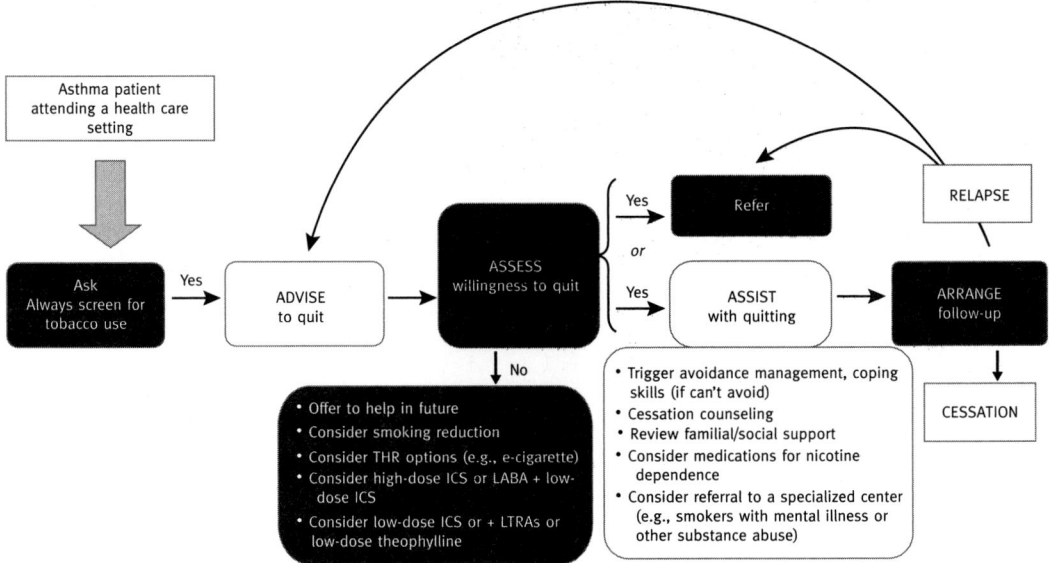

FIGURE 29.2 THR, tobacco harm reduction; LABA, long-acting B2-agonist; ICS, inhaled corticosteroid; LTRA, leukotriene receptor antagonist.

Compared with nonsmoking asthmatic patients, smoking asthmatic patients are at risk for developing more severe symptoms and worse asthma-specific quality of life, with a huge impact on health care resources due to unscheduled doctor visits and frequent hospital admissions.[29] Moreover, cigarette smoking in asthma is associated with a higher frequency of exacerbations, increased number of life-threatening asthma attacks, and greater asthma mortality. Asthma severity is higher and asthma control is worse in asthmatic patients who smoke, the strongest association with more severe disease being observed in those with more than 20 pack-years.[30]

Smoking accelerates decline in lung function and increases severity of airflow obstruction in asthma. It is worth noting that lung function changes can be reversed with smoking cessation.[31]

Smokers with asthma appear to be less sensitive to the beneficial effects of inhaled corticosteroid (ICS) compared with nonsmokers with asthma. Although ICS may relieve, to some extent, unresponsiveness (e.g., β-agonists) in smokers with asthma, decreased responsiveness to ICS continues to be present despite the length of treatment, glucocorticoid molecule, and type of formulation (ICS vs. oral).[32] Few clinical trials studied reversibility of corticosteroid unresponsiveness in asthmatic smokers. A noncontrolled study demonstrates that low-dose theophylline in addition to inhaled beclomethasone improved both lung function and asthma symptoms in 68 asthmatic smokers.[33] A randomized clinical trial suggests that leukotriene antagonists may have a beneficial effect in smokers with mild asthma,[34] but this study has not been replicated. Only one study examined the role of smoking cessation on corticosteroid responsiveness. Progressive improvement in forced expiratory volume in 1 second (FEV_1) and restored corticosteroid responsiveness were reported after 6 weeks of smoking cessation in 21 asthmatic smokers, compared with 11 control smokers.[31]

These findings highlight the importance of smoking cessation in improving many clinical and functional outcomes of asthma. Physicians have the responsibility both to alert their patients with asthma about the additional risks of smoking and to engage in smoking cessation interventions (Figure 29.2).[35]

Alcohol consumption can damage the brain, the liver, and most other body organs (e.g., heart, kidney). Areas of the brain that are especially vulnerable to alcohol-related

Table 29.2. Impact of Alcohol on Asthma

IMPACT	STUDY
Alcohol administered intravenously acts as a bronchodilator	Brown, 1947[40]
Alcohol ingestion improves vital capacity	Herxheimer & Stresemann, 1963[38]
Atopic patients wheeze from alcohol congeners but not pure alcohol	Breslin et al., 1973[41]
Alcohol triggers an immediate irritant response and causes a slow bronchodilator effect	Ayres et al., 1982[39]
Sulfur dioxide in some wines causes wheezing in asthmatic patients	Dahl et al., 1986[42]
Acetaldehyde causes "alcohol-induced bronchial asthma" in some Asians	Shimoda et al., 1996[43]
Aldehyde dehydrogenase type 2 (ALHD2) deficiency has been identified as causing asthma in some Asians	Matsuse et al., 2001[44]

damage are the cerebral cortex, the hippocampus, and the cerebellum (Table 29.2).

Alcohol has been used to treat asthma since antiquity. The earliest indication of alcohol as a treatment for asthma appears on Egyptian papyri from about 2000 B.C.[36]

In the 19th century, Hyde Salter reported self-administration of high amounts of oral alcohol by three of his patients with severe asthma exacerbations and noted improvement of their symptoms.[37] Indeed, the use of alcohol as a treatment was widespread by physicians in the United States well into the early 20th century until Prohibition, when its use was officially renounced by the American Medical Association. Following the repeal of Prohibition in 1933, more rigorous studies using alcohol as a treatment for asthma began to appear.

In 1963, Herxheimer measured lung vital capacity (VC) in normal subjects and asthmatic patients following the ingestion of brandy, vodka, or pure ethanol.[38] Alcohol ingestion did not change the VC in normal subjects but increased VC between 6% and 38% in most of the asthmatic patients and was accompanied by subjective improvement in their asthma symptoms. The VC improvement began about 10 minutes after alcohol ingestion, peaked by 30 minutes, and returned to baseline by 2 hours. The authors concluded that alcohol had an antiasthmatic effect, confirming the findings of Salter from a century before.

Soon thereafter, a small but important clinical study by Ayres examined the effects of drinking alcohol and asthma. Changes in airflow were measured following the ingestion of different concentrations of pure ethanol (diluted in water) in five normal subjects and five patients with asthma.[39] Two of the normal subjects and three of the asthmatic patients had a slight decrease in specific airways conductance with 20% alcohol within 5 minutes of quickly swallowing the whole drink. Higher concentrations of alcohol (60%), when sipped slowly over 5 minutes, resulted in significant increases in airway conductance in four of five of the asthmatic subjects. This study suggests that although alcohol can immediately trigger an initial small upper airway irritant response, a separate slow bronchodilator effect occurs in asthmatic patients.

The first reported use of IV alcohol for the treatment of asthma appeared in 1947 when Brown infused 5% ethanol into children with severe asthma attacks who were unresponsive to conventional asthma therapy.[40] Five of the six patients improved with the alcohol infusion, and no adverse reactions were reported.

The implication that a pure alcohol infusion acted as a bronchodilator and did not worsen asthma was important because some atopic patients report bronchospasm following ingestion of alcoholic beverages. This point was made in a study by Breslin in 1973 of

11 subjects with asthma who reported worsening of their asthma symptoms following the ingestion of an alcoholic beverage.[41] The authors were able to provoke bronchospasm in the laboratory in 6 of the 11 subjects challenged with the offending alcoholic beverage, precipitating a more than 15% reduction in the FEV_1 on spirometry. Importantly, in three of these patients, drink-precipitated bronchospasm was not triggered by an oral ingestion of an equivalent amount of pure alcohol in water, implicating the nonalcohol components of the beverage as the likely asthma trigger. Indeed, treatment with disodium cromoglycate, a drug that inhibits mast cell granule release and is used in the treatment of asthma, prevented bronchospasm to the offending alcoholic beverage. Similar findings were obtained in another study implicating the sulfur dioxide content in red wine as a likely trigger for bronchospasm in asthmatic patients rather than the alcohol itself.[42] These studies indicate that both the purity (pure ethanol vs. an alcoholic beverage) and the route (oral vs. IV) are factors that may determine how alcohol might modify airway function.

Acetaldehyde is produced by the metabolism of ethanol through the action of alcohol dehydrogenases. Acetaldehyde is recognized as a trigger for asthma in Asians and is referred to as "alcohol-induced bronchial asthma."[43] The most susceptible individuals are Asians who have greatly reduced function of the enzyme aldehyde dehydrogenase isoform 2 (ALDH2). They can be identified through genetic testing or ethanol challenge testing.[44] About half of Japanese have inadequate ALDH2 activity and cannot effectively metabolize acetaldehyde. Bronchospasm following alcohol ingestion is closely linked to the ALDH2 genotype.[43] The mechanism for acetaldehyde-triggered bronchospasm in these individuals is thought to occur through a noncholinergic pathway related to degranulation of mast cells triggered by high blood acetaldehyde levels that result in the release of histamine and other bronchoconstricting mediators.[44]

Myou and colleagues found that inhaled ethanol did not trigger bronchospasm in Japanese subjects with alcohol-induced asthma. Indeed, inhaled ethanol attenuated methacholine-induced bronchospasm in these asthmatic patients.[45] This is likely a result of the inability of the airway epithelium to significantly metabolize ethanol into acetaldehyde. This study is consistent with the hypothesis that alcohol, in the absence of acetaldehyde or congeners, does not trigger asthma even in susceptible individuals with impaired ALDH2 function.

Pure ethanol is a moderately effective and transient bronchodilator and likely relaxes airway smooth muscle tone. The mechanisms responsible for alcohol-induced relaxation of airways are poorly understood and may include receptor- and non-receptor-mediated signal transduction pathways involving calcium and/or nitric oxide as second messengers. Many nonalcohol components of alcoholic beverages likely act as triggers for asthma in sensitized individuals and as such are not different from other asthma triggers. Acetaldehyde, the primary metabolite of ethanol, can trigger bronchoconstriction in asthmatic patients with genetically reduced ALDH2 activity and represents a significant trigger for asthma in certain Asian populations.

UNMET, FUTURE RESEARCH NEEDS

1. Further investigations into the pulmonary effects of both acute and chronic substance abuse will result in better methods to treat substance abuse and their complications.
2. Physicians should carefully question their patients about marijuana, tobacco, heroin, cocaine, and alcohol use. These substances place additional burdens on health and the health care system by causing or exacerbating asthma, emphysema, barotrauma, inflammation, and infection.
3. Efforts to prevent and reduce the use of marijuana, tobacco, heroin, cocaine, and alcohol, such as advising patients to quit and providing referrals for support and assistance, will have substantial public health benefits.

CONCLUSION

Asthma and other medical conditions are found at higher rates among patients with substance-related disorders.[5] There is a growing body of evidence that patients with substance-related disorders may receive lower quality care for some medical conditions.[46]

In 2004, a total of 1.8 million emergency department visits, 14.7 million outpatient visits, and 497,000 hospitalizations were attributed to asthma. More than 4,000 people in the United States die from asthma each year.[47] Government health agencies have devoted a great deal of attention to improving the quality of asthma care over the past two decades.[48]

Substance-related disorders may influence rates at which patients achieve standardized asthma care quality measures. Several studies show that patients who abuse drugs may be at increased risk for severe asthma exacerbations or asthma death.[17,18,20,21,25]

Baxter and colleagues[49] demonstrated that patients with substance-related disorders and persistent asthma fill prescriptions for controller medications at lower rates than patients without substance-related disorders. Whether these differences are due to differential access to care, decreased compliance with treatment recommendations, or the receipt of substandard care, these findings still may partially explain the disparities in asthma outcomes observed for these patients. Baxter and colleagues[50] also showed that patients with substance-related disorders are half as likely as patients without these disorders to receive asthma care in outpatient settings and therefore may be less likely to benefit from outpatient-based quality improvement efforts. An integrated approach could lead to effective treatment of these conditions.

REFERENCES

1. American Psychiatric Association. *Diagnostic and Statistical Manual of Mental Disorders*. 4th ed., text revision. Washington, DC: APA; 2000.
2. Substance Abuse and Mental Health Services Administration. *Results from the 2008 National Survey on Drug Use and Health: National Findings*. Rockville, MD: Office of Applied Studies; 2009.
3. Wadland WC, Ferenchick GS. Medical comorbidity in addictive disorders. *Psychiatr Clin North Am*. 2004;27:675–687.
4. Akinbami L. *Asthma Prevalence, Health Care Use and Mortality: United States, 2003–2005*. Hyattsville, MD: Centers for Disease Control and Prevention, National Center for Health Statistics; 2006. Available at www.cdc.gov/nchs.
5. Mertens JR, Lu YW, Parthasarathy S, et al. Medical and psychiatric conditions of alcohol and drug treatment patients in an HMO: comparison with matched controls. *Arch Intern Med*. 2003;163:2511–2517.
6. Matthias P, Tashkin DP, Marques-Magallanes JA, Wilkins JN, Simmons MS. Effects of varying marijuana potency on deposition of tar and delta9-THC in the lung during smoking. *Pharmacol Biochem Behav*. 1997;58: 1145–1150.
7. Tashkin DP. Cannabis effects on the respiratory system. In: Kalant H, Corrigal WA, Hall H, Smart R, eds. *The Health Effects of Cannabis*. Toronto, ON: Centre for Addiction and Mental Health; 1999:311–346.
8. Polen MR, Sidney S, Tekawa IS, Sadler M, Friedman GD. Health care use by frequent marijuana smokers who do not smoke tobacco. *West J Med*. 1993;158:596–601.
9. Gaeta TJ, Hammock R. Association between substance abuse and acute exacerbation of bronchial asthma [Letter]. *Acad Emerg Med*. 1996;3:1170–1172.
10. Tetrault JM, Crothers K, Moore BA, et al. Effects of marijuana smoking on pulmonary function and respiratory complications: a systematic review. *Arch Intern Med*. 2007;167:221–228.
11. Cohen SG. Asthma among the famous: Nathan Tucker (1838–1920), American physician. *Allergy Asthma Proc*. 1997;18:252–255.
12. Waldbott GC. Asthma due to a local anesthetic. *JAMA*. 1932;99:1942.
13. Rubin RB, Neugarten J. Cocaine-associated asthma. *Am J Med*. 1990;88:428–439.
14. Haim DY, Lippmann ML, Goldberg SK, et al. The pulmonary complications of crack cocaine. *Chest*. 1995;107:233–240.
15. Tashkin DP, Kleerup EC, Koyal SN, et al. Acute effects of inhaled and IV cocaine on airway dynamics. *Chest*. 1996;110:904–910.
16. McNagny SE, Parker RM. High prevalence of recent cocaine use and the unreliability of patient self-report in an inner-city walk-in clinic. *JAMA*. 1992;267:1106–1108.
17. Rome LA, Lippmann ML, Dalsey WC, et al. Prevalence of cocaine use and its impact on asthma exacerbations in an urban population. *Chest*. 2000;117:1324–1329.
18. Osborn HM, Tang M, Bradley K, et al. New-onset bronchospasm or recrudescence of asthma associated with cocaine abuse. *Acad Emerg Med*. 1997;4:689–692.

19. Rich JA, Singer DE. Cocaine-related symptoms in patients presenting to an urban emergency department. *Ann Emerg Med.* 1991;20:616–621.
20. Levine M, Iliescu ME, Margellos-Anas H, Estarziau M, Ansell DA. The effects of cocaine and heroin use on intubation rates and hospital utilization in patients with acute asthma exacerbations. *Chest.* 2005;128:1951–1957.
21. Levenson T, Greenberger PA, Donoghue ER, et al. Asthma deaths confounded by substance abuse. *Chest.* 1996;110:604–610.
22. National Institute on Drug Abuse. *Research Report: Heroin Abuse and Addiction.* Publication No. 00-4165. Bethesda, MD: National Institutes of Health, National Institute on Drug Abuse; 1997.
23. Community Epidemiologic Work Group. *Epidemiologic Trends in Drug Abuse.* Vol. 1. Publication No. 00-4529. Rockville, MD: National Institute on Drug Abuse; 1999.
24. Hughes S, Caverly PMA. Heroin inhalation and asthma. *BMJ.* 1988;297:1511–1512.
25. Krantz AJ, Hershow RC, Prachand N, et al. Heroin insufflation as a trigger for patients with life-threatening asthma. *Chest.* 2003;123:510–517.
26. Dixon WE, Brodie TB. Contributions to the physiology of the lungs: Part 1. The bronchial muscles, their innervation, and the action of the drugs upon them. *J Physiol.* 1903;29:171.
27. Withington DE, Patrick JA, Reynolds F. Histamine release by morphine and diamorphine in man. *Anaesthesia.* 1993;48:26–29.
28. Polosa R, Knoke JD, Russo C, et al. Cigarette smoking is associated with a greater risk of incident asthma in allergic rhinitis. *J Allergy Clin Immunol.* 2008;121:1428–1434.
29. Eisner MD, Iribarren C. The influence of cigarette smoking on adult asthma outcomes. *Nicotine Tob Res.* 2007;9(1):53–56.
30. Polosa R, Russo C, Caponnetto P, et al. Greater severity of new onset asthma in allergic subjects who smoke: a 10-year longitudinal study. *Respir Res.* 2011;12:16.
31. Chaudhuri R, Livingston E, McMahaon AD, et al. Effects of smoking cessation on lung function and airway inflammation in smokers with asthma. *Am J Respir Crit Care Med.* 2006;174:127–133.
32. Thomson N, Chaudhuri R. Asthma in smokers: challenges and opportunities. *Curr Opin Pulm Med.* 2009;15:39–45.
33. Spears M, Donnelly I, Jolly L, et al. Effect of low-dose theophylline plus beclomethasone on lung function in smokers with asthma: a pilot study. *Eur Respir J.* 2009;33:1010–1017.
34. Lazarus SC, Chinchilli VM, Rollings NJ, et al. Smoking affects response to inhaled corticosteroids or leukotriene receptor antagonists in asthma. *Am J Respir Crit Care Med.* 2007;175(8):783–790.
35. Polosa R, Caponnetto P, Sands MF. Caring for the smoking asthmatic patient. *J Allergy Clin Immunol.* 2012;130(5):1221–1224.
36. Leake C. *The Old Egyptian Medical Papyri.* Lawrence, KS: University of Kansas Press; 1952.
37. Salter H. On the treatment of asthmatic paroxysm by full doses of alcohol. *Lancet.* 1863;2:558–559.
38. Herxheimer H, Stresemann E. Ethanol and lung function in bronchial asthma. *Arch Int Pharmacodyn Ther.* 1963;144:310–314.
39. Ayres J, Ancic P, Clark TJ. Airways responses to oral ethanol in normal subjects and in patients with asthma. *J R Soc Med.* 1982;75:699–704.
40. Brown EA. The use of intravenous ethyl alcohol in the treatment of status asthmaticus. *Ann Allergy.* 1947;5:193–195.
41. Breslin AB, Hendrick DJ, Pepys J. Effect of disodium cromoglycate on asthmatic reactions to alcoholic beverages. *Clin Allergy.* 1973;3:71–82.
42. Dahl R, Henriksen JM, Harving H. Red wine asthma: a controlled challenge study. *J Allergy Clin Immunol.* 1986;78:1126–1129.
43. Shimoda T, Kohno S, Takao A, et al. Investigation of the mechanism of alcohol-induced bronchial asthma. *J Allergy Clin Immunol.* 1996;97:74–84.
44. Matsuse H, Shimoda T, Fukushima C, et al. Screening for acetaldehyde dehydrogenase 2 genotype in alcohol-induced asthma by using the ethanol patch test. *J Allergy Clin Immunol.* 2001;108:715–719.
45. Myou S, Fujimura M, Nishi K, et al. Effect of ethanol on airway caliber and nonspecific bronchial responsiveness in patients with alcohol-induced asthma. *Allergy.* 1996;51:52–55.
46. Druss BG, Rosenheck RA, Desai MM, et al. Quality of preventive medical care for patients with mental disorders. *Med Care.* 2002;40:129–136.
47. Akinbami L. *Asthma Prevalence, Health Care Use and Mortality: United States, 2003–2005.* Hyattsville, MD: Centers for Disease Control and Prevention, National Center for Health Statistics; 2006. Available at www.cdc.gov/nchs.
48. *Healthy People 2010: Objectives for Improving Health, Part B. Focus Areas 15–28.* Vol II, 2nd ed.

Washington, DC: U.S. Department of Health and Human Services; 2000. Available at www.healthypeople.gov/publications.
49. Baxter JD, Samnaliev M, Clark RE. The quality of asthma care among adults with substance-related disorders and adults with mental illness. *Psychiatr Serv*. 2009;60(1):43–49.
50. Baxter JD, Samnaliev M, Clark RE. Patterns of health care utilization for asthma in adults with substance use disorders. *J Addict Med*. 2008;2:79–84.

SECTION EIGHT

EXERCISE

30

EXERCISE-INDUCED BRONCHOCONSTRICTION AND ASTHMA

COEXISTING

Matteo Bonini, André Moreira, and Sergio Bonini

KEY POINTS

- Exercise-induced bronchoconstriction (EIB) is defined as "the transient narrowing of the airway with increasing airway resistance after exercise."[1]
- EIB may occur in subjects with or without clinical asthma.
- EIB is mainly related to epithelial damage induced by airway cooling and dehydration following hyperventilation associated with exercise.
- Self-reported symptoms of EIB require objective confirmation by pulmonary function tests before and after exercise or other surrogate challenges.
- Exercise-induced laryngeal dysfunction and other exercise-related conditions may mimic EIB and therefore require a differential diagnosis.
- Treatment of EIB is based on reversing bronchial obstruction with short-acting β_2-adrenergic agents.
- Prevention of EIB differs in subjects with or without clinical asthma and includes both pharmacologic and nonpharmacologic options.

INTRODUCTION

Exercise-induced bronchoconstriction (EIB) is defined as "the transient narrowing of the airway with increasing airway resistance after exercise."[1] This chapter, in line with the objective of the book, discusses the relationship between EIB and asthma, with special reference to clinical features, pathophysiologic mechanisms, diagnostic criteria, and treatment and preventive options.

CLINICAL FEATURES

It has long been known that physical exercise may trigger symptoms of asthma. However, the interest for an objective study of this phenomenon dates back 50 years, to when Jones and coworkers[2] focused on the physiologic response to exercise in asthmatic children and named the postexercise airway obstruction after an exercise challenge *exercise-induced asthma* (EIA). Subsequent research defined the different patterns of response to exercise in asthmatic patients; the effect of type, intensity, and duration of challenges; and the influence of antiasthmatic drugs on EIA. In reviewing these studies, Godfrey concluded that, despite "some exceptions," "there has been no evidence that EIA occurs in patients other than asthmatics...and although sporadic cases have been reported where exercise appears to have been the only precipitant of asthma in a patient (usually an adult), careful investigation has usually revealed other clinical and physiological manifestations of bronchial asthma."[3]

Although some authors consider EIA as a distinct asthma phenotype,[4] it is quite evident that exercise may trigger bronchial obstruction and clinical symptoms in almost all asthmatic patients, independently from the causes and mechanisms of the underlying asthma. In fact, EIA has been reported in up to 90% of asthmatic patients, reflecting the level of disease control,[1] with EIA occurring more frequently in more severe and uncontrolled asthmatic patients. Accordingly, asthma guidelines include tolerance to exercise among criteria to establish the level of disease control.[5]

However, the concept that exercise may induce bronchial obstruction in asthmatic patients only is in question. The response to exercise in an unselected population, in fact, distributes along a normal curve, and bronchial obstruction may develop even in subjects without any clinical asthma.[1] This is particularly true in children, athletes, and patients with atopy or rhinitis, or following respiratory infections. It is not easy, however, to report prevalence rates in these populations because they also depend on the type and intensity of exercise, as well as the environmental conditions in which the challenge is performed. Whether these subjects who develop bronchial obstruction after exercise should be considered asthmatic or at risk for developing clinical asthma in future years is still a matter of debate. Certainly, EIB that occurs in athletes without clinical asthma has peculiar clinical and pathologic features and often disappears after discontinuation of intense training.[6]

Exercise-Induced Bronchoconstriction with or without Asthma

To bring some clarity to this still controversial issue, a Practice Parameter, jointly developed by the American Academy of Allergy Asthma and Immunology and the American College of Allergy Asthma and Immunology, proposes abandoning the term EIA (because exercise is not the cause but only a trigger of asthma) and referring to EIB with asthma (EIB_A), the occurrence of bronchial obstruction after exercise in asthmatic patients, and EIB without asthma (EIB_{wA}), the occurrence of bronchial obstruction in subjects without other clinical and functional symptoms and signs of clinical asthma.[1] In this chapter we adopt this nomenclature to address the complex relationships between EIB and asthma.

MECHANISMS

EIB was initially thought to be secondary to a mediator release from mast cells.[3] This hypothesis was also supported by the refractory period observed after a positive exercise challenge, interpreted as the period needed for mast cell recharge, and by the preventive effect offered by mast cell–stabilizing agents, such as sodium cromoglycate.

Although mediator release does contribute to cause EIB, pathophysiologic changes induced by intense exercising are definitely more complex.

At present, it is widely accepted that hyperventilation through the mouth associated with intense exercise causes the need for humidifying and heating large volumes of air during a short period of time. Elegant experiments performed by Anderson and coworkers[7] show that the respiratory water loss and the increase in osmolarity of the airways surface liquid represent the major determinants of EIB (osmotic theory). In fact, the dryer and colder the inspired air and the higher the ventilation, the greater the likelihood of a positive response to exercise,[1] which also explains the higher prevalence of EIB in winter athletes.[8] The vasodilation associated with airways rewarming (thermal theory) may also play a role in inducing bronchial obstruction after exercise.[9]

In EIB_A, the previously mentioned mechanism only represents a trigger of the underlying airway hyperreactivity in subjects with different phenotypes of asthma not under control.

However, in EIB_{wA}, the epithelial damage produced by dehydration and cooling of a large number of airways divisions down to peripheral airways represents the predominant pathogenetic mechanism.[10] In fact, a direct effect of viral and occupational agents and exercise may represent a causal mechanism of asthma, alternative to the classic eosinophilic mast cell–dependent mechanism occurring in allergic asthma.[11]

The role of epithelial damage and of substances released by the epithelium and found in sputum, such as interleukin-8 and leukotrienes,[12,13] and in serum or urine, such as the Clara cell protein CC16,[12,14] may also explain the heterogeneous inflammatory response reported in EIB.[15] The increase of columnar epithelial cells in induced sputum[12] is, in fact, associated with a neutrophilic or mixed eosinophilic–neutrophilic inflammation.[16,17] The importance of aquaporin, expressed by the subepithelial glandular cells, in regulating the water transport through the epithelium,[18] as well as increased mucus production, as shown by the increased expression of MUC5AC in induced sputum,[19] may be important in EIB.

Finally, autonomic dysregulation may also have a role in causing bronchial obstruction in EIB,[20] both through the basal increased parasympathetic tone shown in athletes and through reflex mechanisms induced by exercise.

DIAGNOSIS

Self-reported respiratory symptoms after exercise are not sufficient for a diagnosis of EIB.[21] This requires an objective evaluation of bronchial obstruction through pulmonary function tests before and after a standardized challenge.[1]

Diagnostic Tests

After a careful history and physical examination, an exercise challenge, standardized for duration, intensity, temperature, and water content of the inhaled air,[1,22] represents the first step in the diagnostic algorithm of EIB. An exercise challenge should be performed in subjects with EIB_A only when their baseline forced expiratory volume in 1 second (FEV_1) is more than 70% of normal.

A 10% or greater decrease in FEV_1 at any two consecutive time-point recordings (1 to 3, 5, 10, 15, 20, 25, 30) after 6 to 8 minutes of treadmill or cycloergometer exercise in ambient conditions (20°C to 25°C; relative humidity, <50%), may be considered diagnostic of EIB.[1] The intensity of exercise should be enough to produce a 60% increase in predicted maximum ventilation and an 85% increase in maximal heart rate (HR_{max}, calculated as 220 − age or 208 − [0.7 × age]).

However, standard criteria for laboratory exercise testing may be insufficient to induce a positive response in highly trained individuals. Accordingly, sports-specific on-the-field challenges are also used in athletes. These are more difficult to standardize, as is free regular running, often used as a challenge for children. Other bronchoprovocative tests (BPTs) may be adopted as surrogate diagnostic tools for EIB.[23] However, the correlation between exercise tests and other BPTs is not very high and varies from test to test.

Direct BPTs, such as methacholine and histamine provocation, are accurate to document bronchial hyperreactivity in asthma and in EIB_A. However, indirect tests, such as eucapnic voluntary hyperpnea, hypertonic saline challenge, and mannitol inhaled powder challenge, better reproduce the effects of exercise on the airways and are therefore more accurate to diagnose EIB_{wA}.

Table 30.1. Criteria of the International Olympic Committee to Define a Positive Bronchial Provocation Test in Athletes with Reported EIB_{wA}

METHOD	PROTOCOL	POSITIVITY CRITERIA
Bronchodilation test	FEV_1 before and 15 minutes after inhalation of a standard $β_2$-agonist	FEV_1 increase from baseline ≥200 mL and ≥12% of predicted
Bronchial provocation challenges		
Methacholine test	Provocative dose (PD20) or concentration (PC20) of inhaled methacholine inducing an FEV_1 decrease from baseline ≥20%	PC20 ≤4 mg/mL or PD20 ≤400 μg (cumulative dose) or ≤200 μg (noncumulative dose) in those not taking inhaled corticosteroid (ICS) PC20 ≤16 mg/mL or PD20≤ 1,600 μg (cumulative dose) or ≤800 μg (noncumulative dose) in those taking ICS for at least 1 month
Eucapnic voluntary hyperpnea	FEV_1 before and within 30 min of 6 min dry (or dry and cool) air inhalation at 85% of predicted maximum voluntary ventilation	≥10% decrease in FEV_1 from baseline
Hypertonic saline inhalation	FEV_1 before and after inhaling 22.5 mL of 4.5 g% NaCl	≥15% decrease in FEV_1 from baseline
Mannitol inhalation	Provocative dose of inhaled mannitol inducing an FEV_1 decrease from baseline ≥15% (PD15M)	PD15M ≤635 mg of mannitol
Exercise challenge (field or laboratory)	FEV_1 before and within 30 min of exercise challenge achieving heart rate >85% for at least 4 min	≥10% decrease in FEV_1 from baseline

The International Olympic Committee recommends specific thresholds (Table 30.1) for the various BPTs to document asthma or EIB and to permit the use of antiasthmatic drugs that are controlled or limited by the World Anti-Doping Agency (WADA). Standardized protocols for diagnosis of EIB are reported in detail by Weiler and colleagues.[1]

Differential Diagnosis

The differential diagnosis of EIB should take into account exercise-induced laryngeal dysfunctions, exercise-induced dyspnea and hyperventilation, exercise-induced hypoxemia, dyspnea on exertion in obese or poorly fit individuals, or shortness of breath with exercise due to obstructive, other than asthma, or restrictive lung diseases (Table 30.2).[1,24]

In particular, vocal cord dysfunction and structural glottis abnormalities are increasingly recognized as conditions that may mimic EIB.[25] In vocal cord dysfunction, inspiratory stridor during exercise usually resolves within 5 minutes and is the major differentiating sign, associated with negative BPT result and poor response to antiasthmatic treatment (see Chapter 22).

When EIB is associated with pruritus or an urticarial or systemic reaction, exercise-induced urticaria or exercise-induced anaphylaxis has to be considered.[26,27]

Table 30.2. Most Common Differential Diagnoses for Exercise-Induced Bronchoconstriction

CONDITION	SYMPTOMS	SIGNS	TESTING	TIPS
EIB	Chest tightness, wheezing, cough, shortness of breath, generally occurring within 5 to 30 min after intense exercise (sometimes during exercise)	Expiratory dyspnea Expiratory rhonchi or wheezing	Reversibility on lung function testing Increased airway responsiveness in provocation challenges	Improvement occurs either spontaneously or after inhaled bronchodilator
Vocal cord dysfunction	Throat tightness, shortness of breath, increased inspiratory effort, stridor and wheeze Only during maximal exercise and stopping right after (unless hyperventilation) Most often occurs in well-trained teenager girls	Stridor Audible inspiratory sounds from the laryngeal area without signs of bronchial obstruction	Flattened inspiratory flow–volume loop during stridor	No effect of asthma medication Consider direct fiberoptic laryngoscopy during exercise to check for paradoxical vocal cord movement and to differentiate from laryngomalacia
Exercise-induced arterial hypoxemia	Occurs in well-trained athletes with high VO_{2max}	Respiratory distress	Reduction in arterial oxygen saturation	Primarily due to diffusion limitations and ventilation-perfusion mismatch
Exercise-induced hyperventilation (pseudo-asthma syndrome)	Dyspnea and chest tightness during exercise	Hyperventilation	Increased end-tidal carbon dioxide	Symptoms are not directly related to bronchial obstruction but include hypocapnia and a possible abnormal ventilatory homeostasis during exercise
Poor physical fitness	Dyspnea and muscular stiffness related to expectations and training level	High heart rate after low-grade exercise load	Normal lung function and negative provocation challenges	Exercise rehabilitation or training can improve aerobic fitness and endurance and can shift the lactate/ventilatory threshold so that more work is required before lactate accumulates and ventilation increases Improved aerobic fitness through exercise training can thus decrease the hyperpnea and dyspnea associated with exercise

EIB, exercise-induced bronchoconstriction; VO_{2max}, maximum oxygen uptake.

TREATMENT AND PREVENTION

Treatment of both EIB_A and EIB_{wA} is based on reversing bronchial obstruction with short-acting β_2-agonists (SABA).[1,28]

Nonpharmacologic Prevention

Similar nonpharmacologic preventive measures can be adopted in both EIB_A and EIB_{wA}. These include, whenever possible, avoiding exercise in an at-risk air environment because of temperature, humidity, and pollutants or specific allergens in sensitized subjects. Gradual warming-up and cooling-down periods are always suggested. Some athletes also take advantage of the refractory period after bronchial obstruction deliberately induced by hyperventilation or by an intense exercise challenge. There is some evidence that dietary factors, such as a low sodium intake, omega-3 polyunsaturated fatty acids, or a supplementation of ascorbic acid, may be helpful in reducing the severity of EIB.[1]

Pharmacologic Prevention

Different approaches to pharmacologic prevention should be taken for EIB_A and EIB_{wA}.

Because EIB_A is a sign of poor asthma control, prevention consists of following international guidelines to achieve asthma control.[5] The potential occurrence of EIB, however, should not prevent asthmatic patients from physical exercise, which, on the contrary, should represent part of their treatment.

Several drugs are available to prevent EIB_{wA}. Usually they do not eliminate EIB_{wA} but attenuate it or shift the dose-response relationship so that some submaximal efforts become tolerated. The efficacy of various drugs in preventing EIB depends on their mechanism of action and potential tachyphylaxis, variability of asthma, environmental conditions, type and intensity of exercise, and interpatient variability in responsiveness to the drug.

Special precautions must be taken with respect to WADA rules related to use of medications in competitive sports. It is the athletes' responsibility to know the rules and to abide by them. However, because these guidelines often change, sometimes annually, the physician caring for subjects who are active in sports should also be updated. Table 30.3 presents the most frequently used asthma medications and the 2013 WADA rules and regulations.

The mast cell stabilizers disodium cromoglycate and nedocromil sodium attenuate both EIB_A and EIB_{wA} when inhaled shortly before exercise, but only have a short duration of action.[29]

A similar protective effect is reported for the leukotriene antagonists montelukast and zafirlukast.[30,31] However, protection may not be complete and occurs in approximately 50% of subjects.[32]

Regular use of inhaled corticosteroid (ICS) represents the treatment of choice for asthma control and therefore is a recommended treatment to prevent EIB_A. However, the efficacy of ICS in preventing EIB_{wA}, particularly in athletes, is controversial.[33]

β_2-Adrenergic drugs (both short-acting beta$_2$ agonist [SABA] and long-acting β_2-agonists [LABA]), when given in a single inhaled dose or with intermittent administration 5 to 20 minutes before exercise, are the most useful drugs to prevent both EIB_A and EIB_{wA}.[34] They provide complete protection against exercise (FEV_1 fall <10%) in 68% of the subjects, as shown in a Cochrane review.[35] The effect usually lasts 2 to 4 hours for SABA and up to 12 hours for LABA, which makes this latter group of medications a treatment of choice for prolonged physical activity. Subgroup analysis of the 44 studies reviewed in the previously mentioned Cochrane review shows that the heterogeneity observed in the efficacy of β_2-adrenergic agents to prevent EIB is dependent not on the type of molecule used but rather on the population sample studied, with more variable effects reported in children.[35]

However, the chronic use of SABA and LABA often results in a reduction in the duration and/or magnitude of protection against EIB with cross-reacting tolerance to other β_2-agonists.[34-36] Furthermore, daily use of SABA and LABA may also result in a worsening of EIB. This loss of efficacy seems not to be prevented by ICS.[37] Therefore, chronic administration of LABA should be avoided without concomitant ICS to prevent EIB_A according to the U.S. Food and Drug Administration warning,[38] and both SABA and LABA should be used with caution on a daily basis to prevent EIB_{wA}, without concurrent use of ICS.

Table 30.3. Most Frequently Used Exercise-Induced Bronchoconstriction Medications and 2013 World Anti-Doping Agency Rules

TREATMENT	WADA RULES	NOTES
Controller medication		
Inhaled corticosteroids	Permitted	
Antileukotrienes	Permitted	
Immunotherapy*	Permitted	
Reliever medication		
Inhaled β_2-agonists	*Prohibited except* salbutamol, formoterol, and salmeterol	Salbutamol maximum 1,600 µg over 24 hr, and formoterol maximum 54 µg over 24 hr; the presence in urine of salbutamol >1,000 ng/mL or formoterol >40 ng/mL is presumed not to indicate an intended therapeutic use of the substance and will be considered as an adverse analytical finding
Oral β_2-agonists	*Prohibited*	
Oral corticosteroids	*Prohibited in competition*	TUE approval required
Inhaled or nasal ipratropium bromide	Permitted	

*Depends on appropriate choice of allergen and correct dosage regimens, but its proposal depends on risk-to-benefit ratio and should be performed by trained allergists.
TUE, therapeutic use exemption; WADA, World Anti-Doping Agency.

Ipratropium bromide prevents EIB, although this effect is not consistent among patients and may be variable in the same patient.[39] Whether subjects with EIB_{wA} or with a prevalent autonomic imbalance represent an EIB phenotype more responsive to anticholinergic agents represents an interesting hypothesis still waiting for further experimental testing.[40]

Theophylline, antihistamines, calcium channel blockers, α-adrenergic receptor antagonists, inhaled furosemide, heparin, and hyaluronic acid have been studied to prevent EIB with inconsistent results.[1]

UNMET, FUTURE RESEARCH NEEDS

Research is needed to clarify the following:

1. Whether subjects with EIB_{wA} can be considered asthmatic
2. Whether children with EIB_{wA} are at higher risk for developing clinical asthma with age
3. Whether EIB_{wA} in athletes should be considered an occupational disease due to excessive exercising in inadequate environmental conditions

CONCLUSION

Hyperventilation associated with exercise may induce bronchial obstruction in asthmatic patients. However, using the term EIA to define a specific asthma phenotype does not seem appropriate because exercise is only a trigger and not the cause of a symptom common to all etiologic forms of asthma not under control. EIB may also occur in subjects without clinical asthma. Both EIB_A and EIB_{wA} have peculiar pathogenetic mechanisms, specific diagnostic criteria, and responses to treatment and prevention. Further studies are necessary to better understand the relationship between EIB_{wA} and asthma.

REFERENCES

1. Weiler JM, Anderson SD, Randolph C, et al. Pathogenesis, prevalence, diagnosis, and management of exercise-induced bronchoconstriction: a practice parameter. *Ann Allergy Asthma Immunol.* 2010;105:S1–S47.
2. Jones KS, Buston MH, Wharton MJ. The effect of exercise on ventilator function in the child with asthma. *Br J Dis Chest.* 1962:56:78–86.
3. Godfrey S. Exercise-induced asthma. In: Clark TJH, Godfrey S, eds. *Asthma.* London: Chapman and Hall; 1977:57–58.
4. Wenzel SE. Asthma: defining the persistent asthma phenotypes. *Lancet.* 2006;368:804–813.
5. Global Initiative for Asthma. *Global Strategy for Asthma and Management and Prevention.* National Institutes of Health, Lung and Blood Institute, World Health Organization workshop report. Bethesda, MD; Medical Communication Resources; Revised 2007:16–9. Available from: http://www.ginasthma.org.
6. Helenius I, Rytilä P, Sarna S, et al. Effect of continuing or finishing high-level sports on airway inflammation, bronchial hyperresponsiveness, and asthma: a 5-year prospective follow-up study of 42 highly trained swimmers. *J Allergy Clin Immunol.* 2002;109:962–968.
7. Anderson SD, Daviskas E. The mechanism of exercise-induced asthma is.... *J Allergy Clin Immunol.* 2000;106:453–459.
8. Rundell KW, Spiering BA, Evans TM, Baumann JM. Baseline lung function, exercise-induced bronchoconstriction, and asthma-like symptoms in elite women ice hockey players. *Med Sci Sports Exerc.* 2004;36:405–410.
9. McFadden ER. Hypothesis: exercise-induced asthma as a vascular phenomenon. *Lancet.* 1990;1:880–883.
10. Anderson SD, Kippelen P. Airway injury as a mechanism for exercise-induced bronchoconstriction in elite athletes. *J Allergy Clin Immunol.* 2008;122:225–235.
11. Holgate ST. Epithelial dysfunction in asthma. *J Allergy Clin Immunol.* 2007;120:1233–1244.
12. Chimenti L, Morici G, Paternò A, et al. Bronchial epithelial damage after a half-marathon in non-asthmatic amateur runners. *Am J Physiol Lung Cell Mol Physiol.* 2010;298:L857–L862.
13. Hallstrand TS. New insights into pathogenesis of exercise-induced bronchoconstriction. *Curr Opin Allergy Clin Immunol.* 2012;12:42–48.
14. Romberg K, Bjermer L, Tufvesson E. Exercise but not mannitol increases urinary Clara cell protein (CC16) in elite swimmers. *Respir Med.* 2011;105:31–36.
15. Hallstrand TS, Moody MW, Wurfel MM, Schwartz LB, Henderson WR, Aitken ML. Inflammatory basis of exercise-induced bronchoconstriction. *Am J Respir Crit Care Med.* 2005;172:679–686.
16. Karjalainen E-M, Laitinen A, Sue-Chu M, Altraja A, Bjermer L, Laitinen LA. Evidence of airway inflammation and remodeling in ski athletes with and without bronchial hyperresponsiveness to methacholine. *Am J Respir Crit Care Med.* 2000;161:2086–2091.
17. Bougault V, Loubaki L, Joubert P, et al. Airway remodeling and inflammation in competitive swimmers training in indoor chlorinated swimming pools. *J Allergy Clin Immunol.* 2012;129:351–358.
18. Moreira A, Delgado L, Carlsen K-H. Exercise-induced asthma: why is it so frequent in Olympic athletes? *Expert Rev Respir Med.* 2011;5:1–3.
19. Hallstrand TS, Debley JS, Farin FM, Henderson WR Jr. Role of MUC5AC in the pathogenesis of exercise-induced bronchoconstriction. *J Allergy Clin Immunol.* 2007;119:1092–1098.
20. Filipe JA, Falcao-Reis S, Castro-Correia J, Barros H. Assessment of autonomic function in high level athletes by pupillometry. *Auton Neurosci.* 2003;104:66–72.
21. Rundell KW, Im J, Mayers LB, Wilber RL, Szmedra L, Schmitz HR. Self-reported symptoms and exercise-induced asthma in elite athlete. *Med Sci Sports Exerc.* 2001;33:208–213.
22. Crapo RO, Casaburi R, Coates AL, et al. ATS Guidelines for methacholine and exercise challenge testing—1999. *Am J Respir Crit Care Med.* 2000;161:309–329.
23. Rundell KW, Slee JB. Exercise and other indirect challenges to demonstrate asthma or exercise-induced bronchoconstriction in athletes. *J Allergy Clin Immunol.* 2008;122:238–246.
24. Couto M, Moreira A, Delgado L. Diagnosis and treatment of asthma in athletes. *Breathe.* 2012;8:287–296.
25. Christopher KL, Wood RP, Eckert RC, Blager FB, Raney RA, Souhrada JF. Vocal-cord dysfunction presenting as asthma. *N Engl J Med.* 1983;308:1566–1570.
26. Schwartz LB, Delgado L, Craig T, et al. Exercise-induced hypersensitivity syndromes in recreational and competitive athletes: a PRACTALL consensus report (what the general practitioner should know about sports and allergy). *Allergy.* 2008:63:953–961.

27. Sheffer AL, Austen KF. Exercise-induced anaphylaxis. *J Allergy Clin Immunol.* 1984;73:699–703.
28. Carlsen KH, Anderson SD, Bjermer L, et al. Treatment of exercise-induced asthma, respiratory and allergic disorders in sports and the relationship to doping. Part II of the report from the Joint Task Force of European Respiratory Society (ERS) and European Academy of Allergy and Clinical Immunology (EAACI) in cooperation with GA(2)LEN. *Allergy.* 2008;63:492–505.
29. Spooner CH, Spooner GR, Rowe BH. Mast-cell stabilizing agents to prevent exercise-induced bronchoconstriction. *Cochrane Database Syst Rev.* 2003;4:CD002307.
30. Leff JA, Busse WW, Pearlman D, et al. Montelukast, a leukotriene-receptor antagonist, for the treatment of mild asthma and exercise-induced bronchoconstriction. *N Engl J Med.* 1998;339:147–152.
31. Dahlén B, Roquet A, Inman MD, et al. Influence of zafirlukast and loratadine on exercise-induced bronchoconstriction. *J Allergy Clin Immunol.* 2002;109:789–793.
32. Pearlman DS, van Adelsberg J, Philip G, et al. Onset and duration of protection against exercise-induced bronchoconstriction by a single oral dose of montelukast. *Ann Allergy Asthma Immunol.* 2006;97:98–104.
33. Koh MS, Tee A, Lasserson TJ, Irving LB. Inhaled corticosteroids compared to placebo for prevention of exercise induced bronchoconstriction. *Cochrane Database Syst Rev.* 2007;3:CD002739.
34. Anderson SD, Caillaud C, Brannan JD. Beta$_2$-agonists and exercise-induced asthma. *Clin Rev Allergy Immunol.* 2006;31:163–180.
35. Bonini M, Di Mambro C, Calderon MA, et al. Beta-2 agonists for exercise induced asthma. *Cochrane Database Syst Rev.* 2013;10:CD003564
36. Hancox RJ, Subbarao P, Kamada D, Watson RM, Hargreave FE, Inman MD. Beta2-agonist tolerance and exercise-induced bronchospasm. *Am J Respir Crit Care Med.* 2002;165(8):1068–1070.
37. Salpeter SR, Ormiston TM, Salpeter EE. Meta-analysis: respiratory tolerance to regular beta2-agonist use in patients with asthma. *Ann Intern Med.* 2004;140:802–813.
38. US Food and Drug Administration. www.fda.gov. Accessed on October 30, 2013.
39. Boaventura LC, Araujo AC, Martinez JB. Effects of ipratropium on exercise-induced bronchospasm. *Int J Sports Med.* 2010;31:516–520.
40. Knöpfli BH, Bar-Or O, Araújo CG. Effect of ipratropium bromide on EIB in children depends on vagal activity. *Med Sci Sports Exerc.* 2005;37:354–359.

SECTION NINE

ENVIRONMENTAL AND POPULATION EFFECTS

31

ENVIRONMENTAL PROTECTIVE AND RISK FACTORS IN ASTHMA

COMORBID AND COEXISTING

Tari Haahtela and Ömer Kalayci

KEY POINTS

- Traditionally, environmental exposure has been considered a potential risk factor for the development asthma, and to exacerbate and cause chronicity of the disease. However, environmental risk factors and protective factors exist, and they are not usually exclusive.
- The paradigm shift in thinking recognizes the key roles of environmental exposure and type of lifestyle in enhancing immune tolerance, that is, that essential elements of natural environments can promote health.
- The biodiversity hypothesis is an extension of the hygiene and microbial deprivation (microbiota) hypotheses. Biodiversity loss leads to reduced interaction between environmental and human microbiota. This, in turn, may lead to immune dysfunction, impaired environmental adaptation (tolerance), and clinical disease.
- Building and maintaining immunologic tolerance is an active and lifelong process. The hyporesponsive immune system has not learned or has lost its ability to tell the difference between danger and nondanger, self and nonself.
- Understanding the mechanisms of gene–environment interaction and epigenetics is essential to explain the origin of chronic inflammatory diseases, including asthma and allergies, associated with modern societies.
- Both ambient air and indoor air pollutants are major risk factors that can cause symptoms and worsen disease, but their role in inducing new cases of asthma and allergy is overestimated.
- Warming of the climate system is unequivocal. It increases both outdoor pollens and mold spores and indoor aeroallergens (molds, house dust mites, cockroaches, rodents, and others pests).

- Simple behavioral activities confer some protection against or alleviate asthma and allergy. A healthy diet, physical exercise, and connection with the natural environment and countryside induce and maintain immunologic as well as psychological tolerance. Environmental control and allergen avoidance are essential elements of good asthma care, but better targeting and timing are needed.

INTRODUCTION

Generational analyses show that the incidence of asthma by birth cohort increased progressively among subjects born between 1946 and 1971 and that changes in environmental exposure explain this increased incidence.[1] Sensitization rates against inhalant allergens in birth cohorts born in 1923–1990 show similar trends.[2] The allergy gap between Finnish and Russian Karelia increased in the 10-year period from 1997/98 to 2007. The "allergy epidemic" continued in Finland and was mainly attributable to the "year of birth" effect—that is, the younger the subject, the more allergic. In Russian Karelia, no epidemic was discernible, although a decrease (paradoxically) in total immunoglobulin E (IgE) may indicate a change in more recent environmental exposure.[3] Thus, the "allergy epidemic" may just be beginning in the Russian territory.

Genetic causes predispose to the onset of asthma and allergic diseases, but genome-wide association studies in the search for the origins of the increased incidence of allergic diseases and asthma are disappointing. As the genetic background complexity has become apparent,[4] the focus has turned to critical environmental factors to explain these rapid changes in the occurrence of these diseases in different populations.

Traditionally, environmental exposure has been considered a potential risk factor for the development of asthma and allergy and for their exacerbation and chronic disease. Exposure to common allergens, such as dust mites, pollens, molds, animal dusts, and foods, generates symptoms in sensitized individuals; this is not an initial phenomenon and occurs only in sensitized individuals. The same applies to ambient air and indoor air pollutants. They irritate, aggravate inflammation, worsen symptoms, and increase the burden for asthmatic and allergic patients but are probably not very significant as primary causes of these diseases.

Studies of aboriginal populations, of farming versus urban populations, and of immigrants and observations of epigenetics and gene–environment interactions, especially microbiota studies (e.g., mapping of the gut microbiota), provide compelling evidence that the environment fundamentally modulates immune function. Poorly developed or broken immune tolerance plays a key role in the pathogenesis of asthma and allergy and probably also in many other so-called noncommunicable diseases such as those associated with autoimmunity, cancer, chronic infections, obesity, depression, and spontaneous abortions.[5]

This chapter explores environmental determinants related to asthma and allergic comorbidities, especially IgE-associated conditions, and emphasizes the development of tolerance. Finally, practical advice to improve asthma health is provided.

ENVIRONMENTAL BIODIVERSITY

The biodiversity hypothesis is an extension of the hygiene and microbial deprivation (microbiota) hypotheses.[6] It proposes that biodiversity at the level of macrobiota and microbiota is interrelated. Biodiversity loss of the former is likely to be associated with loss of diversity of the latter. Biodiversity loss leads to reduced interaction between environmental and human microbiota. This, in turn, may lead to immune dysfunction, impaired tolerance, and clinical disease. Globally, population growth, rapid urbanization, changes in food and household water, destruction of natural areas, and deforestation are key factors driving this process.

Hanski and colleagues[7] showed that atopic individuals, compared with healthy adolescents in the Finnish Karelia, had lower environmental biodiversity in the surroundings of their homes in the form of species richness of native flowering plants and the type of land use. The atopic adolescents also had significantly lower generic diversity of gram-negative γ-proteobacteria on their skin. Furthermore, the abundance of the genus *Acinetobacter* in the skin microbiota was positively correlated with the peripheral mononuclear cell expression of interleukin-10 (IL-10), a key antiinflammatory cytokine associated with immune tolerance. γ-Proteobacteria are common in the soil but are particularly dominant in above-ground vegetation, such as flowering plants.

Living in an urban environment with higher exposure to chemicals and with reduced green space and, as a consequence, limited plant, animal, and microbial life is associated with immune dysfunction and impaired tolerance.[8] With urbanization, the perpetual coexistence of environmental microorganisms with humans is severely disturbed. An environment rich in microbes in childhood reduces the risk for developing atopic disease later in life.[9] Continuous stimulation of the innate immunity by commensals and saprophytes is necessary for mucosal homeostasis.[10] Such continuous stimulation of the immune system through the skin, respiratory tract, and gut activates the regulatory network, which is decisive in the development tolerance.

The key issue in tolerance development might well be the diversity of microorganisms in the environment. The microbial quantity and diversity in drinking water and house dust were strikingly higher in Russian versus Finnish Karelia, with much lower allergy prevalence in the Russian territory. The microbial determinants in dust and water were associated with an allergy-protective effect.[11,12] Ege and colleagues[13] showed that children living on farms were exposed to a wider range of dust microbes than were children in the reference group. This exposure explains the substantial fraction of the inverse relationship between asthma and growing up on a farm.

Reduced contact with nature and environmental microbiota appears to be linked with a range of civilization diseases, not only asthma and allergy. Of considerable concern is that chronic inflammatory diseases are becoming increasingly prevalent also in low- and middle-income countries in parallel to their improving economic development and adoption of Western-type urbanization. It is also possible that biodiverse exposure confers protection, not only against chronic inflammatory and possibly malignant diseases[14] but also against infectious diseases.[15]

Novel methodologies now allow accurate determination of microbial communities in various ecosystems. Despite this advance in technology, little is known about the interactions between environmental and indigenous microbiota. For example, how is reduced biodiversity and change in the microorganism profile, found in urban and more affluent environments, reflected in indigenous human microbiota? What are the effects of the biodiversity loss of plants and animals on environmental microbiota?

TOLERANCE—ENVIRONMENTAL ADAPTATION

In allergic individuals, exposure to allergens and bioparticles does not lead to the development of tolerance as occurs in healthy individuals; instead, it results in prolonged inflammatory responses.

It is hypothesized that the dose-response curve for gaining immunologic tolerance to allergens and bioparticles varies from one allergen to another. However, the emerging picture is that a nonlinear bell-shaped dose-response curve is a universal phenomenon, demonstrated at least for endotoxin, fungal 1-3-β-glucans, cat and dog allergens, rat and mouse allergens, and house dust mite allergens.[16] Small doses of allergen cause sensitization, but with increasing doses, tolerance begins to develop.

The concept of inducing immune tolerance is a prime target for the prevention and treatment strategies for many diseases, including allergy, asthma, autoimmunity, organ transplantation, and infertility, in which dysregulation of the immune system plays an essential role. Various modes of allergen-specific immunotherapy and healthy immune response development during high-dose allergen exposure in beekeepers and cat owners have been intensively studied to try to understand the mechanism of allergen tolerance. The crucial players are regulatory

T cells. Mechanisms include changes in the profiles of allergen-specific memory T- and B-cell responses; specific antibody isotypes toward a noninflammatory direction; and decreased activation, tissue migration, and degranulation of mast cells, basophils, and eosinophils.[5] Broken tolerance indicates that there is an imbalance between different T cells. In atopic individuals, the proportion of regulatory T cells is markedly diminished or their function is impaired.[17]

Clinical tolerance, in its broadest terms, comprises not only immunologic tolerance but also tolerance affecting tissues and cells other than those of the immune system, including psychological tolerance. Sensitization or mild allergy can be viewed as a trait or characteristic rather than a state requiring major interventions, regular treatment, or strict instructions for allergen avoidance. Mild allergy does not necessarily worsen with time[18] and often, particularly in children, wanes naturally through childhood and adolescence.

Little attention is devoted in different guidelines and consensus reports to immunologic tolerance and how to strengthen it to prevent and manage asthma and allergic diseases. This is true despite the fact that basic immunologic mechanisms of tolerance have been largely unravelled, and the commonly used strategy to reduce allergen exposure at different stages from the inception of an allergic disease to its lifelong expression (allergen avoidance) is of questionable efficacy. With the possible exception of occupational exposures, effective allergen avoidance is difficult, if not impossible, and the results from trials in which avoidance is attempted are mostly discouraging. Although there is some evidence that multiple allergen reduction strategies are more successful, at least for primary prevention,[19] complex and multifaceted avoidance is not a long-term solution for this common public health problem.[20]

GENE–ENVIRONMENT INTERACTION

The increasing prevalence of allergic diseases cannot be attributed to genes because they have not undergone any major changes in the past 150 years. Compelling evidence indicates, nevertheless, that the expression of many clinical phenotypes is a consequence of a strong interaction between the genes and the environment. This is unequivocally established in both animal and certain epidemiologic studies.[21]

Understanding the mechanisms of gene–environment interaction and epigenetics is essential to explain the origin of chronic inflammatory diseases associated with modern societies. For example, Eastern versus Western environments appear to exert an effect through opposite alleles on the risk for allergic diseases. For both CD14 C-159T and CC16 A38G, the risk allele for atopic phenotypes in Finnish Karelia, surprisingly, was the protective allele in Russian Karelia.[22]

CD14 is a pattern recognition receptor that plays a central role in innate immunity through recognition of bacterial lipoglycans such as endotoxin. Endotoxin constitutes the major portion of the cell membrane of gram-negative bacteria and is ubiquitously present in the environment. Polymorphisms of the CD14 gene are associated with several asthma phenotypes,[23] and at low levels of endotoxin exposure, the C-allele may be a risk factor for the allergic phenotypes, whereas the T-allele may be a risk factor with high levels of exposure.[24]

The same genetic variant can also result in the expression of different clinical phenotypes depending on environmental exposures. For example, Bouzigon and colleagues showed that 11 of the 36 single nucleotide polymorphisms (SNPs) in the 17q21 region were associated with early-onset asthma.[25] However, they observed this significant association with early-onset asthma only in subjects exposed to environmental tobacco smoke in early life. In a birth cohort, a null mutation in the filaggrin gene increased the risk for eczema by a factor of 2.6. However, with a cat in the environment, in addition to filaggrin gene mutation, the risk increased to 11.1.[26]

Exposure to pollutants, such as benzene, toluene, xylene, polycyclic aromatic hydrocarbons, and small particulate matter, is associated in several studies with asthma and a DNA methylation pattern, even when exposure takes place during intrauterine life.[27] Particulate matter alters the DNA methylation in both in vitro and in vivo models, and exposure to benzene in childhood is associated with an increased asthma risk and altered DNA methylation.[28]

Epigenetic Modulation

Epigenetic mechanisms have received much attention during the past few years as a possible explanation for how environmental exposure modulates the immune system. Environmental factors play key roles in activating or silencing genes by altering DNA, histone methylation, histone acetylation, and chromatin structure, which might modify disease susceptibility. These changes in DNA and chromatin structure are noncoding changes but can be inherited by genetic imprinting. Epigenetics is the science that investigates such alterations in the genetic structures in particular diseases.

In general, microbe-rich environments induce both proinflammatory and regulatory circuits early in life, indicating an early activation of the relevant genes. Vuillermin and colleagues[29] suggest that microbial exposure is linked with demethylation (activation) of the interferon-γ (*IFN-γ*) gene in naïve T cells. Thus, microbial deprivation in early life is associated with persistent methylation (silencing) of the *IFN-γ* gene, resulting in reduced IFN-γ production and an increased risk for allergic diseases.

Under helper T-cell type 2 (T_H2)-polarizing conditions, the IL-4 gene promoter is demethylated in activated naïve T cells.[30] Webster and colleagues report that the methylation pattern of the IL-13 promoter varies in naïve and T_H2-polarized cells. In naïve CD4+ T cells, DNA hypomethylation is limited to the *distal* promoter of IL-13, but with T_H2 differentiation, it is the *proximal* IL-13 promoter being preferentially hypomethylated.[31] Janson and colleagues examined the methylation profile of the FoxP3 promoter in the commitment toward the regulatory T-cell lineage. They found that human CD4+, CD25 high regulatory T cells display a demethylated FoxP3 promoter, in contrast to CD4+, CD25 low regulatory T cells, which are only partially methylated.[32] These results suggest that a demethylation pattern is a prerequisite for stable FoxP3 expression and the development of tolerance (suppressive phenotype).

Although early life is crucially important for epigenetic modulation, significant changes also occur later, as shown in a comprehensive study of monozygotic twins.[33] Although the twins appeared to be epigenetically indistinguishable in early life, older monozygotic twins who had different lifestyles and had spent less of their life together had substantial differences in overall content and genomic distribution of methylation and histone acetylation, which probably contributes to discordance in disease susceptibility.

Munthe-Kaas and colleagues[34] showed that CD14 methylation increased significantly from age 2 to 10 years, and of the three SNPs that are associated with sCD14 levels within the first 2 years of life, only one was associated at 10 years. They also showed that the level of methylation is inversely correlated with sCD14 levels at 10 years.

Together, these observations call for even more attention to the role of microbial stimuli in the epigenetic modulation of T cells, particularly regulatory T-cell function.

IMMUNE HYPERRESPONSIVENESS OR HYPORESPONSIVENESS?

It used to be thought that allergy is hyperresponsiveness, that is, too active an immune response, but it is probably just the opposite. Allergy might be caused by epithelial *hyporesponsiveness* to bioparticles as a consequence of poor microbial exposure (training), especially in early childhood. During the birch pollen season, more transcripts show modified expression levels in nasal epithelium in healthy than in allergic subjects.[35] In birch pollen–allergic versus healthy individuals, large amounts of the major allergen in birch pollen (Bet v 1) are rapidly absorbed into the mucosal epithelium with the help of caveolar protein transportation. In healthy subjects, this traffic is actively blocked. The hyporesponsive allergic immune system is not able to tell the difference between danger and nondanger, self and nonself.

The biologic function of the IgE cascade, the basis of atopic asthma, seems to be complementary to other immune responses. It is one of the guardian angels monitoring the borders between human and environment. If poorly "educated," it gets activated by innocuous proteins (allergens) and attaches to the short fragments of polypeptide chains located in the β strands of the epitopes of the allergen molecules. These strands cover a flat area on the allergen surface and may mimic similar pathogen structures such as parasites.[36]

POPULATION EFFECTS

The rise in asthma prevalence, morbidity, and mortality became apparent around 1960 to 1970 in many industrialized countries. This increase was accompanied by an increase in atopic sensitization and allergic conditions, such as rhinitis, which lead to chronic sinusitis, suggesting that there is a systemic (immunologic) component to the inflammation associated with asthma.

The prevalence in different countries varies considerably,[37] but the international differences may be lessening because of the rising prevalence in low- and middle-income countries. Many of these countries have undergone rapid economical and societal changes as well as urbanization over several decades.

Worldwide, aboriginal and farming populations have much less asthma, allergic rhinitis, and allergic sensitization compared with urban populations (Figure 31.1). The racial and ethnic differences in asthma prevalence probably reflect more of a change in lifestyle and the environment than in underlying genetics. This is supported by data of the immune system cross-talk with the human and environmental microbiota being decisive for properly developed tolerance. A dysregulated immune system (i.e., insufficient mucosal homeostasis) may be the common denominator that increases disease risk in susceptible individuals. There are insufficient data to determine the exact causes of these variations of prevalence within and between populations.

The impact of the disease on individuals and the asthma burden are very much dependent on socioeconomic factors. Occurrence of asthma, and especially the burden of the disease on everyday life, is often pronounced, particularly among poor populations. Several factors contribute to this and include polluted residential areas, poor housing conditions with exposure to indoor allergens and pollutants, heavy smoking, lack of healthy and adequate food, lack of health care and essential

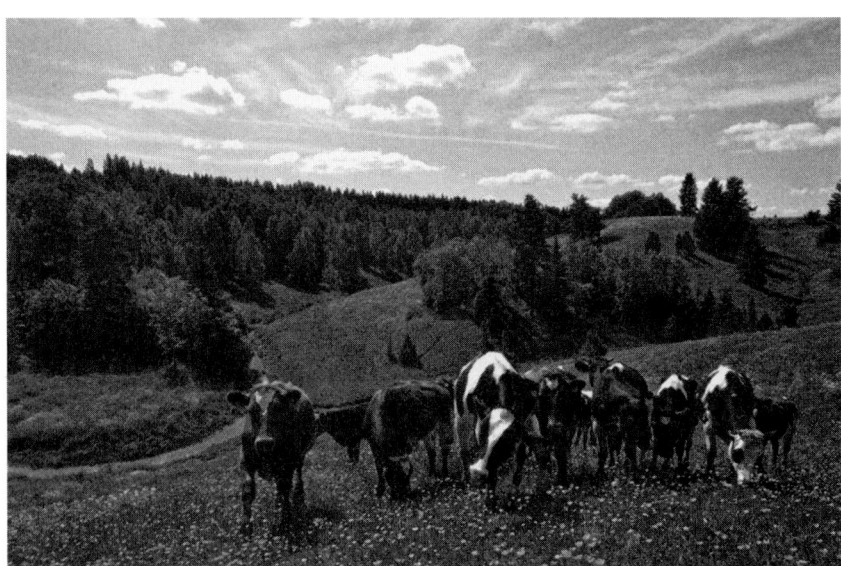

FIGURE 31.1 Traditional lifestyles associated with farming are disappearing in many areas that are experiencing rapid urbanization. (Photo courtesy of Tari Haahtela, South Finland, 2012.)

medications, psychosocial stress with unemployment, and lack of control by the individuals of their lifestyle.[38] Health problems, such as asthma mortality, cannot be solved without understanding the role of psychosocial determinants and environmental inequality.[39] However, change for the better can be achieved in a relatively simple manner; for example, in Bahia, Brazil, with the creation of easy access to inhaled corticosteroids, asthma morbidity declined significantly.[40]

The "inner-city asthma problem" is a complex entity that refers especially to the asthma problem among low-income black populations in large U.S. cities. Since 1991, the National Institute of Allergy and Infectious Diseases (NIAID) has funded research initiatives to investigate this problem.[41] Ambient air and indoor pollution, exposure to mites and cockroaches, respiratory infections, obesity, and psychosocial factors contribute to this high prevalence. However, a key goal of current research is to define mechanisms of immune system deviation and immune tolerance and apply this knowledge to generate improvements in asthma care.

The burden of asthma may have leveled off in high-income countries, although the prevalence is still high. Treatment programs improved with the concept that inflammation plays a central role in asthma pathogenesis. Antiinflammatory medications became first-line treatments, and implementation of national and global guidelines led to earlier detection and more effective management.[42] Asthma control improved, and a change for the better was observed in many countries.[40,43] In addition, in some areas environmental influences associated with modern life may have reached their maximum in inducing symptoms and disease in genetically susceptible individuals. Available data obtained from Canada and non–English-speaking countries in Europe show that the peak in asthma prevalence has reached its zenith at 8% to 12%.[44]

IMMIGRATION RESHAPING IMMUNE REGULATION

Immigrant studies provide invaluable evidence for the immunoregulatory capacity of the living environment (reviewed in Ref. 6). When immigrants move from areas of low prevalence to high prevalence of disease, they are in good health when they arrive (healthy immigrant effect), but this declines thereafter and converges to that of the native population or even becomes worse. Immunomodulatory changes appear to occur within 10 years upon arrival, and these changes are seen not only in young individuals but also in adults. This immunomodulation by "cultural adaptation," which leads to changes in disease susceptibility, appears to be universal and is reported for various inflammatory diseases, including asthma and allergic diseases, autoimmune diseases such as type 1 diabetes and multiple sclerosis, obesity and type 2 diabetes, depression, and cancers of "modern civilization."

Recently arrived individuals may experience a particularly dramatic reduction in health status, even if they are younger than the native residents and earlier immigrants. The relatively rapid change in health status is best explained by dietary factors affecting gut microbiota. In addition to dietary factors and environmental exposures, psychological factors, such as a decrease in socioeconomic status, contribute to stress and depression. These are likely to play a key role in immune modulation observed in these individuals.

AIR POLLUTION

The main air pollutants are derived from fuel combustion from traffic and various industrial sources like power plants and refineries. Fine particulate matter, nitrogen and sulfur compounds (NOx, SOx), are the most important pollutants emitted directly into the atmosphere. Ozone (O_3) is produced by the reaction of sunlight with air containing hydrocarbons and NOx.

Outdoor and indoor pollution is an important environmental risk factor for asthma and other allergic diseases, causing both symptoms and chronic and acute exacerbations. Many of the association studies of air pollution and asthma indicate that there is more asthma in the large urban centers than in the country, resulting in the conclusion that air pollutants are the main reason for this difference. However, these studies are confounded by other environmental factors that are not taken into account—for example, the differences in lifestyles in terms of microbial contacts, through gut, skin, and respiratory tract, which modulate the immune system much more readily than pollutants.

Gowers and colleagues[45] reviewed the evidence addressing an important question, "Does outdoor air pollution induce new cases of asthma?" Although air pollutants are important, they only make a small contribution to this question compared with other factors, and only in a small portion of the population.

Nevertheless, the properly conducted association studies seem to indicate that ambient air pollution is connected to the increased prevalence of asthma, rhinitis, acute respiratory tract infections, the need for asthma medications, and hospital admissions associated with these problems. Air pollution is a global problem, and an especially rapidly growing one in large Asian cities (Figure 31.2). With the rapid economic development over the past decade, the levels of air pollution from both industrial and motor vehicle emissions has increased to intolerable levels. In China, ambient air pollution is estimated to be associated with 300,000 deaths and 20 million cases of respiratory illnesses annually.[46]

The most important sources of indoor air pollutants, in addition to tobacco smoke, are biomass fuels, like wood and coal for heating and cooking, cleaning and washing products, and mold caused by dampness. Conservative estimates indicate that indoor air pollution may be responsible for nearly 2 million deaths per year in developing countries.[47] In a 2012 systematic review of the indoor environment, dampness and mold problems were determinants for developing asthma. The paper concluded that visible mold with a moldy odor increased this risk.[48]

Indoor tobacco smoke is also a major risk factor, but it can be reduced by legislation and education. In Turkey, a tobacco ban initiated in 2009 resulted in a 24% decrease in 1 year in respiratory emergency department visits in Istanbul.[49] The effect of cigarette smoke on human and respiratory health begins with intrauterine life, when its effects are probably strongest, and continues throughout life. Cigarette smoke is a risk factor not only for asthma but also for poor asthma control and increased resistance to the treatment effects of inhaled corticosteroids.[50] It has a direct toxic effect on the bronchial epithelium,[51] triggering release of proinflammatory mediators and cytokines.[52] A major effect of cigarette smoke is oxidative damage to the airways.

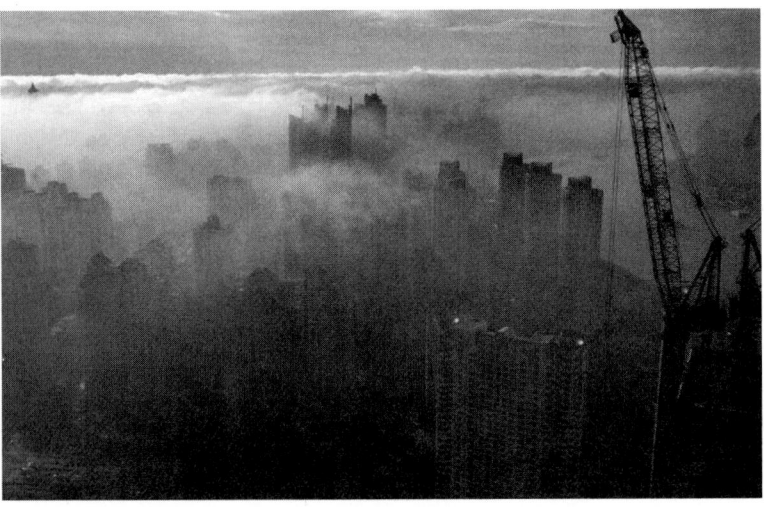

FIGURE 31.2 The growth of mega-cities is exponential. Shanghai, 2011 (23.5 million people, predicted to reach 30 million in 2020). (Photo courtesy of Tari Haahtela.)

Oxidative Stress

The lung, with its direct exposure to the environment, is highly susceptible to oxidant injury. Atmospheric oxygen, cigarette smoke, ozone, diesel exhaust particles, and subpollen particles are all known oxidative insults. Thus, oxidative stress can be an underlying mechanism for a variety of detrimental environmental effects. Reactive oxygen species inactivate antiproteases, induce apoptosis, increase production of chemoattractant molecules, increase vascular permeability, and lead to increased airway reactivity and secretions, which collectively augment the existing inflammation. The human body is equipped with strong enzymatic and nonenzymatic antioxidant defense systems. The enzymatic antioxidants include superoxide dismutases, catalase, and glutathione peroxidase, whereas the majority of nonenzymatic antioxidants of the lungs are glutathione, some specialized proteins such as thioredoxins, and some vitamins such as ascorbic acid, α-tocopherol, and carotenoids, including lycopene and β-carotene.[53]

Increased production of reactive oxygen substances such as superoxide (O_2^-), hydrogen peroxide (H_2O_2), and hydroxyl radical (OH) that lead to an imbalance between the oxidative forces and the antioxidant defense systems are implicated in the pathogenesis of many lung diseases, including asthma.[54]

Interventions to reverse this imbalance might offer promise as an adjunct to the existing treatments for asthma. However, results of trials of various treatment approaches to counteract the oxidant attack are inconsistent, and current guidelines do not include recommendations for asthma treatment with antioxidants. The major reason for this is the lack of a sufficiently efficient and stable antioxidant molecule. Therefore, research focusing on the discovery of such a molecule seems reasonable.

CLIMATE CHANGE

The Intergovernmental Panel on Climate Change (IPCC) defines climate change as a "change in the state of the climate that can be identified (e.g. using statistical tests) by changes in the mean and/or the variability of its properties and that persists for an extended period, typically decades or longer. It refers to any change in climate over time, whether due to natural variability or as a result of human activity." The IPCC further states that warming of the climate system is unequivocal, demonstrated by increases in global air and ocean temperatures in addition to the widespread melting of snow and ice and rising sea levels.[55] Climate change also is resulting in chemical, physical, and biologic health stressors that affect asthma and allergy (reviewed in Ref. 6) (Figure 31.3).

Climate change has a direct impact on pollens and mold spores. Preindustrial CO_2 levels in 1870 were 280 ppm, followed by a steady increase of 35% by 2005 to 379 ppm, with urban areas exhibiting the highest levels.[56] Several studies demonstrate direct correlations between rising CO_2 and increases in both pollen and biomass levels, as well as increased allergenicity of pollens.

Ziska and colleagues[57] tested the hypothesis that ragweed pollen levels were affected by the pre–industrial revolution CO_2 level (280 ppm), current CO_2 level (370 ppm), and CO_2 level (600 ppm) projected for the year 2100. There was a 132% increase in ragweed pollen from preindustrial time to the present, and there will be an additional 90% increase in the pollen level in 2100. In the greater Baltimore

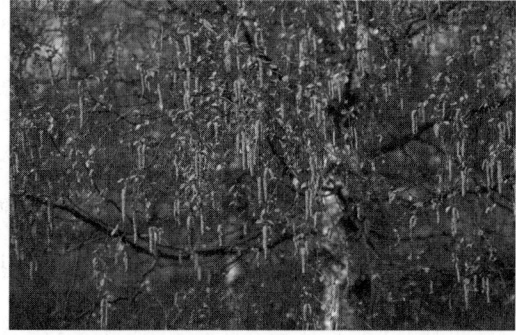

FIGURE 31.3 Global warming is heavily affecting the northernmost areas. Exceptionally intensive and prolonged pollination seasons of birch have been observed in Finland. (Photo courtesy of Tari Haahtela, South Finland.)

area, between 2000 and 2001, Ziska demonstrated that the urban levels of CO_2 were 30% higher and the temperature 2°C higher than in surrounding rural areas. In the urban area, the ragweed plants produced 189% more pollen compared with the surrounding rural area. A fundamental aspect of climate change is the potential shift in flowering phenology and pollen initiation associated with milder winters and warmer seasonal air temperature.[58]

Birch pollen exhibits increased Bet v 1–specific IgE binding in high-CO_2 environments compared with baseline levels.[59] Similar findings are demonstrated with molds, specifically, *Alternaria alternata*, with a significant increase in spore production as well as allergenicity in high- versus low-CO_2 environments.[60]

Correlations among earlier ragweed pollen start dates, prolonged pollination cycles, and increasing latitudes of ragweed growth in North America also are reported, with a nearly linear increase from Oklahoma City with 1 day earlier from 1995 to 2009 to a high of 27 days earlier in Saskatoon, Canada.[61] In addition to the increase in pollen levels and prolonged pollination cycles, there is also evidence of an impact on pollen spatial distribution, dispersal of pollen, and increased allergenicity of the pollens.

D'Amato and colleagues[62] described the potential of climate change to alter atmospheric circulation patterns, which contribute to the long-distance transport of allergenic pollen. Extreme events like thunderstorms and cyclones have an impact on aeroallergens, increasing the risk for sudden exposure.

In Southern Europe, a retrospective study examined 27 years of pollen counts with the prevalence of allergen sensitivity. Significant increases in pollen levels and duration of the pollen season of cypress (+18 days), olive (+18 days), and *Parietaria* species (+85 days) were demonstrated, with no significant change in birch or grass. The percentage of patients sensitized to those pollens significantly increased ($P < .05$), whereas there was no change in the prevalence of dust mite sensitivity (used as a control). The authors examined climate variables, finding significant correlations with rising pollen levels and prolonged seasons with increased temperatures and solar irradiation.[63]

Demain and coworkers[64] reported a retrospective review of the Alaska Medicaid database from 1999 to 2006. It shows increases in medical claims for insect reactions among all regions, with the largest percentage of increases in the most northern areas. The number of insect reactions in Alaska began to rise after increases in annual and winter temperatures were noted, raising the question of a causal relationship.

The impact of climate change on indoor aeroallergens, such as molds, house dust mites, cockroaches, rodents, and other pests, has received less attention than its effect on outdoor allergens. For example, increased relative humidity increases the risk for mold growth, and heavy periodic rainfalls stress the continuity of buildings because of the excessive water flow and possible increased incursion of water associated with this change.

PRACTICAL ACTIONS TO PROMOTE ASTHMA HEALTH

There are no established guidelines for primary prevention of allergic disease or any established methods to nonspecifically induce tolerance in established disease. However, data indicate that simple behavioral activities can confer some protection against or alleviate allergic diseases, providing indirect evidence of their beneficial effects to help induce tolerance. Not unexpectedly, such interventions include a healthy diet, physical exercise, and connection with the natural environment and countryside (Figure 31.4). Allergen immunotherapy, which enhances tolerance, also is important for secondary prevention (Table 31.1).

Chronic inflammatory diseases affect an increasing proportion of the world population. Studies that highlight the antiinflammatory effects of environmental and lifestyle factors are important but are largely lacking at this time.

Healthy Diet

Dietary factors, in addition to microorganisms, have been extensively studied to uncover possible additional factors behind the asthma

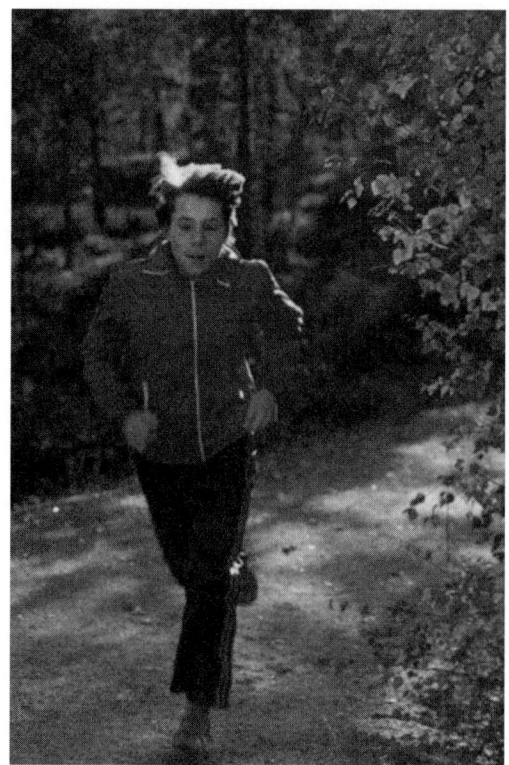

FIGURE 31.4 Exercise in green environments supports health. (Photo courtesy of Tari Haahtela, Southeast Finland.)

and allergy epidemics in modern urban environments, given the modulatory potential of nutrients on epigenetics, intestinal microbiota, and immune function. Although an inverse link between various nutrients or vitamins and occurrence of allergic diseases has been proposed in cross-sectional studies, the results are inconsistent and inconclusive. However, a systematic review based on 62 reports and 11 databases concludes that the epidemiologic evidence supports a beneficial role for increased consumption of more fruits and vegetables that is associated with better asthma and allergy outcomes.[65] For example, a traditional Mediterranean diet confers some protection against persistent wheeze and atopy. It must be also born in mind that at least a part of the beneficial effect of such foods may be mediated by microorganisms, abundantly present on their surfaces.[66]

Vitamin D deficiency is suspected to play a role in the "asthma epidemic" because it may influence genomic programming of fetal development and subsequent disease risk and is tightly linked to diet and exposure to sunlight. This hypothesis is in the process of being tested for the primary prevention of asthma in a large controlled trial in pregnant women and their offspring.[67]

In all little is known of the mechanisms involved in the effects of healthy diets on the origins and progression of asthma and allergy or associated diseases.

Probiotics

The benefits of probiotics to prevent or treat allergic diseases and asthma remain inconclusive. Bacteria-based products hold great promise for allergy prevention, but in the case of probiotics, the most beneficial bacterial strains, doses, duration, and timing of supplementation are not determined.[68] A controlled clinical trial of about 1,000 high-allergy-risk infants indicates that a probiotic mixture for 6 months has some protective effect against IgE-associated (atopic) eczema at 2 years. This effect disappeared at 5 years, but remained in caesarean-delivered children.[69] Probably a more or less continuous stimulation of innate immunity is needed to build up and maintain tolerance, not only intervention for 6 months.

Antibiotics

Antibiotics strongly modulate microbiota, and the effect may be long term. Even a 1-week course affected the gut microbiota for 3 years.[70] A systematic review by Murk and colleagues[71] indicates a slight increase in the risk for asthma when antibiotics are used during pregnancy or in the first year of life. Hill and colleagues[72] showed that in antibiotic-treated mice, commensal-derived signals influence basophil hematopoiesis and susceptibility to T_H2 cytokine-dependent inflammation and allergic disease. Cho and colleagues[73] increased adiposity in young mice by administering subtherapeutic doses of antibiotics. Changes were observed in the gut microbiota as well as in copies of key genes involved in the metabolism of carbohydrates to short-chain fatty acids.

Table 31.1. Practical Advice to Build Up and Improve Tolerance for Primary Prevention and Symptom Prevention (Secondary Prevention) and to Prevent Exacerbations and Attacks (Tertiary Prevention)[84]

PRIMARY PREVENTION	SECONDARY AND TERTIARY PREVENTION

• Support breastfeeding. Solid foods from 4–6 months.
• Do not avoid environmental exposure unnecessarily (e.g., foods, pets).
• Strengthen immunity by increasing connection to natural environments.
• Strengthen immunity through regular physical exercise.
• Strengthen immunity through healthy diet (e.g., traditional Mediterranean or Baltic type).
• Use antibiotics only for true need. The majority of microbes are useful and build up health immune function.
• Probiotic bacteria in fermented food or other preparations may strengthen immune function.
• Do not smoke (e.g., parental smoking increases asthma risk in children).
	• Regular physical exercise is antiinflammatory.
	• Healthy diet is antiinflammatory (e.g., traditional Mediterranean or Baltic type of diet improves asthma control).
	• Probiotic bacteria in fermented food or other preparations may be antiinflammatory.
	• Allergen-specific immunotherapy:
	  - Allergens as in foods
	  - Sublingual tablets or drops (pollens, mites?)
	  - Subcutaneous injections (e.g., insect stings)
	• Hit early and hit hard respiratory, or skin inflammation with medication. Find treatment for long-term control.
	• Do not smoke. Asthma and allergy medications are not fully effective in smokers.

In conclusion, antibiotic manipulation seems to alter metabolic homeostasis, especially in early life, and increases the risk for allergic and other inflammatory conditions. Use of antibiotics should be restricted to those in real need. This is obvious but difficult to implement. Antibiotics should be used only by prescription. The general public needs continuous information on the use and misuse of antibiotics, especially their lack of effectiveness in the most common infections: viral infections of the upper respiratory tract.

Physical Activity

Several outlines of evidence emphasize the risks of a sedentary lifestyle for health. Physical inactivity increases the inflammatory burden independently of obesity, and conversely, exercise programs decrease systemic low-level inflammation in some patient groups and healthy adults. The antiinflammatory effects of physical exercise seem to be mediated by activating the regulatory circuits, including regulatory T cells. For example, in healthy adults, a 12-week program of moderate exercise three times per week significantly improved regulatory T-cell numbers and function.[74] In patients with type 2 diabetes, moderate exercise for 12 weeks significantly decreased HbA1c levels while increasing IL-12 levels and the expression of transcription factors T-bet and Fox3p+, indicating improvements in both the metabolic and the immune systems.[75]

In asthmatic children, a 12-week exercise program decreased total and house dust mite–specific IgE levels.[76] The antiinflammatory effect of exercise also has been demonstrated in a murine model of asthma.[77] Physical activity is an especially important means for primary allergy prevention in children; in particular, those with asthma benefit from moderate physical activity because they have been frequently found to be less active than their nonasthmatic peers.

Connection with the Natural Environment

An urban environment appears to lack elements that apparently are important for the proper development of immune tolerance. The recognition of the (absolute) dependence of humans on both the commensal and environmental microbiota is crucial to unravelling the mechanisms involved.

Concepts such as "ecotherapy," "green exercise," and "forest therapy" have been launched. Urbanization and densification policy continues globally, and within the next 30 years, it is estimated that two-thirds of the world's population and 85% of the population in the developed countries will live in urban areas with little green space.[78]

A large study found that the annual prevalence rate of most disease clusters was lower in environments where people live with more green space (10% or more than the average) within a 1-km radius. This effect was most pronounced for depression and anxiety, but it was also significant for asthma/chronic obstructive pulmonary disease, diabetes, and coronary heart disease.[79]

Green space, including forests and natural areas such as parks, may act as a buffer between stressful life events and health. Aligned to this concept, better self-reported health and lower stress scores also have been reported to be inversely associated with the distance to green space.[80]

A meta-analysis of 10 intervention studies revealed that "green exercise" (activities in natural environments), even of short duration, significantly improved physical and mental health.[81] Of importance, physical activity in a natural environment versus other settings appears to have more beneficial health effects.[82]

Several ongoing studies have examined the health effects of forests. Compared with urban settings, forest environments are associated with lower cortisol levels, lower pulse rates and blood pressures, and higher parasympathetic and lower sympathetic nerve activity in healthy individuals.[83] Exposure to nature, and to forest environments in particular, has the potential to substantially improve human health (Figure 31.5).

The prevalence of inflammatory diseases is likely to increase even more. The health effects of nature and green spaces should be recognized, and measures to limit excessive land use and fragmentation urgently undertaken. There is already a rich literature to

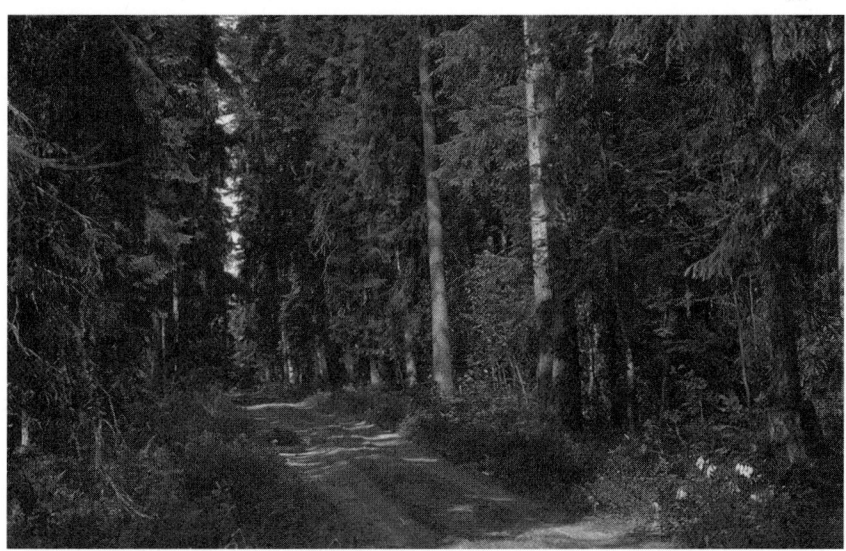

FIGURE 31.5 Population growth and intensive urban and industrial development are causing an escalating loss of habitats and natural environments, especially forests. (Photo courtesy of Tari Haahtela, South Estonia, 2008.)

demonstrate that natural environments are of vital importance to the physical and mental health of humans, and as a consequence, biodiversity should be integrated into the conventional measures of well-being and recognized as a global public good that requires conscious collective choices.

The health effects of natural environments are obvious but difficult to examine experimentally. More data and better understanding of the relevant mechanisms underlying the "nature effect" at the cellular and molecular levels are necessary. Direct asthma-related data are urgently needed.

UNMET, FUTURE RESEARCH NEEDS

1. Key questions on immune tolerance should be explored: What are the hallmarks of "normal" development of immune tolerance? What are the essential factors to maintain tolerance? What breaks up the tolerance?

2. More data and better understanding of the relevant mechanisms underlying the "nature effect" at the cellular and molecular levels are necessary. Direct asthma-related data are needed.

3. Very little is known about the interactions between environmental and indigenous microbiota. How are reduced biodiversity and changes in the microorganism profile, found in urban and more affluent environments, reflected in indigenous human microbiota? What are the effects of the biodiversity loss of plants and animals on environmental microbiota?

4. How should asthma health be promoted? How should patients balance environmental control/allergen avoidance and tolerance-inducing exposure to the environment (e.g., diet, physical activity, connection to natural environments)?

5. The medical community cannot solve the health problems of the rapidly changing and developing societies; collaboration with other scientific communities, including environmental organizations, is necessary. Also, patient organizations should be better involved.

6. A global action plan for asthma and allergy could be a tool for reducing disease burden to individuals and societies as a platform to implement preventive measures.

CONCLUSION

Behavioral activities, including a healthy diet, regular exercise, and exposure to the natural environment and countryside, may confer some protection against or help alleviate asthma, allergy, and other inflammatory diseases. These activities promote immunologic and psychological normalcy. Environmental control and allergen avoidance also are essential elements for optimal asthma care and a healthy lifestyle.

REFERENCES

1. Sunyer J, Anto JM, Tobias A, Burney P, for the European Community Respiratory Health Study (ECRHS). Generational increase of self-reported first attack of asthma in fifteen industrialized countries. *Eur Respir J*. 1999;14:885–891.
2. Isolauri E, Huurre A, Salminen S, Impivaara O. The allergy epidemic extends beyond the past few decades. *Clin Exp Allergy*. 2004;34:1007–1110.
3. Laatikainen T, von Hertzen L, Koskinen JP, et al. Allergy gap between Finnish and Russian Karelia on increase. *Allergy*. 2011;66:886–892.
4. Moffatt M, Gut IG, Demenais F, et al. A large-scale consortium-based genomewide association study of asthma. *N Engl J Med*. 2010;363:1211–1221.
5. Akdis M, Akdis CA. Therapeutic manipulation of immune tolerance in allergic disease. *Nat Rev Drug Discov*. 2009;8:645–660.
6. Haahtela T, Holgate ST, Pawankar R, et al. The biodiversity hypothesis and allergic diseases. WAO Statement. *WAO J*. 2013;6:3.
7. Hanski I, von Hertzen L, Fyhrquist N, et al. Environmental biodiversity, human microbiota, and allergy are interrelated. *Proc Natl Acad Sci U S A*. 2012;109:8334–8339.
8. Rook GAW. 99th Dahlem conference on infection, inflammation and chronic inflammatory disorders: Darwinian medicine and the "hygiene" or "old friends" hypothesis. *Clin Exp Immunol*. 2010;160:70–79.
9. Riedler J, Braun-Fahrländer C, Eder W, et al. Exposure to farming in early life and development of asthma and allergy: a cross-sectional survey. *Lancet*. 2001;358:1129–1133.

10. Rakoff-Nahoum S, Paglino J, Eslami-Varzaneh F, Edberg S, Medzhitov R. Recognition of commensal microflora by Toll-like receptors is required for intestinal homeostasis. *Cell.* 2004;118:229–241.
11. von Hertzen L, Laatikainen T, Pitkänen T, et al. Microbial content of drinking water in Finnish and Russian Karelia—implications for atopy prevalence. *Allergy.* 2007;62:288–292.
12. Pakarinen J, Hyvärinen A, Salkinoja-Salonen M, et al. Predominance of gram-positive bacteria in house dust in the low-allergy risk Russian Karelia. *Environ Microbiol.* 2008;10:3317–3325.
13. Ege M, Mayer M, Normand AC, et al. Exposure to environmental microorganisms and childhood asthma. *N Engl J Med.* 2011;364:701–709.
14. von Hertzen L, Joensuu H, Haahtela T. Microbial deprivation, inflammation and cancer. *Cancer Metast Rev.* 2011;30:211–323.
15. Keesing F, Belden LK, Daszak P, et al. Impacts of biodiversity on the emergence and transmission of infectious diseases. *Nature.* 2010;468:647–652.
16. Platts-Mills TA, Woodfolk JA. Allergens and their role in the allergic immune response. *Immunol Rev.* 2011;242:51–68.
17. Ling EM, Smith T, Nguyen D, et al. Relation of CD4+CD25+ regulatory T cell suppression of allergen-driven T cell activation to atopic status and expression of allergic disease. *Lancet.* 2004;363:608–615.
18. Teppo H, Revonta M, Haahtela T. Allergic rhinitis and asthma have generally good outcome and little effect on quality of life: a 20-year follow-up. *Allergy.* 2011;66:1123–1125.
19. van Schayck OC, Maas T, Kaper J, Knottnerus AJ, Sheikh A. Is there any role for allergen avoidance in the primary prevention of childhood asthma? *J Allergy Clin Immunol.* 2007;119:1323–1328.
20. Asher I, Baena-Cagnani C, Boner A, et al., for the World Allergy Organization. World Allergy Organization guidelines for prevention of allergy and allergic asthma. *Int Arch Allergy Immunol.* 2004;135:83–92.
21. Ober C, Vercelli D. Gene-environment interactions in human disease: nuisance or opportunity? *Trends Genet.* 2011;27:107–115.
22. Zhang G, Khoo SK, Laatikainen T, et al. Opposite gene by environment interactions in Karelia for CD14 and CC16 single nucleotide polymorphisms and allergy. *Allergy.* 2009;64:1333–1341.
23. Sackesen C, Karaaslan C, Keskin O, et al. The effect of polymorphisms at the CD14 promoter and the TLR4 gene on asthma phenotypes in Turkish children with asthma. *Allergy.* 2005;60:1485–1492.
24. Martinez FD. CD14, endotoxin, and asthma risk actions and interactions. *Proc Am Thorac Soc.* 2007;4:221–225.
25. Bouzigon E, Corda E, Aschard H, et al. Effect of 17q21 variants and smoking exposure in early-onset asthma. *N Engl J Med.* 2008;359:1985–1994.
26. Bisgaard H, Simpson A, Palmer CN, et al. Gene-environment interaction in the onset of eczema in infancy: filaggrin loss-of-function mutations enhanced by neonatal cat exposure. *PLoS Med.* 2008;5:e131.
27. Perera F, Tang WY, Herbstman J, et al. Relation of DNA methylation of 5′-CpG island of ACSL3 to transplacental exposure to airborne polycyclic aromatic hydrocarbons and childhood asthma. *PLoS One.* 2009;4:e4488.
28. Bollati V, Baccarelli A, Hou L, et al. Changes in DNA methylation patterns in subjects exposed to low-dose benzene. *Cancer Res.* 2007;67:876–880.
29. Vuillermin PJ, Ponsonby AL, Saffery R, et al. Microbial exposure, interferon gamma gene demethylation in naïve T-cells, and the risk of allergic disease. *Allergy.* 2009;64:348–353.
30. Lee D, Agarwal S, Rao A. Th2 lineage commitment and efficient IL-4 production involves extended demethylation of the IL-4 gene. *Immunity.* 2002;16:649–660.
31. Webster R, Rodriguez Y, Klimecki W, Vercelli D. The human IL-13 locus in neonatal CD41 T cells is refractory to the acquisition of a repressive chromatin architecture. *J Biol Chem.* 2007;282:700–709.
32. Janson P, Winerdal M, Marits P, et al. FOXP3 promoter demethylation reveals the committed Treg population in humans. *PLoS One.* 2008;3:e1612:1–13.
33. Fraga MF, Ballestar E, Paz MF, et al. Epigenetic differences arise during the lifetime of monozygotic twins. *Proc Natl Acad Sci U S A.* 2005;102:10604–10609.
34. Munthe-Kaas MC, Torjussen TM, Gervin K, et al. CD14 polymorphisms and serum CD14 levels through childhood: a role for gene methylation? *J Allergy Clin Immunol.* 2010;125(6):1361–1368.
35. Joenväärä S, Mattila P, Renkonen J, et al. Caveolar traffic through nasal epithelium of birch pollen allergen Bet v 1 in allergic patients. *J Allergy Clin Immunol.* 2009;124:135–142.
36. Niemi M, Jylhä S, Laukkanen ML, et al. Molecular interactions between a recombinant

IgE antibody and the beta-lactoglobulin allergen. *Structure.* 2007;15:1413–1421.
37. Mallol J, Crane J, von Mutius E, Odhiambo J, Keil U, Stewart A, for the ISAAC Phase Three Study Group. The International Study of Asthma and Allergies in Childhood (ISAAC) Phase Three: a global synthesis. *Allergol Immunopathol.* 2013;41(2):73–85.
38. Wright RJ, Sternthal MJ. Socio-economic factors and environmental justice. In: Pawankar R, Canonica GW, Holgate ST, Lockey RF, eds. *WAO White Book on Allergy.* Milwaukee, WI; 2011:91–95.
39. de Souza-Machado C, Souza-Machado A, Cruz AA. Asthma mortality inequalities in Brazil: tolerating the unbearable. *Sci World J.* 2012;2012:625829.
40. Kupczyk M, Haahtela T, Cruz A, Kuna P. Reduction of asthma burden is possible through National Asthma Plans. *Allergy.* 2010;65: 415–419.
41. Togias A, Fenton MJ, Gergen PJ, Rotrosen D, Fauci AS. Asthma in the inner city: the perspective of the National Institute of Allergy and Infectious Diseases. *J Allergy Clin Immunol.* 2010;125:540–544.
42. Global initiative for asthma (GINA). Global strategy for asthma management and prevention. www.ginasthma.org. Updated 2012.
43. Haahtela T, Tuomisto LE, Pietinalho A, et al. A 10 year asthma programme in Finland: major change for the better. *Thorax.* 2006;61:663–670.
44. von Hertzen L, Haahtela T. Signs of reversing trends in prevalence of asthma. *Allergy.* 2005;60:283–292.
45. Gowers AM, Cullinan P, Ayres JG, et al. Does outdoor air pollution induce new cases of asthma? Biological plausibility and evidence; a review. *Respirology.* 2012;17:887–898.
46. Millman A, Tang D, Perera FP. Air pollution threatens the health of children in China. *Pediatrics.* 2008;122:620–628.
47. Maio S, Cerrari S, Simoni M, Sarno G, Baldacci S, Viegi G. Environmental risk factors: indoor and outdoor pollution. In: Pawankar R, Canonica G, Holgate S, Lockey R, eds. *WAO White Book on Allergy 2011–2012.* Milwaukee, WI; World Allergy Organization; 2011:84–90.
48. Quansah R, Jaakkola MS, Hugg TT, Heikkinen SA, Jaakkola JJ. Residential dampness and molds and the risk of developing asthma: a systematic review and meta-analysis. *PLoS One.* 2012;7:e47526.
49. Dagli E, Erdem E, Topuzoglu A, et al. The impact of smoke-free legislation on smoke-related emergency admissions in Istanbul. 21st European Respiratory Society Meeting, Amsterdam, Holland. *Eur Respir J.* 2011;Suppl 55:855s.
50. Stapleton M, Howard-Thompson A, George C, Hoover RM, Self THJ. Smoking and asthma. *Am Board Fam Med.* 2011;24:313–322.
51. Floreani A, Rennard S. The role of cigarette smoke in the pathogenesis of asthma and as a trigger for acute symptoms. *Curr Opin Pulm Med.* 1999;5:38–46.
52. Chalmers G, MacLeod KJ, Thomson L, et al. Smoking and airway inflammation in patients with mild asthma. *Chest.* 2001;120:1917–1922.
53. Birben E, Sahiner UM, Sackesen C, Erzurum S, Kalayci O. Oxidative stress and antioxidant defense. *WAO J.* 2012;5:9–19.
54. Sahiner UM, Birben E, Erzurum S, Sackesen C, Kalayci O. Oxidative stress in asthma. *WAO J.* 2011;4:151–158.
55. IPCC (United Nations Intergovernmental Panel on Climate Change). *Climate Change 2007: Forth Assessment Report (AR4) 2007; Synthesis Report.* Cambridge, UK: Cambridge University Press; 2007. Available at: http://www.ipcc.ch/ipccreports/assessments-reports.htm. Accessed June 4, 2011.
56. Noyes PD, McElwee MK, Miller HD, et al. The toxicology of climate change: environmental contaminants in a warming world. *Environ Int.* 2009;35:971–986.
57. Ziska LH, Gebhard DE, Frenz DA, Faulkner S, Singer BD. Cities as harbingers of climate change: common ragweed, urbanization and public health. *J Allergy Clin Immunol.* 2003;111:290–295.
58. Ziska LH, Knowlto K, Rogers C, et al. Recent warming by latitude associated with increased length of ragweed pollen season in central North America. *Proc Natl Acad Sci U S A.* 2011;108: 4248–4251.
59. Ahlholm JU, Helander ML, Savolainen J. Genetic and environmental factors affecting the allergenicity of birch pollen. *Clin Exp Allergy.* 1998;28:1384–1388.
60. Wolf J, O'Neill NR, Rogers CA, Muilenberg ML, Ziska LH. Elevated atmospheric CO2 concentrations amplify *Alternaria alternate* sporulation and total antigen production. *Environ Health Persp.* 2010;118:1223–1228.
61. Ziska LH, Knowlto K, Rogers C, et al. Recent warming by latitude associated with increased length of ragweed pollen season in central North America. *Proc Natl Acad Sci U S A.* 2011;108: 4248–4251.

62. D'Amato G, Cecchi L, Bonini S, et al. Allergenic pollen and pollen allergy in Europe. *Allergy*. 2007;62:976–990.
63. Ariano R, Canonica GW, Passalacqua G. Possible role of climate change in variations in pollen seasons and allergenic sensitizations during 27 years. *Ann Allergy Asthma Immunol*. 2010;104:215–222.
64. Demain JG, Gessner BD, McLaughlin JB, Sikes DS, Foote JT. Increasing insect reactions in Alaska: is this related to changing climate? *Allergy Asthma Proc*. 2009;30:238–243.
65. Nurmatov U, Devereux G, Sheikh A. Nutrients and foods for the primary prevention of asthma and allergy: systematic review and meta-analysis. *J Allergy Clin Immunol*. 2011;127:724–733.
66. Jawetz F, Melnick JC, Adelberg EA. *Review of Medical Microbiology*. Los Altos, CA: Lange Medical Publications; 1980.
67. Litonjua AA, Weiss ST. Is vitamin D deficiency to blame for the asthma epidemic? *J Allergy Clin Immunol*. 2007;120:1031–1035.
68. Fiocchi A, Burks W, Bahna SL, et al., for the WAO Special Committee on Food Allergy and Nutrition. Clinical use of probiotics in pediatric allergy (CUPPA): a World Allergy Organization position paper. *WAO J*. 2012;5(11):148–167.
69. Kuitunen M, Kukkonen K, Juntunen-Backman K, et al. Probiotics prevent IgE-associated allergy until age 5 years in cesarean-delivered children but not in the total cohort. *J Allergy Clin Immunol*. 2009;123:335–341.
70. Dethlefsen L, Huse S, Sogin ML, Relman DA. The pervasive effects of an antibiotic on the human gut microbiota, as revealed by deep 165 rRNA sequencing. *PLoS Biol*. 2008;6:2383–2400.
71. Murk W, Risnes KR, Bracken MB. Prenatal or early-life exposure to antibiotics and risk of childhood asthma: a systematic review. *Pediatrics*. 2011;127:1125–1138.
72. Hill DA, Siracusa MC, Apt MC, et al. Commensal bacteria–derived signals regulate basophil hematopoiesis and allergic inflammation. *Nat Med*. 2012;18:538–546.
73. Cho I, Yamanishi S, Cox L, et al. Antibiotics in early life alter the murine colonic microbiome and adiposity. *Nature*. 2012;488:621–626.
74. Yeh SH, Chuang H, Lin LW, Hsiao CY, Eng HL. Regular Tai Chi Chuan exercise enhances functional mobility and CD4CD25 regulatory T cells. *Br J Sports Med*. 2006;40:239–243.
75. Yeh SH, Chuang H, Lin LW, et al. Regular Tai Chi Chuan exercise improves T cell helper function of patients with type 2 diabetes mellitus with an increase in T-bet transcription factor and IL-12 production. *Br J Sports Med*. 2009;43:845–850.
76. Moreira A, Delgado L, Haahtela T, et al. Physical training does not increase inflammation in asthmatic children. *Eur Respir J*. 2008;32:1570–1575.
77. Lowder T, Dugger K, Deshane J, Estell K, Schwiebert L. Repeated bouts of aerobic exercise enhance regulatory T cell responses in a murine asthma model. *Brain Behav Immun*. 2010;24:153–159.
78. World Urbanization Prospects: The 2007 Revision Population Database. http://esa.un.org/unup/. Accessed October 14, 2013.
79. Maas J, Verheij RA, de Vries S, Speeuwenberg P, Schellevis FG, Groenewegen PP. Morbidity is related to a green living environment. *J Epidemiol Commun Health*. 2009;63:967–973.
80. Stigsdotter UK, Ekholm O, Schipperijin J, Toftager M, Kamper-Jorgensen F, Randrup TB. Health promoting outdoor environments: associations between green space, and health, health-related quality of life and stress based on a Danish national representative survey. *Scand J Public Health*. 2010;38:411–417.
81. Barton J, Pretty J. What is the best dose of nature and green exercise for improving mental health? A multi-study analysis. *Environ Sci Technol*. 2010;44:3947–3955.
82. Mitchell R, Popham F. Effect of exposure to natural environment on health inequalities: an observational population study. *Lancet*. 2008;372:1655–1660.
83. Park BJ, Tsunetsugu Y, Kasetani T, Kagawa T, Miyazaki Y. The physiological effects of *Shinrin-yoku* (taking in the forest atmosphere or forest bathing): evidence from field experiments in 24 forests across Japan. *Environ Health Prev Med*. 2010;15:18–26.
84. Haahtela T, Valovirta E, Kauppi P, et al., for the Finnish Allergy Programme Group. The Finnish Allergy Programme 2008–2018: scientific basis and practical implementation. *Asia Pacific Allergy*. 2012:2;275–279.

SECTION TEN

AGE

32

ASTHMA OVER 65

A DISEASE ABOUT WHICH LITTLE IS KNOWN

Chelle Pope, Richard D. deShazo, and Monroe James King

KEY POINTS

- Asthma in elderly people is underdiagnosed and undertreated.
- Asthma is an increasing problem in the elderly population.
- Elderly asthmatic patients have been excluded from many clinical trials.
- Asthma in elderly people often presents differently than in the younger population.
- Diagnosis and treatment of asthma in elderly people can be difficult because of coexisting diseases and comorbidities often found in this population.
- Research in every aspect of asthma in elderly people is needed.

INTRODUCTION

With the worldwide increase in the older population and the growing prevalence of asthma, it is no surprise that asthma in elderly people is also an increasing problem. Insufficient data exist to make firm conclusions on many important issues about this condition. Seniors with asthma often have coexisting and comorbid conditions, and the combination of age and illness has precluded, in general, their participation in clinical trials. There are other important variables, including differences in perception, interpretation, and response to the symptoms of airway obstruction in this population. Many patients mistakenly believe that wheeze and dyspnea are normal,[1] and they commonly decrease their activity, a response that can induce further social isolation and a decreased quality of life. Coupled with the challenge of misdiagnosis or underdiagnosis are the potential problems associated with side effects from medications, drug–drug interactions, problems appropriately using medications, and compliance. This

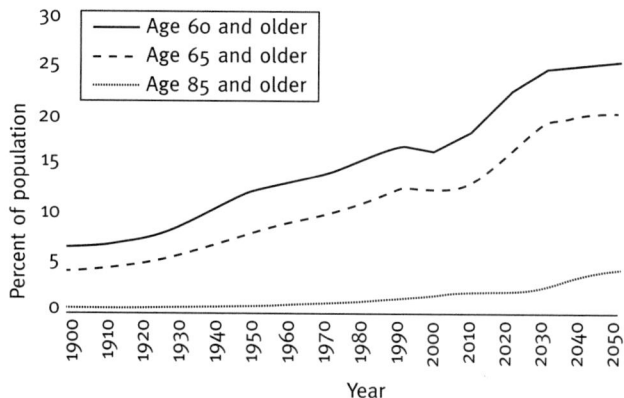

FIGURE 32.1 Population by 2050. The percentage of the U.S. population in all age groups older than 60 years will continue to increase in the near term. (Adapted from Moorman JE, Mannino DM. Increasing US asthma mortality rates: who is really dying? *J Asthma*. 2001;38[1]:65–71.)

chapter identifies the prevalence of asthma, which affects decisions about therapy and the important questions in this age group yet to be answered.

EPIDEMIOLOGY

The proportion of the population older than 60 years is projected to rise to 25% in the United States by the year 2050[2] (Figure 32.1). The prevalence of many chronic diseases, including asthma, will also increase.[3] Asthma in seniors can be characterized as early-onset asthma, present before age 65 years, or late-onset asthma, which manifests as a new health problem after this age, although the proportions of each remain unknown.[4] Asthma prevalence, since 1980, is increasing in all age groups[5,6] and now affects at least 10% of adults older than 60 years.[1,6] This prevalence is most likely underestimated in all groups and particularly in elderly people, in whom it is often underdiagnosed or misdiagnosed.[7]

Not only is the prevalence of asthma high among elderly patients, but also the associated mortality is disproportionately high[8,9] (Figure 32.2). Although most epidemiologic studies are based on death certificates, which probably underestimate asthma prevalence, some data are compelling.[10] Regardless, elderly

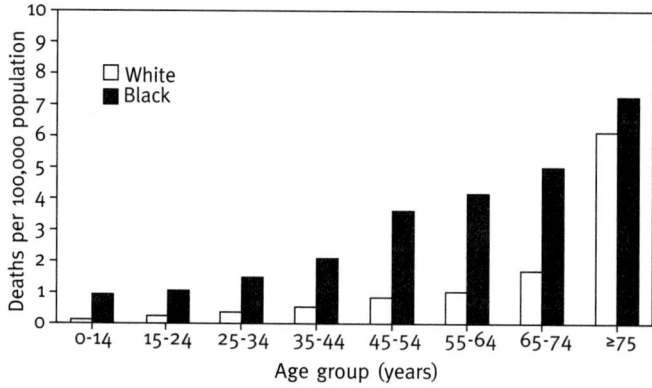

FIGURE 32.2 Death rate from asthma. Asthma death rates in black and Caucasian patients reflect significant health disparities. (Adapted from: QuickStats: Asthma Death Rates, by Race and Age Group—United States, 2007–2009. [2012]. Retrieved October 28, 2013, from http://www.cdc.gov/mmwr/preview/mmwrhtml/mm6117a11.htm?s_cid=mm6117a11_w.)

patients tend to have additional medical problems, always making the determination of an exact cause of death more difficult.[3] One study from the Centers for Disease Control and Prevention (CDC) shows a death rate from asthma that is almost five-fold greater in elderly people compared with the other adult age groups.[6,11] Evidence from a separate 1979 to 1996 CDC study shows that the mortality rate in elderly individuals from asthma is increasing rapidly.[8] Although the cause is unclear, hospitalization (3:1) and mortality (2:1) rates from asthma are higher for older females versus males.[12] Elderly asthmatic patients also have more severe impairment of their quality of life compared with younger patients.[13,14]

The economic challenges of asthma are also greater among elderly patients. They tend to have more emergency department visits and hospitalizations and a longer length of stay than younger adults.[13]

Despite these statistics, asthma in this age group has largely been ignored in the medical community and literature. Studies of asthma, in general, and large clinical trials, in particular, excluded them.[3] Few data on the diagnosis, treatment, and effects of this disease on the quality of life in elderly patients are available, especially compared with the information about pediatric and young adult subjects.

CLINICAL FEATURES

Differences in Presentation

Asthma in elderly people often presents differently than in the younger population[3] (Table 32.1). For example, elderly subjects tend to have a more progressive disease and often fixed airway obstruction at the time of presentation.[15] Seniors also tend to present later than younger asthmatic patients, sometimes years after symptoms begin.[16] Studies suggest a decreased perception of dyspnea as a possible explanation for this observation.[17] Decreased lung compliance, static elastic recoil, and respiratory muscle strength[18] in seniors may lead to a decrease in activity level in order to accommodate for asthmatic symptoms. The sum total of these features likely contributes to the increase in asthma morbidity and mortality in this population.[3]

Table 32.1. Features of Asthma in Elderly Patients

PULMONARY AND THORACIC PATHOPHYSIOLOGIC DIFFERENCES

1. Decreased respiratory muscle strength
2. Decreased lung elastic recoil
3. Decreased lung compliance
4. More progressive, irreversible obstruction
5. Late presentation with more severe disease

NEUROLOGIC AND COGNITIVE DIFFERENCES

1. Decreased perception of bronchoconstriction
2. Decreased perception of air hunger
3. Significantly decreased activity to compensate for symptoms

OTHER DIFFERENCES

1. Fewer allergic triggers
2. Late-onset intrinsic triggers—viral upper respiratory infection, fungal
3. Increased morbidity and mortality

Adapted from Stupka E, deShazo R. Asthma in seniors: Part 1. Evidence for underdiagnosis, undertreatment, and increasing morbidity and mortality. *Am J Med.* 2009;122:6–11.

Natural History

The natural history of asthma is poorly understood, particularly in elderly patients. Increased levels of irreversible airflow obstruction and a more rapid decline in forced expiratory volume in 1 second (FEV_1) are documented.[19] Long-standing asthma contributes to both increased airway smooth muscle mass and declining FEV_1 compared with late-onset asthma.[20] Some data suggest that this may result from structural changes in the airway from higher levels of neutrophils found in the bronchi and sputum of elderly versus younger adults.[19] The inflammatory response, with eosinophilic and neutrophilic influx into the airways, is associated with the presence of oxygen free radicals, proteolytic enzymes, and cytokines that affect extracellular matrix proteins and other airway structural components.[19,21] However, a clear association between the severity of asthma and sputum neutrophilia is not established.[19]

The role of respiratory allergens in the pathogenesis of asthma in elderly versus younger patients is less clear.[4,22] Elderly subjects are less sensitive and have lower levels of specific immunoglobulin E (IgE).[4,22]

Role of Allergic Triggers

There is a functional decline in the innate and adaptive immune systems with aging,[2,23] but how these changes relate to the prevalence of allergic disease in this age group remains unclear. For example, although atopic dermatitis declines with age, there are strong associations among atopic dermatitis, allergic rhinitis, and asthma in seniors,[2,24,25] but the association of IgE sensitization and sensitivity in elderly patients is unclear. Bronchial and nasal allergen challenges have not been performed in seniors who have allergen-specific IgE. Likewise, no studies demonstrate that age-related decreases in IgE affect the severity of asthma.[2,3] One study suggests that late-onset nonallergic (intrinsic without evidence of allergen sensitization) asthma is triggered by upper respiratory tract infection in at least 60% of patients.[26] Respiratory tract infections with rhinovirus, respiratory syncytial virus, influenza, and *Mycoplasma* species are major causes of morbidity and mortality in long-term care facilities.[27] Because many elderly patients live in these facilities, they are the population at risk for these infections.

DIAGNOSIS

Difficulties with Diagnosis

Spirometry that demonstrates a ratio of FEV_1 to forced vital capacity (FVC) that is less than the lower limits of normal, with reversibility defined as a postbronchodilator increase of greater than 12% and more than 200 mL in FEV_1 and/or FVC, can help distinguish asthma from other lung disease, such as chronic obstructive pulmonary disease (COPD). However, the diagnosis and treatment of this population can be challenging and difficult.[5,28] The results of the Respiratory Health in the Elderly Study (SARA), performed in Europe, suggest that only 68 of 128 (53%) elderly subjects known to have asthma were accurately diagnosed.[29] The cause of this is multifactorial. Successful spirometry may be difficult in 10% to 20% of elderly patients because of poor physical and cognitive function.[30,31] Likewise, the number of β-adrenergic receptors in airway smooth muscle decreases with age. This may result in a poor bronchodilator response.[28] Moreover, there is a high prevalence of irreversible airway obstruction in elderly asthmatic patients. Therefore, a 2- to 3-week trial of systemic corticosteroids, such as 20 to 40 mg daily, followed by repeat spirometry with and without a bronchodilator, may be required to confirm the diagnosis.[32]

Diagnostic Approach

Many illnesses in elderly patients can masquerade as asthma, such as cough, wheeze, dyspnea, fatigue, and functional decline, reinforcing the importance of accurate spirometry. COPD, congestive heart failure (CHF), hypersensitivity pneumonitis, sarcoidosis, depression, and "aging" are commonly misdiagnosed as asthma.[7] The initial evaluation of any subject should include a thorough history and physical examination. A history of allergic diseases, such as rhinosinusitis and eczema, makes a diagnosis of asthma more likely. When a diagnosis is in doubt, basic laboratory studies (e.g., hemogram and chemistries, chest radiograph, arterial blood gases, and electrocardiogram) may be helpful. If the history warrants, chest computed tomography can help exclude other diseases, such as pulmonary embolus, sarcoidosis, and neoplasm. A high-resolution computed tomography scan of the chest can be helpful to rule out interstitial lung disease and other problems. Brain natriuretic peptide and echocardiogram may be helpful to rule out CHF.[33]

Asthma–Chronic Obstructive Pulmonary Disease Overlap

Asthma and COPD can be difficult to differentiate in the elderly population, especially since elderly asthmatic patients may present with some fixed airflow obstruction and some patients with COPD have documented FEV reversibility.[15] The responses to treatment of these two diseases are different.[34] COPD is primarily a disease of smokers and is further characterized by its own constellation of clinical characteristics. It typically requires at least a 10 pack-year history of cigarette smoking; however, it can also develop in nonsmokers, including some patients with asthma. It is usually associated with more fixed airway obstruction, lung hyperinflation, decreased pulmonary elastic recoil, and impaired D_{LCO}.[35] Smoking may complicate the asthma, thus making a differential diagnosis between these two diseases more difficult.[35,36] A history of atopy, environmental allergies, and rhinitis is more consistent with asthma than COPD.[5] So, too, is an increased absolute peripheral blood eosinophil count greater than 300/mm^3. COPD versus asthma in younger patients is characterized typically by a high sputum neutrophil versus eosinophil count.[34,37] Elderly patients tend to have higher airway neutrophil counts at baseline, making this feature less helpful in differentiating these diseases. To complicate things, the Lung Health Study shows that in mild to moderate COPD, a methacholine challenge study detects airway reactivity in up to 70% of adult COPD patients, whereas 85% have a bronchodilator response on repeated pulmonary function testing.[5] The common constellation of symptoms, clinical presentation, and pathophysiologic mechanisms in these two diseases can complicate the diagnosis of one versus the other.

Comorbidities

"Frailty" is a term used to describe older individuals who are less robust than their peers. However, a consensus about diagnostic criteria or the utility of using this term has not been reached.[5,38] It is intuitive that having multiple chronic medical conditions is more likely to affect the quality of life and daily activities. Therefore, in some cases, asthma may be a coexisting disease, or, conversely, asthma may coexist with other diseases, the sum total of which contributes to frailty. Thus, in the evaluation of any senior with asthma, comorbid and coexisting diseases must be assessed and addressed for successful outcomes. Likewise, appropriate communication with other consultants as well as primary care physicians is of utmost importance.

Common comorbidities in seniors with asthma include gastroesophageal reflux disease (GERD), obstructive sleep apnea (OSA), obesity, diabetes mellitus, CHF, and rhinosinusitis and others.[35] How GERD may contribute to asthma is unclear, but GERD symptoms can mimic and appear to sometimes worsen asthma symptoms.[5] Many elderly individuals do not have typical GERD symptoms, such as heartburn, nausea, water brash, dysphagia, and odynophagia.[5,39] Likewise, the effect of OSA on systemic and upper airway inflammation and its role in elderly asthma is less clear than in other age groups.[40,41] Weight loss and nocturnal continuous positive airway pressure (CPAP) improve the symptoms and quality of life in patients with asthma and OSA. Whether this is related to improvement in asthma alone or is attributable to the decrease in work of breathing is unclear. One study shows no change in airway responsiveness 6 weeks after initiation of nocturnal CPAP.[42] This suggests that barotrauma associated with CPAP does not adversely affect airway function in patients with airway inflammation associated with asthma. Although obesity increases the risk for new-onset asthma and complicates treatment, studies on the relationship between obesity and asthma in elderly people are limited.[43] Studies demonstrate that increased central adiposity in the elderly population is a risk factor for developing late-onset asthma[44]; however, the relationship between increased visceral fat, a major source of proinflammatory cytokines, and asthma remains unknown.[45]

Lifestyle and Behavioral Modifications

Nonpharmacologic interventions are important in the treatment of asthma. For example, swimming and warm-water exercise are thought to be helpful with asthma management in older patients.[46] Preventative measures, such as immunizations and smoking cessation, are also key to appropriate long-term care.[47,48] Controlling other comorbidities, for example, weight loss in obese asthmatic patients, may help with symptom control. Treatment of GERD and OSA, educational programs that teach self-management, and regular contact with a health care professional with knowledge about this disease are also helpful. Peak flow determinations are especially useful to recognize changes in symptoms that require medical attention.[13]

TREATMENT

Treatment Guidelines

Asthma therapy goals are similar among all age groups[49] and include the prevention of acute exacerbations, maintenance of lung function and normal activity, prevention of emergency department visits and hospitalizations, and a treatment program with minimal or no side effects.[5,34,50,51] The National Institutes of Health and Global Initiative for Asthma (GINA) guidelines are used widely to direct asthma management.[50-52] These guidelines use a physician-directed step-up approach to therapy based on the severity of symptoms.[5] Other approaches include measuring FEV_1 or peak expiratory flow, either at home or in the clinic, and the use of a validated questionnaire to assess symptom control.[32] The use of clinical guidelines to treat asthma in elderly patients is not evidence based as it is for younger age groups and for individuals with mild to moderate asthma.

Use of Clinical Guidelines in Seniors

Elderly asthmatic patients are usually excluded from clinical trials based on their age or coexisting or comorbid conditions.[53] Furthermore, there is a lack of incentive for pharmaceutical companies to perform trials in this age group because elderly patients often are compelled to use generic versus patented medications because of cost. Thus, an evidenced-based approach to asthma management in seniors is not currently possible, and future research is needed to improve the understanding of treating the older asthmatic patient. Extrapolation of treatment from studies of younger populations must be done with caution.[46] Furthermore, use of a symptom-based approach to treatment of elderly asthmatic patients may be suboptimal because symptoms of airway obstruction are often underreported by or unrecognized in this population. Therefore, using pulmonary function testing as a guide for treatment, when possible, may be most appropriate in the elderly asthmatic patient.[16,17,53]

The 2007 National Asthma Education and Prevention Program Expert Panel Report III includes the section "Special Issues for the Elderly Asthmatics," which addresses the difficulty of asthma treatment in seniors.[32] One study shows that 69% of older individuals with asthma had not received any respiratory medications, and only 30% of those who did receive respiratory medications were on short-acting bronchodilators.[47,48] Another study demonstrates that inhaled corticosteroids are underutilized in this age group, and that when they are prescribed, they are often given suboptimal doses.[7,54] Likewise, the potential side effects associated with these medications, and their cost, also play a role in treatment outcomes.

β-Agonists and Corticosteroids

The appropriate use of β-adrenergic agonists and corticosteroids is the cornerstone of asthma treatment. β-Agonists, the mainstay medication for bronchodilation and symptomatic relief, are associated with some controversy.[55] β-Agonists, which stimulate β receptors in skeletal muscle, can be associated with tremor, insomnia, nervousness, and occasional muscle cramps.[5] Hypokalemia, QT prolongation, and tachycardia, although rare, are a potential concern, particularly in this age group. Clinical trials on the use of β-agonists in the elderly population are limited.[56] Long-acting β-agonists have been associated with a small but significant increase in respiratory-related deaths in all age groups when used without an inhaled corticosteroid. This observation particularly applies to African Americans.[32,57]

Many studies show that inhaled corticosteroids are safe and effective to treat persistent asthma. However, none of these studies has targeted elderly asthmatic patients.[5] There is evidence that inhaled corticosteroids improve morbidity and mortality in COPD patients older than 65 years,[58] but no such data exist for patients with asthma. Because inhaled corticosteroid formulations have some systemic absorption, there is always a potential for side effects, especially when using high-dose inhaled corticosteroids over several years. Epidemiologic studies show that there is an increased risk for ocular hypertension, open-angle glaucoma, and cataracts in elderly patients treated with these medications over prolonged periods.[59-61] All patients should therefore be placed on the lowest dose possible to control their symptoms. Despite these side effects, the benefits of inhaled corticosteroids and β-agonists to treat asthma outweigh the risks of their use.[32] Spacer devices can increase oral deposition of inhaled corticosteroids. Rinsing the mouth after their use also seems logical to decrease systemic absorption and the incidence of oral candidiasis. Physicians should also consider that patients on long-term use of any type of corticosteroid, whatever the route, may be at increased risk for osteopenia and osteoporosis. Therefore, appropriate bone densitometry studies and calcium and vitamin D intake are necessary.[32] Systemic corticosteroids are commonly required in elderly patients for 5 days to several weeks to prevent exacerbations as well as to demonstrate the reversibility necessary to make the diagnosis of asthma.[32] Elderly patients may become hyperactive and experience insomnia on oral corticosteroids. Hyperglycemia and hypokalemia are also possible side effects. The long-term use of oral corticosteroids should be avoided, when possible, because of the increased risks for osteoporosis, cataracts, muscle weakness, and other side effects.[5] Physicians should also discuss potential side effects of all medications prescribed.

Anticholinergic Medications

Anticholinergic medications may be considered for elderly asthmatic patients, in particular, because of the associated side effects of $β_2$-agonists. Some studies, none of which exclusively includes patients older than 65 years, show that inhaled anticholinergics provide symptomatic benefit and improve pulmonary function studies compared with a placebo.[62,63] However, in one study, the combination of an inhaled anticholinergic and $β_2$-agonists did not provide additional benefit compared with one or the other for maintenance therapy. This combination, however, did provide benefit in the treatment of acute, moderate to severe exacerbations in an emergency setting. Because elderly patients tend to present with more severe obstruction, anticholinergic agents can be considered for a quick-relief medication in those who do not tolerate short-acting $β_2$-agonists.[32] Tiotropium bromide, a long-acting anticholinergic, improves lung function when used for maintenance therapy in patients with uncontrolled asthma who are already taking inhaled corticosteroids and long-acting β-agonists. Elderly patients were either excluded or not separated from younger adults in these studies.[64,65] Not separating or not including such patients in these studies is problematic in that anticholinergic medications can have serious central nervous system effects, such as insomnia, depression, and headache, and are associated with urinary retention, dry mouth, and constipation, particularly in seniors.

Leukotriene Receptor Antagonists

The role of leukotriene inhibitors in elderly asthmatic patients is unclear. However, in the past, high costs have precluded their use on a regular ongoing basis. Now, some are generic, so this is no longer true. In one study, zarfirlukast decreased asthma symptoms regardless of age, having its greatest beneficial effects in adolescents and adults. It did not alter lung function in older subjects.[66] A limited study from Japan demonstrates that pranlukast is equal in efficacy to inhaled fluticasone and is preferred by elderly patients.[67]

Anti–Immunoglobulin E Therapy

Use of a monoclonal antibody against IgE, omalizumab, is an option to treat difficult-to-control asthma. One review of seven randomized, controlled studies evaluated the effectiveness of omalizumab on asthma exacerbations. Its use was associated with a decrease in asthma exacerbations and emergency department visits only for those asthmatic patients with elevated IgE. Although the benefits were observed among all age groups, the improvements in patients older than 65 years did not reach statistical significance.[68]

Theophylline

Theophylline is a bronchodilator with some antiinflammatory effects, and low-dose theophylline is helpful in treating patients who are not willing or able to tolerate inhaled corticosteroids.[69] However, theophylline toxicity, which may occur at any blood level, particularly when greater than 15 µg/mL, may cause nausea, vomiting, diarrhea, seizures, cardiac arrhythmias, and other side effects. Because of its narrow therapeutic range, side-effect profile, and many drug interactions that affect clearance, theophylline levels must be closely monitored in all age groups, particularly in elderly patients.[5]

Allergen Immunotherapy

Data on the role of allergic triggers in elderly asthmatic patients are conflicting.[4] However, when patients have symptoms on exposure to specific allergens, avoidance is the therapeutic choice.[5] Although there are no controlled trials of allergen immunotherapy in this population, it should be considered in patients who have unavoidable ongoing exposure to the offending allergen to which they have specific IgE and appropriate clinical data supporting the allergen as a trigger for their asthma or rhinitis.[46]

Adherence

Other obstacles, not unique to the elderly population, can make asthma treatment difficult. Correct use of the various inhalation devices can be a significant problem in this population, particularly when there is cognitive impairment.[70] When patients cannot use metered-dose inhalers, nebulized medications are desired. Because of comorbidities and coexisting problems, elderly patients are more likely to be taking medications that may exacerbate their asthma. Common examples include nonsteroidal antiinflammatory drugs, such as aspirin, and β-blockers.[5] Compliance is a particular problem in this age group. The complexity of the treatment regimen, in combination with cognitive, visual, and musculoskeletal impairment, often present in this age group, contributes to noncompliance.[1,5,49,71] Elderly patients also exhibit more concerns about possible side effects associated with the medications, and these concerns contribute to noncompliance.[1,72] Therefore, physicians and other health care professionals should ensure that the patient and family understand the rationale behind using different medications and their possible side effects.[5] Choice of treatment always has to include consideration of comorbid and coexisting conditions, the medications used to treat these diseases, and the costs.[13,72]

UNMET, FUTURE RESEARCH NEEDS

Some important research options regarding asthma in the elderly population (Table 32.2) include the following:

1. Examining the conclusions reached in treatment trials and clinical guidelines for asthma because seniors with asthma have largely been excluded from studies to date
2. Building on the limited data on the natural history of asthma and, in particular, of asthma in elderly people, to better differentiate the asthma phenotype in seniors
3. Understanding the roles of gene–environment interactions and the roles of epigenetic factors in late-onset asthma
4. Determining how the interactions of toll-like receptors and protease-activated receptors function with their antigens to increase smooth muscle contraction and fibrosis, and

Table 32.2. Areas of Future Research

Genetic factors

Immune factors and triggers

Causes and differences of airway inflammation

Relationships among genetics, inflammation, and fixed obstruction

Sensitivity and specificity of pulmonary function and bronchial provocation tests

Differences in severity, comorbidity, emotional status, and cognitive status

Exclusion of elderly people from clinical trials; consideration of confounding variables and comorbidities

Adapted from deShazo R, Stupka E. Asthma in US seniors: Part 2. Treatment: seeing through the glass darkly. *Am J Med.* 2009;122:109–113.

the role they play in the fixed obstruction seen in elderly patients with asthma

5. Studying the role of infectious agents, such as *Pseudomonas aeruginosa, Aspergillus fumigatus,* and adenovirus, in the pathogenesis of late-onset "intrinsic" asthma

6. Determining the role of atopy in the pathogenesis of asthma in the elderly population

7. Determining whether age-related alterations in host biology effect responses to environmental and endogenous triggers for airway inflammation and hyperreactivity

8. Using research funding opportunities to study asthma in older individuals, such as those now offered by the National Institutes of Health

CONCLUSION

The paucity of evidence-based data available on elderly asthmatic patients makes asthma more difficult to recognize and treat in this age group. Seniors with asthma typically present later and with more severe cough, wheeze, dyspnea, and functional limitation than the younger asthmatic population. Clinicians must have a high index of suspicion for asthma in this population, in which asthma and COPD frequently overlap, especially because the airway obstruction may be irreversible. The presence of multiple coexisting and comorbid conditions in the elderly patient can also complicate diagnosis and treatment. Furthermore, drug interactions must be carefully considered before implementing a medical treatment regimen in patients, many of whom are taking multiple medications. The natural history of asthma in elderly people is poorly understood. Despite slow progress in understanding the contributions of infection, genetics, and allergic triggers, there is much to be learned about asthma in this population. Until more clinical information about asthma in elderly people is available, making an accurate diagnosis, providing adequate treatment, and improving quality of life will remain challenging.

REFERENCES

1. Gibson PG, McDonald VM, Marks GB. Asthma in older adults. *Lancet.* 2010;376:803–813.
2. Viswanathan RK, Mathur SK. Role of allergen sensitization in older adults. *Curr Allergy Asthma Rep.* 2011;11(5):427–433.
3. Stupka E, deShazo R. Asthma in seniors: Part 1. Evidence for underdiagnosis, undertreatment, and increasing morbidity and mortality. *Am J Med.* 2009;122(1):6–11.
4. Braman S, Kaemmerlen J, Davis S. Asthma in the elderly: a comparison between patients with recently acquired and long-standing disease. *Am Rev Respir Dis.* 1991;143(2):336–340.
5. Hanania NA, King MJ, Braman SS, et al. Asthma in the elderly: current understanding and future research needs. A report of a National Institute on Aging (NIA) workshop. *J Allergy Clin Immunol.* 2011;128(3 Suppl):S4–S24.
6. Moorman JE, Rudd RA, Johnson CA, et al. National Surveillance of Asthma—United States, 1980–2004. *MMWR Surveill Summ.* 2007;56(8):1–54.
7. Enright PL, McClelland RL, Newman AB, et al. Underdiagnosis and undertreatment of asthma in the elderly. Cardiovascular Health Study Research Group. *Chest.* 1999;116(3):603–613.
8. Moorman JE, Mannino DM. Increasing US asthma mortality rates: who is really dying? *J Asthma.* 2001;38(1):65–71.
9. Bellia V, Pedone C, Catalano F, et al. Asthma in the elderly: mortality rate and associated risk factors for mortality. *Chest.* 2007;132(4):1175–1182.

10. Hunt LW Jr, Silverstein MD, Reed CE, et al. Accuracy of death certificate in a population-based study of asthmatic patients. *JAMA*. 1993;269(15):1947–1952.
11. Evans R 3rd, Mullally DI, Wilson RW, et al. National trends in the morbidity and mortality of asthma in the U.S. Prevalence, hospitalization and death from asthma over two decades: 1965–1984. *Chest*. 1987;91(6 Suppl):65S–74S.
12. Centers for Disease Control and Prevention. National Health Interview Survey. http://www.cdc.gov/nchs/nhis.htm. Accessed October 15, 2013.
13. Jones SC, Iverson D, Burns P, et al. Asthma and ageing: an end user's perspective—the perception and problems with the management of asthma in the elderly. *Clin Exp Allergy*. 2011;41(4):471–481.
14. Adams RJ, Wilson DH, Taylor AW, et al. Coexistent chronic conditions and asthma quality of life: a population-based study. *Chest*. 2006;129(2):285–291.
15. Reed CE. The natural history of asthma in adults: the problem of irreversibility. *J Allergy Clin Immunol*. 1999;103(4):539–547.
16. Vergnenegre A, Antonini MT, Bonnaud F, et al. Comparison between late onset and childhood asthma. *Allergol Immunopathol*. 1992;20(5):190–196.
17. Connolly MJ, Crowley JJ, Charan NB, et al. Reduced subjective awareness of bronchoconstriction provoked by methacholine in elderly asthmatic and normal subjects as measured on a Simple Awareness Scale. *Thorax*. 1992;47(6):410–413.
18. Janssens JP, Pache JC, Nicod LP. Physiological changes in respiratory function associated with ageing. *Eur Respir J*. 1999;13(1):197–205.
19. Ducharme ME, Prince P, Hassan N, et al. Expiratory flows and airway inflammation in elderly asthmatic patients. *Respir Med*. 2011;105(9):1284–1289.
20. Kaminska M, Foley S, Maghni K, et al. Airway remodeling in subjects with severe asthma with or without chronic persistent airflow obstruction. *J Allergy Clin Immunol*. 2009;124(1):45–51.
21. Shaw DE, Berry MA, Hargadon B, et al. Association between neutrophilic airway inflammation and airflow limitation in adults with asthma. *Chest*. 2007;132(6):1871–1875.
22. Burrows B, Barbee RA, Cline MG, et al. Characteristics of asthma among elderly adults in a sample of the general population. *Chest*. 1991;100(4):935–942.
23. Mishto M, Santoro A, Bellavista E, et al. Immunoproteasomes and immunosenescence. *Ageing Res Rev*. 2003;2(4):419–432.
24. O'Conner GT, Sparrow D, Segal MR, et al. Smoking, atopy, and methacholine airway responsiveness among middle-aged and elderly men: the Normative Aging Study. *Am Rev Respir Dis*. 1989;140(6):1520–1526.
25. Ohman JL Jr, Sparrow D, MacDonald MR. New onset wheezing in an older male population: evidence of allergen sensitization in a longitudinal study. Results of the Normative Aging Study. *J Allergy Clin Immunol*. 1993;91(3):752–757.
26. Bauer BA, Reed CE, Yunginger JW, et al. Incidence and outcomes of asthma in the elderly: a population based study in Rochester, Minnesota. *Chest*. 1997;111(2):303–310.
27. Falsey AR, Dallal GE, Formica MA, et al. Long-term care facilities: a cornucopia of viral pathogens. *J Am Geriatr Soc*. 2008;56(7):1281–1285.
28. Pfeifer MA, Weinberg CR, Cook D, et al. Differential changes of autonomic nervous system function with age in man. *Am J Med*. 1983;75(2):249–258.
29. Bellia V, Battaglia S, Catalano F, et al. Aging and disability affect misdiagnosis of COPD in elderly asthmatics: the SARA Study. *Chest*. 2003;123(4):1066–1072.
30. Braman SS. Asthma in the elderly. *Exp Lung Res*. 2005;31(Suppl 1):6–7.
31. Quadrelli SA, Roncoroni A. Features of asthma in the elderly. *J Asthma*. 2001;38(5):377–389.
32. National Asthma Education and Prevention Program. *Expert Panel Report III: Guidelines for the Diagnosis and Management of Asthma*. Bethesda, MD: National Heart, Lung, and Blood Institute; 2007 (NIH Publication No. 08-4051).
33. Morrison LK, Harrison A, Krishnaswamy P, et al. Utility of a rapid B-natriuretic peptide assay in differentiating congestive heart failure from lung disease in patients presenting with dyspnea. *J Am Coll Cardiol*. 2002;39(2):202–209.
34. Di Lorenzo G, Mansueto P, Ditta V, et al. Similarity and differences in elderly patients with fixed airflow obstruction by asthma and by chronic obstructive pulmonary disease. *Respir Med*. 2008;102(2):232–238.
35. Boulet LP. Influence of comorbid conditions on asthma. *Eur Respir J*. 2009;33(4):897–906.
36. Boulet LP, Lemière C, Archambault F, et al. Smoking and asthma: clinical and radiologic features, lung function, and airway inflammation. *Chest*. 2006;129(3):661–668.
37. Gibson PG, Simpson JL. The overlap syndrome of asthma and COPD: what are its

features and how important is it? *Thorax.* 2009;64(8):728–735.
38. Bergman H, Ferrucci L, Guralnik J, et al. Frailty: an emerging research and clinical paradigm—issues and controversies. *J Gerontol A Biol Sci Med Sci.* 2007;62(7):731–737.
39. Räihä I, Impivaara O, Seppälä M, et al. Determinants of symptoms suggestive of gastroesophageal reflux disease in the elderly. *Scand J Gastroenterol.* 1993;28(11):1011–1014.
40. Boulet LP, Hamid Q, Bacon SL, et al. Symposium on Obesity and Asthma, November 2, 2006. *Can Respir J.* 2007;14(4):201–208.
41. Zamarron C, García Paz V, Riveiro A. Obstructive sleep apnea syndrome is a systemic disease: current evidence. *Eur J Intern Med.* 2008;19(6):390–398.
42. Lafond C, Séries F, Lemière C. Impact of CPAP on asthmatic patients with obstructive sleep apnoea. *Eur Respir J.* 2007;29(2):307–311.
43. Lang JE, Hossain J, Dixon AE, et al. Does age impact the obese asthma phenotype? Longitudinal asthma control, airway function, and airflow perception among mild persistent asthmatics. *Chest.* 2011;140(6):1524–1533.
44. Leone N, Courbon D, Berr C, et al. Abdominal obesity and late-onset asthma: cross-sectional and longitudinal results. The 3C Study. *Obesity.* 2012;20:628–635.
45. Song WJ, Kim SH, Lim S, et al. Association between obesity and asthma in the elderly population: potential roles of abdominal subcutaneous adiposity and sarcopenia. *Ann Allergy Asthma Immunol.* 2012;109:243–248.
46. deShazo RD, Stupka JE. Diagnosing asthma in seniors: an algorithmic approach. *J Respir Dis.* 2008;29(10):391–396.
47. Craig BM, Kraus CK, Chewning BA, et al. Quality of care for older adults with chronic obstructive pulmonary disease and asthma based on comparisons to practice guidelines and smoking status. *BMC Health Serv Res.* 2008;8:144.
48. *Global Initiative for Chronic Obstructive Lung Disease. Executive Summary: Global Strategy for the Diagnosis, Management and Prevention of Chronic Obstructive Pulmonary Disease.* Bethesda, MD: National Heart Lung and Blood Institute, National Institutes of Health; 2001:1–30 (NIH Publication No. 2701A).
49. Braman SS, Hanania NA. Asthma in older adults. *Clin Chest Med.* 2007;28(4):685–702, v.
50. National Heart, Lung and Blood Institute National Institutes of Health. *National Asthma Education and Prevention Program: Expert Panel Report 2—Guidelines for the Diagnosis and Management of Asthma.* Bethesda, MD: National Heart, Lung, and Blood Institute; 2007.
51. NAEPP Working Group. *Consideration for Diagnosing and Managing Asthma in the Elderly.* Bethesda, MD: National Institutes of Health; 1996.
52. From the Global Strategy for Asthma Management and Prevention, Global Initiative for Asthma (GINA) 2011. http://www.ginasthma.org/. Accessed October 15, 2013.
53. deShazo RD, Stupka JE. Asthma in seniors: Part 2. Treatment: seeing through the glass darkly. *Am J Med.* 2009;122(2):109–113.
54. Smith AM, Villareal M, Bernstein DI, et al. Asthma in the elderly: risk factors and impact on physical function. *Ann Allergy Asthma Immunol.* 2012;108(5):305–310.
55. Inman WH. Monitoring of adverse reactions to drugs in the United Kingdom. *Proc R Soc Med.* 1970;63(12):1302–1304.
56. Robin ED, McCauley R. Sudden cardiac death in bronchial asthma and inhaled beta-adrenergic agonists. *Chest.* 1992;101(6):1699–1702.
57. Nelson HS, Weiss ST, Bleecker ER, et al. The Salmeterol Multicenter Asthma Research Trial: a comparison of usual pharmacotherapy for asthma or usual pharmacotherapy plus salmeterol. *Chest.* 2006;129(1):15–26.
58. Sin DD, Tu JV. Inhaled corticosteroids and the risk of mortality and readmission in elderly patients with chronic obstructive pulmonary disease. *Am J Respir Crit Care Med.* 2001;164(4):580–584.
59. Leone FT, Fish JE, Szefler SJ, et al. systematic review of the evidence regarding potential complications of inhaled corticosteroid use in asthma: collaboration of American College of Chest Physicians, American Academy of Allergy, Asthma and Immunology, and American College of Allergy, Asthma and Immunology. *Chest.* 2003;124(6):2329–2340.
60. Garbe E, LeLorier J, Boivin JF, et al. Inhaled and nasal glucocorticoids and the risks of ocular hypertension or open-angle glaucoma. *JAMA.* 1997;277(9):722–727.
61. Garbe E, Suissa S, LeLorier J. Association of inhaled corticosteroid use with cataract extraction in elderly patients. *JAMA.* 1998;280(6):539–543.
62. Donohue JF. Therapeutic responses in asthma and COPD: bronchodilators. *Chest.* 2004;126(2 Suppl):125S–137S.
63. Westby M, Benson M, Gibson P. Anticholinergic agents for chronic asthma in adults. *Cochrane Database Syst Rev.* 2004;(3):CD003269.

64. Kerstjens HA, Disse B, Schröder-Babo W, et al. Tiotropium improves lung function in patients with severe uncontrolled asthma: a randomized controlled trial. *J Allergy Clin Immunol.* 2011;128(2):308-314.
65. Kerstjens HA, Engel M, Dahl R, et al. Tiotropium in asthma poorly controlled with standard combination therapy. *N Engl J Med.* 2012;367(13):1198-1207.
66. Korenblat PE, Kemp JP, Scherger JE, et al. Effect of age on response to zafirlukast in patients with asthma in the Accolate Clinical Experience and Pharmacoepidemiology Trial (ACCEPT). *Ann Allergy Asthma Immunol.* 2000;84(2):217-225.
67. Horiguchi T, Tachikawa S, Kondo R, et al. Comparative evaluation of the leukotriene receptor antagonist pranlukast versus the steroid inhalant fluticasone in the therapy of aged patients with mild bronchial asthma. *Arzneimittelforschung.* 2007;57(2):87-91.
68. Bousquet J, Cabrere P, Berkman N, et al. The effect of treatment with omalizumab, an anti-IgE antibody, on asthma exacerbations and emergency medical visits in patients with severe persistent asthma. *Allergy.* 2005;60(3):302-308.
69. The American Lung Association Asthma Clinical Research Centers. Clinical trial of low-dose theophylline and montelukast in patients with poorly controlled asthma. *Am J Respir Crit Care Med.* 2007;175(3):235-242.
70. Ho SF, O'Mahony MS, Steward JA, et al. Inhaler technique in older people in the community. *Age Ageing.* 2004;33(2):185-188.
71. King MJ, Hanania NA. Asthma in the elderly: current knowledge and future directions. *Curr Opin Pulm Med.* 2010;16(1):55-59.
72. Goeman DP, Douglass JA. Understanding asthma in older Australians: a qualitative approach. *Med J Aust.* 2005;183(1 Suppl):S26-S27.

SECTION ELEVEN

FOOD

33

ATOPIC DERMATITIS, FOOD ALLERGY, AND ANAPHYLAXIS

COMORBID AND COEXISTING

Julie Wang, Hugh A. Sampson, Alessandro Fiocchi, and Scott Sicherer

KEY POINTS

- More than 40% of children with atopic dermatitis develop asthma, and approximately 30% to 40% of children with moderate to severe atopic dermatitis have concurrent food allergy.
- Coexisting atopic dermatitis and food allergy are associated with increased asthma morbidity.
- New theories suggest that allergen exposure through a disrupted skin barrier can lead to sensitization and thus influence the development of food allergies and asthma.
- Optimal management of these comorbid atopic disorders is essential for improved outcomes.

INTRODUCTION

Asthma, food allergy, and atopic dermatitis are common disorders affecting children that commonly coexist. Children can develop atopic dermatitis in infancy and later develop food allergies as new foods are introduced. In these highly atopic children, respiratory symptoms can also develop. This pattern of allergic disease progression has been termed the "atopic march." Allergic (helper T-cell type 2 [T_H2] biased) inflammation and allergen sensitization are underlying mechanisms of these disorders, and control of one disease may affect the outcomes of the other disorders. Therefore, an understanding of the relationship between these allergic entities is important.

ATOPIC DERMATITIS

Atopic dermatitis is a chronic inflammatory skin disorder characterized by pruritus and chronic, relapsing eczematous lesions. Atopic dermatitis affects 10% to 20% of children and

1% to 3% of adults.[1] Symptoms present in the first 5 years of life in about 80% of affected children. The symptoms manifest as a result of the interplay between xerosis, scratching, and colonization and infection with *Staphylococcus aureus*.[1]

Diagnosis of atopic dermatitis is made based on clinical history of a pruritic skin rash that may include erythema with edema, papules, vesicles, and serous exudate in the acute stages, and lichenification in the chronic stages.[1] The cheeks and extensor surfaces of the arms and legs are generally affected in young infants, whereas the flexor surfaces, hands, and feet are more commonly affected in teenagers and young adults.[2] Exacerbating factors can include temperature, humidity, food or environmental allergens, irritants, and infections.

Other skin problems that present similarly and must be considered include seborrheic dermatitis in infants, keratosis pilaris, psoriasis, ichthyoses, infections (e.g., scabies, dermophytosis), malignancies (e.g., cutaneous T-cell lymphoma, Letterer-Siwe disease), immunologic disorders (e.g., dermatitis herpetiformis, dermatomyositis, hyper–immunoglobulin E [IgE] syndrome), and nutritional deficiencies (e.g., zinc or niacin deficiency).[1] Often these conditions will not respond to standard atopic dermatitis management. In cases in which the diagnosis is uncertain, skin biopsy can be helpful.

FOOD ALLERGY

Food allergies affect up to 8% of children.[3] Most present early in life, with immediate symptoms triggered by specific foods. Exposures to food allergens can induce cutaneous symptoms, including urticaria, angioedema, and rash, as well as gastrointestinal, respiratory, and cardiovascular symptoms. In severe reactions, life-threatening anaphylaxis can occur. The foods accounting for more than 90% of serious food allergies are milk, egg, wheat, soy, peanut, tree nuts, fish, and shellfish.

The diagnosis of food allergy relies on a complete history: the timing of exposure to the onset of symptoms, the types of symptoms, the quantity of food that triggered the reaction, prior exposures to the triggering food or related foods, and association of cofactors such as exercise and concurrent medications. A history of symptoms following exposure to the triggering food and lack of symptoms when the food is excluded are highly suggestive of allergy. For infants who are breastfed, the maternal diet can be informative because food allergen exposures can occur through breast milk.[4]

DIAGNOSTIC TESTS

The identification of allergic triggers for atopic dermatitis and food allergies is based on a suggestive history and detection of allergen-specific IgE through skin prick tests (SPTs) and/or measurement of serum allergen-specific IgE concentrations.

SPTs provide rapid detection of IgE sensitization with high sensitivity. Glycerinated extracts of allergens are placed on the skin along with positive (histamine) and negative controls (saline), and the skin is pricked with an appropriate needle to allow access to cutaneous mast cells. If the patient has IgE antibodies to the allergen being tested, a wheal will develop at the site. Although this test has a high negative predictive value (negative tests effectively exclude IgE-mediated allergy), the positive predictive value is less than 50% for foods; thus an isolated positive test is not diagnostic for food allergy.[5-7] However, when a positive test to a food is used in conjunction with a highly suggestive history, the SPT can serve to confirm the diagnosis of food allergy. Of note, intradermal testing is not recommended for the evaluation of food allergy because it has been associated with severe systemic reactions and has no better positive predictive accuracy than SPTs.[5]

Specific IgE testing is a quantitative measure of allergen-specific IgE antibody levels in serum. It is preferred for patients with dermatographism or severe skin disease, and for those who cannot discontinue use of antihistamines. With regard to food allergies, larger SPT results and higher levels of specific IgE indicate an increased likelihood of an allergic reaction with exposures.[8] However, there are no diagnostic tests that can predict the severity of any given food allergic reaction.

For food allergy diagnosis, the gold standard is a double-blind, placebo-controlled oral food challenge in which the potential food allergen is gradually fed in increasing doses under supervision.[9] In clinical practice, single-blind or open challenges are more often performed. Challenges are considered diagnostic when no symptoms develop (negative challenge) or when objective allergic symptoms develop that are consistent with the medical history (positive challenge). Because there is a risk for anaphylactic reaction, food challenges should be performed by experienced medical staff, and emergency equipment should be readily available.

A comprehensive literature review and expert panel report on diagnostic testing for food allergies was recently published.[9]

ATOPIC DERMATITIS, FOOD ALLERGY, AND ASTHMA—COEXISTING

Atopic dermatitis and food allergies are common comorbid conditions in asthmatic patients. More than 40% of children with atopic dermatitis develop asthma,[10] and approximately 30% to 40% of children with moderate to severe atopic dermatitis have concurrent food allergy.[9] Children with both atopic dermatitis and egg allergy are at significant risk for developing asthma.[11] Not only does having atopic dermatitis and food allergies increase a child's risk for having asthma, but there is evidence to suggest that the severity of asthma symptoms may be affected by the presence of underlying atopic dermatitis and food allergies.[12-15] In a study of 500 patients with asthma with or without atopic dermatitis, subjects with atopic dermatitis had more severe asthma than those without atopic dermatitis.[12] In birth cohorts, atopic children with early food allergy and concomitant respiratory symptoms have an increased risk for persistent asthma by age 7 years.[16] In addition, children with cow's milk allergy display a longer duration of the disease in the presence of early respiratory symptoms.[17] Large epidemiologic studies demonstrate a high rate of food sensitization (a likely food allergy) in asthmatic children and its association with increased asthma severity. Results from the National Cooperative Inner City Asthma Study (NCICAS), which enrolled children with asthma from inner cities in the United States and collected serum samples, show that the prevalence of food sensitization is surprisingly high, with 45% of the asthmatic children having detectable food-specific IgE to at least one of the six most common food allergens (milk, egg, wheat, soy, peanut, or fish).[13] Data from the National Health and Nutrition Examination Survey (NHANES) show that patients with asthma and evidence of food sensitization (likely food allergy) are more likely to have had a severe asthma exacerbation compared with asthmatic patients without food sensitization (odds ratio [OR], 6.9; 95% confidence interval [CI], 2.4 to 19.7).[14] Although these studies examine food sensitization based only on serologic test results, several studies observe a link between clinical food allergy and increased asthma morbidity. In a study comparing children with life-threatening asthma exacerbations (requiring ventilation) and those with non–life-threatening asthma exacerbations, those with more severe asthma are more likely to have a history of food allergy (OR, 8.58; 95% CI, 1.85 to 39.71).[15] Another study demonstrates that asthmatic children with peanut allergy have higher rates of hospitalization and use of systemic corticosteroids compared with asthmatic patients without peanut allergy.[18] Similar findings are reported in the adult population. Berns and colleagues determined that adults who self-reported allergies to more than one food have increased rates of asthma-related hospitalization, emergency department visits, and use of oral corticosteroids.[19]

The relationship between atopic dermatitis, food allergy, and asthma has been further explored in several studies using objective measurements of lung dysfunction. In a study of 43 children with atopic dermatitis, bronchial hyperresponsiveness (BHR) is seen in both children who have a diagnosis of asthma and those with no clinical history of asthma symptoms.[20] In a prospective study of unselected children, cow's milk allergy is a predictor of BHR and airway inflammation later in life.[21] Young children with IgE-mediated milk allergy, confirmed by oral food challenge, have an increased risk for elevated BHR (measured by histamine challenge) and increased exhaled nitric oxide levels when evaluated at 8 years of age. In another study, BHR (measured by methacholine challenge) is increased in food-allergic children compared with healthy children without food allergy.[22] These children with increased BHR did not have clinical diagnoses of asthma or allergic rhinitis. Although presence of atopic dermatitis or food allergy appears to increase the risk for BHR, the clinical relevance of these findings is unclear.

ATOPIC DERMATITIS, FOOD ALLERGY, AND ASTHMA—PATHOPHYSIOLOGIC LINK?

The relationship between atopic dermatitis, food allergies, and asthma is believed to be due to the altered skin barrier function present in atopic dermatitis, which predisposes to cutaneous allergen sensitization. Using a murine model, Kondo and colleagues demonstrate that tape-stripped mice exposed epicutaneously to allergen develop sensitization, indicating that in the setting of disrupted skin barrier function, allergen exposure can trigger systemic IgE and T_H2 cytokine production.[23] Spergel and colleagues show that not only does epicutaneous exposure to allergen induce systemic T_H2 responses, but airway hyperreactivity is also induced.[24] BALB/c mice were sensitized to ovalbumin through either the epicutaneous (EC) or intraperitoneal (IP) route. EC-sensitized mice had increased ovalbumin-specific IgE production, higher than in those that underwent IP sensitization. Skin biopsy of the exposed site of EC mice revealed dermatitis with T-cell and eosinophil infiltration. In addition, EC-sensitized mice that were challenged with inhaled ovalbumin had increased sensitivity to methacholine challenge, and bronchoalveolar lavage samples showed increased eosinophils.

Given the high heritability of allergic diseases, there is great interest in identifying genes associated with these disorders. Studies have identified a molecular basis for the skin barrier dysfunction in some atopic dermatitis patients as being due to mutations in the filaggrin gene, a protein that plays an important role in epidermal differentiation, desquamation, and barrier function.[25] Mutations in the filaggrin gene lead to barrier dysfunction, allowing allergens to be transferred across the skin to Langerhans cells leading to induction of a T_H2 immune response with IgE production by B cells.[26,27] Patients with the filaggrin null mutation are at a 1.2- to 13-fold increased risk for having atopic dermatitis.[28] Moreover, functional deficits in filaggrin can be induced by T_H2 inflammation of the skin,[29] and treatment of active lesions with antiinflammatory agents can reverse the reduced filaggrin expression.[30]

Although filaggrin is not expressed on respiratory epithelia,[31] asthmatic patients with filaggrin mutations have more difficult-to-manage asthma, with more frequent exacerbations.[32] Research is ongoing in this area to determine how and why filaggrin gene mutations can increase the risk for asthma, aside from predisposing to systemic allergen sensitization, as well as to identify other defects that are involved, because not all patients with atopic dermatitis have filaggrin gene mutations.

The link between cutaneous exposures to allergen and development of food allergies has been examined. Using a cohort of more than 13,000 children enrolled in the Avon Longitudinal Study of Parents and Children, Lack and colleagues collected data regarding peanut allergy as well as detailed retrospective information by interviewing the parents of children with peanut reactions and parents of children from two control groups.[33] The results indicate that peanut allergy is significantly associated with rash over joints and skin creases (OR, 2.6; 95% CI, 1.4 to 5.0) and oozing, crusted rash (OR, 5.2; 95% CI, 2.7 to 10.2). Interview data demonstrate a significant association between peanut allergy and history of using topical preparations containing peanut oil (OR, 6.8; 95% CI, 1.4 to 32.9). Additionally, a dose-response effect is seen between environmental peanut exposure and the development of peanut allergy in a questionnaire-based case-control study of children with and without peanut allergy.[34] Another study has found an association between peanut allergy and filaggrin loss-of-function mutations, suggesting that filaggrin may play a key role in food allergies for children with atopic dermatitis.[35] Further research in this area should elucidate the interrelationship between these atopic diseases and potentially identify additional factors that may be important in skin barrier function, because many have atopic dermatitis without evidence of filaggrin gene mutations.

CLINICAL IMPACT OF THESE DIAGNOSES

Despite these studies showing an association between food allergy and asthma, these diagnoses should be pursued only with a relevant clinical history. For example, respiratory symptoms are known to occur during food allergic reactions, but food allergy is generally not associated with chronic or isolated respiratory symptoms.[36] Food challenge data from 279 asthmatic patients with a history of food-induced wheezing demonstrate that 40% of the positive double-blind, placebo-controlled oral food challenges (DBPCFCs) had wheezing as one of several symptoms.[37] However, only five subjects had wheezing without other symptoms during food challenges. In another large study of more 300 patients with both food allergy and atopic dermatitis, 27% of the positive DBPCFCs had respiratory symptoms as part of the allergic reaction. Of these, only 17% was wheezing, and very few patients had isolated wheezing.[38] Thus, isolated wheezing or respiratory symptoms unrelated to food ingestion in a patient with food allergies should prompt an independent investigation for possible asthma. However, a patient with uncomplicated asthma alone should not lead to an indiscriminate search for food allergies without a convincing history of food reaction.

Patients with diagnoses of both food allergy and asthma are at risk for poor outcomes. For example, studies have found that the presence of asthma is a predictor for persistent cow's milk allergy.[38–40] More important, asthma is a risk factor for fatal food-induced anaphylaxis.[41] In a study of anaphylaxis prevalence in the United Kingdom, food-allergic patients with asthma had significantly higher rates of anaphylaxis compared with those without asthma.[42] Similar findings are reported in a northern California managed care organization, which found a five-fold higher risk for anaphylactic shock due to food allergies in asthmatic patients compared with those without asthma.[43] The risk for anaphylaxis is notably higher in those with severe asthma (hazard ratio, 8.23; 6.59 to 10.27) than those classified as having nonsevere asthma (hazard ratio, 5.05; 4.39 to 5.80). Moreover, suboptimally controlled asthma has been reported to be a risk factor for adverse reactions during oral immunotherapy to peanut.[44] In summary, patients with both food allergies and asthma should be managed aggressively.

MANAGEMENT STRATEGY

There is ample evidence that children with concurrent atopic dermatitis, food allergy, and asthma are at risk for poor outcomes. Therefore, management of all conditions should be optimized to prevent potential morbidity and mortality. Ensuring the accurate diagnoses of atopic dermatitis and food allergies in a patient who has asthma are the first steps. Food allergies should be investigated if there is clinical suspicion based on history, and elimination diets should be instituted only when specific food allergens are identified because there is a risk for developing acute allergic reactions upon reexposure or accidental exposure after prolonged avoidance in those without previous reactions.[45] In certain cases of acute life-threatening asthma with no identifiable triggers or severe, treatment-resistant asthma outside the typical season for viral infections, food allergy may be considered even without a history suggestive of acute reactions to foods. Furthermore, a food allergy evaluation may be indicated for highly atopic children with severe persistent asthma resistant to medical treatment in whom a history of food-associated respiratory symptoms may not be reliable because of fragmented care (e.g., children in foster care).[46]

Table 33.1. Management of Atopic Dermatitis

TREATMENT MODALITY	EXAMPLES
General skin care	• Improve skin barrier function—hydration, emollients, wet wraps
	• Identification and avoidance of allergic triggers
Antiinflammatory agents	• Corticosteroids, calcineurin inhibitors
Antimicrobial therapy	• Topical or oral antibiotics, antiviral medications
Adjuvant therapies	• Control pruritus—oral antihistamines
	• Refractory atopic dermatitis—phototherapy, systemic immunosuppressants

Management of atopic dermatitis entails restoration of skin barrier function, use of antiinflammatory medications, and identification and avoidance of allergic triggers[1] (Table 33.1). Skin barrier function is improved with hydration and use of emollients. Wet wraps are another effective option for hydrating the skin. Topical corticosteroids are effective antiinflammatory treatments for most cases. The potency of the medication is selected based on the severity and location of the affected areas. Topical calcineurin inhibitors (tacrolimus and pimecrolimus) are safe and effective alternatives to corticosteroids.[1] Allergen avoidance is based on a suggestive history and supportive testing (SPT and/or serum-specific IgE levels). Because pruritus is a key factor in perpetuating the symptoms of atopic dermatitis, use of oral antihistamines may be beneficial (e.g., hydroxyzine at bedtime). Patients with atopic dermatitis are often colonized and infected with *S. aureus*; therefore, topical and oral antibiotics may be necessary when infection is a concern. Viral skin infections, including herpes simplex, warts, and molluscum contagiosum, can be complicating factors requiring appropriate treatment. In severe cases of atopic dermatitis, systemic corticosteroids or immunosuppressants, such as cyclosporine and interferon-γ, may be required to control symptoms. Phototherapy has also been shown to be effective as adjunctive treatment for refractory atopic dermatitis.[1]

For food allergies, education about dietary avoidance of the food allergens and emergency management of acute allergic reactions are the mainstays of treatment.[9] Avoidance of food allergy triggers is essential to minimize the risk for reactions. However, avoidance is difficult, and accidental exposures are common.[47] Patients and their families need to understand how to read ingredient labels and to be educated in issues related to cross-contamination in food processing and preparation.[48] Dietary counseling can be helpful, particularly when multiple food allergens need to be avoided. There is evidence that food allergen avoidance reduces the severity of atopic dermatitis in appropriately diagnosed individuals. However, it is uncertain whether food allergen avoidance can alter the natural course of atopic dermatitis or asthma.[9] When food allergen exposure occurs, allergic reactions are likely and of unpredictable severity. The acute management of a food allergic reaction is dictated by its severity. For mild reactions, use of oral antihistamines is appropriate.

For anaphylaxis, a severe allergic reaction that is rapid in onset and potentially life threatening, intramuscular epinephrine is the drug of choice.[9] Epinephrine for self-injection and written emergency action plans should be prescribed to any individual at risk for food-induced reactions, particularly to those who have asthma and are at high risk for anaphylaxis and poor outcomes. Epinephrine autoinjectors are preferred, when affordable and available (i.e., Adrenaclick [Amedra, Middlesex, NJ]; Auvi-Q [Sanofi, Paris, France]; EpiPen [Dey Pharma, Basking Ridge, NJ]; Jext [ALK-Abello, Horsholm, Denmark]). Some anaphylaxis action plans include an area to identify a food-allergic individual as having comorbid asthma, thereby alerting the caretaker to the higher risk for a severe reaction (Figure 33.1). Optimal management of coexisting asthma with controller medication is essential. In addition, these individuals require particular attention because food-allergic reactions can sometimes be confused with acute asthma exacerbations. If the clinical suspicion for

FARE — FOOD ALLERGY & ANAPHYLAXIS EMERGENCY CARE PLAN

Name: _____ D.O.B.: _____
Allergy to: _____
Weight: _____ lbs.   Asthma: [ ] Yes (higher risk for a severe reaction) [ ] No

PLACE STUDENT'S PICTURE HERE

For a suspected or active food allergy reaction:

FOR ANY OF THE FOLLOWING SEVERE SYMPTOMS

[ ] If checked, give epinephrine immediately if the allergen was definitely eaten, even if there are no symptoms.

- **LUNG**: Short of breath, wheezing, repetitive cough
- **HEART**: Pale, blue, faint, weak pulse, dizzy
- **THROAT**: Tight, hoarse, trouble breathing/swallowing
- **MOUTH**: Significant swelling of the tongue and/or lips
- **SKIN**: Many hives over body, widespread redness
- **GUT**: Repetitive vomiting or severe diarrhea
- **OTHER**: Feeling something bad is about to happen, anxiety, confusion
- **OR A COMBINATION** of mild or severe symptoms from different body areas.

NOTE: Do not depend on antihistamines or inhalers (bronchodilators) to treat a severe reaction. **Use Epinephrine.**

1. **INJECT EPINEPHRINE IMMEDIATELY.**
2. **Call 911.** Request ambulance with epinephrine.
- Consider giving additional medications (following or with the epinephrine):
  » Antihistamine
  » Inhaler (bronchodilator) if asthma
- Lay the student flat and raise legs. If breathing is difficult or they are vomiting, let them sit up or lie on their side.
- If symptoms do not improve, or symptoms return, more doses of epinephrine can be given about 5 minutes or more after the last dose.
- Alert emergency contacts.
- Transport student to ER even if symptoms resolve. Student should remain in ER for 4+ hours because symptoms may return.

NOTE: WHEN IN DOUBT, GIVE EPINEPHRINE. MILD SYMPTOMS

[ ] If checked, give epinephrine immediately for ANY symptoms if the allergen was likely eaten.

- **NOSE**: Itchy/runny nose, sneezing
- **MOUTH**: Itchy mouth
- **SKIN**: A few hives, mild itch
- **GUT**: Mild nausea/discomfort

1. **GIVE ANTIHISTAMINES, IF ORDERED BY PHYSICIAN**
2. Stay with student; alert emergency contacts.
3. Watch student closely for changes. If symptoms worsen, **GIVE EPINEPHRINE.**

MEDICATIONS/DOSES

Epinephrine Brand: _____
Epinephrine Dose: [ ] 0.15 mg IM   [ ] 0.3 mg IM
Antihistamine Brand or Generic: _____
Antihistamine Dose: _____
Other (e.g., inhaler-bronchodilator if asthmatic): _____
_____

PARENT/GUARDIAN AUTHORIZATION SIGNATURE   DATE   PHYSICIAN/HCP AUTHORIZATION SIGNATURE   DATE

FORM PROVIDED COURTESY OF FOOD ALLERGY RESEARCH & EDUCATION (FARE) (WWW.FOODALLERGY.ORG) 8/2013

FIGURE 33.1A This panel provides an example of a food allergy action plan with general recommendations concerning response. (©2013, Food Allergy Research & Education. Used with permission.)

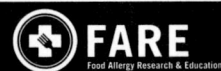

FOOD ALLERGY & ANAPHYLAXIS EMERGENCY CARE PLAN

EPIPEN® (EPINEPHRINE) AUTO-INJECTOR DIRECTIONS
1. Remove the EpiPen Auto-Injector from the plastic carrying case.
2. Pull off the blue safety release cap.
3. Swing and firmly push orange tip against mid-outer thigh.
4. Hold for approximately 10 seconds.
5. Remove and massage the area for 10 seconds.

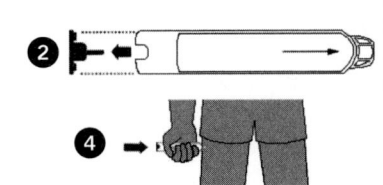

AUVI-Q™ (EPINEPHRINE INJECTION, USP) DIRECTIONS
1. Remove the outer case of Auvi-Q. This will automatically activate the voice instructions.
2. Pull off red safety guard.
3. Place black end against mid-outer thigh.
4. Press firmly and hold for 5 seconds.
5. Remove from thigh.

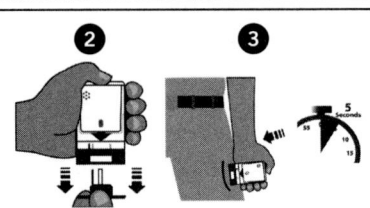

ADRENACLICK®/ADRENACLICK® GENERIC DIRECTIONS
1. Remove the outer case.
2. Remove grey caps labeled "1" and "2".
3. Place red rounded tip against mid-outer thigh.
4. Press down hard until needle penetrates.
5. Hold for 10 seconds. Remove from thigh.

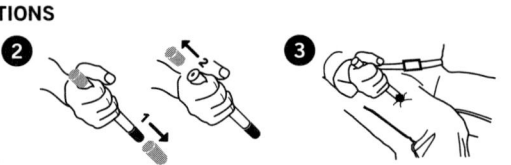

OTHER DIRECTIONS/INFORMATION (may self-carry epinephrine, may self-administer epinephrine, etc.):

Treat student before calling Emergency Contacts. The first signs of a reaction can be mild, but symptoms can get worse quickly.

EMERGENCY CONTACTS — CALL 911

RESCUE SQUAD: _____

DOCTOR: _____ PHONE: _____

PARENT/GUARDIAN: _____ PHONE: _____

OTHER EMERGENCY CONTACTS

NAME/RELATIONSHIP: _____

PHONE: _____

NAME/RELATIONSHIP: _____

PHONE: _____

PARENT/GUARDIAN AUTHORIZATION SIGNATURE _____ DATE _____

FORM PROVIDED COURTESY OF FOOD ALLERGY RESEARCH & EDUCATION (FARE) (WWW.FOODALLERGY.ORG) 8/2013

FIGURE 33.1B This panel provides an example of a food allergy action with recommendations concerning the use of autoinjector epinephrine. (©2013, Food Allergy Research & Education. Used with permission.)

food-induced anaphylaxis is high, injectable epinephrine is the treatment of choice; short-acting bronchodilators should not be relied on in this situation.

Periodic reevaluation of these disorders is advised to ensure that appropriate management continues. Timing of reevaluation and adjustments in medications for asthma and atopic dermatitis are determined based on the age of the patient and interval history. Because many food allergies can be outgrown, repeat testing will guide decision making as to when food reintroductions or oral food challenges may be appropriate.

UNMET, FUTURE RESEARCH NEEDS

Epidemiologic studies have clearly shown an association between these common childhood conditions, and data are lending support to the hypothesis that skin barrier dysfunction associated with atopic dermatitis plays a key role in the development of allergic sensitization leading to food allergies and allergic asthma. Therefore, treating young children with atopic dermatitis to restore their skin barrier function may be a strategy to reduce the risk for allergic sensitization, asthma, and food allergies. For example, Iikura and colleagues report that infants with atopic dermatitis, but no history of wheezing, who were randomized to receive ketotifen had a significantly lower prevalence of asthma compared with the placebo-treated children after 1 year.[49] This effect was seen only in children who had elevated total IgE levels at baseline. In another study, children with atopic dermatitis were treated with cetirizine (which has been shown to inhibit allergen-induced eosinophil trafficking to the skin, nose, and lung) as a method of asthma prevention.[50] Although no difference between the active and placebo-treated groups was seen after 18 months of treatment, a significantly lower rate of asthma was observed in the active groups when examining the subset of children with allergic sensitization to grass and/or dust mite. This finding is not confirmed by a prospective study focusing on grass- and/or dust mite–allergic children.[51]

With greater understanding of the immunologic mechanisms underlying allergic diseases, novel therapies using monoclonal biologics increasingly are being explored. A treatment that could potentially target atopic dermatitis, food allergies, and asthma simultaneously is anti-IgE antibody. Omalizumab (Xolair, Genentech) is approved by the U.S. Food and Drug Administration for the treatment of moderate to severe, persistent, allergic asthma in patients 12 years or older. Various published case reports suggest the potential benefits of anti-IgE in the treatment of recalcitrant atopic dermatitis.[52,53] In an open-label, pilot study of adults with severe asthma, with and without concomitant atopic dermatitis, treatment with omalizumab for 1 year (in addition to standard asthma and atopic dermatitis treatment) resulted in significant improvement in quality of life for patients with atopic dermatitis as well as decreased topical and oral steroid use in those with concomitant disease.[54] Anti-IgE treatment in food allergy has also been explored with encouraging results. In a double-blind, randomized, dose-ranging trial of TNX-901, another anti-IgE formulation, 84 peanut-allergic patients underwent 4 months of treatment.[55] Those receiving the highest dose experienced significant decreases in symptoms after peanut challenge compared with the placebo-treated group. The median threshold of sensitivity to peanut increased from 178 mg of peanut protein (equivalent to one peanut) to almost 9 peanuts (2.8 g). Although 25% of subjects were able to tolerate more than 20 peanuts after treatment, another 25% failed to develop any improvement in tolerance, indicating that the treatment response can be highly variable. Another study using omalizumab for the treatment of peanut allergy was initiated but was discontinued because of safety concerns related to the pretreatment peanut challenges.[56] Analysis of data from the 14 patients who had completed the post-treatment food challenge before the termination of the study indicated increased tolerance to peanut at the post-treatment food challenge in the omalizumab-treated group compared with the placebo-treated group. Additional studies in larger groups of patients are needed to assess whether anti-IgE treatment can confer significant benefits in patients with these comorbid diseases.

CONCLUSION

Coexisting atopic dermatitis, food allergy, and asthma are common in atopic children, and these individuals are at higher risk for morbidity and mortality. A greater understanding of the interrelationship between these entities may allow for the development of prevention and treatment strategies. In the meantime, accurate diagnoses and close management of these patients are necessary to provide optimal care.

REFERENCES

1. Leung DY, Nicklas RA, Li JT, et al. Disease management of atopic dermatitis: an updated practice parameter. Joint Task Force on Practice Parameters. *Ann Allergy Asthma Immunol.* 2004;93(3 Suppl 2):S1–S21.
2. Hanifin JM, Rajka G. Diagnostic features of atopic dermatitis. *Acta Derm Venereol Suppl (Stockh).* 1980;92:44, 45–47.
3. Gupta RS, Springston EE, Warrier MR, et al. The prevalence, severity, and distribution of childhood food allergy in the United States. *Pediatrics.* 2011;128(1):e9–e17.
4. Sorva R, Makinen-Kiljunen S, Juntunen-Backman K. Beta-lactoglobulin secretion in human milk varies widely after cow's milk ingestion in mothers of infants with cow's milk allergy. *J Allergy Clin Immunol.* 1994;93(4):787–792.
5. Bock SA, Buckley J, Holst A, May CD. Proper use of skin tests with food extracts in diagnosis of hypersensitivity to food in children. *Clin Allergy.* 1977;7(4):375–383.
6. Sampson HA, Albergo R. Comparison of results of skin tests, RAST, and double-blind, placebo-controlled food challenges in children with atopic dermatitis. *J Allergy Clin Immunol.* 1984;74(1):26–33.
7. Eigenmann PA, Sampson HA. Interpreting skin prick tests in the evaluation of food allergy in children. *Pediatr Allergy Immunol.* 1998;9(4):186–191.
8. Sampson HA. Utility of food-specific IgE concentrations in predicting symptomatic food allergy. *J Allergy Clin Immunol.* 2001;107(5):891–896.
9. Boyce JA, Assa'ad A, Burks AW, et al. Guidelines for the diagnosis and management of food allergy in the United States: summary of the NIAID-sponsored Expert Panel Report. *J Allergy Clin Immunol.* 2010;126(6 Suppl):1105–1118.
10. Gustafsson D, Sjöberg O, Foucard T. Development of allergies and asthma in infants and young children with atopic dermatitis: a prospective follow-up to 7 years of age. *Allergy.* 2000;55(3):240–245.
11. Tariq SM, Matthews SM, Hakim EA, et al. Egg allergy in infancy predicts respiratory allergic disease by 4 years of age. *Pediatr Allergy Immunol.* 2000;11(3):162–167.
12. Buffum WP, Settipane GA. Prognosis of asthma in childhood. *Am J Dis Child.* 1966;112(3):214–217.
13. Wang J, Visness CM, Sampson HA. Food allergen sensitization in inner-city children with asthma. *J Allergy Clin Immunol.* 2005;115(5):1076–1080.
14. Liu AH, Jaramillo R, Sicherer SH, et al. National prevalence and risk factors for food allergy and relationship to asthma: results from the National Health and Nutrition Examination Survey 2005–2006. *J Allergy Clin Immunol.* 2010;126(4):798–806.
15. Roberts G, Patel N, Levi-Schaffer F, et al. Food allergy as a risk factor for life-threatening asthma in childhood: a case-controlled study. *J Allergy Clin Immunol.* 2003;112(1):168–174.
16. Illi S, von Mutius E, Lau S, et al. The natural course of atopic dermatitis from birth to age 7 years and the association with asthma. *J Allergy Clin Immunol.* 2004;113(5):925–931.
17. Fiocchi A, Terracciano L, Bouygue GR, Veglia F, Martelli A, Restani P. Incremental prognostic factors associated with cow's milk allergy outcomes in infant and child referrals: the MiCMAC study. *Ann Allergy Asthma Immunol.* 2008;101(2):166–173.
18. Simpson AB, Glutting J, Yousef E. Food allergy and asthma morbidity in children. *Pediatr Pulmonol.* 2007;42(6):489–495.
19. Berns SH, Halm EA, Sampson HA, Sicherer SH, Busse PJ, Wisnivesky JP. Food allergy as a risk factor for asthma morbidity in adults. *J Asthma.* 2007;44(5):377–381.
20. Salob SP, Laverty A, Atherton DJ. Bronchial hyperresponsiveness in children with atopic dermatitis. *Pediatrics.* 1993;91(1):13–16.
21. Malmberg LP, Saarinen KM, Pelkonen AS, et al. Cow's milk allergy as a predictor of bronchial hyperresponsiveness and airway inflammation at school age. *Clin Exp Allergy.* 2010;40(10):1491–1497.
22. Krogulska A, Dynowski J, Wasowska-Królikowska K. Bronchial reactivity in schoolchildren allergic to food. *Ann Allergy Asthma Immunol.* 2010;105(1):31–38.
23. Kondo H, Ichikawa Y, Imokawa G. Percutaneous sensitization with allergens through barrier-disrupted skin elicits a Th2-dominant cytokine response. *Eur J Immunol.* 1998;28(3):769–779.
24. Spergel JM, Mizoguchi E, Brewer JP, Martin TR, Bhan AK, Geha RS. Epicutaneous sensitization with protein antigen induces localized allergic dermatitis and hyperresponsiveness to methacholine after single exposure

to aerosolized antigen in mice. *J Clin Invest.* 1998;101(8):1614–1622.
25. Flohr C, England K, Radulovic S, et al. Filaggrin loss-of-function mutations are associated with early-onset eczema, eczema severity and trans-epidermal water loss at 3 months of age. *Br J Dermatol.* 2010;163(6):1333–1336.
26. Dubrac S, Schmuth M, Ebner S. Atopic dermatitis: the role of Langerhans cells in disease pathogenesis. *Immunol Cell Biol.* 2010;88(4):400–409.
27. Irvine AD, McLean WH, Leung DY. Filaggrin mutations associated with skin and allergic diseases. *N Engl J Med.* 2011;365(14):1315–1327.
28. Brown SJ, Irvine AD. Atopic eczema and the filaggrin story. *Semin Cutan Med Surg.* 2008;27(2):128–137.
29. Howell MD, Kim BE, Gao P, et al. Cytokine modulation of atopic dermatitis filaggrin skin expression. *J Allergy Clin Immunol.* 2007;120(1): 150–155.
30. Jensen JM, Pfeiffer S, Witt M, et al. Different effects of pimecrolimus and betamethasone on the skin barrier in patients with atopic dermatitis. *J Allergy Clin Immunol.* 2009;124(3 Suppl 2):R19–R28.
31. Ying S, Meng Q, Corrigan CJ, Lee TH. Lack of filaggrin expression in the human bronchial mucosa. *J Allergy Clin Immunol.* 2006;118(6): 1386–1388.
32. Palmer CN, Ismail T, Lee SP, et al. Filaggrin null mutations are associated with increased asthma severity in children and young adults. *J Allergy Clin Immunol.* 2007;120(1):64–68.
33. Lack G, Fox D, Northstone K, Golding J, for the Avon Longitudinal Study of Parents and Children Study Team. Factors associated with the development of peanut allergy in childhood. *N Engl J Med.* 2003;348(11):977–985.
34. Fox AT, Sasieni P, du Toit G, Syed H, Lack G. Household peanut consumption as a risk factor for the development of peanut allergy. *J Allergy Clin Immunol.* 2009;123(2):417–423.
35. Brown SJ, Asai Y, Cordell HJ, et al. Loss-of-function variants in the filaggrin gene are a significant risk factor for peanut allergy. *J Allergy Clin Immunol.* 2011;127(3):661–667.
36. James JM. Respiratory manifestations of food allergy. *Pediatrics.* 2003;111(6 Pt 3):1625–1630.
37. Bock SA. Respiratory reactions induced by food challenges in children with pulmonary disease. *Pediatr Allergy Immunol.* 1992;3(4):188–194.
38. James JM, Bernhisel-Broadbent J, Sampson HA. Respiratory reactions provoked by double-blind food challenges in children. *Am J Respir Crit Care Med.* 1994;149(1):59–64.
39. Saarinen KM, Pelkonen AS, Mäkelä MJ, et al. Clinical course and prognosis of cow's milk allergy are dependent on milk-specific IgE status. *J Allergy Clin Immunol.* 2005;116(4): 869–875.
40. Skripak JM, Matsui EC, Mudd K, et al. The natural history of IgE-mediated cow's milk allergy. *J Allergy Clin Immunol.* 2007;120(5): 1172–1177.
41. Bock SA, Muñoz-Furlong A, Sampson HA. Fatalities due to anaphylactic reactions to foods. *J Allergy Clin Immunol.* 2001;107(1):191–193.
42. González-Pérez A, Aponte Z, Vidaurre CF, et al. Anaphylaxis epidemiology in patients with and patients without asthma: a United Kingdom database review. *J Allergy Clin Immunol.* 2010;125(5):1098–1104.
43. Iribarren C, Tolstykh IV, Miller MK, et al. Asthma and the prospective risk of anaphylactic shock and other allergy diagnoses in a large integrated health care delivery system. *Ann Allergy Asthma Immunol.* 2010;104(5):371–377.
44. Varshney P, Steele PH, Vickery BP, et al. Adverse reactions during peanut oral immunotherapy home dosing. *J Allergy Clin Immunol.* 2009;124(6):1351–1352.
45. Flinterman AE, Knulst AC, Meijer Y, Bruijnzeel-Koomen CA, Pasmans SG. Acute allergic reactions in children with AEDS after prolonged cow's milk elimination diets. *Allergy.* 2006;61(3):370–374.
46. Maloney JM, Nowak-Wegrzyn A, Wang J. Children in the inner city of New York have high rates of food allergy and IgE sensitization to common foods. *J Allergy Clin Immunol.* 2011;128(1):214–215.
47. Fleischer DM, Perry TT, Atkins D, et al. Allergic reactions to foods in preschool-aged children in a prospective observational food allergy study. *Pediatrics.* 2012;130(1):e25–e32.
48. Sicherer SH, Vargas PA, Groetch ME, et al. Development and validation of educational materials for food allergy. *J Pediatr.* 2012;160(4):651–656.
49. Iikura Y, Aspitz CK, Mikawa H, et al. Prevention of asthma by ketotifen in infants with atopic dermatitis. *Ann Allergy.* 1992;68(3): 233–236.
50. Warner JO, for the ETAC Study Group. Early treatment of the atopic child. A double-blinded, randomized, placebo-controlled trial of cetirizine in preventing the onset of asthma in children with atopic dermatitis: 18 months' treatment and 18 months' posttreatment follow-up. *J Allergy Clin Immunol.* 2001;108(6):929–937.

51. Simons FE, for the Early Prevention of Asthma in Atopic Children (EPAAC) Study Group. Safety of levocetirizine treatment in young atopic children: an 18-month study. *Pediatr Allergy Immunol.* 2007;18(6):535–542.
52. Ramírez del Pozo ME, Contreras Contreras E, López Tiro J, Gómez Vera J. Omalizumab (an anti-IgE antibody) in the treatment of severe atopic eczema. *J Invest Allergol Clin Immunol.* 2011;21(5):416–417.
53. Fernández-Antón Martínez MC, Leis-Dosil V, Alfageme-Roldán F, Paravisini A, Sánchez-Ramón S, Suárez Fernández R. Omalizumab for the treatment of atopic dermatitis. *Actas Dermosifiliogr.* 2012;103(7):624–628.
54. Velling P, Skowasch D, Pabst S, Jansen E, Tuleta I, Grohé C. Improvement of quality of life in patients with concomitant allergic asthma and atopic dermatitis: one year follow-up of omalizumab therapy. *Eur J Med Res.* 2011;16(9):407–410.
55. Leung DY, Sampson HA, Yunginger JW, et al. Effect of anti-IgE therapy in patients with peanut allergy. *N Engl J Med.* 2003;348(11):986–993.
56. Sampson HA, Leung DY, Burks AW, et al. A phase II, randomized, double-blind, parallel-group, placebo-controlled oral food challenge trial of Xolair (omalizumab) in peanut allergy. *J Allergy Clin Immunol.* 2011;127(5):1309–1310.

INDEX

NOTE: Page numbers followed by t indicate a reference to a table on the designated page. Italicized page numbers indicate a figure on the designated page

AAT deficiency. see α_1-antitrypsin (AAT) deficiency
ABPA. see allergic bronchopulmonary aspergillosis (ABPA)
ABRS. see acute bacterial rhinosinusitis (ABRS)
absent sympathetic vasoconstriction (Horner's syndrome), 253t
achondroplasia, and OSA in childhood, 50t
acinic cell carcinoma, 141t
acquired immunodeficiency syndrome (AIDS), 33
acute bacterial rhinosinusitis (ABRS), 249t, 263, 264, 265–266
acute epiglottitis, 142
acute rhinosinusitis (ARS)
  in children, 266
  clinical features, 264
  complications, 265–266
  diagnosis, 264–265
  epidemiology, 264
  lifestyle modification strategies, 265
  pathophysiology
    acute bacterial rhinosinusitis, 264
    postviral rhinosinusitis, 264
  pharmacologic treatment, 265
  surgical treatment, 265
acute-onset dyspnea, 144
acute/recurrent bacterial rhinosinusitis, 249t, 263
Addison's disease, 335, 339–340, 342, 349t

adenoid systic carcinoma, 141t
adenomas of salivary gland-type tumors, 141t
adenotonsillar hypertrophy, 50t, 51, 59
adult cardiac conditions, 193–201
adult-onset asthma, 172, 173–174, 176, 184–185
adults with asthma
  allergic sensitization role in, 335
  GER prevalence in, 303–306, *304*, *307*
    treatment decisions, 313–315
  hiatal hernia prevalence in, *307*
  HRQoL in, 382–383
  obesity and, 329, 330
  viral respiratory tract infections and, 262
age, over 65, and asthma. see elderly people with asthma
air pollution, 238, 263, 264, 270, 427–429
airflow obstruction, irreversible. see chronic obstructive pulmonary disease (COPD), and irreversible airflow obstruction
airway obstruction
  in ANCA-positive vasculitis, 18
  defined, 81–82, 82t
  in hypersensitivity pneumonitis, 8
  irreversible, in COPD patients, 80
    diagnosis, 82
    lifestyle/behavior modification strategies, 85

airway obstruction (Cont.)
    in nonsmoking asthma patients, 85
    in smoking asthma patients, 85
    in OSA/OSAS, 50, 51, 52, 53, 57, 59.68, 70, 72
    reversibility, in asthma, 4t
AIT. see allergen immunotherapy (AIT)
alcohol and asthma, 395, 397t, 399–402, 401t
alexithymia, 379, 381–382, 381t, 385, 388, 389t, 391
allergen immunotherapy (AIT), 166, 232, 236, 430, 448
allergic angiitis with granulomatosis (AAG), 13
allergic bronchopulmonary aspergillosis (ABPA), 21–30, 94–95, 95, 96t
    asthma subtype comorbidity, 26–27
    background information, 21–22
    with bronchiectasis, 96t
    clinical features, 22, 22
    complications, 22
    diagnosis, 23–26, 23t, 24
    differential diagnosis, 27
    future research needs, 29
    lifestyle/behavior modification strategies, 27–28
    pharmacologic treatment, 25–26, 28–29
    prevalence in chronic asthma, 98
    stages, 25, 26t, 28
allergic bronchopulmonary aspergillosis with central bronchiectasis (ABPA-CB), 23, 23t, 24, 25, 26
allergic fungal sinusitis, 274–275
allergic rhinitis (AR)
    ABPA and, 22, 27
    in asthmatic children, 57
    background information, 231–232
    bronchiolitis and, 107t
    comorbidities, 237, 238
        acute/chronic sinusitis, 240–241
        asthma, 237–240
        conjunctivitis, 237
        sleep issues, 240
    diagnosis, 232
    future research needs, 241
    mimicking conditions, 33
    OSA and, 50, 50t, 51, 52, 56t
    pathophysiology of, 232–233
    pharmacologic treatment, 166
        allergen immunotherapy, 236
        anticholinergic drugs, 235
        antihistamines, 233
        combinations, 236
        cromolyn sodium, 235
        decongestants, 233–234
        leukotriene modifiers, 235–236
        systemic corticosteroids, 235
        topical intranasal glucocorticosteroids, 234–235
Allergic Rhinitis and its Impact on Asthma (ARIA) guidelines, 232
allergy epidemic, in Finland, 422
α_1-antitrypsin (AAT) deficiency
    asthma comorbidity, 134
    with bronchiectasis, 96t
    description, 115
    diagnosis
        lifestyle/behavior modification, 135
        screening, 134–135
    epidemiology, 128
    pathophysiology
        bronchiectasis, 134
        clinical features, 128
        emphysema, 128, 134
    treatment, pharmacologic
        augmentation therapy by inhalation, 136
        intravenous human plasma-derived augmentation therapy, 135
        lung transplantation, 136
        recombinant augmentation therapy and synthetic elastase inhibition, 136
    treatment, surgical
        lung transplantation, 136
        lung volume reduction surgery, 136
α-antitrypsin level and cystic fibrosis conductance regulator gene mutation analysis, 95–96
Ambrisentan in Pulmonary Arterial Hypertension (ARIES)-1 trial, 224
Ameille, J., 183
American Academy of Allergy Asthma and Immunology (AAAAI), 410
American College of Allergy Asthma and Immunology (ACAAI), 410
American College of Chest Physicians, 82, 172
American College of Rheumatology, 17
American Thoracic Society-European Respiratory Society Task Force
    AAT deficiency screening recommendations, 134
    airway obstruction defined, 82t
    bronchodilator reversibility defined, 83t
amyloidosis, 140
Anderson, S. D., 411
antibody deficiency disorders
    common variable immunodeficiency, 40
    congenital agammaglobulinemia, 40
    laboratory findings, 39t
    selective immunoglobulin A deficiency, 41
    specific antibody deficiency, 40
    transient hypogammaglobulinemia of infancy, 40–41
antineutrophil cytoplasmic antibody (ANCA)-positive vasculitis, 12–19
    background information, 12–13
    clinical characteristics, 14–16
    diagnosis, 16–18
    etiology, 14
    future research needs, 19
    pharmacologic treatment, 18–19, 19t
    vasculitis/classifications, 15t
Apert's syndrome, and OSA in childhood, 50t
apnea-hypopnea index (AHI), 52–53, 58–59, 64, 65t, 67, 71
AR. see allergic rhinitis (AR)
ARS. see acute rhinosinusitis (ARS)
Aspergillus species, 21–29, 42, 94–95, 142
asthma, coexisting conditions
    adult cardiovascular disease, 193–201
    antineutrophil cytoplasmic antibody-positive vasculitis, 12–19
    atopic dermatitis, food allergy, and anaphylaxis, 455–463
    bronchiectasis, 92–101
    bronchiolitis, 103–112
    congestive heart failure, 144
    COPD and irreversible airflow obstruction, 80–88
    cough, 161–169
    endocrine disorders, 334–342
    environmental protective and risk factors, 421–434
    food allergy, 455–463
    genetic disorders, 115–136
    hypersensitivity pneumonitis, 3–9
    immunodeficiency: innate, primary, secondary, 32–45
    obesity, 321–330
    osteopenia, osteoporosis, 345–361
    pediatric cardiac conditions, 204–212

pneumonia, 148–158
pregnancy, 367–374
psychological factors, 379–391
pulmonary hypertension, 215–224
sleep apnea in children, and the upper airway, 49–60
substance abuse, tobacco use, 395–403
valvular heart disease, 144
vocal cord dysfunction, 288–295
asthma, comorbid conditions
   allergic bronchopulmonary aspergillosis, 21–30
   allergic rhinitis, 231–241
   antineutrophil cytoplasmic antibody-positive vasculitis, 12–19
   atopic dermatitis, food allergy, and anaphylaxis, 455–463
   bronchiectasis, 92–101
   bronchiolitis, 103–112
   cardiovascular disease, 194t
   COPD and irreversible airflow obstruction, 80–88
   cough, 161–169
   endocrine disorders, 334–342
   environmental protective and risk factors, 421–434
   exercise-induced bronchoconstriction, 409–415
   food allergy, 455–463
   gastroesophageal reflux, 299–315
   immunodeficiency: innate, primary, secondary, 32–45
   infectious, in the upper airway, 260–276
   nasal polyps, 280–282
   nonallergic rhinopathies, lower airway syndromes, 244–256
   obesity, 321–330
   occupational asthma, 172–185
   occupational rhinitis, 183–184
   osteopenia, osteoporosis, 345–361
   pneumonia, 148–158
   pregnancy, 367–374
   psychological factors, 379–391
   sleep apnea in children, and the upper airway, 49–60
   substance abuse, tobacco use, 395–403
   vocal cord dysfunction, 288–295
asthma, mimicking conditions
   acute infectious diseases, 142–143
   bronchiectasis, 33t, 34
   bronchiolitis, 33t
   carcinoid syndrome, 143
   COPD, 33t, 34
   dyspnea
      acute-onset, 144
      functional/sighing, 145
   follicular bronchiolitis, 144
   idiopathic pulmonary fibrosis, 144
   interstitial lung disease, 33t, 34, 144
   lymphangioleiomyomatosis, 143, 144
   pneumonia, 33t, 34
   pneumothorax, 145
   pulmonary conditions, 33t
   systemic mastocytosis, 143
   upper airway obstruction, 139
Asthma Insights and Reality in Europe (AIRE) study, 380
Asthma Symptom Checklist scale., 382
asthma-specific psychological factors, 380, 381t
"Asthmatics Have More Frequent Life-Threatening Reflux Symptoms Than Non-Asthmatics, and They Are Related to Bed-Time Eating" study, 313–315
ataxia-telangiectasia, 42
atopic cough, 161, 162, 163t
atopic dermatitis, 455–463
   allergic rhinitis and, 444
   background information, 455–456
   in children, 455, 457
   coexistence with food allergy, asthma, 457–458
      clinical impact of diagnoses, 459
      emergency care plan, 461–462
      pathophysiologic link, 458–459
   diagnosis, 107t, 456–457
   food allergy triggers, 456–457
   future research needs, 463
   management strategy, 459–463, 460t
atypical mycobacteria, in hypersensitivity pneumonitis, 6–7
Aurelianus Caelius (Roman physician), 300
autosomal recessive agammaglobulinemia (ARAG), 35t, 39t, 40
Avon Longitudinal Study of Parents and Children, 458

Bafadhel, M., 83
Barach, A., 70
Barrett's esophagus, 305, 306
basaloid squamous cell carcinoma, 141t
behavioral modification strategies. see lifestyle/behavioral modification strategies
Behçet's disease, 15t
Belsey, R., 301
BENARS. see blood eosinophilic nonallergic rhinitis syndrome (BENARS)
Berkson's Fallacy, 302
β-blocker therapy, 196–197, 208, 211
Blanc, P. D., 174
blood eosinophilic nonallergic rhinitis syndrome (BENARS), 248, 249t
BMI (body mass index)
   airway hyperresponsiveness and, 67, 68
   leptin hypothesis and, 67
   Manchester Asthma and Allergy Study, 335
   obesity data, 64, 322
BOLD program. see Burden of Obstructive Lung Disease (BOLD) program
Bosentan Randomized trial of Endothelin Antagonist THErapy (BREATHE)-1, 224
Bray, G. W., 301
Brenner, B. E., 337
bronchial anthracofibrosis, 142
bronchiectasis, 92–101
   background information, 92–93
   clinical features, 93–94
      allergic bronchopulmonary aspergillosis, 94–95
   commonality in PIDDs, 37
   comorbid diseases
      AAT deficiency, 134
      ABPA, 98
      asthma, 97–98
      COPD, 98
      GERD, 98
   definition, 37–38
   diagnosis
      α-antitrypsin level and cystic fibrosis conductance regulator gene mutation analysis, 95–96
      blood tests, 95
      chest X-ray, 96–97
      HRCT, 97
      immunoglobulins, 95
      pulmonary function tests, 97
      sputum analysis, 96
   differential diagnosis, 97–98
   diseases associated with, 96t
   future research directions, 100
   Kartagener's syndrome of, 249t
   management

bronchiectasis (*Cont.*)
  antibiotics, 100
  bronchial hygiene, 99
  inhaled corticosteroids, 99
  inhaled-β-agonists, 99
  oral corticosteroids, 99–100
  mimicking of asthma by, 33*t*, 34
  pathogenesis of, 93
  subdivisions, 93
bronchiolitis, infectious, 103–112
  asthma exacerbations, development of, 109–110
  asthma/wheezing, development in children, 107–109, 108*t*
  background information, 103–104
  clinical features, 105
  diagnosis, 105
    age-related, for wheezing, 106*t*
  differential diagnosis, 106–107
  etiologies/epidemiology, 104–105
  immune response, 109–110
  lower respiratory tract infection in, 103–105, 107, 108, 111
  mimicking of asthma by, 33*t*
  treatment, 110
bronchiolitis, viral, 104, 105
bronchiolitis obliterans, 27, 104, 110–111, 136, 143, 145, 179–180
bronchiolocentric lymphocytic interstitial pneumonitis., 6
bronchodilator reversibility, 34, 35*t*, 82–83, 83*t*, 84, 162
bronchodilator-induced GER, 308, *309*, 310
bronchomalacia, with bronchiectasis, 96*t*
Broughton, W. A., 71
Burden of Obstructive Lung Disease (BOLD) program, 85
Burkholderia cepacia, 22, 42
Burrows, B., 222
Busino, R. S., 59
Buteyko breathing method, 182

Candida, 42
Candida albicans, 234
capillary hemangioma, 141*t*
carcinoid syndrome, 143
carcinoid tumor, typical or atypical, 141*t*, 143
cardiac asthma
  bronchial asthma comparison, 197*t*
  CHF and, 195, 207
  common symptoms with asthma, 193
cardiac conditions. *see* adult cardiac conditions
cardiac dysfunction
  chronic asthma and, 204, 210–211
    pharmacologic treatment, 211–212
  in OSAS, 72, 72–73
  making improvements, 73
cardiovascular disease (CVD), 193–201. *see also* pediatric cardiac conditions
  asthma comorbidity, 194*t*
    medication side effects, 198*t*
    systemic inflammation markers, 198–199
    vascular complications, 199
  asthma treatment and, 197–198, 198*t*, 200, 208, 211
  cardiac-/bronchial asthma differential diagnosis, 197*t*
  COPD/CHF, 194–196
  future research directions, 200–201
  left heart disease, 219, 220, 221–222
  lifestyle/behavior modification strategies, 199–200
  prevalence, in asthma, 193
  pulmonary hypertension, 196
  risk factors, 194

Carr, D. T., 70
Centers for Disease Control and Prevention reports
  asthma-related costs, 322
  asthma-related death rates, 443
  gender-related hospitalizations, 336
  morbidity data, 395–396
  mortality data, 395–396, 443
  obesity rates (US), 64
central-type sleep apnea, 52
cerebral palsy, and OSA in childhood, 50*t*
CGD. *see* chronic granulomatous disease
Chapel Hill Consensus Conference (1994), 17
Chen, C-C, 240
Cherry, J., 301
children. *see also* obstructive sleep apnea (OSA), in children
  acute rhinosinusitis in, 266
  asthma-pneumonia comparison, 155*t*
  atopic dermatitis in, 455, 457
  chronic rhinosinusitis in, 273–274
  congestive heart failure in, 207–208
  DiGeorge syndrome in, 41
  etiology of neurosis in, 386
  infectious bronchiolitis in, 107–110, 108*t*
  infectious rhinitis in, 262
  LRTI, suggested approach, *108*
  MBL deficiency in, 43
  medication nonadherence issues, 384, 385*t*
  nasal polyps in, 123
  obesity and OSA in, 49, 50, 50*t*, 51, 58, 67–70
  pediatric cough, 166
  SCID in, 36, 38, 40
  sleep apnea, upper airway, 49–60
  transient hypogammaglobulinemia of infancy, 40–41
  upper airway resistance syndrome in, 50, 53
  wheezing/age-related differential diagnosis, 106*t*
children with asthma
  allergic rhinitis in, 57*t*
  cognitive function abnormalities, 387–388
  food allergies in, 457
  GER prevalence in, 306–308
    treatment decisions, 313–315
  obesity in, 57*t*, 322–326, *323*, 328–329
  oral glucocorticoid study, 350
  osteoporosis risks, 360
  physical activity response in, 410, 432
  pneumonia in, 151
  SDB prevalence in, 49, 53, 56
  vitamin D levels in, 328
Chlamydophila pneumoniae, 148, 149*t*, 150
cholinergic rhinitis, 253*t*
chondroma, chondrosarcoma, 141*t*
Chromobacterium, 42
chronic cough, 38, 93, 123
  asthma syndrome and, 162
  in cystic fibrosis, 124*t*
  management, 166–167
  NAEB and, 162
  nonasthmatic, 163–165
  pediatric chronic cough, 161
chronic graft-versus-host disease, 37
chronic granulomatous disease (CGD), 42, 96*t*
chronic inflammation-induced osteoporosis, 351–352
chronic invasive fungal rhinosinusitis, 275
chronic obstructive pulmonary disease (COPD), and irreversible airflow obstruction, 80–88
  airway obstruction
    defined, 81–82, 82*t*
    diagnosis, 82

lifestyle/behavior modification strategies, 85
  in nonsmoking asthma patients, 85
asthma/COPD and, 194–196
background information, 80–81
BOLD program report, 85
bronchodilator reversibility, 82–83, 83t
clinical features, 83–84
differential diagnosis, 179
"Dutch hypothesis," 81
in elderly asthmatics, 445
future research directions, 86–87
genes associated with development of, 88t
infectious rhinitis comorbidity, 262
lifestyle/behavior modification strategies, 85
mimicking of asthma by, 33t
pharmacologic treatment, 86
phenotypes (irreversible airflow obstruction)
  in COPD patients, 84–85
  in nonsmoking asthma patients, 85
  in smoking asthma patients, 85
PLATINO study, 84–85
pneumonia with, 157
chronic rhinosinusitis (CRS), 260. *see also* chronic rhinosinusitis with nasal polyps; chronic rhinosinusitis without nasal polyps
in children, 273–274
clinical features, 268
comorbidities
  aspirin intolerance, 270
  links with asthma, 269–270
diagnosis, 268–269
epidemiology, 269
lifestyle and burden of, 282–283
lifestyle modification strategies, 270
with nasal polyps, 266–267, 267
pathophysiology, 266–268
pharmacologic treatment, 270–273
surgical treatment, 273
without nasal polyps, 266, 267
chronic rhinosinusitis with nasal polyps (CRSwNP)
in Asian people, 280
asthma comorbidity, 269–270, 281
clinical features, 268, 282
CRS$_s$NP comparison, 269
diagnosis, 268–269, 269, 282
differential characteristics, 280
differential diagnosis, 282
eosinophilic type, 267
inflammatory/remodeling parameters, 267
lifestyle and burden of, 282–283
pathogenesis, 281
pharmacologic treatment
  evidence-based medicine, 285t
  intranasal corticosteroids, 283
  long-term antibiotics, 284
  short-/intermediate-term antibiotics, 284
  systemic corticosteroids, 283
  topical corticosteroids, 272
Staphylococcus aureus influence in, 260, 267, 281
surgical treatment, 273, 284
chronic rhinosinusitis without nasal polyps (CRSsNP)
aspirin intolerance in, 270
characteristics, 266
clinical features, 268
CRSwNP comparison, 269
diagnosis, 268
differential characteristics, 280
inflammatory/remodeling parameters, 267

lifestyle and burden of, 282–283
pharmacologic treatment, 270–271
Staphylococcus aureus influence in, 281
surgical treatment, 273
chronic thromboembolic pulmonary hypertension (CTEPH), 220, 223
Churg-Strauss Syndrome, 13, 14–16
ANCA profile, 18t
diagnosis, 17t
differential diagnosis, 27, 95, 155, 245t, 249t
with eosinophilic granuloma, 249t
nasal polyps in, 269
skin biopsy, 18
skin rash, 15
ciliary dyskinesia (primary and secondary), with bronchiectasis, 96t
Cimbollek, S., 375
Cincinnati Irritant Index Scale, 247
cleft palate, repaired, and OSA in childhood, 50t
climate change, 391t, 429–430
clinical features
  of ABPA, 22, 22
  of acute rhinosinusitis, 264
  of α_1-antitrypsin (AAT) deficiency, 128
  of ANCA-positive vasculitis, 14–16
  of bronchiectasis, 93–95
  of chronic rhinosinusitis, 268
  of CRSwNP, 268, 282
  of elderly people with asthma, 443–444
  of exercise-induced bronchoconstriction, 410
  of hypersensitivity pneumonitis, 4t, 5
  of infectious rhinitis, 262
  of nonallergic rhinitis, 246
  of occupational asthma, 174–176
  of primary ciliary dyskinesia, 116
  of pulmonary hypertension, 216, 216–218, 217, 218t
  of vocal cord dysfunction, 292
cocaine and asthma, 395, 397–399, 397t
cold dry air-induced rhinorrhea (skier's rhinitis), 253t
Collins, L. C., 340
common variable immunodeficiency (CVID), 37, 40
community-acquired methicillin-resistant *S. aureus* (CA-MRSA), 157
community-acquired pneumonia (CAP), 148
  clinical features, 150–151
  diagnosis, 151–154
    blood specimen, 152–153
    invasively collected specimens, 153–154
    pleural fluid, 153
    sputum specimen, 153
    urine specimen, 153
  differential diagnosis, 154–155, 155t
  etiologic agents, 149t, 150
  future research directions, 157–158
  lifestyle/behavior modification strategies, 155–156
  pharmacologic treatment, 156–158
    considerations for asthma patients, 157
congenital agammaglobulinemia, 40
congenital complement deficiency, 15t
congestive heart failure (CHF), 144
  cardiac asthma and, 193, 195, 196, 197t, 207
  in children, 207–208
    left ventricular dysfunction, 208
    left-to-right shunts, 207–208
  in elderly people with asthma, 444
  management of, 196
conjunctivitis, 237
constrictive bronchiectasis, 93, 179–180

COPDGene Study, 85, 88
Corrao, W. M., 162
corrosive occupational rhinitis, 249t
cough, 161–169. *see also* chronic cough
   ABPA and, 22, *24*, 26
   ANCA-positive vasculitides and, 13
   ataxia-telangiectasia and, 42
   atopic cough, 161, 162, 163t
   bronchiectasis and, 92–94
   bronchiolitis and, 36, 105, 106
   bronchiolitis obliterans and, 111
   chronic ILD and, 37
   COPD and, 81
   cystic fibrosis and, 122, 123, 124t
   future research directions, 167–168
   HP and, 3, 5
   lifestyle modifications, 166
   mechanisms, epidemiology, measurement, 161–162
   nonasthmatic, differential diagnosis
      GERD, 163–164
         psychogenic cough, 165
         rhinitis/rhinosinusitis, 164–165
         unexplained/idiopathic cough, 165
   PCD and, 118, 119t, 120
   pediatric cough, 161, 166
   pharmacologic treatment, 99
   pneumonia and, 36, 148, 150–151
   suppression therapies, 167–168
   upper airway obstruction and, 140, 142
cough-asthma syndromes, 162, 163t
cough-variant asthma, 162
CPAP (continuous positive airway pressure) therapy, 58, 63, 65–67, 69–73
   anti-acid reflux effect of, 72
   antiinflammatory effects, 71
   asthma, positive influences on, 65
   benefits, 67–68
   diagnosis, 81–83
   for elderly people with OSA, 445
   heart function improvements, 73
   mechanical, neuromechanical effects, 69–70, 73
   pathological features impacted by, 63, 66t
craniofacial abnormalities, and OSA in childhood, 50t
cricoarytenoid arthritis, 142
Crouzon's syndrome, and OSA in childhood, 50t
cylindrical bronchiectasis, 93
cysteinyl leukotrienes, 49, 56–57, 57t, 60
cystic fibrosis (CF). *see also* cystic fibrosis (CF), clinical presentations
   ABPA and, 21
   asthma comorbidity, 126–128
   background information, 121
   with bronchiectasis, 96t
   diagnosis
      criteria, 124
      general process recommendations, 125–126
      mutation analysis, 124–125
      nasal potential difference measurements, 125
      phenotypic features, 123, 124t
      sweat test, 124
   genetic mutations in, 115
   nasal polyps in, 124t, 249t, 269
   pharmacologic treatment, 128
      new/modified, 132t–133t
      past/recently available, 129t–131t
cystic fibrosis (CF), clinical presentations
   adolescents and adults, 123
   infancy and childhood

      gastrointestinal tract, 123
      lower respiratory tract, 123
      upper respiratory tract, 123
   neonatal
      growth failure, 122
      jejunal atresia, 122
      liver disease, 122
      meconium ileus, 122
      meconium plug syndrome, 122
      pulmonary manifestations, 122
   prenatal
      fetal intestinal obstruction, 122
      high-risk pregnancies, 121–122

Denjean, A., 69
diagnosis
   of ABPA, 23–26, 23t, *24*
   of acute rhinosinusitis, 264–265
   of allergic rhinitis, 232
   of ANCA-positive vasculitis, 16–18
   of asthma in pregnancy, 369
   of atopic dermatitis, 456–457
   of bronchiectasis, 95–97
   of chronic granulomatous disease, 42
   of chronic rhinosinusitis, 268–269
   of CRSwNP, 268–269, *269*, 282
   of elderly people with asthma, 444–445
   of hypersensitivity pneumonitis, 4t, 5–6
   of infectious rhinitis, 263
   of nasal polyps, 268
   of nonallergic rhinitis, 246–248
   of OSA in children, 52–53
   of osteoporosis, 353
   of panic disorder, 182
   of primary ciliary dyskinesia, 116–118
   of psychological factors in asthma, 388–391, 389t, 390t–391t
   of pulmonary hypertension, 218–220
   of upper airway obstruction, 142
   of vocal cord dysfunction, 292–293
"Diagnosis and Management of Work-Related Asthma" consensus statement (American College of Chest Physicians), 172
Diagnostic and Statistical Manual of Mental Disorders (DSM)
   panic disorder criteria, 182
   substance abuse disorders, 395
dietary-induced osteoporosis, 351
differential diagnosis
   of ABPA, 27
   of adult cardiac conditions, 193–201
   of adult-onset asthma, 176
   of allergic bronchopulmonary aspergillosis, 27
   of asthma during pregnancy, 370
   of bronchiectasis, 92–101
   of bronchiolitis, 103–112
   of Churg-Strauss Syndrome, 27, 95, 155, 245t, 249t
   of COPD/irreversible airflow obstruction, 80–88, 194
   of cough, 161–169
   of eosinophil-predominant rhinopathies, 249t
   of exercise-induced bronchoconstriction with asthma, 412, 413t
   of genetic disorders, 115–136
   of hormonal/drug-related rhinopathies, 252t
   of hypersensitivity pneumonitis, 8
   of infectious rhinitis, 263
   of nasal structural anomalies, 251t
   of neurologic rhinopathies, 253t
   of neutrophil-predominant rhinopathies, 249t
   of nonallergic rhinitis, 245, 248–253

of occupational asthma, 172–185
of rhinitis, 245t
of rhinopathies with complex cellular infiltrates or temporal evolution of inflammation, 250t
of vocal cord dysfunction, 177, 178t, 289, 294t
diffuse panbronchiolitis, 96t
DiGeorge syndrome (22q11.2 deletion), 41
diphtheria, 143
The Diseases of Children and Their Remedies (Rosenstein), 300
double-blind, placebo-controlled oral food challenges (DBPCFC), 459
Down syndrome, and OSA in childhood, 50t
drug-induced osteoporosis
  glucocorticoids, 347, 349–351
    dose-response effect, 350–351
    kinetics, 350
    pathophysiology, 349–350
  other drugs, 351
Duchenne's muscular dystrophy, and OSA in childhood, 50t
"Dutch hypothesis," 81
dysfunctional breathing group
  hyperventilation syndrome, 181–182
  panic disorder, 182
  work-related laryngeal dysfunction, 180–181

Ehlers-Danlos syndrome, with bronchiectasis, 96t, 348
elderly people with asthma, 441–449
  clinical features, 443t
    natural history, 443–444
    presentation differences, 443
    role of allergic triggers, 444
  diagnosis
    approach, 444
    comorbidities, 445
    COPD overlap, 445
    difficulties with, 444
  epidemiology, 442–443
  future research needs, 448
  immunodeficiency disorders, 33
  infectious bronchiolitis, 104
  lifestyle/behavioral modifications, 445–446
  medication nonadherence issues, 384, 385t
  memory/psychological factors, 383
  nasal structural anomalies, 251
  pneumonia, 149–151, 155–156
  pulmonary hypertension, 219
  treatment
    adherence issues, 448
    allergen immunotherapy, 448
    anti-immunoglobulin E therapy, 448
    β-agonists, corticosteroids, 446–447
    guidelines, 446
    leukotriene receptor antagonists, 447
    theophylline, 448
  virus susceptibility, 150
emphysema, with α_1-antitrypsin (AAT) deficiency, 128, 134
endobrachial adenocarcinoma, invasive adenocarcinoma, 141t
endobrachial small cell carcinoma, 141t
endobrachial squamous cell carcinoma, 141t
endocrine disorders and asthma, 334–342
  Addison's disease, 335, 339–340, 342, 349t
  background information, 334–335
  clinical practice guidelines, 342t
  exogenous hormonal treatment findings, 338t
  future research needs, 342
  gender influence on asthma, 335–336, 336t
  hyperthyroidism, 234, 334, 335, 338–339, 338–339, 341
  hypothyroidism, 64t, 248, 251, 252t, 338–339

low testosterone, 340
menstrual cycle, 336–338, 338t
treatment strategies, 341–342
vitamin D deficiency, 340–341
Endothelin Antagonist Trial in Mildly Symptomatic Pulmonary Arterial Hypertension Patients (EARLY) Study, 224
environmental protective and risk factors in asthma, 421–434
  AAT deficiency and, 135
  air pollution, 238, 263, 264, 270, 427–429
  allergic rhinitis and, 237, 237, 238, 239, 241
  background information, 421–422
  bronchiolitis and, 105, 107
  climate change, 391t, 429–430
  COPD and, 80, 81, 87.88, 179
  coughing and, 166
  environmental biodiversity, 422–423
  exercise-induced bronchoconstriction and, 410, 414–415
  gene-environment interaction, 421, 422, 424–425
  health-promoting actions, 430–434
    antibiotics, 431–432
    healthy diet, 430–431
    natural environment connection, 433–434
    physical activity, 432
    probiotics, 271t, 431
  hypersensitivity pneumonitis and, 4, 5, 6, 8–9
  immune hyper-/hyporesponsiveness, 425–426
  immunodeficiencies and, 43
  nonallergic rhinitis and, 244, 246–247, 250
  pneumonia and, 156
  population effects, 426–427
  tolerance/environmental adaptation, 423–424
  upper airway infectious comorbidities, 261, 263, 281t
  vocal cord disorders and, 292
eosinophil predominant rhinopathies, 249t
eosinophilia syndrome, 248
eosinophilic bronchitis, 179
eosinophilic granulomatosis with polyangiitis (EGPA). *see* Churg-Strauss Syndrome
epidemiology
  of acute rhinosinusitis, 264
  of α_1-antitrypsin (AAT) deficiency, 128
  of chronic rhinosinusitis, 269
  of cough, 161–162
  of cystic fibrosis, 128
  of elderly people with asthma, *442*, 442–443
  of hypersensitivity pneumonitis, 4–5
  of immune deficiency, 33–34
  of infectious bronchiolitis, 104–105
  of infectious rhinitis, 262
  of vocal cord dysfunction, 291
epiglottitis, 142–143
epithelial tumors, benign and malignant, 141t
erythema nodosum, 15t
Essex, H. E., 70
etiology
  of ABPA, 127
  of acute rhinosinusitis, 265
  of allergic fungal sinusitis, 274
  of ANCA-positive vasculitis, 14, 19
  of asthma, 173
    cardiac asthma, 197t
  of bronchiectasis, 95, 99
  of bronchiolitis, 103, 111
  of chronic interstitial lung disease, 37
  of congestive heart failure, 196
  of cough

etiology (Cont.)
 chronic, 162, 166
 idiopathic, 165
 of neurosis in children, 386
 of pneumonia, 148, 149t, 150–151, 156–157
 of primary immunodeficiency diseases, 33
 of pulmonary hypertension, 219
 of vocal cord dysfunction, 291–292
European Antimicrobial Resistance Surveillance Network (EARS-Net), 157
European Community Respiratory Health Survey (ECRHS), 248, 335
European Network for Understanding Mechanisms of Severe Asthma (ENFUMOSA), 336
European Position Paper on Rhinosinusitis and Nasal Polyps (EP²OS), 265
European Respiratory Society (ERS), 82
eustachian tube dysfunction, 239, 262
excessive daytime sleepiness, in children with OSA, 52
exercise-induced arterial hypoxemia, 413t
exercise-induced asthma (EIA), 289, 410
exercise-induced bronchoconstriction with asthma (EIB_{wA})
 defined, 409
 diagnosis, 411–412
 differential diagnosis, 412, 413t
 future research needs, 415
 International Olympic Committee criteria, 412t
 mechanisms, 410–411
 prevention, nonpharmacologic, 414
 prevention, pharmacologic, 414–415, 415t
 with/without asthma, 410
exercise-induced hyperventilation (pseudo-asthma syndrome), 413t
extrinsic allergic alveolitis. *see* hypersensitivity pneumonitis

Feldman, J. M., 382
fibroconnective tissue tumors (benign or malignant), 141t
fibrosing mediastinitis, 142
Field, S. K., 303
Finnish Karelia, 422–424, 434
follicular bronchiolitis, 144
food allergies
 ABPA and, 22
 atopic dermatitis, anaphylaxis and, 455–464
 children with CF and, 122
 dietary-induced osteoporosis and, 351
 nonallergenic rhinitis and, 247
 WAS and, 41
 Wiskott-Aldrich syndrome (WAS) and, 41
free-base cocaine. *see* cocaine and asthma
Friedman, G. D., 306
Fujimura, M., 162
functional dyspnea, 145
fungal ball, 274
fungal rhinosinusitis
 fungi as causative of all chronic rhinosinusitis, 275
 invasive
  chronic invasive fungal rhinosinusitis, 275
  granulomatous invasive fungal rhinosinusitis, 275
 noninvasive
  allergic fungal sinusitis, 274–275
  fungal ball, 274
fungal sinusitis syndromes, 250t
future research needs
 of allergic bronchopulmonary aspergillosis, 29
 of allergic rhinitis, 241
 of ANCA-positive vasculitis, 19
 of atopic dermatitis, 463

 of elderly people with asthma, 448
 of endocrine disorders, 342
 of exercise-induced bronchoconstriction with asthma, 415
 of gastroesophageal reflux, 315
 of hypersensitivity pneumonitis, 9
 of immunodeficiencies, 45
 of nonallergic rhinitis, 255
 of obesity, 329–330
 of osteoporosis, 361
 of pediatric cardiac conditions, 212
 of pregnancy, 374
 of psychological factors in asthma, 391
 of pulmonary arterial hypertension, 223
 of substance abuse, 402

Gaeta, T. J., 398
gastroesophageal reflux (GER), 299–315
 asthma (defined), 303
 asthmatic children, prevalence in, 306–308
 background information, 299–300
 bronchodilator effects on, 308, *309*, 310
 documentation methods, *303*
 effects of therapy on pulmonary symptoms, 310–311, *311*
 future research needs, 315
 GER-Asthma Theory, 313
 idiopathic pulmonary fibrosis and, 311–313
 interstitial lung disease and, 311–312
 legends, myths, possibilities, 300
 obesity and, 71
 OSAS and, 71–72, *72*
 pre-bedtime eating study, 313–315, *314*
 prevalence in pulmonary patients
  coexistence studies, 302
  studies with adequate data, 302–303
  study designs, sampling procedures, 302
 surgical treatment, 299
 symptoms, 300
 treatment decisions, 313–315, *314*
 twentieth-century research, 301–302
gastroesophageal reflux (GER), in asthmatic adults, 303–306, *304*
 in elderly people, 445
 GER defined as presence of abnormal acid reflux, 304, *305*
 GER defined as presence of esophageal mucosal disease, 304–305, *306*
 GER defined as presence of hiatal hernia, 305–306, *307*
 GER defined as presence of reflux symptoms, 303–304
gastroesophageal reflux disease (GERD)
 CPAP's anti-acid reflux effect, 72
 defined, 303
 OSAS and, 71–72, *72*
 treatment, 98
gender
 asthma differences, 335–336, 336t
 cardiovascular diseases, 193, 194
 female asthma frequency data, 335
 and HIV-associated asthma, 34
 hormonal differences, 325, 336–338
 nonallergenic rhinitis, 247, 248
 obesity/asthma risk factors, 322–323
 OSA and, 51–52, 58
 RSV/asthma risk factors, 108
 systemic inflammation, 326
 underreporting in girls, 335
gene-environment interaction, 421, 422, 424–425
genetic disorders, 115–136. *see also* α_1-antitrypsin (AAT) deficiency; cystic fibrosis (CF); primary ciliary dyskinesia (PCD)

GERD-induced vocal cord dysfunction, 292
Gibbs, C. J., 336
Glauser, F. L., 162
GLILD. see granulomatosis-lymphocytic interstitial lung disease (GLILD)
Global Allergy and Asthma Network of Excellence (GA$_2$LEN), 269
Global Initiative for Asthma (GINA), 382, 446
Global Initiative for Chronic Obstructive Lung Disease (GOLD), 82, 110
Global Strategy for the Diagnosis, Management, and Prevention of Chronic Obstructive Pulmonary Disease
  airway obstruction definition, 81t
  bronchodilator reversibility definition, 82t
glomus tumor, 141t
glucocorticoid-resistant allergic rhinitis (mixed rhinitis), 246
Godfrey, S., 410
Grammer, L. C., 173
granular cell tumor, 141t
granulomatosis vasculitis group, 15t
granulomatosis with polyangiitis (GPA). see Wegener's granulomatosis
granulomatosis-lymphocytic interstitial lung disease (GLILD), 37
granulomatous invasive fungal rhinosinusitis, 275
Green, B. T., 71
Green, M., 340
gustatory rhinitis, 253t

Haemophilus influenzae, 33, 38, 96, 142, 148, 149, 166, 264
Hamada, K., 222
hamartoma, 141t
Hammock, R., 398
Harris, P. W., 340
Hashimoto's thyroiditis, 340
Hastie, A. T., 83
Hatha yoga, 182
Heberden, William, 300
Helicobacter pylori infection, 264
hemangiosarcoma (Kaposi's sarcoma), 141t
Henoch-Schönlein purpura (HSP), 15t
hereditary angioedema, 42–43
heroin and asthma, 395, 397–399, 397t
The History and Cure of Diseases (Heberden), 300
HIV (human immunodeficiency virus) infection, 33, 38
Holzmann, D., 240
hormonal/drug-related rhinopathies, 252t
hormone replacement therapy (HRT) and asthma., 338
Horner's syndrome (absent sympathetic vasoconstriction), 253t
HP. see hypersensitivity pneumonitis (HP)
human rhinovirus (HRV) bronchiolitis, 103–105, 107–110, 148
hydrocodone and asthma, 399
hyperactive behavior, in children with OSA, 52
hyperactive cholinergic parasympathetic function with excessive mucous exocytosis, 253t
hyper-immunoglobulin E (IgE) syndrome, 42
hypersensitivity pneumonitis (HP), 3–9
  background information, 3–4
  with bronchiectasis, 96t
  diagnosis
    clinical manifestations, 4t, 5
    criteria, 5–6
    pathogenesis/histopathology, 6
    radiographic findings, 6
  differential diagnosis, 8, 179
  epidemiology, 4–5
  exposures and causes, 7t
    atypical mycobacteria, 6–7
    chemicals, 8
    fungi, 7
    thermophilic bacteria, 7–8
  future research needs, 9
  major presenting features, 4t
  management, prognosis, 8–9
  risk factors, 7t
hypersensitivity vasculitis group, 15t
hyperthyroidism, 234, 334, 335, 338–339, 341
hyperventilation syndrome (HVS) with asthma, 180, 386–387
  assessment of, 387
  causes/symptoms, 386
  differential diagnosis, 177, 178t
  symptoms, 181–182
hypogammaglobulinemia (acquired and congenital), 96t, 249t
hypothyroidism, 64t, 248, 251, 252t, 338–339
hypovitaminosis D-induced osteoporosis, 351

idiopathic nonallergic rhinopathy (iNAR), 244, 248, 252–255
idiopathic pulmonary arterial hypertension (IPAH), 220
idiopathic pulmonary fibrosis (IPF), 96t, 144, 311–313
IIOA. see irritant-induced occupational asthma (IIOA)
immune hyper-/hyporesponsiveness, 425–426
immunodeficiencies, 32–45. see also primary immunodeficiency diseases (PIDDs)
  background information, 32–33
  clinical evaluation, 43, 44t
  epidemiology of, 33–34
  future research needs, 45
  innate immunity, 34t, 35t
  pharmacologic treatment, 44–45
  primary immunodeficiency diseases
    comorbidity considerations, 36–38
    etiology of, 33
    evaluation, 36–37
    forms of, 34
    IUIS classification of, 34t
    pharmacologic treatment, 44–45
    therapy, 37
    U.S. prevalence, 34
  secondary immunodeficiencies, 33, 34, 37
immunodeficiencies, specific, with predominant pulmonary disease
  antibody deficiency disorders
    common variable immunodeficiency, 40
    congenital agammaglobulinemia, 40
    laboratory findings, 39t
    selective immunoglobulin A deficiency, 41
    specific antibody deficiency, 40
    transient hypogammaglobulinemia of infancy, 40–41
  ataxia-telangiectasia, 42
  chronic granulomatous disease, 42
  combined T-cell/B-cell deficiencies, 38, 40
  DiGeorge syndrome, 41
  hyper-immunoglobulin E syndrome, 42
  mannose-binding lectin deficiency, 43
  Wiskott-Aldrich syndrome, 41
immunologically mediated occupation asthma (IMOA), 173
infectious rhinitis
  in children, 262
  clinical features, 262
  complications, 263
  diagnosis, 263
  differential diagnosis, 263

infectious rhinitis (Cont.)
  epidemiology, 262
  links with asthma, COPD, 262–263
  pathophysiology, 261–262
  treatment
    pharmacologic, 263–264
    prevention, 263
inflammatory bowel disease, 96t
inflammatory pseudotumor, 141t
innate immunity, 34t, 35t
insulin resistance
  and arginine metabolism, 326–328, 327
  asthma/obesity and, 324t, 337
  CPAP and, 66t
  menopausal women and, 338
  OSAS/weight gain and, 67–70, 321
  PCOS and, 337, 341
International Asthma Patient Insight Research (INSPIRE) study, 380
International Union of Immunological Societies (IUIS), 33–34, 34t
interstitial lung disease (ILD), 33t, 34, 144
  chronic, 37
  GER and, 311–312
  invasive, 36
  mimicking of asthma by, 33t, 34
invasive fungal rhinosinusitis, 275
IPAH. see idiopathic pulmonary arterial hypertension (IPAH)
irritable larynx syndrome, 142
irritant rhinitis, 253t
irritant-induced occupational asthma (IIOA), 173

Joint United Nations Programme on HIV/AIDS (UNAIDS), 34
Jones, R. S., 410

Karelia, Finnish and Russian, 422–424, 434
Kartagener's syndrome, 249t
Kawasaki disease, 15t
Kheirandish-Gozal, L., 59
Klebsiella ozaenae, 252
Klebsiella pneumoniae, 151
Klebsiella rhinoscleromatis, 142
Krantz, A. J., 399

Lack, G., 458
large cell carcinoma, 141t
large cell neuroendocrine carcinoma, 141t
Larrain, A., 310
Latin American Project for the Investigation of Obstructive Lung Disease (PLATINO), 84–85
Lavoie, K. L., 182
left heart disease, 219, 220, 221–222
Legionella species, 148, 150–152, 154, 156–157
leiomyoma, 141t
leiomyosarcoma, 141t
leptin hypothesis, 66–67
Levenson, T., 399
Levine, M., 398–399
lifestyle/behavioral modification strategies
  for ABPA, 27–28
  for acute rhinosinusitis, 265
  for chronic rhinosinusitis, 270
  for COPD/irreversible airflow obstruction, 85
  for cough, 166
  for CVD and asthma, 199–200
  for elderly people with asthma, 445–446
  for endocrine conditions, 341
  for nonallergic rhinitis, 253
  for OSA in children, 57
  for pneumonia, 155–156
Lim, K. H., 340
lipoma, liposarcoma, 141t
Litonjua, A. A., 68
low testosterone, 335, 340
low-dose irritant asthma, 175
lower respiratory tract infection (LRTI)
  in infectious bronchiolitis, 103–105, 107, 108, 111
  Klebsiella pneumoniae LRTI, 150
  in pneumonia, 158
  suggested approach, in children, 108
LRTI. see lower respiratory tract infection (LRTI)
Lung Health Study, 85, 445
lymphangioleiomyomatosis, 143, 144
lymphomatoid granulomatosis, 15t

Maimonides, Moses, 300, 301
malignant lymphoma of bronchial-associated lymphoid tissue, 141t
Manchester Asthma and Allergy Study (UK), 335
mandibular distraction osteogenesis, 59
mandibular hypoplasia, marked, and OSA in childhood, 50t
mannose-binding lectin (MBL) deficiency, 43
Margulies, S. I., 301
marijuana and asthma patients, 395, 396, 397t
McNagny, S. E., 398
menstrual cycle, 336–338
metastatic endobronchial carcinoma, 141t
microscopic polyangiitis (MPA), 13–19, 15t
Miedinger, D., 183
migraine-related rhinorrhea, 253t
Millon Clinical Multiaxial Inventory (MCMI), 182
mixed rhinitis (glucocorticoid-resistant allergic rhinitis), 246
mixed-type sleep apnea, 52
Modified Asthma Predictive Index, 107t
monomorphic adenoma, myoepithelioma, 141t
Moore, W. C., 85
Moraxella catarrhalis, 38, 166, 264
morphine and asthma, 399
Mounier-Kuhn syndrome (tracheomegaly), 96t, 142
mucoepidermoid carcinoma, 141t
mucopolysaccharidoses, and OSA in childhood, 50t
mucosal barrier, 260, 261, 274
mucous gland adenoma, 141t
multiple chemical sensitivity syndrome, 177
Munthe-Kaas, M. C., 425
Mycoplasma pneumoniae, 148, 149t, 150, 151–152, 153, 158

Nadel, J. A., 69
NAEB. see nonasthmatic eosinophilic bronchitis (NAEB)
Nager's syndrome, and OSA in childhood, 50t
NAR. see nonallergic rhinitis (NAR)
nasal eosinophilia, 248
nasal mucosa edema, 51
nasal nitric oxide (NNO), 117–118, 119t
nasal polyps (nasal polyposis). see also chronic rhinosinusitis with nasal polyps (CRSwNP); chronic rhinosinusitis without nasal polyps (CRSsNP)
  background information, 279–280
  comorbidities
    asthma, 280–282
    Churg-Strauss syndrome, 269
    cystic fibrosis, 124t, 249t, 269
  diagnosis, 268
  differential diagnosis, 249t
  EP²OS guidelines, 265

in infancy/childhood, 123
NSAID intolerance in, 270
pharmacologic treatment, 273
nasal septum deviation, 51
National Asthma Education and Prevention Program Expert Panel Report 3 (NAEPP-ERP3), 63, 65, 81
  airway obstruction definition, 82t
  asthma therapy guidelines, 110, 111b
National Cooperative Inner City Asthma Study (NCICAS), 457
National Health and Nutrition Examination Survey (NHANES), 64, 457
National Heart Lung Blood Institute Expert Panel Report, 14
National Institutes of Health-National Heart Lung and Blood Institute Asthma Phenotype Workshop, 82
neuroma, neurosarcoma, 141t
neutrophil-predominant rhinopathies, 249t
Nijmegen Questionnaire, 182
Nocardia, 42, 142
nociceptive rhinitis, 253t
nonallergic rhinitis (NAR), 166, 244
  background information, 245–246
  clinical features, 246
  diagnosis, 246–248
  differential diagnosis, 245, 248–253
  future research needs, 255
  lifestyle/behavioral modification strategies, 253
  pharmacologic treatment, 244–245, 253–254
nonasthmatic eosinophilic bronchitis (NAEB), 162
noninvasive fungal rhinosinusitis
  allergic fungal sinusitis, 274–275
  fungal ball, 274
nonspecific interstitial pneumonitis, 144–145
nontuberculosis atypical mycobacterium (NTM), 36

obesity
  defined, 322
  GER and, 71
  leptin hypothesis, 66–67
  and OSA in childhood, 50t, 51, 58
    adenotonsillar hypertrophy, 49, 50, 50t, 51
    stepwise treatment approach, 58
    weight gain mechanisms, 67–70
  osteoporosis and, 352
  pediatric heart conditions and, 204, 211
  pulmonary hypertension and, 220
obesity and asthma, 321–330
  in adults, 329, 330
  background information, 321–322
  in children, 57t, 322–326, 323, 328–329
  epidemiologic studies
    of asthma, 322
    asthma-obesity association, 322–323, 324t
    of obesity, 322
  future research needs, 329–330
  mechanisms, management implications
    arginine metabolism, 327, 327–328
    atopy/eosinophilic inflammation, 326
    comorbidities, 324–325
    decreased medication response, 328–329
    genetic determinants, 328
    hormonal differences, 325–326
    insulin resistance, 326–327
    lung mechanics, 323–324
    respiratory physiology, 323–324
    systemic inflammation, 326
    vitamin D, 328
    weight loss, asthma control, 329

obstructive hyperventilation, 50, 53
obstructive sleep apnea (OSA)
  apnea-hypopnea index, 52–53, 58–59, 64, 65t, 67, 71
  in elderly people with asthma, 445
obstructive sleep apnea (OSA), in children, 49–60
  asthma and
    coexistence with, 53
    epidemiologic studies, 54t–55t
    pathogenetic linking mechanisms, 56–57, 57t
    similarities/differences, 53, 56t
    treatment effectiveness considerations, 59
  background information, 49–50
  behavioral consequences, 52
  causes, 49
  clinical features
    diurnal symptoms, 51
    nocturnal symptoms, 51
    OSA-related morbidity, 51–52
    physical exam findings, 51
  cysteinyl leukotrienes and, 49, 56–57, 57t, 60
  defined, 52
  diagnosis, 52–53
  future research directions, 60
  lifestyle/behavior modification strategies, 57
  predisposing conditions, 50t, 51
  treatment
    specific modalities, 58–59
    stepwise approach, 58
  types of, 52
obstructive sleep apnea syndrome (OSAS) and asthma, 63–74
  background information, 63–66
  cardiac dysfunction in, 72–73
  CPAP therapy, 58, 63, 65–67
    anti-acid reflux effect of, 72
    antiinflammatory effects, 71
    heart function improvements, 73
    mechanical effects, 69–70
    mechanics of, 73
    neuromechanical effects, 69–70
    pathological features impacted by, 66t
  diagnosis
    history, physical exam, lab features, 64t
    OSA confirmation, 65t
    severity grading, 65t
  epidemiologic studies, 54t–55t
  future research directions, 73
  symptoms provoking evaluation, 65t
  VEGF and airway angiogenesis, 70–73
    anti-acid reflux effect of CPAP, 72
    anti-inflammatory effects of CPAP, 71
    cardiac dysfunction, 72–73
    gastroesophageal reflux, 71–72, 72
  weight gain mechanisms in, 67–70
    airway smooth muscle, 68
    local airway inflammation, 68
    neural receptors, mechanical effects, 68–69
    obesity/leptin hypothesis, 66
    serum leptin level reductions, 67
obstructive sleep disordered breathing (SDB), 50
occupational asthma, 172–185
  adult-onset asthma and, 172, 173–174, 176, 184–185
  background information, 172–174
  classification scheme, *174*
  clinical features, 174–176
  common agents/related jobs, 174t
  comorbid/coexisting disease, 182–184

occupational asthma (*Cont.*)
  diagnosis of, *175*, 176–177
  differential diagnosis
    asthma-like symptoms, 178*t*
    bronchiolitis, 179–180
    COPD, 179
    eosinophilic bronchitis, 179
    HP, 179
    hyperventilation syndrome, 181–182
    OILD, 177
    panic disorder, 181–182
    work-related laryngeal dysfunction, 180–181
    work-related rhinitis, 180
  future research directions, 184
  WEA distinction from, 178*t*
occupational immunologic lung disease (OILD), 173, 177, 178*t*
occupational rhinitis, 183–184
  with eosinophilia, 250*t*
OILD. *see* occupational immunologic lung disease (OILD)
oligomenorrhea, 337
oncocytoma, 141*t*
opioid drugs and asthma, 399
oral contraceptive pill (OCP) use, 337, 342
Orie, N.G.M., 81
OSAS. *see* obstructive sleep apnea syndrome (OSAS) and asthma
Osler, William, 300–301
osteoporosis, 345–361
  asthma-specific risks, 361
  background information, 345–346
  diagnosis
    absolute fracture risk calculator, 353
    clinical exam features, 353
    densitometry screening, 353
    fracture/bone loss (defined), 346–347
  future research needs, 361
  glucocorticoid management, 359–360
  nonpharmacologic prevention and treatment
    exercise, 353–354
    smoking cessation, 354
  nutritional and pharmacologic prevention and treatment, 354–359
    bisphosphonates, 357
    calcitonin, 357, 359
    calcium, vitamin D, 355, 357, 358*t*
    hormone replacement therapy, 359
    parathyroid hormone, 357
    RANK-L antagonist, 359
  risk reduction/assessment, in underdeveloped regions, 361
  thyroid disorders and, 338
osteoporosis, risk factors
  modifiable, 348*t*
    chronic inflammation-induced osteoporosis, 351–352
    dietary-induced osteoporosis, 351
    drug-induced osteoporosis: glucocorticoids, 347, 349–351
    drug-induced osteoporosis: other drugs, 347, 349–351
    obesity, sedentary lifestyle, 352
    smoke-induced osteoporosis, 352
  nonmodifiable, 348*t*–349*t*, 352
  potentially modifiable, 349*t*
osteosarcoma, 141*t*
otitis media, recurrent, 41
oxycodone and asthma, 399

panic disorder
  differential diagnosis, 177, 178*t*
  symptoms/diagnosis, 182
papillomas, 141*t*
paradoxical vocal fold motion disorder (PVFMD). *see* vocal cord dysfunction (VCD)
parainfluenza, 34
paroxysmal nocturnal dyspnea, 195, 197*t*
pathogenesis
  of acute/chronic sinusitis, 240
  of adenotonsillar hypertrophy, 49, 60
  of ANCA-positive vasculitis, 14, 19
  of asthma, 67, 71, 158, 328, 330, 340
    adult-onset, 334, 337
    atopic, in children, 154
    bronchial, 70
    elderly population, 449
    hyperventilation syndrome, 387
    inflammation factors, 427
    psychological factors, 379, 389, 390*t*
    respiratory allergens, 444
  of bronchiectasis, 93
  of chronic rhinosinusitis with nasal polyps, 281
  of COPD, 81
  of hypersensitivity pneumonitis, 6
  of mannose-binding lectin deficiency, 43
  of obstructive SDB, 52
  of pneumococcal invasive infections, 156
  of pulmonary hypertension, 216, 223
  of sleep apnea in children, 49
  of viral rhinitis, 250
  of vocal cord dysfunction, 291
pathophysiology
  of ABPA, 26
  of acute rhinosinusitis, 264
  of allergic rhinitis, 232–233, 241
  of α_1-antitrypsin (AAT) deficiency, 134, 136
  of chronic rhinosinusitis, 241, 266, 269
  of COPD, 194
  of infectious rhinitis, 261–262
  of nasal polyps, 267, 279
  of nonallergic rhinitis, 254
  of OSAS, 68
  of osteoporosis, 347, 349
    glucocorticoid-induced, 357
  of upper airway diseases, 281
  of vocal cord dysfunction, 290
Paulson, D. L., 301
PCD. *see* primary ciliary dyskinesia (PCD)
pediatric cardiac conditions, 204–212
  asthma, coexisting conditions
    cardiac tamponade, 210
    chest pain, 210
  asthma/pharmacologic treatment effects, 211–212
  asthma-related dysfunction, 210–211
  background information, 204
  congestive heart failure, 207–208
    left ventricular dysfunction, 208
    left-to-right shunts, 207–208
  differential diagnosis, 205–207
    aortic aneurysm, 207
    congenital heart disease associated with bronchial compression of bronchomalacia, 205
    pseudoaneurysm, 207
    pulmonary artery sling, 207
    pulmonary atresia with ventricular septal defects, aortopulmonary collaterals, 206
    pulmonary hyperinflation, 207
    tetralogy of Fallot with absent pulmonary valve syndrome, 205

vascular rings, 206–207
future research needs, 212
postoperative single ventricle patients, 209
pulmonary venous hypertension, 208–209
suggestive clinical features, 209t
wheezing-related anatomy, physiology, 205t
Perkner, J. J., 181
Perrin-Foyalle, M., 303
pertussis, 143
Pfeiffer's syndrome, and OSA in childhood, 50t
PH. *see* pulmonary hypertension (PH)
pharmacologic treatment
  of ABPA, 28–29
  of acute rhinosinusitis, 265
  of allergic rhinitis, 166, 233–236
  of α_1-antitrypsin (AAT) deficiency, 136
  of ANCA-positive vasculitis, 18–19, 19t
  of atopic dermatitis, 460–461
  of bronchiectasis, 99–100
  of CGD, 42
  of chronic rhinosinusitis
    CRSsNP, 270–271
    CRSwNP, 272–273
  of COPD and irreversible airflow obstruction, 86
  of CRSsNP, 270–271
  of CVD, 197–198, 198t, 200
    asthma medication side effects, 198t
  of cystic fibrosis (CF), 128
    new/modified, 132t–133t
    past/recently available, 129t–131t
  of elderly people with asthma, 446–448
  of exercise-induced bronchoconstriction with asthma, 414–415, 415t
  of GERD, 98
  of hereditary angioedema, 43
  of immunodeficiencies with asthma, 44–45
  of infectious bronchiolitis, 110
  of infectious rhinitis, 263–264
  of nasal polyps, 273
  of nonallergic rhinitis, 244–245, 253–254
  of pneumonia, 148, 156–158
  of pregnancy and asthma, 371–373
  of primary ciliary dyskinesia, 118–121
  of primary immunodeficiency diseases, 44–45
  of psychological factors in asthma, 384–385
  of pulmonary arterial hypertension, 223
  of pulmonary infections, in immunocompromised patients, 37
  of UACS, 166–167
PIDDs. *see* primary immunodeficiency diseases (PIDDs)
Pierre Robin sequence
  and OSA in childhood, 50t
PLATINO study. *see* Latin American Project for the Investigation of Obstructive Lung Disease (PLATINO)
pleiotropic carcinomas with sarcomatoid elements, blastoma, 141t
pleomorphic adenoma (benign mixed tumor), 141t
Pneumocystis carinii pneumonia, 157
Pneumocystis jiroveci pneumonia, 34, 36
pneumonia
  asthma comorbidity, 34, 35t, 36
  background information, 148
  bacterial, 41
  clinical features, 150–151
  diagnosis, 151–154
    blood specimen, 152–153
    invasively collected specimens, 153–154
    pleural fluid, 153

    sputum specimen, 153
    urine specimen, 153
  differential diagnosis, 154–155, 155t
  etiologic agents, 148, 149t, 150
  future research directions, 157–158
  lifestyle/behavior modification strategies, 155–156
  mimicking of asthma by, 33t, 34
  pharmacologic treatment, 148
  symptoms, 148
Pneumonia Severity Index, 151
pneumothorax, 145
pollution-induced neutrophilic mucositis, with epithelial and ciliary dysplasia, 249t
polyarteritis nodosa (PAN), 15t
polychondritis, recurring, 142
polycystic ovary syndrome (PCOS), 337
polyps, 51
Prader-Willi syndrome, and OSA in childhood, 50t
pregnancy and asthma, 367–374
  asthma control assessment, 370t
  asthma's effects on, 367–369
  diagnosis, 369
  dyspnea differential diagnosis, 370
  education and adherence, 370–371
  future research needs, 374
  hormonal/drug-related rhinopathies and, 252t
  nasal obstruction and, 251
  pharmacologic treatment
    cromolyn, 373
    inhaled β-agonists, 372–373
    inhaled corticosteroids, 371–372
    leukotriene modifiers, 373
    oral corticosteroids, 373
    theophylline, 373
  physician treatment reluctance, 368
  severity assessment, 369–370, 369t
primary ciliary dyskinesia (PCD)
  asthma comorbidity, 118
  background information, 115–116
  clinical features, 116
  diagnostic strategies
    approach, 118, 119t
    ciliary motility, 116–117
    ciliary ultrastructure, 116
    gene mutation analysis, 117, *117*
    mucociliary clearance measurement, 118
    nasal nitric oxide, 117
  pharmacologic treatment
    adjunctive measures, 121
    antibiotics, 120
    anti-inflammatories, 120
    monitoring, 118–120
    mucus clearance, 120
    otologic/sinus disease management, 120
primary immunodeficiency diseases (PIDDs)
  comorbidity considerations
    bronchiectasis, 37–38
    bronchiolitis/pneumonia, 36–37
    chronic interstitial lung disease, 37
    GLILD, 37
    pharmacologic treatment, 44–45
  etiology of, 33
  evaluation, 36–37
  IUIS classification of, 34t
  therapy, 37
  U.S. prevalence, *34*
primary nocturnal enuresis, 51
primary pulmonary melanoma, 141t

PRIME-MD interview, 182–183
The Principles and Practice of Medicine (Osler), 300
probiotics, 271t, 431
Pseudomonas aeruginosa, 22, 93, 96, 264
psychogenic cough, 165
psychological factors in asthma, 379–391
   asthma-specific, 380, 381t
   background information, 379–380
   clinical features, patient perceptions
      alexithymia, 379, 381–382, 381t, 385, 388, 389t, 391
      comprehension, memory, 382–383
      coping strategies, 382–383
   future research needs, 391
   hyperventilation syndrome, 386–387
   pharmacologic treatment
      adherence issues, 384–385
      non-patient-dependent nonadherence, 385t
   premorbid personality and social maladaption in asthmatic patients, 386
   psychoneurovegetoimmune abnormalities, 379, 387–388
   psychosomatic disorders
      diagnosis, prevention, 388–391, 389t
      emotional state, 385
      psychotherapeutic treatment, 389, 390t
psychoneurovegetoimmune abnormalities in asthma, 379, 387–388
psychosomatic disorders
   diagnosis, prevention, 388–391, 389t
   emotional state, 385
   psychotherapeutic treatment, 389, 390t
pulmonary arterial hypertension (PAH), 220–221
   bronchial asthma and, 197t
   characteristics, 215
   chest radiograph, *216*
   future research needs, 224
   idiopathic, 220
   pharmacologic treatment, 223
pulmonary hypertension (PH), 215–224
   asthma-related symptoms, 196
   background information, 215
   in children, 210
   clinical features, *216*, 216–218, *217*, 218t
   comorbidities
      chronic thromboembolic disease, 220, 222
      left heart disease, 219, 220, 221–222
      lung disease, 222
      pulmonary arterial hypertension, 215, *216*, 220–221
   diagnosis, 218–220
   HP and, 5
   OSA and, 52, 58, 64t
   sleep-disordered breathing and, 220, 222
Pulmonary Hypertension Connection registry, 221
pulmonary thromboemboli, 144
pulmonary venous hypertension
   in children, 208–209
   left atrial hypertension mimicking of, 209
   left heart disease and, 221
pursed-lip breathing, 182

reactive airways dysfunction syndrome (RADS), 173, 174, 178t
   diagnostic features, 175t
   low-dose, 172, 175
Registry to Evaluate Early and Long-term PAH Disease Management (REVEAL), 221
respiratory syncytial virus (RSV), 34, 104, 148
rhabdomyosarcoma, 141t
rheumatoid arthritis, 142
   with bronchiectasis, 96t
   with follicular bronchiolitis, 144
rhinitis. *see* allergic rhinitis (AR); infectious rhinitis; nonallergic rhinitis (NAR); work-related rhinitis (WRR)
rhinitis medicamentosa, 251, 252t
rhinopathies with complex cellular infiltrates or temporal evolution of inflammation, 250t
rhinosinusitis. *see* acute bacterial rhinosinusitis; chronic rhinosinusitis; chronic rhinosinusitis with nasal polyps (CRSwNP); chronic rhinosinusitis without nasal polyps (CRSsNP); fungal rhinosinusitis
rhinosinusitis (UACS-post-nasal drip syndrome), 164–165
Rome, L. A., 398
Rosenstein, Nicholas Rosen von, 300
Roth, H. P., 384
Russian Karelia, 422–424, 434

S. aureus, 42
Sabin, B. R., 173
saccular/cystic bronchiectasis, 93
Saito, H., 59
Savolainen, S., 240
selective immunoglobulin A (IgA) deficiency, 41
Serratia, 42
serum sickness, 15t
Severe Asthma Research Program (SARP), 88
severe combined immune deficiency (SCID), 33, 36, 38, 40
Shivaram, U., 70
sighing dyspnea, 145
65 years of age (and older) and asthma. *see* elderly people with asthma
Sjögren's syndrome
   with bronchiectasis, 96t
   with follicular bronchiolitis, 144
sleep apnea. *see* apnea-hypopnea index; central-type sleep apnea; hypopnea; mixed-type sleep apnea; obstructive sleep apnea (OSA), in children; obstructive sleep apnea syndrome (OSAS) and asthma
sleep-disordered breathing (SDB), 220
   epidemiological studies, 54t–55t
   pulmonary hypertension and, 220, 222
   treatment modalities, 58–59
smoking-induced osteoporosis, 352
snoring, in children with obstructive SDB, 51, 53
soft tissue tracheal tumors, 141t
Sontag, S., 302, 303
Spechler, S. J., 310–311
specific antibody deficiency (SAD), 40
squamous cell carcinoma, papillary variant, 141t
squamous cell papillomas, papillomatosis, 141t
Staphylococcus aureus, 96, 260, 267–268
Stickler's syndrome, and OSA in childhood, 50t
Streptococcus milleri, 151
Streptococcus pneumoniae, 33, 38, 96, 148, 149, *150*, 166, 264
Streptococcus viridans, 151
Strongyloides stercoralis, 27
Subpopulations and Intermediate Outcome Measures in COPD Study (SPIROMICS), 88
substance abuse
   alcohol and asthma, 395, 397t, 399–402, 401t
   asthma frequency rates, 396
   commonly used/abused drugs, *396*, 397t
   future research needs, 402
   heroin and asthma, 397–399, 397t
   marijuana and asthma, 396, 397t
   opioid drugs and asthma, 399
   tobacco smoking and asthma, 395, 397t, 399–402, *400*

summer-type pneumonitis, 7
superantigen rhinitis with neutrophilia, 249t
surgical treatment
   of acute rhinosinusitis, 265
   of α_1-antitrypsin (AAT) deficiency, 136
   of chronic rhinosinusitis, 273
   of CRSsNP, 273
   of CRSwNP, 273, 284–285
Svanes, C., 337
Swenson, P., 70
synovial sarcoma, 141t
systemic amyloidosis, 140
systemic inflammation
   asthma and markers of, 198–199
   CPAP and, 71
   obesity association, 66
   OSAS and, 70, 72
systemic mastocytosis, 143

Takayasu's arteritis, 15t
Tashkin, D. P., 398
T-cell lymphopenia, 41, 42
temporal arteritis (giant cell arteritis), 15t
testosterone, low, 335, 340
thermophilic bacteria, in hypersensitivity pneumonitis, 7–8
tobacco smoking and asthma, 395, 397t, 399–402, 400
Toren, K., 174
tracheobronchomalacia, 142
tracheomalacia, 142
tracheomegaly (Mounier-Kuhn syndrome), 142
transient hypogammaglobulinemia of infancy (THI), 40–41
Treacher Collins syndrome, and OSA in childhood, 50t
Treatise on Asthma (Maimonides), 300
treatment. *see* lifestyle/behavioral modification strategies; pharmacologic treatment; surgical treatment
Tucson Children's Assessment of Sleep Apnea Study, 52
Tucson Children's Respiratory Study, 335
Tucson Epidemiologic Study of Obstructive Lung Disease, 248

UACS-post-nasal drip syndrome, 164–165, 166
"united airways" disease, 245, 260–261
upper airway cough syndrome (UACS), 163
   chronic cough and, 166
   pharmacologic treatment, 166–167
   -post-nasal drip syndrome, 164
upper airway obstruction, 139–142
   asthma's mimicking of, 139
   CPAP and, 73
   diagnosis, 142
   OSA and, 53, 57
   presenting symptoms, 140
   sleep disordered breathing and, 50, 51, 52, 53, 57
   soft tissue tracheal tumors, 141t
upper airway resistance syndrome, 50, 53
Urschel, H. C., 301
U.S. Centers for Disease Control and Prevention, 336
U.S. Nurse Health Study, 337
U.S. Office of National Drug Control Policy, 398
usual interstitial pneumonia, 144

Valipour, A., 71
valvular heart disease, 144
vascular endothelial growth factor (VEGF) and airway angiogenesis, 70–73
   anti-acid reflux effect of CPAP, 72
   anti-inflammatory effects of CPAP, 71
   cardiac dysfunction, 72–73
vasculitis, associated with infections, 15t
vidian neurectomy, 253t
viral papillomatosis, 140
virus-induced infectious rhinitis, 260
vitamin D
   for ABPA patients, 29
   for comorbid conditions, 330
   cystic fibrosis and, 124t
   deficiency of, and asthma, 324t, 328, 340–341
   hypovitaminosis D-induced osteoporosis, 351
   obesity and, 324t
   in osteoporosis treatment, 355, 357
vocal cord dysfunction (VCD), 106t
   anatomy/function (of vocal cord), 290–291, *293*
   background information, 288
   clinical features, 292
   comorbidity with asthma, 142
   diagnosis, 292–293
   differential diagnosis, 177, 178t, 289, 413
   epidemiology, 291
   etiology, 291–292
   GERD-induced VCD, 292
   historical perspective, nomenclature, 289–290, *290*
   management, 293, 294t
   mimicking of asthma, 142
   nomenclature, 289–290
   pathogenesis, 291
   presentation in asthma, 289
   prognosis, 294–295
   symptoms, 181, 289t
   triggers of, 165, 289t
Vuillermin, P. J., 425

Wang, L., 69
WEA. *see* work-exacerbated asthma (WEA)
Wegener's granulomatosis, 13, *13*, 15t, 142
weight gain mechanisms in OSAS, 67–70
   airway smooth muscle, 68
   local airway inflammation, 68
   neural receptors, mechanical effects, 68–69
   obesity/leptin hypothesis, 66
   serum leptin level reductions, 67
weight loss and asthma control, 329
   in children with OSA, 57, 59, 60, 67–68
   in COPD, 85, 88
   in obese individuals, 321, 329
Widdicombe, J. G., 69
Wiskott-Aldrich syndrome (WAS), 41
work-exacerbated asthma (WEA), 172, 174, 178
work-related asthma (WRA). *see* occupational asthma; work-exacerbated asthma (WEA)
work-related laryngeal dysfunction (WRLD), 177
work-related rhinitis (WRR), 177, 180, 184

X-linked agammaglobulinemia (XLA), 40

Yacoub, M. R., 182–183
yellow nail syndrome, 96t
Young's syndrome, 96t, 249t

Zimmerman, J. L., 337